Advanced Practice Nursing

ESSENTIAL KNOWLEDGE

FOR THE PROFESSION

Edited by

Anne M. Barker, EdD, RN
Professor of Nursing
Sacred Heart University
Fairfield, CT

JONES AND BARTLETT PUBLISHERS
Sudbury, Massachusetts
BOSTON   TORONTO   LONDON   SINGAPORE

World Headquarters
Jones and Bartlett Publishers
40 Tall Pine Drive
Sudbury, MA 01776
978-443-5000
info@jbpub.com
www.jbpub.com

Jones and Bartlett Publishers
Canada
6339 Ormindale Way
Mississauga, Ontario L5V 1J2
Canada

Jones and Bartlett Publishers
International
Barb House, Barb Mews
London W6 7PA
United Kingdom

Jones and Bartlett's books and products are available through most bookstores and online booksellers. To contact Jones and Bartlett Publishers directly, call 800-832-0034, fax 978-443-8000, or visit our website www.jbpub.com.

Substantial discounts on bulk quantities of Jones and Bartlett's publications are available to corporations, professional associations, and other qualified organizations. For details and specific discount information, contact the special sales department at Jones and Bartlett via the above contact information or send an email to specialsales@jbpub.com.

The authors, editor, and publisher have made every effort to provide accurate information. However, they are not responsible for errors, omissions, or for any outcomes related to the use of the contents of this book and take no responsibility for the use of the products and procedures described. Treatments and side effects described in this book may not be applicable to all people; likewise, some people may require a dose or experience a side effect that is not described herein. Drugs and medical devices are discussed that may have limited availability controlled by the Food and Drug Administration (FDA) for use only in a research study or clinical trial. Research, clinical practice, and government regulations often change the accepted standard in this field. When consideration is being given to use of any drug in the clinical setting, the health care provider or reader is responsible for determining FDA status of the drug, reading the package insert, and reviewing prescribing information for the most up-to-date recommendations on dose, precautions, and contraindications, and determining the appropriate usage for the product. This is especially important in the case of drugs that are new or seldom used.

Production Credits
Executive Editor: Kevin Sullivan
Acquisitions Editor: Emily Ekle
Acquisitions Editor: Amy Sibley
Editorial Assistant: Patricia Donnelly
Production Director: Amy Rose
Production Editor: Renée Sekerak
Production Assistant: Julia Waugaman
Associate Marketing Manager: Rebecca Wasley
Associate Marketing Manager: Ilana Goddess
Manufacturing and Inventory Supervisor: Amy Bacus
Composition: Paw Print Media
Cover Design: Anne Spencer
Cover Images: © Taewoon Lee/ShutterStock, Inc.
Printing and Binding: Malloy, Inc.
Cover Printing: Malloy, Inc.

Library of Congress Cataloging-in-Publication Data

Advanced practice nursing : essential knowledge for the profession / edited by Anne M. Barker.
    p. ; cm.
  Includes bibliographical references and index.
  ISBN 978-0-7637-4899-9 (pbk.)
 1. Nursing. 2. Nursing—Study and teaching. I. Barker, Anne M.
  [DNLM: 1. Nursing—trends. 2. Education, Nursing, Graduate--trends. 3. Leadership. 4. Nurse Administrators—trends.
5. Nurse Clinicians—trends. WY 16 A2437 2008]
  RT41.A363 2008
  610.73—dc22

                    2007034621

6048

Printed in the United States of America
12 11 10 09 08   10 9 8 7 6 5 4 3 2

Contents

CONTRIBUTORS   xv
INTRODUCTION   xix

Part I   *Professional Roles for Advanced Nursing Practice* 1

Chapter 1   The Slow March to Professional Practice   7
Karen A. Wolf

Chapter Objectives	7
Introduction	7
Nursing as a Profession: Key Ideas for Integration	7
Roots of Nursing Contradictions	9
Nursing Takes Root in the United States	10
The Changing Organization of Work	12
Instability in the Nursing Labor Force	13
Militancy Rocks the Hospital Boat	14
Nursing Is Not Alone: The National Crisis in the Quality of Work Life	15
Patient-Centered Care and the Emergence of Primary Nursing	16
The Missing Links: Shared Governance and Recognition	17
The Attraction of Magnet Hospitals	19
Professional Nursing and Nurse Staffing: Chicken or Egg?	19
Conclusion	20
Discussion Questions	20
References	20

Chapter 2   Advanced Practice Nursing:
            Moving Beyond the Basics   23
            Joyce Pulcini

            Chapter Objectives   23
            Introduction   23
            Educational Standards   26
            Theoretical Issues and Challenges   27
            Conclusion   29
            Discussion Questions   29
            References   30

Chapter 3   The Evolution of Doctoral Education
            in Nursing   31
            Michael Carter

            Chapter Objectives   31
            Introduction   31
            A Brief History of Doctoral Education   32
            Doctoral Programs in and for Nursing   34
            Clinical Doctoral Programs   36
            Future Doctoral Education   38
            Conclusion   39
            Discussion Questions   40
            References   41

Chapter 4   Leadership Development Through Mentorship
            and Professional Development Planning   43
            Anne M. Barker

            Chapter Objectives   43
            Introduction   43
            Mentorship Model   43
            Stages of the Mentor–Mentee Relationship   45
            Mentorship versus Networking   48
            A Model of Career Development   48
            Process for Career Development Planning   50
            Discussion Questions   52
            References   52

Chapter 5   Managing Personal Resources:
            Time and Stress Management   53
            Anne M. Barker

            Chapter Objectives   53

Introduction 53
Time Management 53
Stress Management 62
Discussion Questions 64
References 64

Part II   The Health Care Delivery System and Health Care Policy . . . . , , , , , ... 65

Chapter 6   A Distinctive System of Health Care Delivery 71
Leiyu Shi and Douglas A. Singh

Chapter Objectives 71
Introduction 71
An Overview of the Scope and Size of the System 72
A Broad Description of the System 72
Basic Components of a Health Services
    Delivery System 75
A Disenfranchised Segment 77
Transition from Traditional Insurance to
    Managed Care 78
Primary Characteristics of the U.S. Healthcare
    System 79
Trends and Directions 87
Significance for Healthcare Practitioners and
    Policy Makers 88
Conclusion 89
Discussion Questions 90
References 90

Chapter 7   Beliefs, Values, and Health 93
Leiyu Shi and Douglas A. Singh

Chapter Objectives 93
Introduction 93
Significance for Managers and Policy Makers 94
Basic Concepts 94
Health Promotion and Disease Prevention 99
Developmental Health 101
Public Health 101
Health Protection 102
Quality of Life 104
Determinants of Health 104

Lifestyle 108
Heredity 108
Medical Care 109
Overarching Factors and Implications for
    Healthcare Delivery 109
A Social Model of Health 111
Equitable Distribution of Health Care 112
Justice in the U.S. Health Delivery System 116
Equity in the U.S. Healthcare Delivery System 117
Integration of Individual and Community Health 119
Conclusion 124
Discussion Questions 125
References 125

Chapter 8 The Evolution of Health Services in the
            United States 129
            Leiyu Shi and Douglas A. Singh

Chapter Objectives 129
Introduction 129
Medical Services in Preindustrial America 130
Medical Services in Postindustrial America 135
Medical Care in the Corporate Era 155
Conclusion 158
Discussion Questions 160
References 160

Chapter 9 Financing Health Care 163
            Harry A. Sultz and Kristina M. Young

Chapter Objectives 163
Introduction 163
Healthcare Expenditures in Perspective 164
Components of Healthcare Expenditures 169
Sources of Healthcare Payment 170
Evolution of Health Insurance:
    Third-Party Payment 171
Self-Funded Insurance Programs 174
Government as a Source of Payment 175
Medicare 176
The Balanced Budget Act of 1997 185

The Medicare Prescription Drug, Improvement,
and Modernization Act of 2003   191
Medicaid   192
Other Services Funded by Government   197
The Future: Continuing Change   197
Conclusion   198
Discussion Questions   198
References   199

Chapter 10   Managing Financial Resources   203
Dori Taylor Sullivan

Chapter Objectives   203
Introduction   203
The Healthcare Environment: Deciding
Whether Health Care Is a Right or a Privilege   204
Financial Management for Advanced
Practice Nurses   209
Financial Results and Quality Outcomes   216
Conclusion   217
Discussion Questions   217
References   218

Chapter 11   Managed Care   219
Harry A. Sultz and Kristina M. Young

Chapter Objectives   219
Introduction   219
Managed Care Fundamentals   221
HMO Act of 1973   223
The Evolution of Managed Care   225
Emerging Developments in Managed Care   228
Medicare and Medicaid Managed Care   232
Managed Care Organizations and Quality   234
The Future of Managed Care   237
Discussion Questions   238
References   238

Chapter 12   The Future of Health Services Delivery   241
Leiyu Shi and Douglas A. Singh

Chapter Objectives   241
Introduction   241
Trends in Private and Public Health Insurance   242

Future Options in Financing and Insurance 246
Future Challenges for Managed Care 249
Comprehensive Reform: If and When It Occurs 250
National and Global Challenges 254
Bioterrorism and the Transformation of
 Public Health 258
The Future Outlook for U.S. Hospitals 260
The Future of the Healthcare Workforce 261
Work Organization 264
Enhanced Focus on Customer Service 265
New Frontiers in Clinical Technology 266
The Era of Evidence-Based Health Care 267
Conclusion 269
Discussion Questions 270
References 271

Chapter 13   Advanced Practice Nurses and Public
        Policy, Naturally 275
    Jeri A. Milstead

    Chapter Objectives 275
    Introduction 275
    Changes in the Practice of Nursing 275
    The Emerging Political Role of Nurses 278
    Finding a Foundation in Theory and Research 280
    A New Organizational Paradigm 282
    The Changing Paradigm in Health Care 284
    What Is Public Policy? 288
    An Overview of the Policy Process 291
    A Bright Future 295
    Conclusion 300
    Discussion Questions 301
    References 301

Chapter 14   Making the Political Process Work 305
    Catherine J. Dodd

    Chapter Objectives 305
    Introduction 305
    Ten Universal Commandments of Politics and
     Reasons to Obey Them 306

Conclusion 314
Discussion Questions 315
References 315

Part III   *Quality and Information for Advanced*
Nursing Practice *317*

Chapter 15   Health Care Quality 323
Dori Taylor Sullivan

Chapter Objectives 323
Introduction 323
Introduction of Continuous Quality
     Improvement to Health Care 324
Tools and Techniques for Improving Quality
     and Performance 328
What Makes Quality Improvement Successful? 335
Clinical Process Improvement and
     Evidence-Based Practice 336
Accreditation and Regulatory Focus on Quality 339
Conclusion 343
Discussion Questions 344
References 344

Chapter 16   Contributions of the Professional, Public, and
     Private Sectors in Promoting Patient Safety 347
Evelyn D. Quigley

Chapter Objectives 347
Introduction 347
Responses by Professional Associations 348
First Institute of Medicine Report and Responses 349
Second IOM Report and Responses 353
Nursing's Role 355
Conclusion 357
Discussion Questions 357
References 358

Chapter 17   Information Technology for Advanced
     Nursing Practice 361
Michelle Godin

Chapter Objectives 361

Introduction   361
Basic Computer Concepts   362
Information Privacy and Confidentiality Issues   364
Hospital Information Systems   365
Clinical Systems   366
Administrative Systems   368
Educational Applications   370
Conclusion   371
Discussion Questions   371

*Part IV   Theoretical Foundation and Research for
           Advanced Nursing Practice* *373*

Chapter 18   Theory-Based Advanced Nursing Practice   379
             Janet W. Kenney

Chapter Objectives   379
Introduction   379
Relevance of Theory-Based Practice in Nursing   380
Issues Related to Theory-Based Nursing Practice   381
Structure of Nursing Knowledge and Perspective
    Transformation   383
Models and Theories Applicable in Advanced
    Nursing Practice   385
Selection of Relevant Models and Theories   389
Guidelines for Selecting Models and Theories for
    Nursing Practice   391
Application of Theory-Based Nursing Practice   392
Conclusion   394
Discussion Questions   395
References   396

Chapter 19   Values-Based Practice and Evidence-Based
             Care: Pursuing Fundamental Questions
             in Nursing Philosophy and Theory   399
             William K. Cody

Chapter Objectives   399
Introduction   399
Value-Laden Theory and the Fallacy of
    Value-Free Science   401
The Clarion Call for Evidence-Based Practice   402

Understanding Praxis   403
Practice as Praxis   404
Care   404
Differentiating Practice and Care   405
Values-Based Practice and Evidence-Based Care   406
Discussion Questions   407
References   407

Chapter 20   Fundamental Patterns of Knowing in Nursing   409
             Barbara A. Carper

             Chapter Objectives   409
             Introduction   409
             Identifying Patterns of Knowing   409
             Using Patterns of Knowing   416
             Discussion Questions   417
             References   418

Chapter 21   Patterns of Knowing: Review, Critique,
                 and Update   419
             Jill White

             Chapter Objectives   419
             Introduction   419
             Empirics: The Science of Nursing   420
             Ethics: The Moral Component   422
             Personal Knowing   424
             Esthetics: The Art of Nursing   427
             Sociopolitical Knowing: Context of Nursing   429
             Discussion Questions   431
             References   431

Chapter 22   Multiple Paradigms of Nursing Science   433
             Elizabeth J. Monti and Martha S. Tingen

             Chapter Objectives   433
             Introduction   433
             The Nature of Paradigms   434
             Paradigms in Nursing   435
             Criticisms of Empiricism   439
             The Interpretative Paradigm   440
             Criticisms of the Interpretative Paradigm   441
             Is Nursing Science a Mature Science?   442
             Single or Multiple Paradigms?   443

Implications of Multiparadigmism for
Nursing Science 446
Summary 447
Discussion Questions 448
References 448

Chapter 23 Research: How Health Care Advances 451
Harry A. Sultz and Kristina M. Young

Chapter Objectives 451
Introduction 451
The Focus of Different Types of Research 452
Research in Health and Disease 452
Epidemiology 453
Experimental Epidemiology 454
Health Services Research 454
Quality Improvement 458
Medical Errors 461
Evidence-Based Medicine 461
Outcomes Research 462
Patient Satisfaction 464
Research Ethics 464
Future Challenges 465
Discussion Questions 468
References 468

Chapter 24 Knowledge Development in Nursing: Our
Historical Roots and Future Opportunities 471
Susan R. Gortner

Chapter Objectives 471
Introduction 471
The Early Years 472
The Transition Years 475
Nursing Research Becomes Nursing Science 478
Nursing Science Comes of Age 479
Future Opportunities 482
Acknowledgment 483
Discussion Questions 483
Notes 484
References 484

Part V Other Core Knowledge for the Advanced Practice of Nursing *487*

Chapter 25 Moving Toward a Culturally Competent
            Profession   491
Deborah Washington

    Chapter Objectives   491
    Introduction   491
    Background   492
    The Diaspora   492
    Culture and Western Health Care   494
    Culturally Competent Care   496
    The Substance of Nursing: Theory and Culture   498
    Conclusion   501
    Discussion Questions   502
    References   502

Chapter 26 Race, Race Relations, and the Emergence of
            Professional Nursing, 1870–2004   505
Patricia St. Hill

    Chapter Objectives   505
    Introduction   505
    The Civil War Era   506
    The Segregation Laws and Nursing   506
    Lowering the Racial Barriers   509
    The Nursing Shortage and Minority Considerations   511
    Facing the Challenges of Tomorrow   513
    Discussion Questions   514
    References   514

Chapter 27 Introduction to Ethics   517
George D. Pozgar

    Chapter Objectives   517
    Introduction   517
    Ethics   517
    Ethical Theories   522
    Code of Hammurabi   525
    Principles of Healthcare Ethics   525
    Morality   531

Virtues and Moral Values   531
Situational Ethics   537
The Final Analysis   537
Discussion Questions   540
Notes   540
References   540

Chapter 28   The Role of Codes of Ethics in Nursing's
             Disciplinary Knowledge   543
             John G. Twomey

Chapter Objectives   543
Introduction   543
Views of Ethics for Nursing   544
A Code of Ethics for Nursing   545
The ANA Code of Ethics   550
Alternative Codes   555
Conclusion   556
Discussion Questions   556
References   557

Index   559

Contributors

Anne M. Barker, EdD, RN
Professor of Nursing
Sacred Heart University
Fairfield, Connecticut

Barbara A. Carper, RN, EdD

Michael Carter, DNSc, APRN, BC, FAAN
Dean Emeritus
College of Nursing
The University of Tennessee, Memphis
Memphis, Tennessee

William K. Cody, RN, PhD, FAAN
Director
Presbyterian School of Nursing
Queens University of Charlotte
Charlotte, North Carolina

Catherine J. Dodd, RN, MSN, FAAN

Michelle Godin, RN, EdD, BC, CNA
Saint Mary's Hospital
Waterbury, Connecticut

Susan R. Gortner, MN, PhD, FAAN
Professor Emeritus
University of California, San Francisco
San Francisco, California

Janet W. Kenney, RN, PhD

Elizabeth J. Monti, MSN, CRNA

Jeri A. Milstead, PhD, RN, FAAN
Professor and Dean
College of Nursing
The University of Toledo
Toledo, Ohio

George D. Pozgar, MBA, CHE
Consultant and Hospital Surveyor
Gp Health Care Consulting, International
Annapolis, Maryland
Surveyor
The Joint Commission
Oakbrook Terrace, Illinois

Joyce Pulcini, PhD, RNCS, PNP, FAAN
Associate Professor
School of Nursing
Boston College
Chestnut Hill, Massachusetts

Evelyn D. Quigley, RN, MN
Senior Executive and Chief Nursing Officer
    and CO-Clinical Patient Safety Officer
MeritCare Health System
Fargo, North Dakota

Leiyu Shi, DrPH, MBA, MPA
Professor
Johns Hopkins School of Public Health
Co-Director
Johns Hopkins Primary Care Policy Center for
    the Underserved
Johns Hopkins University
Baltimore, Maryland

Douglas A. Singh, PhD, MBA
Associate Professor
School of Public Health and Environmental
    Affairs
Indiana University, South Bend
South Bend, Indiana

Patricia St. Hill, PhD, RN, MPH
Associate Professor
Hunter-Bellevue School of Nursing
Hunter College of the City University of New
    York (CUNY)
New York, New York

**Dori Taylor Sullivan, PhD, RN, CAN,
    CPHQ**
Chair and Associate Professor
Department of Physical Therapy and Human
    Movement Science
Sacred Heart University
Fairfield, Connecticut

Harry A. Sultz, DDS, MPH
Professor Emeritus
School of Preventitive Medicine
School of Medicine and Biomedical Sciences
Dean Emeritus
School of Health Related Professions
State University of New York at Buffalo
Buffalo, New York

Martha S. Tingen, PhD, RN, ANP, CS

John G. Twomey, PhD, RN
Associate Professor
MGH Institute of Health Professions
Boston, Massachusetts

Deborah Washington, RN, MSN
Director
Diversity, Patient Care Service
Massachusetts General Hospital
Boston, Massachusetts

Jill White, RN, RM, MEd, PhD
Dean
Faculty of Nursing
Midwifery and Health
University of Technology
Sydney, Australia

Karen A. Wolf, PhD, APRN, BC
Clinical Associate Professor and Chair of
    Generalist Level Nursing
Graduate Program in Nursing
MGH Institute of Health Professions
Boston, Massachusetts

Kristina M. Young, MS
Instructor
Department of Social and Preventative
    Medicine
School of Public Health and Health
    Professions
University of Buffalo, State University of New
    York
Buffalo, New York
President
Kristina M. Young & Associates, inc.
Buffalo, New York

Introduction

This book was conceived in response to a need to present graduate core curriculum content based on the American Association of Colleges of Nursing's *The Essentials of Master's Education for Advanced Practice Nursing* (1996) in a comprehensive, introductory format in a graduate nursing program. The faculty searched for a book that comprehensively addressed all the core curriculum content requirements of the *Essentials* since each of the content areas cannot be covered in separate courses due to credit limitations. In addition, a book that addressed an audience of nurses in a variety of advanced practice nurse roles, not just those providing direct clinical care, was needed. No such book existed. Thus, the editor, Anne M. Barker, and publisher, Jones and Bartlett, embarked on producing a book that would compile select chapters from already existing books in the Jones and Bartlett collection. The strength of this approach is that experts in each of the content areas author each chapter in the book.

The goal of the book is to provide core knowledge that nurses in advanced practice roles require regardless of their specialty or functional focus. This knowledge can then be built upon as graduate students proceed into their specialty. The content for the book was selected by first using the *Master's Essentials*. The content was then cross-referenced with *The Essentials of Doctoral Education for Advanced Nursing Practice* (American Association of Colleges of Nursing, 2006). The task force that developed the *Doctoral Essentials* built their work on the *Master's Essentials*. Table I–1 displays the essential core curriculum content for both the master's and doctoral programs. In the last column, the chapters in this book that address this content are listed.

In preparing the book, we compared the *Master's Essentials* and *Doctoral Essentials,* not only by the difference in the depth of the content, but also across time. The two documents were written 11 years apart, and the *Doctoral Essentials* reflects changes in health care and nursing since 1996. Specifically, new content and focus are evidence-based practice, quality improvement and patient outcomes, and information and technology. This content is essential to both levels of graduate preparation and are therefore included in this book.

Table I–1 COMPARISON OF MASTER'S AND DOCTORAL ESSENTIALS AND BOOK CONTENT

Master's Essentials	*Doctoral Essentials*	*Book*
I. Research	III. Clinical scholarship and analytical methods for evidence-based practice	Chapters 23–24
II. Policy, organization, and financing of health care	II. Organizational systems leadership for quality improvement and systems thinking	Chapters 6–14
	V. Healthcare policy for advocacy in health care	
III. Ethics		Chapters 27–28
IV. Professional role development	VI. Interprofessional collaboration for improving patient and population health outcomes	Chapters 1–5
	VIII. Advanced nursing practice	
V. Theoretical foundations of nursing practice	I. Scientific underpinnings for practice	Chapters 18–24
Human diversity and social issues		Chapters 25–26
Health promotion and disease prevention	VII. Clinical prevention and population health for improving the nation's health	Chapters 6, 7, 12
	IV. Information systems/ technology and patient care technology for the improvement and transformation of health care	Chapters 15–17

Unsurprisingly, the *Doctoral Essentials* has more depth and sophisticated application in each of the content areas than the *Master's Essentials*. However, the book can be used in both master's and postbaccalaureate doctoral programs in the beginning core courses to lay a foundation for advanced nursing practice. As with any textbook, additional scholarly readings, especially research- and evidence-based articles, will enhance the content.

There is confusion about the terminology *advanced nursing practice* and *advanced practice nursing*. Over time, the terms *advanced practice nursing/nurses* have commonly been used to indicate master's-prepared nurses who provide direct clinical care and include the roles of clinical nurse specialist, nurse practitioner, certified nurse–midwife, and certified registered nurse anesthetist, the last three roles requiring a license beyond the basic RN license to practice. This book has adopted a broader, more inclusive definition (AACN, 2004), which reflects the current thinking about advanced practice. Advanced practice nursing is:

> *Any form of nursing intervention that influences health care outcomes for individuals or populations, including direct care of individual patients, management of care for individuals and populations, administration of nursing and health care organizations, and the development and implementation of health policy. (p. 2)*

Thus for this book, nurses in advanced practice will be defined as any nurse who holds a master's degree or higher in nursing and whose role is consistent with this definition. *Advanced practice nursing/nurses* and *advanced nursing practice* are used interchangeably throughout the book.

Currently, there are two major professional forces that are influencing graduate education in nursing and will have dramatic impact on nursing education presently and into at least the next decade. These include:

1. The introduction of a new role in nursing, the clinical nurse leader (CNL). This role was designed to address many of the problems currently evident in health care including the nursing shortage, patient safety and medical errors, and fragmentation of the healthcare system. The AACN (2007) provides this definition of the CNL:

> *The CNL functions within a microsystem and assumes accountability for healthcare outcomes for a specific group of clients within a unit or setting through the assimilation and application of research-based information to design, implement, and evaluate client plans of care. The CNL is a provider and a manager of care at the point of care to individuals and cohorts. The CNL designs, implements, and evaluates client care by coordinating, delegating and supervising the care provided by the health care team, including licensed nurses, technicians, and other health professionals. (p. 6)*

CNLs are considered generalists and will be prepared at the master's level and require the same core curriculum knowledge as do other master's-prepared nurses.

2. The mandate to have the clinical doctorate, designated as a doctor of nursing practice (DNP), as the entry to advanced nursing practice (see the Introduction to Part I for more details).

In both the *Master's Essentials* and *Doctoral Essentials* documents, the AACN lays out the foundation for core knowledge needed by all graduate nursing students. This book provides in one manuscript a foundation for this core knowledge. It does not address any of the specific content needed by the specialties. Further, this is foundational content that should be further integrated and applied throughout the rest of the curriculum.

References

American Association of Colleges of Nursing. (1996). *The essentials of master's education for advanced practice nursing.* Washington, DC: Author.

American Association of Colleges of Nursing. (2004). *AACN position statement on the practice doctorate.* Washington, DC: Author.

American Association of Colleges of Nursing. (2006, August 21). *The essentials of doctoral education for advanced nursing practice.* Washington, DC: Author.

American Association of Colleges of Nursing. (2007, February). *White paper on the education and role of the clinical nurse leader.* Washington, DC: Author.

Part 1

Professional Roles for Advanced Nursing Practice

In Part I of this book, we will consider the role of the advanced practice nurse from a historical, present-day, and future perspective. This content is intended to be a general introduction to select issues in professional role development for the advanced practice of nursing. As students progress in the educational process and develop greater knowledge and expertise, role issues and role transition should be integrated throughout the entire program.

In Chapter 1, Wolf presents a brief history of nursing and its progress towards professional practice. Although not specific to the role of the advanced practice nurse, the information presented in this chapter will assist the advanced practice nurse to have a broader perspective on nursing and health care organizations and their future. This will set the foundation for a deeper understanding of the historical development, current practice, and future opportunities for advanced practice in nursing.

In Chapter 2, Pulcini defines advanced practice nursing from a traditional perspective and traces the history of the roles. Traditionally, and as discussed by Pulcini, advanced practice has been limited to *clinical* roles and includes clinical nurse specialist, nurse practitioner, certified nurse midwife and certified registered nurse anesthetist, the last three roles requiring a license beyond the basic RN license to practice. However, as discussed in the foreword, this book uses an expanded definition of the advanced practice nursing that reflects current thinking. As you read this chapter, keep in mind this expanded definition and at the same time appreciate the development of the advanced clinical roles for nursing practice.

Since Pulcini's work in 2004, much has transpired related to the role and education of nurses for advanced practice. Most revolutionary is the mandate to have the clinical doctorate as the requirement for advanced clinical practice nursing by 2015 (American Association of Colleges of Nursing, 2007). With this change, many master's programs for advanced practice nurses will transition to the doctoral level. The rationale for this position by the American Association of Colleges of Nursing (AACN) was based on several factors, including:

- Current master's degree programs often require credit loads equivalent to doctoral degrees in other healthcare professions
- The changing complexity of the healthcare environment
- The need for the highest level of scientific knowledge and practice expertise to assure high quality patient outcomes

In an effort to clarify the standards, titling, and outcomes of clinical doctorates, the Commission on Collegiate Nursing Education (CCNE), the accreditation arm of AACN, has decided that only practice doctoral degrees awarding a Doctorate of Nursing Practice (DNP) will be eligible for accreditation. In addition, the AACN has published *The Essentials of Doctoral Education for Advanced Nursing Practice,* which sets forth the standards for the development, implementation and program outcomes for Doctorate of Nursing Practice programs.

Needless to say, this recommendation has not been fully supported by the entire profession. For instance, the American Organization of Nurse Executives (AONE, 2007) does not support *requiring* a doctorate for managerial or executive practice based on expense, time commitment, and the cost benefit of the degree. It also suggests nurses may migrate toward a master's in business, social sciences, and public health in lieu of nursing. Further, AONE suggests there is a lack of evidence to support the need for doctoral education across all aspects of the care continuum. However doctoral and master's education for nurse managers and executives is encouraged.

For other advance practice roles, including the clinical nurse leader, nurse educator, and nurse researcher, a different set of educational requirements exist. The clinical nurse leader as a generalist will remain as a master's program. For nurse educators, the position of AACN, although not universally accepted within the profession as demonstrated by the existence of master's programs in nursing education, is that didactic knowledge and practical experience in pedagogy is additive to advanced clinical knowledge. Nurse researchers will continue to be prepared in PhD programs. Thus, there will only be two doctoral programs in nursing, the DNP and the PhD. It will be important for readers to keep abreast of this movement as the profession further develops and debates this issue for implications for their own practice and professional development and within their own specialty. The best resource for this is the AACN Web site and the Web site of specialty organizations.

In Chapter 3, Carter reviews the historical development of doctoral programs, which provides an important background for how the profession has arrived at the aforementioned decisions. Of particular note is his discussion of the controversy around the development of the clinical doctoral programs. He traces the roots of the PhD for research and clinical doctorate for practice. As doctorates in nursing developed in the later part of the last century, there was diversity in titling and role expectations, which called for clarity and direction for the profession.

The last two chapters of Part I take a different perspective on the role of the advanced practice nurse and look at personal development of the reader for assuming a new role and leadership in the profession. In Chapter 4, Barker presents the importance of having a mentor and suggests how to select a mentor and how the relationship develops over time. Use of a checklist for selecting a mentor is a helpful tool for the reader as are the tools used to identify professional development needs and develop a written plan to achieve them.

Conventional wisdom for all leaders is that in order to be successful the individual needs to lead a balanced life. In order to achieve this goal, both time and stress management are central. Chapter 5 suggests strategies for both and offers tools to assist readers in assessing their own skill and developing strategies to capitalize on one's strengths and note opportunities for improvement.

References

American Association of Colleges of Nursing. (2007). Doctor of Nursing Practice. Retrieved July 14, 2007, from http://www.aacn.nche.edu/DNP/ DNPPositionStatement.htm

American Organization of Nurse Executives. (2007). Consideration of the Doctorate of Nursing Practice. Retrieved November 4, 2007, from http://www.aone.org/aone/docs/PositionStatement 060607.doc

Part

I

Professional Roles for Advanced Nursing Practice

CHAPTER 1   The Slow March to Professional Practice

CHAPTER 2   Advanced Practice Nursing: Moving Beyond the Basics

CHAPTER 3   The Evolution of Doctoral Education in Nursing

CHAPTER 4   Leadership Development Through Mentorship and Professional Development Planning

CHAPTER 5   Managing Personal Resources: Time and Stress Management

The Slow March to Professional Practice

Karen A. Wolf

CHAPTER OBJECTIVES

1. Define professionalism.
2. Discuss the development of nursing as a profession over the last century.
3. Consider future trends in nursing that have the potential to positively affect the profession of nursing.

Introduction

Nursing's quest for professionalism has shaped nursing education and practice, past and present, in the United States and abroad. The emergence of professional practice models over the past quarter century represents the latest in professionalizing trends. This effort by nurses and healthcare managers to restructure the workplace and nursing work highlights the evolution of nursing from a simple matter of tasks to the complexity of knowledge-based practice in rapidly changing healthcare organizations. The current healthcare environment is faced with a wide range of regulatory and financial pressures. These include demands to justify healthcare service outcomes, the drive to maintain biomedical and technological currency, and a recurrent nursing shortage.

Looking back through nursing history, one can see that crises in the healthcare system create opportunities for nursing. Too often, nursing's responses to crises have not created outcomes that serve both the interests of the profession and the public. Today, as nurses once again find themselves in the midst of a crisis, there is an opportunity to renegotiate the organizational realities of health care and to advance the contribution of professional nursing to healthcare outcomes.

Nursing as a Profession: Key Ideas for Integration

What makes work professional work? Nursing has struggled with this question throughout its history. For most of the 20th century, nursing

7

was considered a semiprofession or a profession in progress by sociologists (Bucher & Strauss, 1961; Etzioni, 1969). The attention that nursing leaders have given to professional development is manifest in the push for control over educational standards, efforts to develop a theory base for nursing practice, the growth of professional organizations and journals, and, more recently, the reorganization of nursing work within professional nursing practice models. The nature of professional nursing work differs today from what it did for the sacred three professions of medicine, law, and the clergy in 1900. The autonomous solo professional serving the public with expert knowledge and skill is now a rare phenomena. Few occupations can claim pure professional autonomy, because the reach of corporate and institutional control now dominates most sectors of the economy.

Autonomy, a hallmark of professionalism, can be differentiated into autonomy of decision making relative to the client and/or patient care and autonomy from the employing institution (Manthey, 1991). Autonomous practitioners are those who have direct lines of access to clients, who are responsible for their own practice decisions, and who are accountable to clients, peers, and professional organizations, as well as to the courts, for their conduct (Marram, Schlegel, & Bevis, 1974). The nursing profession has struggled with the idea of autonomy because most nurses are employed and subordinated to the authority of organizations such as hospitals (Ashley, 1976; Reverby, 1987; Wolf, 1993). The claim to autonomy with regard to the freedom to make decisions about patient care has advanced over the past few decades, fueled by the development of primary nursing models (Hegyvary, 1982). More recently, health services research studies have integrated the concept of

nursing autonomy. For example, a recent study by Aiken, Clarke, Sloane, Sochalski, and Silber (2002) suggested that increasing nursing autonomy and control over the practice setting was associated with improved patient care outcomes.

Nursing can no longer be viewed as a subsidiary function of medicine that is proscribed by doctors' orders; nursing care now reflects a patient-centered approach based on nursing theory and shaped by a nursing process of reasoning. Current legal and professional regulations legitimate this nurse-driven process of practice. The body of statutory and case law that governs nursing practice holds nurses accountable to a definition of practice that recognizes and codifies practice in accordance with current nursing knowledge and clinical practice standards. Accountability is inherent to autonomy. By definition, accountability calls for professionals to accept responsibility or to account for their actions (Merriam-Webster, 2006). The demand for professional accountability has been spurred on by the health-outcomes movement and patient safety concerns.

Professionalism should and does benefit the public. However, professionalism also arises out of self-interest and provides a means by which occupational groups exert influence to advance their own interests in society. The interest may reflect a desire for greater societal power and/or an increase of rewards or benefits for the group. As such, the quest for professional status by nursing reflects an attempt to access and achieve mobility. Professionalism, by reflecting the underlying meritocratic values of our society, offers a rational system for distributing status and rewards.

Professionalization provides access to social mobility. According to Hughes (1971), there are two types of mobility. The first is the rise of the individual by entering an occupation of high prestige or by achieving special success in his or her profession. The second is the collective effort of an organized occupation to improve its place and increase its power in relation to other occupational groups. In the case of nursing, mobility has traditionally been measured against or referenced to other groups, such as physicians.

Since the 1970s, interest in professionalizing nursing work has emerged in healthcare organizations as a means to provide a substitute motivation for workers with blocked access to structures of mobility. The ideological draw of professionalism is that it offers the promise of higher status and control. A crucial issue that arises out of the trend to professionalize work is the struggle of workers, including nurses, to exercise control over the context (environment) and content of their work. The ability to exercise control, however tentative, appears to mediate individual and collective tensions that arise from the heightened expectations of a more educated nursing workforce. By professionalizing the workplace, management seeks to counter more traditional collective action, such as unionism. Educated to be professionals in colleges and universities, nurses now expect to exercise their knowledge and skills without organizational or bureaucratic constraint. The heightened expectations of nurses is a double-edged sword, offering a challenge to traditional hierarchical controls and opportunity for institutional enhancement.

As hospitals and other healthcare institutions confront the increasing complexity in health care, the application of professional knowledge and skills becomes essential to institutional functioning. That professional knowledge and skills serve institutional goals to solve institutional problems is now embraced by healthcare administrators as an asset, rather than a threat to traditional authority. Perrow (1972) observed in his classic treatise on bureaucracy that professionals, far from antithetical to institutional bureaucracy, are in fact readily harnessed to serve the needs and problems of organizations. Nurses have historically highlighted this phenomenon. More recently, other traditional professions (physicians, lawyers) have become organizational professions. Yet, despite nurses' central role in healthcare services, they have struggled to develop, assert, and be recognized for their professional expertise. Imbued with managerialism, nursing work in hospitals has evidenced a professional paradox (Fourcher & Howard, 1981). The application of nursing knowledge and skill in managing patient care in hospitals has a long history of being subjugated to nursing and hospital administration. Nursing expertise has more often than not been invisible and undervalued, and autonomy of practice has been absent.

Roots of Nursing Contradictions

The concept and actual practice of nursing work has evolved dramatically over the past 100 years. But like many evolutionary paths, old or outdated conceptions of nursing persist. As a result, both popular and professional conceptions of nursing are riddled with contradictory views. Prior to Florence Nightingale's reforms in England, nursing was largely women's work. Nursing was viewed as an extension of motherhood, midwifery, or religious duty. By the late 19th century, women working as nurses began to fill a role in the administration of poverty. Because health care and nursing care of the sick was intertwined with poverty, caring for the sick was largely caring for the poor. Nursing was commonly carried out by impoverished women who worked as nurses in almshouses caring for the poor, the sick, and the destitute. These untrained, able-bodied paupers worked for room and board. The harsh reality was that these nurses were viewed as part of the chaotic environments in which they worked. The Dickinsonian image of Sairey Gamp, a low-class drunkard and disheveled woman, was reflective of the persistent stigma that Nightingale sought to escape with the formal education of a higher class of women (Dean & Bolton, 1980; Williams, 1980).

Although some few nurses saw their work as a religious service, the role of religious values waned with the disintegration of church-based nursing orders with the rise of Protestantism in England. Hospitals, lacking the support of religious nursing orders, struggled to provide nursing care that was haphazard at best. Nurses lacked a systematic set of skills, a knowledge base, or training. Nightingale sought to modernize nursing by developing a trained nursing labor force composed of a higher class of women.

Nightingale also sought to link nursing education with the more formalized development of hospitals. Influenced by her experiences in the Crimea, Nightingale recognized that nursing care was the major determinant of hospital outcomes. A brilliant and politically astute woman, she took on nursing reformation with a passion born of her religious beliefs and desire to reform social expectations for women. Nightingale advanced her case for training nurses based on data. Nightingale contributed some of the earliest biostatistical data of hospital conditions and outcomes, drawing connections between the environments of care and the contribution of nurses (Dossey, 1999).

Despite Nightingale's innovative ideas to systematize the education of nurses, the origins of modern nursing were seeded with social constraints. Nightingale (1866) wrote to a friend that "the whole reform in nursing both at home and abroad has consisted of this: to take all power over the nursing out of the hands of men and put into the hands of one female trained head and making her responsible for everything. . ." (p. 25). Nightingale and her contemporaries purposely overlooked the traditions of men in nursing, such as the work of the Knights Templar (Bullough & Bullough, 1984). The concept of nursing discipline projected by Nightingale, as well as by nursing leaders in the 20th century, held nursing to conventional standards of female subservience within a hierarchy of a moral female authority. Nursing was embraced as a feminine endeavor that was to be the singular focus of the nurse's life. Imbued with inherent religious values, nursing was viewed as a selfless act, and the reward for nursing work was deemed intrinsic to the work itself. Nightingale, although a feminist and supporter of women's suffrage, struggled with contradictions of class and gender as she advanced her campaigns for nursing and health. Despite Nightingale's political opinions, modern nursing was reconceptualized as a woman's calling, and hence doubly subordinated to the paternalism of society.

Nursing Takes Root in the United States

The universal traditions and nursing functions of caring for the sick have existed for centuries. The power of Nightingale's reforms to formalize and reshape nursing has been evident in their global reach. In the United States, as in many other countries, the importation of the Nightingale schools of nursing legitimated nursing work as an occupation for women. Hospital-based schools of nursing offered women access to education and the potential for employment, creating an option for a sustainable livelihood. Employment as a head nurse or private duty nurse was a welcome alternative to agrarian domesticity or mill work.

The demand for nursing grew in response to hospital growth. As industrialization spurred the growth of larger communities, hospitals proliferated and became a central feature of community life (Rosenberg, 1989). Social reformism was a major force because it spurred the development of both public health and hospital-based services to provide health care to the growing industrial labor force (Rosenberg, 1989; Starr, 1982). From 1875 to 1924, the number of hospitals grew from just over 170 to more than 7,000 (Rosner, 1989). However, as noted by Stevens (1989), the central role that health care would take in American society was being shaped by the growing power of medicine. A benevolent paternalism pervaded the structure of healthcare services and harnessed the potential of nursing to support the role of medicine and hospitals (Ashley, 1976). By the early 1900s, the growth of hospitals in the United States generated an unprecedented demand for nurses. The growth of technology from basic advances such as X-rays and anesthesia fueled excitement in hospital investment. Physicians invested their money and technology into hospitals, securing power in their communities as well. Hospitals became a focal point of community life, and hospitals became both a symbol of the prosperity of a community and a focus for social reformism.

The thirst for a cheap and rapidly produced labor supply overshadowed concerns over standards of quality education. From 1900 to 1920, the nursing profession grew "from one in which

there were more than 10 times as many physicians as nurses, to one in which there was less than one physician for every nurse" (Burgess, 1928, p. 43). As hospitals grew, schools of nursing were created to provide a labor force for the hospitals, often at the expense of adequate education (Ashley, 1976). As Dock and Stewart (1938) noted in their history of nursing, "the excess of poor schools and poorly prepared nurses was attributed in large measure to the apprenticeship system that prevailed, with its overemphasis on practice service at the expense of education" (p. 183). Formal studies of nursing education, such as the Goldmark report (1923) and the grading committee report of the National League for Nursing Education (1926), addressed the issue of raising standards for nursing education. Dock and Stewart (1938) suggested that despite the many recommendations for reform, "the system was too deeply rooted and the funds for putting nursing schools on a sound economic and education basis were simply not generally available" (p. 183). Despite forward movement with the establishment of university schools of nursing at Columbia, Yale, and Western Reserve, the push to establish college entrance as a requirement for practice was eclipsed by the hospital training schools. The fundamental professional goal to control the entry into the profession was overridden by hospitals' needs for a cheap labor supply.

The rapid expansion of a nursing labor force occurred with little regard for educational quality. Hospital administrators recognized the economic benefit of using student labor, and physicians began to appreciate the good nursing care offered by graduates of such training. But by the 1930s, concerns about overproduction of nurses emerged and was underscored by the Great Depression. A third of all hospital schools of nursing closed between 1929 and 1939. Nurses, no longer able to secure private duty work, sought employment in hospital wards for hourly or group nursing work. But as Reverby (1979) noted, hospitals were slow to hire graduates as staff nurses, despite admonishments by the nursing leaders and the American Nurses Association. Modified grouped private duty nursing efforts transitioned the development to staff nursing. The dire economic conditions of the Depression reshaped nursing work and healthcare services. Nursing shifted away from private freelance work to organized nursing services in hospitals and public health. As nursing became embedded in hospitals, the primacy of the nurse–patient relationship, a characteristic of private duty nursing, eroded, and the nurse became subordinated to the paternalism of the hospital (Ashley, 1976; Dock & Stewart, 1938).

The Changing Organization of Work

The organizational culture of hospitals, characterized by strong gender-based roles and a hierarchical authority structure, was fertile ground for the application of industrial management methods. The ideas of scientific management made an easy leap from factory floor to hospitals in the first half of the 20th century. Frederick Taylor, the architect of many scientific management ideas, was of a new breed of industrial engineers. His primary concerns were enhancing worker productivity and limiting the threats of unions in order to advance profit from capitalism. Scientific methods were intended to extract labor from workers at the shop-floor level by dividing work into discrete tasks to be done by individual workers. "Taylorism" spread to hospitals and was embraced by nursing leaders, and the quest for efficiency in hospital operations mirrored the factory push toward mechanistic functioning. The application of Taylor's scientific management methods to hospitals included division of labor, the task orientation of functional nursing, and standardized and proscriptive procedure manuals. Hospitals were in a unique position to maximize the control and the execution of nursing work, because they were often both the diploma schools for training nurses and the employer. The hospital culture was able to secure the loyalty of nurses through both school ties and training (Wolf, 1993).

Management in hospitals emerged largely at the ward level. Mobility in nursing became tied to the management structure. Nursing leadership embraced managerialism, because it offered the potential for mobility and status recognition for women. Subordinated to physicians, nurses were unable to gain control over access to patients, use of technology, or application of knowledge. Nursing leader Isabel Stewart attempted to advance scientific nursing, which she thought could be employed in conjunction with industrial methods for standardization and efficiency of hospital care to wrest control from hospitals. However, her academic approach to building a scientific basis for practice was viewed skeptically by nurses and never gained sufficient financial support (Reverby, 1987). Nurses continued to follow orders under a system where work conception was clearly separate from execution.

That the adage "a nurse is a nurse is a nurse" was born in this period reflects the view that nurses were considered an interchangeable part of the hospital machine. Although many nurses preferred to work as private duty nurses, the changing economics of the Great Depression made this an unstable option by the 1930s (Reverby, 1999). As a result of application of scientific management methods to nursing, patient care became fragmented, task oriented, and management focused. Case-based nursing, rooted in the tradition of private duty nursing, fell victim to what was viewed as progress. New models of care, such as group nursing and functional nursing, reflected the pooling of scarce nursing labor resources to meet the needs of the organization, not the patient.

Following World War II, team nursing became the common model of nursing care organization. The team nursing concept was influenced by wartime experiences and the emerging human relations school of management. The goal was to create a team of nursing care providers led by a professional nurse. Emphasis was placed on effective communication and delegation to enhance team functioning. However, nursing shortages often resulted in team leaders struggling to provide care with inadequately trained staff. The result of the team approach was more a functional approach to care, with emphasis on task completion rather than patient care (Hegyvary, 1982). Because of tradition and nursing shortages, remnants of mechanistic task performance continued to permeate the work culture of hospitals and counter professionalization attempts. Nursing leader Lydia Hall, a fierce opponent of team nursing, challenged nursing to put its rhetoric of professionalism to the test of practice. In 1963, she instituted a system of professional nursing practice at the Loeb Center, Montefiore Medical Center, in New York City. The Loeb model of care emphasized nursing autonomy and accountability, giving the nurse responsibility for providing care and making care decisions for his or her patients during the full duration of their hospital stay (Hall, 1969). Her visionary efforts planted ideas for change; however, few hospitals adopted her model.

Instability in the Nursing Labor Force

Despite the emphasis on efficiency and rationality in hospital management, the nursing labor force continued to be wracked by instability. Recurrent nursing shortages during the 1940s and 1960s led to the policies that increased the production of more nurses—short-training nurses in particular. These nursing shortages set the pattern for subsequent policy initiatives dominated by hospital interests (Grando, 1998). Hospital administrators and nursing leaders first encouraged licensed practical nurses and then associate degree nurses. In the midst of the shortages, attempts to fill nursing positions were like filling a leaking bucket. Nurses were clearly unhappy with work conditions and compensation. Shortages of nurses left team nurse leaders working alone as captains of understaffed nursing teams. While hospital nursing administrators struggled with the outflow of nurses, nursing educators struggled with the quest to professionalize nursing. The development of nursing knowledge and skills took on renewed urgency at mid-century. Nursing scholars such as Virginia Henderson (1966) sought to reclaim the primacy of the nurse–patient relationship and expand the focus of nursing care beyond efficiency to a process-oriented effectiveness.

The post–World War II period led to increased federal funding for nursing and health care. Along with the funding came a new closer scrutiny of hospital costs. As the federal government became more involved with funding hospital care, the drive to disentangle educational costs from nursing care costs took force.

By the late 1960s, funding of nursing education began to move away from the hospital training schools to colleges and universities. Early doctoral programs (see Chapter 3) developed as hybrid degrees, between nursing and fields such as education, sociology, psychology, and biology. These graduate programs had as their primary focus the development of a pool of nursing educators. But within a few years, collegiate nursing education institutions expanded programs in nursing administration and clinical specialization. Graduate education became the primary incubator for nursing theory and the growth of professional knowledge and values.

By the 1970s, a culture of professionalism emerged in nursing, fueled by the growth of nursing scholarship. This resulted in a gap between nurses' expectations and the experiential reality of nursing work. This gap, or reality shock (Kramer, 1974), was evidenced by the rapid turnover in staff nursing and nurses' growing discontent. Despite the move to a more efficient hospital functioning, the nursing labor force continued to be wracked by instability. Once again, nursing shortages led to the increased production of nurses, in particular short-training nurses. Hospital administrators and nursing leaders encouraged the addition of associate degree nurse production as a solution.

Nursing education, long tied to hospitals through the tradition of hospital diploma schools, began to break free in the 1960s. The federal government took up more of the financial burden for nursing education. But as nursing education moved into colleges, the trade-off was the loss of nurses' loyalty to hospitals, a central characteristic of hospital-diploma-school nurses. While hospital administrators struggled with the outflow of nurses, the growth of college-based programs at the baccalaureate and associate degree levels infused nursing with a new drive for professional status. As the development of nursing knowledge and skills took on more status and legitimacy, the predominance of nursing management as the primary means of career mobility came to an end (Wolf, 1993).

Militancy Rocks the Hospital Boat

Discontent with the reality of nursing work reflected the changing values and expectations of nurses. With rising expectations of professionalism, nurses' desires for control over their work were influenced by the new social realities of women's employment. Nursing was no longer viewed as a transient occupation for women to keep them busy until they married. The growing careerism sharpened nurses' lenses to workplace realities. Turnover rates in hospitals reflected the discontent with working conditions and benefits. Nurses, college educated and empowered by the emerging women's movement, were no longer willing to bow to the paternalism of hospital administrators.

At various points in nursing history, nurses had discussed or attempted the use of collective action or unionism. The rate of nurses organizing for collective bargaining began to increase in the 1960s, but it was not until 1974, with the addition of amendments to the federal Taft-Hartley Act, that the potential impact of collective bargaining was realized (Foley, 1993). These amendments provided federal protection to nurses and other healthcare employees of non-profit healthcare institutions with regard to the right to organize. The operational structure of the amendments emphasized that nurses were to be a separate and distinct bargaining unit.

The potential of the nursing labor force to be a catalyst for the unionization of the entire hospital labor force was clearly recognized by hospital administrators and union busting consultants. This, in turn, resulted in the idea of requiring hospital employees to organize into separate bargaining groups. Nurses were courted initially by professional nursing organizations, such as the ANA-affiliated state nursing organizations. Within a few years, more traditional industrial and trade unions, such as the United Auto Workers (UAW) and the American Federation of Teachers (AFT) joined efforts to organize nurses and other healthcare workers. The ANA-associated state nursing organizations were viewed as the lesser of two evils because the professionalism inherent in the nursing leadership tempered the militancy.

Hospital administrators explored a variety of means to fight the spread of hospital unionism (Kohles, 1994). Treating various types of hospital workers as contract workers was common, but this approach was neither cost- nor outcome-effective for nursing. Another approach was to create a new work culture and structure that would divide nurses from other hospital employees. This served a double purpose. First, it helped to insulate other hospital workers from nursing collective action. Second, it held the potential to curb the militancy. To effectively bridge the reality gap that had led to nurse militancy, nursing and hospital administrators needed to realistically grapple with the roots of nurses' frustration. The long-standing paternalism was no longer an effective means of controlling nurses.

Nursing Is Not Alone: The National Crisis in the Quality of Work Life

By the late 1970s, professionalism, long viewed as an unnecessary extravagance, was to become a mantra for nursing management. The growing belief that creating a more professional work climate could mitigate the potential for workplace militancy shaped efforts to restructure nursing work in hospitals. As hospital administrators and nursing grappled with what was perceived to be an issue of militancy versus professionalization, the issue was reflected in broader discussions of an emerging national crisis in workplace relations. Nationally, as concerns over decreases in worker productivity grew, labor experts debated the origins and solutions to worker discontent across a wide range of occupations and professions. The U.S. Department of Health, Education, & Welfare (1973) funded a study— "Work in America"—that asked the question, "What do workers want?" The study yielded the following answers: interesting work, enough help and equipment to get the job done, enough information to get the job done, enough authority to get the job done, good pay, opportunities to develop special abilities, job security, and the ability to see the results of one's work. National labor and management experts debated innovations such as worker control programs and work restructuring. However, the long-standing dominance of industrial labor skewed the perspective of labor experts who were slow to recognize the power and problems of the emerging service sector, and specifically the healthcare labor force.

By the mid-1970s, the nursing profession was in the midst of a collective feminist consciousness raising (Wolf, 1993). Nursing's perspective on nurses' discontent with their work held that the conditions nurses faced were unique and were often viewed within the context of gender and professionalism. Jo Ann Ashley (1996), a feminist nursing historian, offered the most vocal of the feminist perspectives. She described nurses' perceived powerlessness to change their situations as a consequence of their unique socialization as a female-gendered occupation and a result of the cultural barriers to the exercise of the power of nursing within paternalistic institutions.

Caught in a rapid current of cultural change, nursing and hospital administrators were pushed by nurses and pulled by larger social, economic, and political currents to face change in healthcare organizations. Collegiate nursing education, which had begun to embrace the notion of nurses as change agents, contributed to a new professional consciousness. The power to change nursing realities was slowly unleashed.

The unfreezing of hospital nursing to change was rapidly catalyzed as the potential threat of collective bargaining became evident to nursing and hospital industry management. Nurses, like workers in other industries and service sectors, wanted control over their work and a more equitable and open system of resource allocation and rewards. Control involved complex problems of achieving and sustaining authority and ensuring accountability for nursing practice. The potential scope of control ranged from specific day-to-day patient care decision making to participation in organizational governance, such as goal setting and finance (Siriani, 1984; Witte, 1972). Hospital decision making is typically viewed as hierarchical, with organizational control at the top and bedside or patient-care issues at the bottom. But in reality, the arenas of decision making are overlapping and interconnected within hospital organizations.

Patient-Centered Care and the Emergence of Primary Nursing

As the workplace reforms movement moved forward in the 1970s, the desire for control over patient care took precedence in most organizations. This reflected the growing necessity for greater nursing decision making given the rapidly increasing complexity of the patient care. The most influential development was primary nursing. According to Marram, Schlegel, and Bevis (1974), primary nursing was a developmental step in professional practice development that supported "the distribution of nursing so that the total care of an individual patient is the responsibility of one nurse, not many nurses" (p. 1). Many of the ideas inherent in primary nursing were previously noted by Lydia Hall (1969) at the Loeb Center. Influenced by the wave of quality in work life ideas in the contemporary management literature, primary nursing was invented as an approach to job redesign. This job-redesign approach had been applied successfully in industrial management in Europe and Japan. The primary nursing model offered hospital management a way to counter worker complaints about deskilling. The work of nursing was restructured and enlarged to make nurses accountable for the whole of patient care rather than just for specific tasks. Primary nursing was also ideologically imbued with professionalism.

The association between primary nursing and enhanced professional orientation was noted in many studies beginning in the 1970s (Marram, Schlegel, & Bevis, 1974). Manthey (1980), an early proponent of primary nursing, noted that primary nursing reflected a philosophical commitment to decision making at the level of action. Primary nursing, drawing on professionalism, sought increased accountability by the nurse for patient care, a rational system of care provided by the nurse who is most knowledgeable about the patient, individualized and personalized patient care, and increased equality among nursing staff (Marram, Schlegel, & Bevis, 1974). To support the initiation of primary nursing, registered nurses had to be reskilled, and hospitals sought to increase the staffing levels of registered nurses while decreasing the employment and roles of licensed practical nurses and nursing assistants. In most instances, this necessitated increased funding or significant reallocation of funds, made possible in the late 1970s by government and private support to hospitals.

Primary nursing provided a process by which patient-centered care could be individualized yet applied within a standardized nursing process. However unique each patient-care situation might be, the process of nursing judgment and discretion became predictable. The application of the nursing process as a method of solving nursing care problems became central to nursing education and practice in the 1970s. The development of professional nursing standards for care by the ANA further codified this process orientation. However, the growing complexity of patient care and the increasing body of nursing theory would soon shift nursing's emphasis to critical thinking.

Despite the shift in control over nursing education from hospitals to academic institutions, the reality was that most nursing graduates were going to be employed by hospitals. Nursing educators faced pressure to produce a product nurse that met the hospital labor market needs in terms of skill, as well as price.

As legal and regulatory pressures for greater accountability mounted, new demands for documentation shaped the day of hospital nurses. Nurses expressed a sense of being pushed into documentation at the expense of being pulled away from patient care. As one primary nurse noted, "Make sure your patient care is your priority, but don't forget your paperwork" (Wolf, 1993, p. 115). The strain of competing demands between the work of nursing and the documentation of the work emerged as a recurring theme underlying alienation and nurse dissatisfaction. As nurses grappled with the potential of primary nursing to provide rewards, the reality of the system's constraints and the contextual issues of organizational control became more apparent.

The Missing Links: Shared Governance and Recognition

The initiation of shared governance in healthcare institutions in the 1980s highlights an attempt to ease the tensions between administrative controls and professional work. Primary nursing, while restructuring nursing work, was quickly found to be limited in its scope. The work of nurses was embedded in the organizational context and was shaped by decisions that were often removed from their sphere of action. From staffing to equipment choice, these decisions often impacted patient care, leaving nurses frustrated, which compounded problems of turnover and militancy. Just as American industry struggled with the push to expand worker control without sacrificing managerial prerogatives, the push for workplace participation in decision making grew. Genuine participation was made difficult by the complex hospital authority structure, which kept nurses trapped between the dual hierarchies of medicine and the hospital administration.

The climb by nurses out from between these two systems of control generated both a threat and an opportunity for the reallocation of power in hospitals. Nursing leaders such as Manthey (1991) cautioned that in order for the reallocation of power to occur, a major change was required in the structure and operation of nursing departments. Change would require a major dismantling of the hospital hierarchy, beginning with the nursing departments. As Porter-O'Grady (2001) noted, "Implementing an empowered format such as shared governance means that the relationships, decisions, structures, and processes will be forever changed at every level of the system and that all the players in the organization will be different and behave differently as a result" (p. 5). The changes in patterns of communication and behaviors extended across relationships, not only nurse–nurse or nurse–patient, but also nurse–physician. Many physicians were initially ambivalent and threatened by shared governance (Wolf, 1993).

In the 1980s and 1990s, many hospitals moved toward flatter management structures in an effort to move toward shared governance. Work, previously viewed as a management prerogative, was typically distributed across the flattened structure to involve staff nurses as well as administrators in decision-making processes at the committee level. Nurse participation was concentrated at the committee level. A study by Jenkins (1988) observed that the expanded committee structure resulted in more time spent in meetings and an overall drop in hours per full-time employee. For example, Massachusetts

General Hospital provides a wide range of committees in its governance structure, including such foci as patient-care quality, diversity, and staff recruitment (Erickson, 1996). Participation is based on an application; it is a selective process that draws from a pool of dedicated full- and part-time nursing staff who give generously of their time and expertise.

A parallel concern to expanded decision making has been the need to recognize nurses for their efforts (McCoy, 1999). Hospital nursing is complex and difficult work. Keeping experienced nurses at the bedside improves the quality of patient care and reduces recruitment and orientation costs. The challenge has been to find a way to reward nurses for a career in direct care rather than management. Career ladders typify the development of new reward systems. Career ladders provide a hierarchical system of rewarding professional behaviors, such as advanced education; scholarship; and contributions to the institution, such as committee work or clinical projects. This system provides the semblance of mobility by recognizing those nurses who choose to stay at the bedside. Given the recurrent stresses of nursing shortages, career ladders have provided another mechanism to attract and retain clinically expert nurses. The career ladder system has codified the job enlargement of the professional nurse, while stimulating nurse productivity in a variety of areas, such as quality assurance, practice policy development, hospital public relations, and nurse recruitment (Wolf, 1993). However, the linking of remuneration with career-ladder progression historically has been problematic for many hospitals. The hospital budget process and pressures to control nurse salaries has thwarted career-ladder development efforts in some hospitals. Many senior nurses find themselves hitting the glass ceiling with new hires rapidly gaining more compensation. Healthcare organizations have also adopted nonmonetary systems of nurse recognition, such as the professional nurse of the month awards. These symbolic rewards, while recognizing clinical excellence, divert attention away from the concrete contextual realities of practice.

The Attraction of Magnet Hospitals

In the early 1980s, the American Academy of Nursing launched an effort to recognize hospitals for their ability to attract and retain nursing staff (Upenickes, 2003). The Magnet Hospital program was launched based on a study that identified hospitals having low staff turnover, high nurse job satisfaction, and low staff nurse vacancy rates. The initial recognition went to some 41 hospitals. The results of the early magnet hospital studies highlighted the importance of organizational factors, such as participatory structures and processes, perceived autonomy of nurses, and empowering leadership (Scott, Sochalski, & Aiken, 1999). The characteristics of these hospitals paralleled many of the recommended changes of the quality of work life advocates. Policy reports by the Institute of Medicine (1981) and the National Commission on Nursing (1981) report by the American Hospital Association gave added legitimacy to the move to restructure hospitals to better attract and retain nursing staff. Some 20 years after the initial magnet studies, a body of research has been collected to justify continuing support for the restructuring of systems

of care. Current efforts focus on validating outcomes of care in magnet hospital systems, but a better understanding of the relationship between outcomes and nurses' autonomy is needed (Havens & Aiken, 1999; Ritter-Teital, 2002; Scott et al., 1999).

Professional Nursing and Nurse Staffing: Chicken or Egg?

How well hospitals are able to sustain professional models is dependent on the political and economic climate of the healthcare market. Past nursing shortages generated greater leverage for nursing stakeholders. Yet as tensions in labor ease or are overcome by greater organizational pressure to contain or depress labor costs, the potential for backpedaling on professional nursing gains increases. Nursing has a greater potential to enhance quality outcomes by maximizing the use of professional expertise. As has been noted in recent studies, sustaining adequate nurse staffing may be one of the most important key factors in patient care outcomes (Aiken et al., 2002; Cho, Ketefian, Barkauskas, & Smith, 2003). Such research further underscores the importance of continuing professional models of development as they support the recruitment and retention of staff. For too long the value of nursing has been hidden in health care by data collection and information systems that give primacy to medicine. Emerging advances in nursing informatics will hopefully add to nursing's visibility and support continued vitality. A firm investment in professional models will also call for healthcare organizations to effectively match nursing education and talents with the complexity of the work. The corporatization of hospitals provides a relative opportunity for nursing to gain power in the healthcare organization. It is time for nursing to cease its dependence on the good will of institutions and to demand full participation in institutional policy making.

Conclusion

Throughout the history of nursing, professionalization has been a driving force for change. From the earliest innovations of Nightingale to the most recent nursing shortage, the work culture of nursing has been reshaped to meet the needs of society or managerial interests, often in the midst of crises. The slow march toward professional practice continues as models of nursing practice offer a powerful ideological hold. Nursing has been influenced by ideas drawn from sociology, management, and industry, resulting in workplace reforms reframed within a professional lens. The power of professionalization has contributed significantly to the success of this reform, offering benefits to both healthcare institutions and nurses. However, nursing shortages remain. Challenging questions for the future include the following: To what extent are professional models of practice sustainable in the face of economic uncertainty? Can institutional control truly be ceded to nurses without a fundamental revolution in the overall restructuring of healthcare financing and service structure?

Discussion Questions

1. In this chapter, the author argues that nursing's role in hospitals is imbued with managerialism, causing a paradox (Fourcher & Howard, 1981). The application of nursing knowledge and skill in managing patient care in hospitals has a long history of being subjugated to nursing and hospital administration. Nursing expertise has more often than not been invisible and undervalued, and autonomy of practice has been absent. Reflecting on this statement, do you agree or disagree?
2. How has societal and healthcare policy affected the development of nursing?
3. What are the pros and cons of unionization in nursing?
4. How will the Magnet Hospital program, shared governance, and mandated staffing ratios affect nursing in the future?

References

Aiken, L. H., Clarke, S. P., Sloane, D. M., Sochalski, J., & Silber, J. H. (2002). Hospital nurse staffing and patient mortality, nurse burnout, and job satisfaction. *Journal of the American Medical Association, 288*, 1987–1993.

Ashley, J. (1976). *Hospitals, paternalism, and the role of the nurse.* New York: Columbia University Press.

Ashley, J. (1996). This I believe about power in nursing. In K. Wolf (Ed.), *Selected readings of Jo Ann Ashley* (pp. 23–34). New York: NLN Press/Jones and Bartlett.

Bucher, R., & Strauss, A. (1961). Professions in progress. *American Journal of Sociology, 66*(4), 325–334.

Bullough, V., & Bullough, B. (1984). *The history, trends, and politics of nursing.* Norwalk, CT: Appleton Century Crofts.

Burgess, M. (1928). *Nurses, patients, and pocketbooks.* New York: Committee on the Grading of Nursing Schools.

Cho, S. H., Ketefian, S., Barkauskas, V. H., & Smith, D. G. (2003). The effects of nurse staffing on adverse events, morbidity, mortality, and medical costs. *Nursing Research, 52,* 71–79.

Dean, M., & Bolton, J. (1980). The administration of poverty and the development of nursing practice in nineteenth-century England. In C. Davies (Ed.), *Rewriting nursing history* (pp. 76–101). London: Croom Helm.

Dock, L., & Stewart, I. (1938). *A short history of nursing.* New York: G. P. Putnam's Sons.

Dossey, B. (1999). *Florence Nightingale: Mystic, visionary, healer.* Springhouse, PA: Springhouse Corporation.

Erickson, J. I. (1996). Our professional practice model. *MGH Patient Care Services, Caring Headlines, 2*(23).

Etzioni, A. (1969). *The semi-professions and their organization.* New York: Free Press.

Foley, M. (1993). The politics of collective bargaining. In D. Mason, S. Talbot, & J. Leavitt (Eds.), *Policy and politics for nurses* (2nd ed., pp. 282–302). Philadelphia: W. B. Saunders.

Fourcher, L., & Howard, M. (1981). Nursing and the managerial demiurge: Social Science and Medicine, Part A. *Medical Sociology, 15*(Pt. 3), 299–306.

Goldmark, J. (1923). *Nursing and nursing education in the U.S. Report of the committee for the study of nursing education.* New York: Macmillan.

Grando, V. T. (1998). Making do with fewer nurses in the United States, 1945–1965. *Image: Journal of Nursing Scholarship, 30*(2), 147–149.

Hall, L. E. (1969). The Loeb Center for Nursing and Rehabilitation, Montefiore Medical Center, Bronx, New York. *International Journal of Nursing Studies, 16,* 215–230.

Havens, D., & Aiken, L. (1999). Shaping systems to promote desired outcomes: The magnet hospitals model. *Journal of Nursing Administration, 29*(2), 14–20.

Hegyvary, S. T. (1982). *The change to primary nursing.* St. Louis, MO: C. V. Mosby.

Henderson, V. (1966). *The nature of nursing.* New York: MacMillan.

Hughes, C. E. (1971). *The sociological eye.* Chicago: Aldine.

Institute of Medicine. (1981). *The study of nursing and nursing education.* Washington, DC: National Academy of Science Press.

Jenkins, J. (1988). A nursing governance and practice model: What are the costs? *Nursing Economics, 6*(6), 302–311.

Kohles, M. K. (1994). Commentary on union election activity in the health care industry. *Health Care Management Review, 19*(1), 18–27.

Kramer, M. (1974). *Reality shock: Why nurses leave nursing.* St. Louis, MO: C. V. Mosby.

Manthey, M. (1980). *The practice of primary nursing.* Boston: Blackwell Scientific Publications.

Manthey, M. (1991). Delivery systems and practice models: A dynamic balance. *Nursing Management, 22*(1), 28–30.

Marram, G., Schlegel, M., & Bevis, E. O. (1974). *Primary nursing: A model for individualized care.* St. Louis, MO: C. V. Mosby.

McCoy, J. M. (1999). Recognize, reward, retain. *Nursing Management, 30*(2), 41–43.

Merriam-Webster's Collegiate Dictionary, 4th ed. (2006). p. 8.

National Commission on Nursing. (1981). *Summary of public hearings.* Chicago, IL: The Hospital Research and Educational Trust.

National League for Nursing Education. (1926). *The grading committee report of the National League for Nursing Education.* New York: NLNE.

Nightingale, F. (1866). Letter to Mary Jones. Cited on p. 25 in B. Abel-Smith, *A history of the nursing profession* (1960). London: Heinman.

Perrow, C. (1972). *Complex organizations: A critical essay.* Glenview, IL: Scott Foresman.

Porter-O'Grady, T. (2001). Is shared governance still relevant? *Journal of Nursing Administration, 31*(10), 467–473.

Reverby, S. (1979). The search for the hospital yardstick. In S. Reverby & D. Rosner (Eds.), *Health care in America* (pp. 206–225). Philadelphia: Temple University Press.

Reverby, S. (1987). *Ordered to care, the dilemma of American nursing, 1850–1945*. Cambridge, England: Cambridge University Press.

Reverby, S. (1999). Neither for the drawing room nor for the kitchen: Private duty nursing in Boston, 1873–1914. In J. Waltzer Leavitt (Ed.), *Women and health in America* (pp. 460–474). Madison: University of Wisconsin Press.

Ritter-Teital, J. (2002). The impact of restructuring on professional nursing practice. *Journal of Nursing Administration, 32*(1), 31–41.

Rosenberg, C. (1989). Community and communities: The evolution of the American hospital. In D. Long & J. Golden (Eds.), *The American general hospital* (pp. 3–17). Ithaca, NY: Cornell University Press.

Rosner, D. (1989). Doing well or doing good: The ambivalent focus of hospital administration. In D. Long & J. Golden (Eds.), *The American general hospital* (pp. 157–169). Ithaca, NY: Cornell University Press.

Scott, J. G., Sochalski, J., & Aiken, L. (1999). Review of magnet hospital research: Findings and implications for professional nursing practice. *Journal of Nursing Administration, 29*(1), 9–19.

Siriani, C. (1984). Participation, opportunity, and equality: Towards a pluralist organization model. In F. Ficher & C. Siriani (Eds.), *Critical studies in organization & bureaucracy* (pp. 482–503). Philadelphia: Temple University Press.

Starr, P. (1982). *The social transformation of American medicine*. New York: Basic Books.

Stevens, R. (1989). *In hospitals and in wealth. American hospitals in the twentieth century*. New York: Basic Books.

Upenickes, V. (2003). Recruitment and retention strategies: A magnet hospital prevention model. *Nursing Economics, 21*(1), 7–13, 23.

Williams, K. (1980). From Sarah Gamp to Florence Nightingale: A critical study of hospital nursing systems from 1840 to 1897. In C. Davies (Ed.), *Rewriting nursing history* (pp. 41–75). London: Croom Helm.

Witte, J. (1972). *Democracy, authority and alienation in work*. Chicago: University of Chicago Press.

Wolf, K. A. (1993). *The professionalization of nursing work: The case of nursing at Mill City Medical Center*. Dissertation microfilms PUZ9322364. Ann Arbor: University of Michigan.

U.S. Department of Health, Education & Welfare. (1973). *Work in America, HEW report*. Cambridge, MA: MIT Press.

Chapter 2

Advanced Practice Nursing: Moving Beyond the Basics

Joyce Pulcini

CHAPTER OBJECTIVES

1. Define *advanced practice nursing* and explain how the term is currently expanding and evolving.
2. Articulate the history, similarities, and differences of each of the traditional roles categorized as advanced practice nursing.
3. Consider how the roles of entry-level nurses through advanced practice nurses should be conceptualized for the future.

Introduction

According to the American Heritage Dictionary (1980), the term *advanced* means "ahead of contemporary thought or practice or at the highest level of difficulty." Practice is defined as "the exercise of an occupation or profession." Nursing has been defined as "The diagnosis and treatment of human responses to actual and potential health problems" (ANA, 1995).

In the last century, nursing has undergone many changes that have reshaped and expanded what is considered to be basic nursing. As nursing's role has evolved, so has its scope of practice. Many of today's nursing functions were originally within the realm of medicine or other disciplines. This metamorphosis has been part of the profession's gradual evolution and maturity over time.

Advanced practice nursing is defined by Hamric, Spross, and Hanson (2005) as "the application of an expanded range of practical, theoretical, and research-based competencies to phenomena experienced by patients within a specialized clinical area of the larger discipline of nursing" (p. 89). The term *advanced practice nursing* was coined to encompass four major roles within nursing: clinical nurse specialist (CNS), nurse practitioner (NP), certified nurse midwife (CNM), and certified registered nurse anesthetist (CRNA). The term distinguishes these nurses with advanced skills from those who practice as more traditional staff nurses and allows for a distinction between the nurse functioning at a more specialized level than the registered nurse. These roles also have been considered to be equally complex or at the same level of advanced practice. A common characteristic of these roles is the application of a greater breadth of knowledge and complexity of decision making to the problems of nursing care. Although each of these roles is distinct with regards to the specific areas of knowledge and skills that they draw on, they all require high levels of critical thinking, independence, and decision making.

Finally, the term *advanced practice* allowed for legislative changes to proceed with a minimum of confusion over how advanced practice and staff nurses differed. This distinction created opportunities for advanced practice nurses (APNs), but it also established a new class of nurse who seemed to some to be more privileged than their peers.

Each of these roles evolved a bit differently. The CNM evolved from the historical role of the midwife, who even today can be a nonnurse. The CRNA role evolved from the experiences of nurses in the Civil War who provided pain relief for soldiers (Hamric, Spross, & Hanson, 2005).

The CNS began to flourish in the 1950s and 1960s due to interest in promoting the highest level of nursing practice that coincided with the strong evolution of nursing theories and frameworks. This early CNS role had its roots in psychiatric nursing in the late 19th century and in specialist nursing roles in the early 1900s (Hamric, Spross, & Hanson, 2005). Initially, the CNS tended to work in hospitals or chronic care facilities caring for ill patients with specific health conditions. A major focus was the performance of indirect roles in nursing, such as

consultation, research, staff education, and patient/family education. Although not exclusive, much of the practice was also directed toward care coordination or institutional management of care. This specialty practice often dealt with symptom management or diagnosis of responses to illness rather than health promotion, and it focused on a unique set of problems emanating from illness. CNSs are highly competent nurses with a specialty focus who effectively meet the needs of patients in an increasingly complex healthcare system.

However, as cost-containment concerns became paramount and hospitals had to begin to cut costs in the 1980s, many of these CNS positions were eliminated even as staff nurses began to deal with sicker patients who had shorter stays in hospitals. In contrast, an increasing demand for nursing care in the community and long-term settings led to new opportunities for CNSs in home health care or specialized care for persons with HIV/AIDS or other chronic illnesses. At that time, CNSs began to function in community and long-term care settings as shortened hospital stays led to the quicker and sicker discharge of patients from hospitals or tertiary care facilities. In the past 10 years, the CNS has reemerged as an important component of patient care. The renewed interest in the CNS role has been fueled by regulatory and professional concerns. Pressures to demonstrate outcomes of care and to reduce risks such as patient injury or financial loss have generated a demand for the advanced practice knowledge and skills offered by the CNS (Heitkemper & Bond, 2004).

The NP role evolved from a shortage of primary care medical providers in underserved areas in the 1960s. Efforts to train NPs were spurred by progressive legislation of the Great Society era. As the federal government expanded financial access to care funded by Medicare, Medicaid, and community health center legislation, the need for more primary care providers became acute. The efforts to expand nursing practice were viewed by some in both medicine and nursing as a way for doctors to extend their care for patients using this new care provider.

This early concept of the NP role led many nurse educators to reject the idea of an advanced practice nurse and to close many avenues to university education. Thus, in the beginning years of NP role preparation, the majority of NP educational programs evolved outside of traditional nursing education in continuing education programs rather than in traditional master's programs. These early programs reflected the collaborative intent of nurses and more progressive doctors to create a new role for primary care practice. Through the NP role, the nurse's scope of practice expanded into realms that were previously only within the scope of medical practice, such as health assessment, medical diagnosis, and treatment of common and chronic illnesses. Most NPs functioned within the realm of primary care or generalist care, adding a strong health-promotion focus, while substituting for physicians who were not numerous enough to meet client needs. As the role has evolved, NPs have assumed greater responsibility in the management of more complex and chronic illnesses, and some have branched into specialty areas such as oncology, cardiology, or emergency care. When the NP role emerged, health promotion and disease prevention were being emphasized as an important component of primary care in all sectors of the healthcare system. As a result, NPs have a very strong foundation in direct patient care rather than in indirect nursing roles (Hamric & Hanson, 2003).

By the 1980s, the original community or public health focus of advanced practice was diluted as medical care became more individually focused and health financing failed to address public health needs. In this period, containment of healthcare costs was paramount in the minds of health policy makers, and the country was on the brink of replacing a public health focus with a system dominated by managed care. One exception was the community health CNS who continued to work in community settings such as Visiting Nurse Associations or home care agencies.

As more patients were discharged from the hospital due to shortened stays and prospective payment methodologies, the need for home care skyrocketed, and an entirely new sector of the healthcare system emerged. Cost-containment efforts of the 1980s were also a major force in the realignment of nursing roles. Diagnosis-related groups (DRGs) and cost-containment efforts led the public, insurers, and policy makers to demand more cost-efficient care. This changed the face of hospital nursing forever. Demands on nurses in inpatient settings increased exponentially. These developments led to nursing shortages and to periodic staffing crises, as were seen in 1989 and 2001.

Several occurrences led to fundamental changes in the mix of roles and the level of independence in nursing and to increasing difficulties in differentiating the various roles for nursing. An overarching factor was the women's movement, which reached its peak in the 1960s and 1970s, because it influenced the increased desire by nurses to have autonomy from other providers, such as physicians. This had a major effect on the nursing profession.

In the 1980s and 1990s, the NP role was viewed as a potentially cost effective option to the growing need for healthcare services. It also received an enormous amount of attention in the public and professional press. Another important change was the increased movement of NPs into acute care and medical specialties from primary care settings. As NP education began to be housed in universities, the distinction between the NP and the CNS was blurred.

In the 1980s, the CNS role was seen as too costly by hospital administrations because of reduced reimbursements from Medicare and shrinking hospital budgets. Thus, many CNS positions were lost across the country as hospitals eliminated any position viewed as providing indirect care. Education for the CNS specialty suffered from a lack of consistency across programs and confusion over the definition of terms. Educational programs reflected this confusion by using the designations NP and CNS interchangeably or by creating blended roles. The blended role was intended to combine the best of both roles, but it also confused those credentialing or hiring these advanced practice nurses (Hamric & Hanson, 2003; Hamric, Spross, & Hanson, 2005). Currently, the predominant view is that the CNS and the NP role are distinct from one another and should have separate educational programs (Hamric & Hanson, 2003; NACNS, 2004).

Since the inception of advanced practice nursing, health policy and regulatory advances enabling practice have moved forward with unprecedented swiftness and congruity. These advanced practice roles seem to have captured the imagination and interests of nurses who want more independent decision making and relief from what has been an increasingly stressful hospital environment. Barriers to practice for advanced practice nurses have decreased greatly over the past 20 years as legislative reforms have swept the nation. Third-party reimbursement for services and legislation for prescriptive privileges are now almost universal for NPs, CNMs, and CRNAs. These regulatory reforms have been far-reaching and now have been adopted by virtually every state (Pearson, 2004; Towers, 2004).

The role of advanced practice nurses has expanded well beyond initial expectations, and demands on practice continue to increase. For example, prescription writing now is virtually universal, and the types and breadth of prescribing has increased across all categories of NPs (Pulcini & Vampola, 2002; Pulcini, Vampola, & Levine, 2005). These authors also speculate that practice barriers may be lowest in rural areas or other areas where there is a greater need for healthcare services.

Educational Standards

Educational standards have evolved in different ways for each specialty. CNMs and CRNAs took the lead in establishing national standards for certification and program accreditation. The American Association of Nurse Anesthetists (AANA) established its own separate certification process in 1945 and an accreditation process in 1952 (AANA, 2004). The American College of Nurse Midwives (ACNM) established its certification process in 1971 and its own separate accreditation process in 1982 (ACNM, 2004). These efforts enabled these specialties to evolve with a consistency not seen in either NP or CNS educational programs, which expanded with less consistency and homogeneity.

Yet regulatory changes and reimbursement efforts for CNSs have lagged behind and are surrounded by controversy, such as whether prescribing should be part of the role (Lyons, 2004). Recently, CNSs have organized under the National Association of Clinical Nurse Specialists (NACNS) and have begun to standardize their education, regulations, and practice, publishing their landmark document, *Statement on Clinical Nurse Specialist Practice and Education* (2004).

Master's degree education preparation for NPs became the norm by the mid-1980s. Educational programs for NPs have become more congruent as a result of the National Organization of Nurse Practitioner Faculties' (NONPF) *Advanced Nursing Curriculum Guidelines and Program Standards for Nurse Practitioner Education* (1995), the *Domains and Competencies of Nurse Practitioner Practice* (2000), the *Criteria for Evaluation of Nurse Practitioner Programs* (2002a), and the *Nurse Practitioner Competencies in Specialty Areas* (2002b). As more NPs entered master's programs, the indirect-role (e.g., consultation, education, research) content in NP programs increased. Currently, more than 90% of NPs are master's prepared, and virtually all NPs are educated in graduate-level programs (Berlin, Stennett, & Bednash, 2004). The concept of the NP tipped in the mid-1990s, to use Malcolm Gladwell's (2000) term, and is now mainstream within nursing education. Currently, 330 graduate programs in nursing offer NP programs, with a total of 706 tracks, and 60% of master's program graduates are enrolled in NP programs (Berlin et al., 2004).

A final factor to consider is the new master's entry option that is popular in nursing education today. This option, which allows a person with a nonnursing degree to earn a master's in nursing as an NP or CNS in 2–3 years, increased threefold in graduate nursing programs from 1990 to 2002 (AACN, 2003). This development is important because originally most advanced practice nurses had experience in nursing before entering the advanced roles.

Theoretical Issues and Challenges

This last shift has been an important factor in the current nursing environment. The key issue is that there are now entry-level advanced practice nurses. However, our understanding of *advanced* has not moved with this paradigm shift. What has occurred is that many of the skills involved in advanced practice roles have moved into the mainstream. Most new nurses see these distinct skills as basic rather than within advanced practice. For example, many baccalaureate nursing programs now integrate physical assessment, pathophysiology, pharmacology, and health promotion, similar to advanced practice program curricula. Currently, the CNS, the CRNA, and the CNM are still viewed within the advanced practice role in the United States. But in many countries, a clear precedent has been set for basic nurses to have the skills of the nurse-midwife.

Internationally, the advanced practice role is evolving in diverse ways depending on the historical, political, and social factors that have shaped the nursing role and educational programs in each country. The definition of advanced practice nursing being adopted by the International Council of Nurses (2002) is as follows:

> The Nurse Practitioner/Advanced Practice Nurse (NP/APN) is a registered nurse who has acquired the expert knowledge base, complex decision-making skills and clinical competencies for expanded practice, the

characteristics of which are shaped by the context and/or country in which s/he is credentialed to practice. A Master's degree is recommended for entry level.

Many countries are beginning to develop advanced practice nursing programs. This role advancement is built on the strong role that nurses have in developing nations. The International Nurse Practitioner/Advanced Practice Nursing Network (INP/APNN), which is affiliated with the International Council for Nurses, has been instrumental in publishing definitions and scope and standards statements to guide nations in the development and expansion of advanced practice nursing. The challenge is to standardize practice definitions and educational standards while building and honoring the traditions of individual countries.

How do we, in 2008, reconceptualize the concept of advanced practice, given the current state of nursing education for APNs both in the United States and internationally? Is our old concept of advanced practice out of date? Can we reconceptualize what we consider to be the skills necessary for entry into nursing practice? If we have been operating with an outdated definition of advanced practice, what are the skills or competencies of advanced practice nurses that can be expected on entry into the profession? Does one need a specified number of years of experience before being called advanced, or are the skills that we once called advanced really mainstream or entry-level skills? If the latter is true, then we need to rethink the skills and competencies necessary for entry-level versus expert practice.

Grypdonck, Schuurmans, Gamel, and Goverde (2004) reconceptualize advanced practice nursing by making a distinction between nursing science and nursing practice. These authors point out that nursing science and nursing practice operate in different spheres and ways of thinking. For example, scientists base their decisions on the greatest possible degree of certainty, and clinicians deal with uncertainty every day. They say that expert advanced practice nurses effectively bridge that gap through their advanced education and practice experience. This is where the practice doctorate may really begin to fit into this complex continuum of advanced practice nurses (see Chapter 3 by Michael Carter).

In nursing, we have placed a great deal of weight on experience and position rather than on a specific level of knowledge. As we replace our current cadre of nurses with younger individuals, we would do best to see knowledge acquisition on a continuum, beginning with a set of basic practice skills and moving to expert practice that integrates scientific principles and research skills with ongoing teaching, mentoring, and expert consultation.

In the last 12 years, the cadre of generic master's programs or accelerated master's programs has grown threefold, and in many master's programs, these students comprise the majority of graduates. We must welcome these relatively young nurses into the fold of advanced practice nurses rather than exclude them and continue to operate in old ways.

In our reconceptualization of advanced practice, we might consider some way to recognize advanced practice through internships or other mechanisms of recognition. We may want to reconsider career ladders or Benner's levels of novice to expert practice. An expert advanced practice nurse should effectively use and incorporate research-based practice with a goal toward independent or collaborative research. Requirements for advanced practice nurses to precept, teach, or mentor newer nurses could be part of the certification credential. High-level skills such as consultation or clinical teaching require a body of expert knowledge and mastery of the content and are clearly in the realm of expert advanced practice nursing. Certification itself could be reframed to recognize entry-level versus expert practices, as was its original intent.

As we progress in redefining advanced practice, new technologies and knowledge, such as genetics and informatics, will increasingly enhance the patient-centered approach. Clinicians now are guided by state-of-the-art knowledge, which can be at the clinician's fingertips at any moment in practice through technology. In this new paradigm, the needs and demands of knowledgeable patients as well as scientific evidence-based guidelines will guide practice.

Conclusion

The nursing profession is now in a period of change, a paradigm shift. Nursing educators and policy makers must recognize this shift in order to plan for the future. As in the past, societal healthcare needs will shape the future direction of advanced practice nursing, and it will be up to our profession to change to meet those needs (Thompson & Watson, 2003). Our profession's ability to manage change and to move to a new conceptualization of advanced practice nursing will determine our success or failure in meeting societal needs. It is time to revisit even basic documents, such as the *Essentials of Master's Education for Advanced Practice Nursing* (AACN, 1996) and the *Essentials of Baccalaureate Education for Professional Nursing Practice* (AACN, 1998), which set the baseline definition of levels of nursing education. Our challenge now is to redefine *advanced* and recognize what is truly basic to all nursing practice.

Discussion Questions

1. Using the definitions of advanced practice nursing, should nursing administration, education, and research be considered advanced practice nursing?
2. List the similarities and differences between each of the roles discussed in this chapter.
3. What is the policy in your state related to licensure, reimbursement, and MD supervision for advanced practice nursing?
4. How can we reconceptualize what we consider to be the skills and knowledge needed for entry into practice as compared to those needed for advanced practice?

References

American Association of Colleges of Nursing. (1996). *The essentials of master's education for advanced practice nursing*. Washington, DC: Author.

American Association of Colleges of Nursing. (1998). *The essentials of baccalaureate education for professional nursing practice*. Washington, DC: Author.

American Association of Colleges of Nursing. (2003). *Accelerated programs: The fast-track to careers in nursing*. Retrieved September 19, 2007, from http://www.aacn.nche.edu/Publications/issues/Aug02.htm

American Association of Nurse Anesthetists, Council on Accreditation of Nurse Anesthesia Programs. (2004). *List of Recognized Educational Programs by Council on Accreditation of Nurse Anesthesia Educational Programs*. Retrieved September 19, 2007, from http://www.aana.com/WorkArea/linkit.aspx?LinkIdentifier=ID&ItemID=118

American College of Nurse Midwives, Division on Accreditation. (2004). *Division of accreditation*. Retrieved September 19, 2007, from http://www.midwife.org/about.cfm?id=54

American Heritage dictionary of the American language. (1980). Boston: Houghton-Mifflin.

American Nurses Association. (1995). *Nursing's social policy statement*. Washington, DC: Author.

Berlin, L., Stennett, J., & Bednash, G. (2004). *Enrollment and graduations baccalaureate and graduate programs in nursing*. Washington, DC: American Association of Colleges of Nursing.

Gladwell, M. (2000). *The tipping point: How little things make a big difference*. Boston, MA: Little Brown Co.

Grypdonck, M., Schuurmans, M., Gamel, C., & Goverde, K. (2004). *Uniting both worlds: Nursing science and advanced nursing practice*. Presented at the International Nurse Practitioner/Advanced Practice Nursing Network Conference, Groningen, The Netherlands.

Hamric, A., & Hanson, C. (2003). Educating advanced practice nurses for practice reality. *Journal of Professional Nursing, 19*(5), 262–268.

Hamric, A., Spross, J., & Hanson, C. (2005). *Advanced practice nursing: An integrative approach*. St. Louis, MO: Elsevier Saunders.

Heitkemper, M., & Bond, E. (2004). Clinical nurse specialists: State of the profession and challenges ahead. *Clinical Nurse Specialist, 18*(3), 135–140.

International Council of Nurses. (2002). Health policy/nurse practitioner/advanced practice: Definitions and characteristics of the role. Retrieved September 19, 2007, from http://www.aanp.org/INP%20APN%20network/practice%20issues/role%20definitions.asp

Lyons, B. (2004). The CNS regulatory quagmire: We need clarity about advanced nursing practice. *Clinical Nurse Specialist, 18*(1), 9–13.

National Association of Clinical Nurse Specialists. (2004). *Statement on clinical nurse specialist practice and education*. Harrisburg, PA: Author.

National Organization of Nurse Practitioner Faculties. (1995). *Advanced nursing practice curriculum guidelines and program standards for nurse practitioner education*. Washington, DC: Author.

National Organization of Nurse Practitioner Faculties. (2000). *Domains and competencies of nurse practitioner practice*. Washington, DC: Author.

National Organization of Nurse Practitioner Faculties. (2002a). *Criteria for evaluation of nurse practitioner programs*. Washington, DC: Author.

National Organization of Nurse Practitioner Faculties. (2002b). *Nurse practitioner competencies in specialty areas*. Washington, DC: Author.

Pearson, L. (2004). Sixteenth annual legislative update: How each state stands on legislative issues affecting advanced nursing practice. *The Nurse Practitioner, 29*(1), 26–51.

Pulcini, J., & Vampola, D. (2002). Tracking NP prescribing trends. *The Nurse Practitioner, 29*, 10.

Pulcini, J., Vampola, D., & Levine, J. (2005). NPACE nurse practitioner practice characteristics, salary, and benefits survey: 2003. *Clinical Excellence for Nurse Practitioners, 9*(1), 49–58.

Thompson, D., & Watson, R. (2003). Advanced practice nursing: What is it? *International Journal of Nursing Practice, 9*, 129–130.

Towers, J. (2004). Region one meeting of the American Academy of Nurse Practitioners, Portsmouth, NH, October 2004.

Chapter 3

The Evolution of Doctoral Education in Nursing

Michael Carter

CHAPTER OBJECTIVES

1. Discuss the history of doctoral education in general and nursing doctoral programs in particular.
2. Differentiate between the different titles and structures for doctoral degrees in nursing.
3. Discuss some of the controversies surrounding the pros and cons of doctoral degrees in nursing
4. List different approaches that will influence the future of nursing doctorates.

Introduction

One of the most important aspects of any profession is the appropriate educational preparation of the leaders of the discipline. Almost without exception, the professions require that their leaders must hold doctoral degrees. The broad purposes of doctoral educational programs are to provide preparation that leads to careers in government, business, and industry, as well as academia (CAGS, 1990). Doctoral programs have been in existence since the Middle Ages, but it was during the 20th century that the United States saw a dramatic proliferation of doctoral educational programs in almost every

academic field. The model of education that was created in the United States was built on earlier models from European universities. However, doctoral programs in the United States took on their own unique characteristics.

Nursing doctoral programs began in the later part of the 20th century, after their development in most other fields. Perhaps this delay was because of nursing's unique history among the professions. Nursing in the United States began outside the mainstream of higher education and was located almost exclusively in hospitals. These hospitals, and the later universities where nursing educational programs moved, were controlled by administrative structures that are best described as highly paternalistic. These paternalistic organizations, in juxtaposition with the fact that most nurses were and still are women, may have delayed the profession from adopting doctoral degrees as the required credential for professional leadership. The profession adopted the master's degree early as the appropriate degree for leaders, and this may have been a disservice to the profession. Currently, nursing is far from having a unified approach to doctoral education.

The purpose of this chapter is to briefly discuss the history of doctoral education in general and nursing doctoral programs in particular. Clearly, this discussion is not exhaustive but is intended to provide an introduction to understanding doctoral education. Other, better historical overviews are available on the general topic of doctoral degrees (Harris, Troutt, & Andrews, 1980). This chapter also includes discussion of some of the controversies that are swirling about how doctoral degrees in nursing should be titled and structured and concludes with some ideas that may portend the future of nursing doctorates.

A Brief History of Doctoral Education

The academic degrees that we see today are an outgrowth of the trade guilds and teaching guilds that flourished in Europe during the Middle Ages (U.S. DHEW, 1971). These early programs were often a product of the educational institutions that were either controlled or heavily dominated by the Catholic Church. Higher education was designed for the elite and certainly not for the general masses. Given this early tie with the Church, we can understand

that many of the symbols, traditions, and rituals of the modern university emerged from the Church's influence on these schools. The doctoral gowns and hoods worn at graduation can be traced back to the garb worn by the priests.

The English word *doctor* comes from the Latin word *doctus*, the past participle of *docere*, which means "to teach" (Webster's New Collegiate Dictionary, 1979). Italian schools awarded formal doctoral degrees by 1219. This was the only degree offered by the schools, because they were preparing teachers. French schools used a slightly different approach and chose the name *masters*, from the Latin word *magister*, for their college graduates. Graduates from these schools were awarded the respective title and were admitted to the guild of teachers (Martin, 1989). Obtaining a degree meant that the graduate was fully qualified to serve as a teacher and did not need additional evaluation to begin this profession.

In the United States, the early colleges were established to prepare clergy and for the most part were built on the English and German systems of higher education. Harvard College was founded in 1636, and from that time until the Civil War, a little over 200 years later, the only degree that could be earned in the United States was the Bachelor of Arts. Alumni who paid fees were able to obtain the master's degree without further collegiate work. Scientists who wished to obtain additional education had to receive this training in Europe (U.S. DHEW, 1971).

Following the Civil War, American colleges began to change. Yale awarded the first PhDs in the United States in 1861 (Martin, 1989). For the first time, there was an emerging emphasis on graduate education and the underlying research that is a part of graduate education today. Many of the faculty had obtained their graduate degrees at German universities. The German graduate school model did not usually include required class attendance or examinations. Rather, students studied under the direction of a major professor, conducted an original piece of research, and were expected to successfully defend their work before the standing faculty of the university in order to be granted the degree. However, because graduate education was embedded in undergraduate colleges, graduate students in the United States were often required to earn grades and attend lectures.

In the later half of the 1800s, several professional associations were formed to advance their respective professions. One of their early activities was to persuade state legislatures that the professional services offered by the various disciplines would be greatly improved by creating licensure or certification requirements. As a part of this effort, educational programs that led to the professional doctorate, including the doctor of medicine (MD) and the doctor of dental surgery (DDS) were developed. New medical schools began to offer limited instruction in allopathic or homeopathic medicine. Although offering a doctoral degree, most of these early schools were little more than diploma mills with few, if any, paid faculty, very limited instruction, and substantial reliance on clerkships with practicing physicians. By the late 1800s, there were many different types of professional schools, but there were no accreditation standards. Most had limited faculty and questionable curricula. Seldom were these programs more than a year in length, and admission depended more on the student's economic achievements than on the student's prior academic achievements (U.S. DHEW, 1971).

Efforts to standardize curricula began at the turn of the century and continued well into the 1900s. Calls went out to improve professional education as well as the quality of the PhD. By 1900, approximately 50 universities in the United States offered the PhD, but there was almost no quality control. At the best universities, the PhD was awarded after about 2 years of postbaccalaureate study. There were a number of calls to improve this situation. For example, Abraham Flexner (1930) argued that the American universities had become misguided by their focus on preparing PhD graduates for practice and not for pure learning. He contended that this had diminished the quality of the education. His work in graduate education came on the heels of his work on the reform of allopathic medical education. By 1935, a fairly standardized model for PhD education was in place, and the emergence of various accrediting bodies ensured that quality standards were met. Many PhD programs were closed or merged because their quality did not meet emerging national standards.

Following World War II, a clear link developed between building the knowledge base for a specialized field and the award of the PhD in that field. For the first time, the U.S. government allocated funds to the building of the research needed to create new knowledge. A large portion of this new money was directed toward science as a part of the country's national defense efforts (Berelson, 1960).

In the early 1950s, a new debate emerged over whether the PhD should be the degree for the professions or whether the professions should use a professional degree such as the doctor of education (EdD), the doctor of business administration (DBA), the doctor of public health (DPH), or the doctor of nursing science (DNSc). The professions believed that the PhD was the standard and was well understood and aspired toward that degree. Arts and sciences faculty believed that awarding a PhD with a specialty in the professions would diminish the degree. In general, the professions prevailed in this argument, and the PhD was selected as the appropriate degree. This degree did carry with it the concomitant requirement that the completion of a satisfactory piece of research was required for its award (Berelson, 1960).

Professions that wished to prepare their practitioners without this research requirement awarded a professional degree such as the doctor of osteopathy (DO), the doctor of medicine (MD), the doctor of dental surgery (DDS), the doctor of dental medicine (DMD), the doctor of pharmacy (PharmD), the doctor of veterinary medicine (DVM), the doctor of optometry (OD), the doctor of chiropractic medicine (DC), and the doctor of podiatric medicine (DPM). These professional programs were not considered graduate programs because few of them required an undergraduate degree for admission and most did not build on undergraduate learning in a specific discipline to prepare for the profession (CAGS, 1966).

Doctoral Programs in and for Nursing

Stevenson and Woods (1986) identified four phases in nursing doctoral programs. Doctoral programs in nursing can be thought of as having four generations. The first phase was between 1900 and 1940, in which the doctor of education (EdD) or another functional degree was available. The second phase was between 1940 and 1960, when the degree could be obtained in a basic or social science discipline with no nursing content. The third phase was between 1960 and 1970, when a basic or social science PhD was available with a minor in nursing. The fourth phase began around 1970 with the rapid proliferation of the DNSc and nursing PhD programs.

The first research-focused doctoral programs in the United States were in various areas of science and did not seek to recruit nurses specifically. Nurses, as well as any other student, could be considered for admission if they possessed the necessary prerequisites. The problem was that few nurses at the beginning of the 20th century held an undergraduate degree. Basic nursing education was hospital based and did not award degrees.

The first doctoral programs that specifically recruited nurses were at Columbia University and New York University. These began in the 1920s and 1930s in education departments and were tailored to prepare nursing faculty. The programs awarded the PhD or EdD, but offered little, if any, coursework in nursing.

In the 1940s and 1950s, baccalaureate programs in nursing were created at a number of universities. Along with this move came important questions about the qualifications of the faculty. Faculty qualifications were a minor issue when the program was located in a hospital, but most universities held rather strict standards for faculty. Few nurses held baccalaureate degrees, and even fewer held master's degrees. Almost none held doctoral degrees, and the doctoral degree was the standard for university faculty positions.

This change in locus of nursing education gave rise to often acrimonious discussions among faculty at several schools of nursing about the need for doctoral education. These discussions often raised the following questions: Should the program of study be focused on the discipline of nursing or a science-related discipline? Should the degree not be in education, since most of the graduates would be educators? Would the master's degree not be sufficient, particularly if the focus of the master's degree was clinical nursing? If the new doctoral programs were to focus on nursing, from where would the faculty be drawn, as the number of nurses with doctorates in nursing was not sufficient for one school faculty let alone many schools?

Several schools did begin doctoral programs in nursing in the 1950s and 1960s. While the program at Teachers College continued in nursing education and nursing administration, the program at New York University reconfigured the curriculum to focus on nursing as the science of unitary humans (Rogers, 1966). Boston University designed the first program to deal with the clinical practice of nursing and created the doctor of nursing science degree, with the first graduate in 1963. The University of California at San Francisco and the Catholic University of America followed Boston University's lead and established doctor of nursing science programs shortly thereafter. The University of Pittsburgh created a PhD in clinical nursing around this same time. The University of Alabama at Birmingham developed a doctor of science in nursing (DSN) shortly thereafter, and it was designed similarly to the DNSc (Kelly, 1978).

A serious problem remained, however, in that many of the key players concluded that nursing science was not of sufficient maturity to justify the PhD. Of course, no measure of scientific maturity was advocated. Perhaps this problem grew from the fact that most nurses with doctorates at this time had obtained their degrees in another discipline. Those disciplines had the

appearance of maturity because they offered a doctorate. These nurses had not spent their doctoral study in nursing because such doctoral study was not widely available. Further, some of the writings of the period display a rather romantic and narrow view of what constituted science. Nursing research texts proposed that science was logical and orderly, when in practice this is seldom the case. Some called for nursing practice to be derived from science, and yet few scientists would argue that practice is derived from science (McManus, 1960).

Funds from the federal government helped a number of nurses to obtain doctoral degrees, which may have contributed to the continuing debate over whether the doctoral degree should be in nursing or a different field. In 1955, the United States Public Health Service started funding doctoral study through the federal Predoctoral Research Fellowship Program. Funds were awarded directly to the doctoral student, and several aspiring faculty members were able to fund their education through this mechanism. Between 1955 and 1970, 156 nurses were supported by Division of Nursing fellowships (Grace, 1978). Almost none of these were in nursing.

Beginning in 1959, the Division of Nursing also funded the Faculty Research Development Grants Program. The purpose of these grants was to increase the research capabilities of faculty in graduate nursing programs by providing seed money. Eighteen institutions qualified for these grants between 1959 and 1968. Of these 18 programs, only three offered doctoral programs in nursing during the grant-funding period (1 PhD, 1 EdD, and 1 DNSc) (Martin, 1989).

In another attempt to increase the number of nurses with doctoral degrees, the Division of

Nursing began to fund the nurse scientist graduate training grants. The intent of this program was to build a cadre of nurses with doctoral degrees at universities and to increase the number of nursing doctoral programs. Funding was designed to assist nurses in obtaining doctoral degrees in fields that were viewed as related to nursing. These fields included such areas as sociology, psychology, anthropology, biology, and physiology, with the expectation that there would be coursework or a minor in nursing. Nine universities representing 34 different departments received these grants. Four of the nine universities had doctoral programs in nursing at the time, but these were not eligible for receipt of this funding (Martin, 1989).

Beginning in the early 1970s, several new doctoral programs in nursing emerged. These new programs were most often in the older, more established schools of nursing. Growth continued through the 1980s and 1990s, with several new programs opening each year. The pace of new program development was often faster than the available faculty would have predicted would be the case. In 1970, there were 20 programs, but by 2000 there were 78 (AACN, 2002). Most of the research being conducted in these schools was done by students. Funding for nursing research in these schools was rare. The most common degree offered was the PhD, but several schools offered the DNSc or the DSN. Doctoral education in nursing became widely available throughout the United States during this time.

New approaches to delivery of the curriculum became available as well. Some schools offered a summers option, in which courses were scheduled during the summer months when faculty in nursing schools who needed the doctoral degree could participate. Other schools offered

weekend programs, and Web-based distance learning programs emerged as well. Interestingly, the rapid increase in the number of programs and the development of creative ways to deliver the curriculum did little to increase the number of graduates each year.

This rapid growth and creativity in curriculum delivery were partly responsible for the development of new standards for doctoral programs. The American Association of Colleges of Nursing created a set of quality indicators for research-focused doctoral programs in nursing (AACN, 1993). These indicators became the standard for evaluation of these programs.

The rapid proliferation of programs did not create a concomitant increase in the number of graduates. The new programs were small (averaging six graduates per year), and the length of time to obtain the degree continued to be long, primarily because of the number of part-time students. Even though the number of programs had increased from 20 to 78, there were only 200 more graduates in 1998 than in 1989, and most of that growth occurred prior to 1992 (AACN, 2003). Clearly, these research-focused doctoral programs could not be expected to meet the needs for nursing faculty because of the small numbers and the fact that all graduates did not assume faculty positions after graduation. Also, the median age of the graduates at completion of the doctorate was over 45 years.

Clinical Doctoral Programs

In 1979, the Frances Payne Bolton School of Nursing at Case Western Reserve University began a new approach to doctoral education in nursing (Standing & Kramer, 2003). Originally conceived as a first professional degree, the doctor of nursing (ND) was open to college graduates and prepared them to be nurses at a level similar to other health professional doctoral programs, such as medicine, veterinary medicine, dentistry, optometry, and others. The creation of this clinical program at the very time that nursing was struggling with building the research enterprise and research-focused doctorates was not accepted with universal agreement. Of some concern was how this program would be different from the DNSc. Up to this time, there had been the assumption that the PhD was to focus on scholarly research and the DNSc was to be the practice-oriented, clinical degree. Yet, studies had shown that the DNSc could not be distinguished from the PhD on the basis of admission standards, curriculum, or dissertation topics (Flaherty, 1989). For the first time, nursing had a doctoral degree that was open to nonnurses and that prepared the beginning clinician at the doctoral level.

Additional clinical doctoral programs were developed at Rush University, the University of Colorado, and the University of South Carolina. Today, most of these programs provide multiple entry points reflective of the diverse nature of nursing practice. Each of these programs prepares the clinician at the doctoral level to exert leadership in evidence-based practice, health policy, and management or education. These new programs created quite a stir, and one that the profession has yet to resolve. In 1963, when the first DNSc was awarded, the profession had assumed that the first clinical doctorate had arrived. But close inspection of the program showed that the DNSc curriculum required mastery within a field of knowledge and demonstrated ability to perform scholarly research— the very characteristics of the PhD (Standing &

Kramer, 2003). The ND, on the other hand, focused exclusively on preparing a clinical leader, not a researcher.

The clinical doctoral programs to some extent reflected the tremendous changes that were taking place in the clinical practice of nursing. The early beginning of the nurse practitioner and clinical nurse specialist movements had taken place. New master's programs were opening each year, and the major thrust of these programs was on advanced nursing practice. State laws were changing, and advanced practice nurses were obtaining greatly expanded scopes of practice and prescriptive privileges. Most of these new master's programs were between 18 months and 2 years in length.

Concern among some faculty was building that the length and rigor of these master's programs needed to be improved and that the graduate should earn a doctorate. Yet, the doctorate needed to be focused in clinical practice. This position was consistent with the Council on Graduate Schools' position that "the professional doctor's degree should be the highest university award given in a particular field in recognition of completion of academic preparation for professional practice" (CAGS, 1966, p. 3). The schools that created the ND programs were noted for their outstanding clinical master's programs. This new degree could be viewed as a logical extension of their programs.

Nursing educators have not universally accepted the ND program. As Standing and Kramer (2003) point out, reviews of nursing doctoral graduates published in the literature almost always ignore the graduates of such programs even though nearly 700 nurses hold this degree. The basis for ignoring or discounting these programs is not clear. The need for the clinical doctorate is clearly documented, and the demand for the scarce slots in these programs is also clear.

Recently, the University of Kentucky began a new clinical doctoral program, the doctor of nursing practice (DNP). On close inspection, this program shares many of the same curricular components as the ND programs. An additional planning group has met for several years to build a consensus for the development of additional doctor of nursing practice programs at senior universities. However, the distinctions between the doctor of nursing practice and the doctor of nursing are far from clear.

Future Doctoral Education

The future of research-based doctoral programs in nursing is not likely to be much different from the recent past. No mechanisms are in place to determine how many programs there should be or to enforce quality standards at these programs. The demand for nursing faculty in the future is acute, and this will likely drive the creation of many more programs. Nursing has not been susceptible to the requirement seen in other disciplines that the faculty should be engaged in funded research prior to offering a research degree. Most schools offering the nursing PhD cannot be considered research-intensive schools.

The decision of a school to offer the PhD versus the DNSc often has been primarily a political decision. The PhD is often governed by the rules of the graduate school in addition to the nursing school, and this may mean that approval would be more problematic. Some schools (such as the University of California at San Francisco, the University of Pennsylvania,

and Indiana University) began their doctoral programs as DNSc programs and later converted them to the PhD. Only two schools have begun PhD programs and then added DNSc programs—the University of Tennessee Health Science Center and Johns Hopkins University. In general, faculty prefer the PhD; therefore, it will likely continue to be the preferred degree in the future.

However, the world of clinical doctorates is quite different. The other major health professions have offered the clinical doctor's degree for a number of years. For example, pharmacy is the most recent profession to mandate the doctorate as the single degree for its professional practice. Nursing, the largest health profession, continues to prepare its beginning practitioners at less than the baccalaureate level. Attempts to alter this situation, even in light of important evidence of the value of higher education, have failed. What is emerging, however, is a de facto second license for nursing, the advanced practice license. This new license may accelerate the development of the clinical doctorate.

Nursing chose the master's degree as the minimum preparation for advanced practice. The master's degree in the United States has always been an unusual degree—more than the baccalaureate but less than the doctorate, and usually discipline specific. This degree is uncommon in the major health professions, at least as a professional degree. This degree designation is used for the master of public health and the master of hospital administration, but the other health professions use a nondegree, postdoctoral training period to prepare their specialists. Reasons as to why nursing adopted the master's degree are somewhat obscure, but are likely related to political considerations.

Nursing's history of hospital-based education rather than degree-based education meant that much of nursing was left out of the advances in higher education during the 20th century. While medicine, dentistry, and to some extent, pharmacy, were able to strengthen their educational programs within the university tradition, nursing was still knocking at the door. Few women were able to obtain a college education until well after World War II. The idea that nursing should have a clinical doctoral degree similar to the other health fields would not have entered the minds of most academics, and certainly not most nurses, until recently.

Today, however, we see advanced practice nurses in roles that were unthinkable just a few years ago. Independent nursing practices in institutions and communities are making substantial changes in the way health care is delivered. The kind of education that these clinicians will need for the future cannot be achieved in today's master's programs. The future advanced practice nurses will need a minimum of a clinical doctoral degree and most likely will require substantial postdoctoral training in narrow specialties.

Not every school that currently offers the master's degree will have the faculty, clinical material, or other requisite resources to offer the clinical doctoral program. These programs are faculty intense, require interdisciplinary coursework with the other major health professions, and are costly to operate. Schools of nursing must have a substantial clinical practice operation to be able to mount such a program. These new programs will prepare highly competent clinicians for such roles as primary care provider for cross-site practice; midwifery practice that includes surgical abilities to perform cesarean sections; anesthesia providers to administer all forms of anesthesia, including intrathecal approaches; as well as national and international leaders in policy formulation, complex organizational administration, and master clinical teachers. These roles cannot be achieved by obtaining a research-focused doctoral degree, and certainly not by way of the master's degree.

Conclusion

Doctoral education in the United States underwent dramatic changes during the 20th century and will likely continue to evolve over the next century. Nurses were once educated outside the mainstream of higher education, but following World War II the locus of nursing education was moved to the university. This has brought with it the need for a faculty commensurate with that of the rest of the university. For the arts and sciences, that meant the PhD degree; for the professional schools, that has meant the clinical doctorate.

Nursing was a bit slow to embrace the idea that nursing faculty would need the research doctorate. But once the idea was adopted, many schools—some would argue too many schools—rapidly developed these programs. There is still a reluctance to move to the development of the clinical doctorate on a broad scale. The potential for this degree to alter the power and political relationships between nursing and other professions, however, is substantial.

The clinical doctorate can provide a skill and science base for the graduate that cannot be achieved in today's educational programs. This level of expertise will be critical as the nation focuses on improving patient care and the safety of the systems that deliver health care. Clearly, the clinical doctorate will bring with it a level of independent practice that cannot be achieved at less than the doctoral level. For the first time, nursing would have parity in educational preparation with other healthcare disciplines.

Nursing is the most comprehensive of all the health professions. Clinical practice demands of nursing clinicians an understanding of the human condition, the environments in which clients live, the systems of care delivery, and the political milieu of care. Preparation of clinical leaders fundamentally requires a doctoral degree. The time is now for the discipline to move to the clinical doctorate to complement the many substantial accomplishments that have taken place by the creation of the research-focused doctorates.

Discussion Questions

1. Visit the Web site of the American Association of Colleges of Nursing and specialty organizations. Read the most recent update on the clinical doctorate. Visit the sites of several universities and compare and contrast the similarities and differences of doctoral programs throughout the United States.
2. What are the pros and cons of requiring doctoral education for advanced practice in nursing? Include personal, professional, healthcare, and societal perspectives.

References

American Association of Colleges of Nursing (AACN). (1993). *AACN position statement: Indicators of quality in doctoral programs in nursing*. Washington, DC: Author.

American Association of Colleges of Nursing (AACN). (2002). *Indicators of Quality in Research-Focused Doctoral Programs in Nursing*. Retrieved September 19, 2007, from http://www.aacn.nche.edu/Publications/positions/qualityindicators.htm

American Association of Colleges of Nursing (AACN). (2003). Indicators of quality in research-focused doctoral programs in nursing. *Journal of Professional Nursing, 18*(5), 289–294.

Berelson, B. (1960). *Graduate education in the United States*. New York: McGraw-Hill.

Council of Graduate Schools (CGS) in the United States. (1966). *The doctor's degree in professional fields*. A statement by the Association of Graduate Schools and the Council of Graduate Schools in the United States. Washington, DC: Author.

Council of Graduate Schools (CGS) in the United States. (1990). *The doctor of philosophy degree: A policy statement*. Washington, DC: Author.

Flaherty, M. J. (1989). The doctor of nursing science degree: Evolutionary and societal perspectives. In S. E. Hart (Ed.), *Doctoral education in nursing: History, process, and outcome* (pp. 17–31). New York: National League for Nursing.

Flexner, A. (1930). *Universities: American, English, German*. New York: Oxford University Press.

Grace, H. (1978). The research doctorate in nursing. In *Proceedings of the 1978 Forum on Doctoral Education in Nursing* (pp. 40–59). Chicago: Rush University.

Harris, J., Troutt, W., & Andrews, G. (1980). *The American doctorate in the context of new patterns in higher education*. Washington, DC: Council on Post Secondary Accreditation.

Kelly, J. (1978). The professional doctorate in nursing from the viewpoint of nursing service. In

Proceedings of the 1978 Forum on Doctoral Education in Nursing (pp. 10–39). Chicago: Rush University.

Martin, E. J. (1989). The doctor of philosophy degree: Evolutionary and societal perspectives. In S. E. Hart (Ed.), *Doctoral education in nursing: History, process and outcome* (pp. 1–16). New York: National League for Nursing.

McManus, L. (1960). Doctoral education in nursing: A nurse educator responds. *Nursing Outlook, 8,* 543–546.

Rogers, M. (1966). Doctoral education in nursing. *Nursing Forum, 5*(2), 75–82.

Standing, T. S., & Kramer, F. M. (2003). The ND: Preparing nurses for clinical and educational leadership. *Reflections on Nursing Leadership, 29*(4), 35–37, 44.

Stevenson, J. S., & Woods, N. F. (1986). Nursing science and contemporary science: Emerging paradigms. In G. E. Sorensen (Ed.), *Setting the agenda for the year 2000: Knowledge development in nursing* (pp. 6–20). Kansas City, MO: American Academy of Nursing.

U.S. Department of Health, Education, and Welfare (U.S. DHEW). (1971). *Future directions of doctoral education for nurses.* (U.S. DHEW Publication No. [NIH] 72–82). Bethesda, MD: Author.

Webster's New Collegiate Dictionary. (1979). Springfield, MA: Merriam-Webster.

Leadership Development Through Mentorship and Professional Development Planning

Anne M. Barker

CHAPTER OBJECTIVES

1. Discuss the benefits of having a mentor.
2. List the issues to consider when selecting a mentor.
3. List the phases of the mentor–mentee relationship.
4. Distinguish between mentoring and networking.
5. Identify professional development needs and make a plan to achieve them.

Introduction

The mentor–mentee relationship is a very special one between two individuals. The benefits of having a mentor, or more than one, are well documented and one should consider them as one decides to find a mentor or enhance the role a mentor plays in one's career. This chapter can help readers evaluate the mentoring relationship and provide a structure for working with a mentor.

Research regarding mentorship shows that individuals who have a mentor, as compared to those not having a mentor, have:

- Increased job satisfaction.
- Higher salaries.
- Enhanced self-esteem and confidence.

- Greater opportunities for promotion and advancement.
- Enhanced role socialization.
- A definitive career plan (Grindell, 2003).

Chapter 4

Mentorship Model

From the many definitions of a mentor, for this chapter the classic definition proposed by Vance (1982) is used. She defines a mentor as an experienced person who guides and nurtures a less experienced person (the mentee). The mentor is someone who inspires, instructs, nurtures, and encourages the mentee. Vance states that the mentoring relationship is a helping relationship that is special, emotional, intense, and enduring

Figure 4–1 The Barker-Sullivan Model of Mentor Partnerships

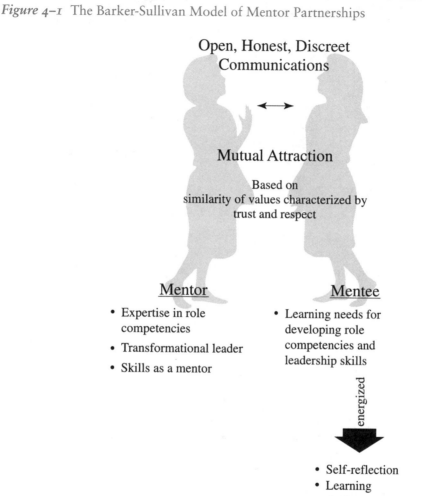

Open, Honest, Discreet
Communications

←——→

Mutual Attraction

Based on
similarity of values characterized by
trust and respect

Mentor

- Expertise in role competencies
- Transformational leader
- Skills as a mentor

Mentee

- Learning needs for developing role competencies and leadership skills

energized

- Self-reflection
- Learning
- Action

as opposed to shorter term and less intense relationships such as preceptor, sponsor, role model, or peer.

Figure 4–1 illustrates the Barker-Sullivan model of mentorship, which was devised through a review of the literature and through personal experiences of having a mentor and being a mentor. The relationship between the mentor and mentee can best be described as a partnership. In

this partnership there is a congruency between the expertise and organizational connections of the mentor and the learning needs of the mentee. As a result of the relationship and interactions between the two, the mentee is energized for self-reflection, learning, and action, leading to professional role development and growth.

At the heart of this relationship there must be mutual trust and respect and open communications

(Klein, 2000). The mentee will be disclosing sensitive information, exposing weaknesses, and discussing lack of skills and competence in job-related areas. Thus, the mentee must feel that he or she can be open and honest and, in return, expect confidential, nonjudgmental, and sensitive feedback from the mentor.

Stages of the Mentor–Mentee Relationship

The mentor–mentee relationship ideally exists over a long period of time and therefore goes through several stages (Anderson et al., 2002). Each stage is discussed next. Readers can use this information to understand what to expect from a mentor–mentee relationship, or, for those who already have a mentor, use the information to assess their relationship.

Stage One: Selecting a Mentor and Determining Expectations

Mentee–mentor relationships are formed in healthcare organizations in one of two ways, formally or informally. Some organizations have formal, structured mentorship programs established to assist new employees in developing their role. The benefit of a formal mentorship program is that it provides structure and well-defined expectations for both parties, as well as deploying organizational resources, particularly time, for the ongoing development of the relationship (Anderson et al., 2002).

Having a formal mentorship program does not preclude the mentee from initiating other informal mentor relationship(s). In fact, informal mentor relationships are often the best

ones because at the heart of the mentor–mentee relationship is an attraction of both people whose personality and values fit. Informal mentor–mentee relationships happen because both the mentor and mentee wish to work together and share mutual respect and admiration. This may or may not happen when one is assigned a mentor in a formal program.

There are many considerations as one decides who to ask to be a mentor. We offer several guidelines to assist in identifying appropriate individuals. First, one may find that there are several people to consider as mentors. Each of these individuals can bring something different to one's professional growth and development; therefore, no one should rule out having more than one mentor.

Second, we do not recommend choosing a direct supervisor or a potential supervisor. There are several reasons for this, the most important being that since the supervisor serves as an evaluator, the mentee may be reluctant to be vulnerable and share what he or she sees as weaknesses for fear that they will turn up on an official evaluation. However, to be an effective advanced practice nurse, the nurse does need to establish an effective and appropriate relationship with his or her supervisor. Having a mentor can help with this relationship and contribute to professional growth and learning.

A third consideration is whether to ask someone within or outside the organization to serve as a mentor. The pros of having an internal mentor are that the person knows the organization, can help make connections, can observe behaviors and outcomes, and may get indirect feedback about the mentee's performance from others. On the other hand, a mentor external to an organization can offer new insights and different ways of doing things and can help make connections outside the organization.

A final consideration is whether to use a peer mentor or someone in an advanced position other than the supervisor position. The advantages of having a mentor from among peers are that they are experiencing the issues and needs of the role in a similar way. Their network of connections may be more appropriate. A mentor at a higher level in the organization, however, can provide a broader view of the organization and a different level of connections with others.

In summary, it is worth considering having more than one mentor representing other disciplines, both genders, cultural and generational diversity, and professionals who work in other organizations. Table 4–1 is a checklist for you to use in selecting someone as a mentor. The first six questions focus on the person's leadership skills and role expertise. If the answer is "no" to any of these questions, then we recommend reconsidering the person as a mentor. However, that person might have several important skills the mentee wishes to learn and the assessment might make it clear of what the potential mentor can and cannot offer. The last five questions relate to the person's ability to be an effective mentor.

After selecting a mentor(s), the next step is to establish ground rules. Borges and Smith (2004) provide a set of strategies to set up expectations for the relationship in this very early stage. First, they suggest setting up the details of when, where, and how long meetings will take place and what other forms of communication, such as e-mail, should be used. Second, the mentee should write down long-term career goals/visions and use this as a starting point for discussion and planning. The last strategy is to develop specific professional learning goals and personal goals. In the next section we discuss tools for assessing developmental needs and a form for documenting plans for meeting these

needs and progress toward goals. In this process the mentee should also consider life goals such as salary, health, family, spiritual needs, and so forth. We believe that an advanced practice nurse must lead a balanced and happy life to be effective. A mentor can help set and pay attention to personal goals and help balance them with professional goals.

Stage Two: Development of Role Competencies

In stage two, the mentee works on developmental goals by engaging in specific learning activities, with the guidance and support of the mentor. The mentor serves as teacher, advisor, facilitator, coach, and sounding board (Anderson et al., 2002). During this time the mentor connects the mentee to appropriate people both inside and outside the organization and helps the mentee develop the skills, knowledge, and attitudes to be effective.

Stage Three: Growing Independence

As time progresses, the mentee grows in confidence, gains the necessary knowledge and skills to be an effective advanced practice nurse, and demonstrates the attainment of the role competencies. At this point the mentee begins to seek independence, and the mentor role changes to consultant, giving advice only when asked (Anderson et al., 2002).

Stage Four: The Dissolution of the Relationship

In the last stage, the mentee is ready to move on from the relationship and no longer needs the mentor's advice and support. However, often an

Table 4-1 Mentor Selection Checklist

Name of Potential Mentor:
Brief explanation of why you are considering this person:

Desired Characteristic	Yes	No	Don't Know
1. Does the person have the expert knowledge and skills in the competencies that you need to develop?			
2. Is the person a leader by action and by example?			
3. Does this person have the ability to guide, coach, and teach you?			
4. Is the person respected in the organization?			
5. Does the person have access to important organizational information and can he or she help you to direct attention on important issues?			
6. Does the person have a network of influential people and is he or she willing to assist you to be visible, credible, and accepted by others in the organization?			
7. Is the person willing to work collaboratively with you?			
8. Is the person willing to spend the time and energy required for the development of this relationship?			
9. Are you comfortable with this person and do you trust him or her to hold confidentiality?			
10. Is the person able to provide you with negative as well as positive feedback?			
11. Can the person help you identify what you need to learn and provide the structure for learning activities?			
Summary statement:			

enduring friendship and colleagueship evolves and is maintained over the course of many years (Anderson et al., 2002).

Mentorship versus Networking

Networking is interacting with individuals within and outside the organization to share ideas, information, and experiences, and to give and get advice. In contrast to mentoring, networking has less sustained interactions with others and is less structured. Having a network of people is as important for professional development as it is to have a mentor.

For networking to be effective, one needs to reflect on networking needs and set up processes to ensure that one interacts with people who can contribute to professional growth and development. First of all, one should think about people in the organization who can provide good insights about the organization, whose personality and values are similar to one's own, whose communication style is compatible, and who might be willing to share. In turn, the advanced practice nurse should think about people in the organization with whom he or she could share experiences and ideas. He or she should think about this broadly and include other disciplines and peers. Next, he or she simply needs to make contact with these people by asking them for coffee or lunch, or to stay after a meeting for a few minutes just to talk or to ask for their advice about a specific issue. As nurses establish a relationship with others, phone calls and e-mail will assist them in maintaining contact even when they are busy. The key here is to be attentive about developing the networks, rather than just letting the relationships emerge. Further, the nurse and the person he or she networks with should establish guidelines for confidentiality, being clear what information can and cannot be shared.

Besides having a network within the organization, everyone should also establish a network of contacts outside the organization. Most often this occurs through professional organizations and meetings. The same thought process put into establishing an internal network should be used for establishing a network of people outside the organization. Contact with others should be made, and the contact should be maintained over time.

A Model of Career Development

In the next section of this chapter, we will discuss a process for assessing career development needs and planning for continual growth. These activities should provide a structure for a mentor and mentee to begin their initial work together. Our goal in this activity is for people to develop certain capabilities, including:

- Engaging in self-reflection and self-awareness.
- Enhancing self-confidence.
- Learning to take a broad systematic view of health care and one's organization.
- Learning to work effectively within an organization and with others.
- Developing the ability to think critically and creatively.
- Engaging in experimental learning.

Klein (2002) presents a model of career development that provides a useful framework for reflecting on career development needs. Most

Table 4–2 MODEL OF CAREER DEVELOPMENT

	Internal	External
Individual	**Quadrant 1** **Self** • Values • Purposes • Personal meaning	**Quadrant 2** **Your Behaviors** • Competencies • Skills • Knowledge • Leadership traits
Collective	**Quadrant 3** **Organizational** **Culture** • Vision • Shared values • Shared purpose • Relationships	**Quadrant 4** **The Environment** • Organizational structures and systems • Technology • The healthcare delivery system

Source: Klein, E. (2002, First Quarter). Missing something in your career? *Reflections on Nursing Leadership*, 41–42. Used with permission.

professional development programs place an emphasis on the development of individual skills and competencies and learning how the organization works while ignoring the vision and values of the individual and the organization. This model presents a more holistic view; the tools presented here were developed using this framework.

Table 4–2 has four quadrants to consider in looking at career development. Individual and collective aspects are placed along the vertical axis while internal and external aspects are placed along the horizontal axis. Individual aspects are things to consider about oneself whereas collective aspects deal with the organization and the larger world.

Quadrants 1 and 2 list individual aspects of career, internal and external, respectively. Quadrant 1 is the internal or self aspects. In this area nurses reflect on their individual values, purposes, and the personal meaning that leadership and their profession have for them. In quadrant 2, the external individual aspects of

career development (behaviors) reside and include the competencies and skills needed to perform a job or to obtain advanced positions.

Quadrants 3 and 4 attend to the collective aspects of one's career, both internal and external. In quadrant 3, the internal collective aspects of organizational culture include consideration of the shared values, shared purposes, and relationships that affect how one relates to others in the organization. Quadrant 4, the environment, includes the organizational structures and systems, policies and procedures, and technology in the organization.

It is useful to study Table 4–2 to gain a full understanding of career development needs. No one quadrant stands on its own. For instance, values and beliefs as an individual must be consistent with the values and purposes of the organization. Likewise, the external competencies and skills one develops must be pertinent to and useful for the work environment. These activities can maximize the chances of a good fit between the nurse and the organization, increasing role satisfaction.

Process for Career Development Planning

Using the career development model, we suggest a four-step career development planning process (Donner & Wheeler, 2001). Tables 4–3 and 4–4 give two tools to integrate these steps with the model:

- Scan the environment (Table 4–3).
- Complete a self-assessment (Table 4–3).
- Create a career vision (Table 4–3).
- Develop a career plan (Table 4–4).

The first section of Table 4–3 asks individuals to scan the environment and look at the organizational culture and the environmental

considerations (quadrants 3 and 4 of Table 4–2) discussed in the model. This will help nurses to understand their developmental needs in a broad context of the overall environment of health care and professional nursing.

The second section of Table 4–3 is a self-assessment (quadrants 1 and 2 of Table 4–2) in which users are asked to assess their values and beliefs, skills, and knowledge needed for advanced practice.

In the third section of Table 4–3, users are asked to write down their overall career goal and vision. This will serve as a starting point in initiating conversations with a mentor about goals and learning needs.

Professional Development Plan

Based on the self-assessment, Table 4–4 can be used to develop an individualized professional

---

Table 4–3 SELF-ASSESSMENT OF ADVANCED PRACTICE NURSING DEVELOPMENT NEEDS

Section 1: Scan the Environment

1. What are the current realities about advanced practice nursing in your organization, your state, and in the nation and what are the future trends?
2. How do you see your strengths and weaknesses related to the needs of the healthcare environment and the organization and your role as an advanced practitioner?
3. What are the organization's vision and shared values, and how do you contribute to moving them forward?

Section 2: Self-Assessment

1. What are your personal values about your profession and about health care? How do you find meaning and purpose in your career and in your personal life?
2. What strengths/experiences/knowledge do you have to build on?
3. What new experiences or knowledge do you need for the future?
4. What are your limitations?

Section 3: Career Vision

1. Where do you see yourself going?
2. What is stopping you? What are you doing about it?

Table 4-4 PROFESSIONAL DEVELOPMENT PLAN

Goals	Plans	Timelines	Resources

development plan. Space is provided for goals, plans, timelines, and the resources to be used.

It is easy to pass over these activities and exercises, because one already has them in mind, but one of the keys to success is having written goals and plans and reviewing and revising them periodically. Completing these activities and exercises will help one to select a mentor who can assist with learning needs. Further, this self-assessment and plan should be reviewed and revised with a mentor at planned intervals and/or when the mentee has completed a significant accomplishment.

The benefits of goal setting are:

- The individual will feel that his or her future is positive and that he or she has control over where he or she is headed.

- The individual knows what he or she wants and how to get there.

- The individual has clear targets to focus on and to guide each day's actions and commitments.

- Daily actions will build into personal successes over time.

Discussion Questions

1. Who are some individuals you currently know who may be a good mentor for you? Using Table 4–1, assess whether you should approach these persons about mentoring you.
2. Complete Tables 4–3 and 4–4 and discuss the similarities and differences of your plan with your peers.

References

Anderson, M., Kroll, B., Luoma, J., Nelson, J., Sheman, K., & Surdo, J. (2002). Mentoring relationships. *Minnesota Nursing Accent, 74*(4).

Borges, J. R., & Smith, B. C. (2004, June). Strategies for mentoring a diverse nursing workforce. *Nurse Leader*, 45–48.

Donner, G. J., & Wheeler, M. M. (2001). Career planning and development for nurses: The time has come. *International Nursing Review, 48*(2), 79–86.

Grindell, C. G. (2003). Mentor managers. *Nephrology Nursing Journal, 30*(5), 517–522.

Klein, E. (2002). Missing something in your career? *Reflections on Nursing Leadership, 30*(1), 41–42.

Vance, C. (1982). The mentor connection. *Journal of Nursing Administration, 12*(4), 7–13.

Managing Personal Resources: Time and Stress Management

Anne M. Barker

CHAPTER OBJECTIVES

1. Discuss the benefits of managing time and stress.
2. List strategies to management time and stress that can enhance work life.

Introduction

One of the recurring themes in the literature about nursing and the nursing shortage is the need for nurses to lead a balanced life. As one advances his or her career and expertise, this skill becomes even more vital especially when pursuing new goals and developing new expertise. By completing the exercises and assessments in this chapter, the reader should gain a better understanding of his or her strengths and weaknesses regarding time and stress management.

Time Management

Time is one of the most precious resources that we have and one we can control. To be effective and efficient in one's role as an advanced practice nurse, one needs to manage time in order to spend it in professional activities that are mean-

ingful and effective while at the same time gaining satisfaction and enjoyment in the role.

Chapter 5

Benefits of Managing Time

The traditional view of time management is that time is a precious resource that must be managed. However, there is more to time management than only thinking of it as a resource. The most important benefits of time management are (Barker, 1992):

- Having clarity of mind. When a nurse manages time well, he or she can have a clear, calm mind when confronted with the multiple demands of his or her role. In the confusion and disorder of daily activities and crises, nurses still must pay attention to the most important aspects of the job. If they are struggling to accomplish daily tasks and to keep on top of their workload, they will not have the peace of mind to reflect on their own practice, be there for others, and act proactively.

- Conserving personal energy. Nurses have a limited amount of energy to use for the achievement of professional and personal goals, no matter how vigorous and energetic they are. Another goal of managing time is to minimize the number of demands on themselves at any one time to assure that they have adequate energy at all times.

- Nonverbal messaging about significance. How nurses spend their time sends a message to others about what they think is important and what they do not think is important. It is in essence "walking the talk" or spending time on important activities.

- Contributing to feelings of well-being and happiness. When an individual manages his or her time, he or she will feel more in control of his or her life, less stressed, and be less likely to experience burnout. In fact, personal success can be measured by how a person spends his or her time and if he or she is spending it on activities that bring meaning, satisfaction, and joy to his or her life.

Consequences of Poor Time Management

The consequences of not managing time well include:

- Being unable to manage oneself.
- Negatively impacting others. Others in the workplace can be negatively affected

if someone does not complete his or her work and projects on time. People often rely on others' input and work to complete their work. It is simply unfair to others not to be timely in submission of one's own work (Barker, 1992).

Time Management: Self-Assessment

In this section, two approaches to assess time management skills are presented. Those who are experiencing any one of the following should pay particular attention to this section:

- Regularly exceeding the number of required hours spent on the job
- Regularly taking work home and working in the evenings and on weekends
- Feeling resentful about the amount of time that one must devote to his or her position
- Not having clarity of mind
- Constantly feeling rushed and out of control
- Not having time for personal reflection and growth

The good news is that people can gain control over their time. Time management experts believe that people waste on average 2–3 hours per day as a result of ineffective use of time (Davenport, 1982). When an individual assesses how he or she uses time and by adopting the suggested techniques, he or she should be able to capture some of this wasted time for more meaningful and important activities.

We suggest engaging in two activities to assess time management strengths and weaknesses. The first is to do a brief self-assessment (see Table 5–1). After completing the assessment,

Table 5–1 ASSESSMENT TOOL FOR TIME MANAGEMENT

Use the following scoring system for each answer below.
Place an X in the appropriate column.
1 = Never
2 = Rarely
3 = Occasionally
4 = Usually
5 = Always

	1	2	3	4	5
I feel calm and in control of my time.					
I am aware of fluctuations in my energy level and perform my most challenging tasks when my energy level is at its highest.					
I spend the majority of my time in meaningful work that contributes to the positive work on my clinical unit.					
I spend the majority of my time in activities that I find satisfying.					
I complete my paperwork and projects on time.					
I follow through on promises I make to my staff, boss, and others.					
I have written daily goals.					
I delegate tasks to others in my clinical unit.					
I assess tasks for their importance and their urgency.					
I keep a "to do" list and schedule time to complete the tasks on the list.					
I set aside time each week to complete paperwork and other tasks.					
I am able to control interruptions.					
I embrace the philosophy "do today instead of putting off until tomorrow."					
I set aside time each day for planning.					
I have written long term goals.					

those who score a 3 or less in any area should pay particular attention in their reading about those areas.

The second way for someone to assess how he or she is spending time is to keep a time log for at least 1 week. This is a more detailed assessment but is well worth the effort. It is best to keep a time management log for both organizational time and personal time, since the goal is to have a balance between both aspects of life.

Table 5–2 is a time log format that can be used for completing this activity. Column 1 is used to indicate the begin and end time for an activity. There should be an entry for every activity switch. In column 2, the individual completing the log should state what the activity is and who is involved in this activity with him or her. In column 3, he or she should state the purpose of the activity. (This is to help determine if he or she is spending time in activities that he or she deems important for the leadership of the unit versus mundane and even unmeaningful tasks.) The user should indicate his or her energy level in column 4: L for low, M for medium, and H for high. (The purpose of reflecting on energy level is to analyze if the individual is doing his or her most important work when his or her energy level is highest.) In column 5, the individual should note if he or she was interrupted while completing the activity and make notes about who interrupted and the reason for the interruption. Each interruption can be rated as very important (VI), important (I), or of little importance (LI). The last column is provided to make notes about the effectiveness of how the individual spent his or her time as soon as possible after the event or at the end of the day. Questions that one might ask oneself when completing this column are:

- Was this activity directly related to my role in the organization and/or assuring positive patient outcomes?
- Could the task have been done in a better way or delegated?
- Did I spend too much or not enough time on the activity? Was I able to complete the task?
- Was the task performed at the right time in relationship to my energy level?

Table 5–2 TIME MANAGEMENT LOG

Time	Activity/ People	Purpose	Energy Level	Interruptions	Effectiveness of the Time Spent

At the end of the week, the nurse should perform an analysis of the entire week. Besides the questions above, other questions to ask himself or herself are:

- What percentage of my time is spent in work, family, home, social, spiritual, and physical activities? Do I have the balance of these that I want?
- What percentage of my time do I spend in activities that are important or urgent?
- Who am I spending time with and are they the most appropriate people to help me reach my goals?
- What are my main interruptions? Assess the percentage of time they fall into each of the categories: very important, important, little importance. How can I decrease the number of unimportant interruptions?
- What are my biggest time wasters?
- Are there any activities I can reduce or eliminate?
- Is there anything I can delegate to others or simplify?
- Can I save time by grouping related tasks?
- Were there any tasks that I had put off and then felt pressure to complete?

This activity can be completed annually or more often if a time management tune-up is needed. This will help show areas of improvement and what else can be done in the future. Time management is not easy, and everyone will experience setbacks and days when they will not feel they have managed their time well. It takes constant care and attention to be a good manager of time.

Strategies for Managing Time

Based on the self-assessment and the findings from the time management log, several of the strategies discussed in the following pages will provide leverage in managing time. The conventional wisdom is that it is using these strategies collectively, not in isolation of one another, that will give the best results (Seaward, 2004).

Goal Setting and Planning

Most time management experts agree that goal setting and planning are the premier time management strategies. In this section, ways to plan for goal achievement are suggested.

First, individuals should write down their goals. Once they have written goals, they should carry them in a day planner, personal digital assistant (PDA), or a handheld computer. They should do two complementary things with these written goals. First, they should look at their goals daily to keep them fresh in their mind. By doing this, they will be more sensitive to opportunities that will help them reach their goals.

At the beginning of each day they should have a list of activities to accomplish that day to move toward their written goals. It is not easy to set realistic daily goals; at first it is common to plan more than one can accomplish, but as time progresses most people will get better at doing this. Most important, people should not get frustrated if they don't accomplish every task every day. In fact, one time management principle suggests that a task will consume the time that has been allotted for it. Therefore, planning an aggressive schedule is a good strategy as long as one does not get frustrated that one did not accomplish everything he or she set out to do.

Barker (1992) suggests a number of guidelines to follow when setting goals:

- Goals should include all aspects of life, including work, family, social, financial, spiritual, physical, and psychological areas.
- Goals should be measurable and achievable, yet challenging.
- In determining realistic goals, organizational constraints, resources, and personal strengths and skills should be considered.
- Time frames for goal completion should be realistic but should not allow for procrastination. Timelines can be reassessed and new deadlines set, and new goals can be added or old ones dropped when appropriate.
- Individuals should reward themselves upon completion of goals.
- People should pursue goals with enthusiasm, even when they are not feeling enthusiastic.

Scheduling

Nurses should have a calendar/day planner/PDA in which to schedule meetings, make plans for time to accomplish tasks, keep goals, and have an ongoing to do list. Each day when they review their goals, they should also review their schedule and block in time to accomplish daily tasks and work on long-term goals.

They need to see not only what the schedule for each day is, but they need a broader view of the week and month. They can put deadlines into the planner and block out times to work on projects or paperwork to accomplish them in a timely manner. There are two benefits to doing this: it assures they have a plan to get their work completed on time and they do not have to worry needlessly about when and how they are going to accomplish it.

Prioritizing Tasks: Urgent Versus Important

A useful way of prioritizing a daily list of goals and tasks is to consider whether the task is important or not important and if it is urgent or not urgent. Figure 5–1 provides a template to assess importance and urgency of tasks to help prioritize daily activities accordingly. On the vertical axis is a rating of urgency from low to high, and on the horizontal axis is a rating of importance from low to high. The grid prioritizes tasks by importance first and urgency second. The user should place each activity in one of the four quadrants. He or she should first complete the tasks in quadrant I—those that rate a high urgency and high importance score. Next, he or she should complete the activities in quadrant II, which are high importance and low urgency. Next, he or she should complete the activities in quadrant III, which are low importance and high urgency. Finally, he or she should complete those tasks low in urgency and importance.

Another complementary way to prioritize daily activities is to understand the Pareto principle, also known as the 80/20 rule. This principle suggests that 80% of positive, satisfying outcomes are a result of just 20% of the time spent. Or in other words, paying attention to important tasks will give 80% of the results. This principle is useful for assigning importance to each task in the grid. This principle also shows that minor changes to time management skills can produce dramatic results.

Figure 5–1 Assessing Tasks for Importance and Urgency

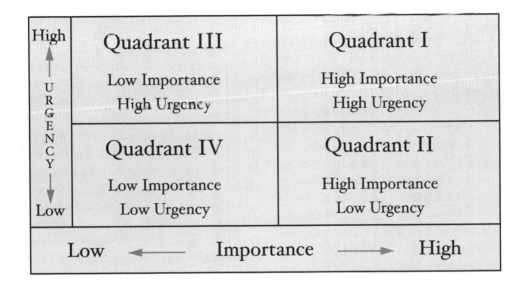

Delegation

Delegation is an important skill for being able to accomplish one's work and goals. But before a nurse can successfully delegate to others, he or she needs to think about his or her attitude and values about delegating. Here are some useful ways to think positively about delegation:

- Delegation is a trust-building activity.
- Delegation builds the confidence and self-esteem of others.
- Delegation unburdens one from routine, mundane tasks to provide the time for important activities and relationship building.
- Delegation helps others to grow, learn, and become leaders as they see more of the big picture.

- Delegation is an important tool in succession planning.
- Delegation can match the right person with the right expertise to the right job.

The process of delegation involves looking at the task(s) a nurse plans to delegate and the people to whom she or he will delegate. Some tasks should not be delegated. These include organizational functions and meetings that the nurse attends or leads, or personnel matters including rewarding people, conflict management, and so forth if they fall within the purview of his or her job. This leaves him or her with a substantial number of routine tasks that he or she might possibly delegate.

The next step is to consider the individuals to whom he or she might delegate. He or she should judge the expertise, strengths, knowledge, interests, skills, and attitudes of the staff. These should match the job to be done. When delegating, one needs to be sensitive to the workload of the person to whom one is delegating. Giving the person the ability to negotiate what they will do and when it will be done and the appropriate time to complete the delegated task is essential for success.

The process used to delegate is important. First, the person who is being assigned a task needs to understand its importance, why it is being delegated, and what the requirements and guidelines are. He or she will need appropriate information and resources such as time, space, and money to complete the task. He or she should be aware of dates for task completion and periodic evaluation if the task extends over a long time period. As difficult as this may be to delegate, the results of the assignment are more important than the means by which the person completes them, as long as he or she completes the task consistent with organizational policies and works with others in a positive manner.

Throughout the process of task completion, the person who assigned the task must be available to give advice, support, and guidance. Once the task is completed an appropriate reward needs to be given.

Allowing Oneself Private Time

An oft-spoken value for which nurses take great pride is having an open-door policy. There is a difference between having an open-door policy and having the door open all the time. One of the most effective time management strategies is to schedule and set aside time every week to close your door and to get required paperwork and tasks completed. Everyone should review their calendar and find a time when they do not

have meetings and book in private time for 2–4 hours per week in one to two blocks of time for the next 6 months.

Controlling Interruptions

On average, we experience one interruption every 8 minutes or approximately seven per hour. In an 8-hour day, that totals around 50–60 interruptions in the day. The average interruption takes approximately 5 minutes. If someone has 50 interruptions in the day and each takes 5 minutes, that totals 250 minutes, or 50% of the workday. Moreover, most people will discover that only about 20% of their interruptions are important or very important. Thus, if an individual experiences 250 minutes of interruptions in a day and 80% have little value, then 3 hours per day are being consumed by interruptions that are not worthy of his or her time (Wetmore, 1999).

This math shows how one can capture time. People should go back over their time logs and try to identify patterns in their interruptions, the time they spend dealing with them, and if there are people who tend to take more of their time than others. After this analysis, they can then set some strategies to decrease their interruptions. For example, if one person interrupts more than others, it might be necessary to schedule time with this person periodically and ask them to have a list of items to discuss rather than ask for time on the fly.

Procrastination and Perfectionism

Procrastination, putting off what needs to be done until the last minute, is often referred to as "putting off until tomorrow what I should have done today." Procrastination can take several forms, including knowingly doing something other than what needs to be done, starting to work on a project, then stopping work on it only to have to complete it at the last minute, or doing less difficult tasks rather than the required one (Seaward, 2004). Being aware of a tendency toward procrastination is important in understanding time management skills and strategies. Scheduling, maintaining to do lists, and adhering to them can help break this habit.

A different but parallel problem is being a perfectionist. Perfectionists generally get caught up in the details and never see the whole picture; thus they waste time (Seaward, 2004). Further, believing that one should and can be perfect is detrimental to one's self-esteem. No one can be perfect. When an individual holds himself or herself up to a standard of perfection and does not meet this standard, he or she then feels as if he or she failed. Recognizing a tendency to want to be perfect and moderating it is important not only to time management but also to self-esteem.

One way to reduce a need to be perfect is to consider what is good enough. To do this, one must make a judgment about the level of perfection/accuracy required for the specific task.

Managing Communications

Reading and responding to e-mail can consume a large portion of time. Here are several hints for making the task more meaningful and less time consuming:

- One should read e-mail one to two times per day depending on one's schedule and the volume received. One should not have e-mail constantly on and interrupting.
- Individuals should set up folders for e-mails from important people, about meetings, or tasks to be done.

- E-mail users should keep the inbox uncluttered by reading and responding to messages, then moving those e-mails to an appropriate folder if they need to keep them for the future. Otherwise, they should immediately delete e-mails that do not need to be saved.
- Everyone should respond immediately to e-mails that need short responses (2 minutes or less) and then move the e-mails or delete them.
- One should read e-mails that are marked as urgent first.
- Nurses should sort e-mail by sender and read e-mails from their boss and other important contacts in the organization next.
- If an e-mail cannot be responded to quickly and one does not have time to answer it, schedule time for a response at a later time. One should print the e-mail as a reminder to follow up.

Managing phone calls is another important time management technique. Phone conversations can be much more pertinent and personal than e-mails, but everyone should learn to keep their calls to less than 5 minutes. The downside of phone calls is that we often find ourselves playing phone tag, which can be a time waster. When someone leaves a person voice mail, he or she should specify a good time for the person to return the call in order to increase the possibility of being available when the person calls.

A nurse who has a support person who answers the phone should give instructions for how to handle phone calls. Whoever is taking calls should be able to screen calls and refer the caller to the appropriate person. The support person can find out when a convenient time is to return the call or can even schedule a phone appointment if the person keeps the nurse's calendar. The nurse can also instruct on how to communicate availability. For example, saying that "she is not on the unit" is a different message than saying "she is at *x* meeting and I expect her back in an hour."

Stress Management

As health care professionals, nurses should already be familiar with the physiology of stress and stress-related diseases. Stress management is a life skill and although it is important to success as an advanced nurse practitioner, much stress management occurs outside the workplace. No doubt nurses already use many different techniques to reduce their stress. In this section we look briefly at occupational stressors and provide some stress management techniques.

Occupational Stress

The National Safety Council (Seaward, 1994) lists many causes of job stress. How someone experiences and reacts to these stressors varies from person to person. Table 5–3 can be used to assess job-related stress based on the reasons identified by the National Safety Council. After an individual completes the assessment, he or she should look closely at items that he or she rated 3 or more before reading the next section.

A Stress Management Model

People have many ways of dealing with stress. Those who read this section should note the techniques that appeal to them. Using a mix of techniques can help readers be more effective in dealing with stress. These techniques fall into three categories: altering behaviors to deal more

effectively with stress, avoiding stress, or accepting stress (Tubesing & Tubesing, 1983). We recommend selecting at least one strategy from each category as a beginning point. Some of the techniques require behavioral approaches to managing stress while others require a change of thinking.

The purpose of stress management is to adopt coping skills. Coping is defined as the process of managing demands that are perceived by the person as demanding or exceeding the individual's resources. The purpose of coping skills can be to reduce the harmful effects of the stressor, to be able to better tolerate or adjust to negative events, to maintain a positive self-image, and to keep emotional equilibrium while maintaining satisfying relationships with others (Lazarus, 1999).

Altering Techniques

Many stressors cannot be eliminated, but there are techniques to alter how one deals with stress. These include:

- Problem solving
- Communication
- Having the right information
- Time management, priority setting, and planning
- Conflict management (Tubesing & Tubesing, 1983; Seaward, 2004)

Avoidance Techniques

A second set of strategies to deal with stress suggests avoiding stress, rather than altering one's reactions to it as just discussed. These strategies include:

- Using an assertive communications style
- Saying no and walking away
- Letting go

Table 5–3 ASSESSMENT TOOL FOR OCCUPATIONAL STRESS

Use the following scoring system for each answer below.
Place an X in the appropriate column.
1 = Never
2 = Rarely
3 = Occasionally
4 = Usually
5 = Always

	1	2	3	4	5
I have too much responsibility with little or no authority.					
The organization sets unrealistic expectations and deadlines that I am unable to meet.					
I do not feel adequately trained for my position.					
I do not feel appreciated.					
I am not able to voice concerns.					
I have too much to do with too few resources.					
I lack a clear understanding of what is expected of me.					
I have a difficult time keeping pace with technology.					
The physical environment in which I work has poor lighting, a lot of noise, and poor ventilation.					
There is the possibility of workplace violence.					
People in the organization have experienced sexual harassment and racial discrimination.					
The organization has recently downsized or restructured.					
Creativity and autonomy are not valued.					

- Delegating tasks
- Being aware of personal limitations and energy (Tubesing & Tubesing, 1983)

Acceptance Techniques

These acceptance techniques fall into two different categories. The first are techniques to build up resistance to stress, and the second are cognitive approaches to change one's perception of the stress.

Building Resistance to Stress: These techniques are probably most familiar as stress management techniques. They include such things as diaphragmatic breathing, meditation, yoga, music, massage, progressive muscular relax-ation, nutrition, physical exercise, engaging in creative activities or hobbies, humor, and prayer.

Changing Perceptions of Stress: A second set of techniques are cognitive ones that help one deal more effectively with stress by changing one's perceptions of both oneself and one's reactions to stress. This set of techniques includes:

- Being optimistic and positive, rather than negative
- Using visualization and affirmation, including positive self-talk
- Journal writing for self-expression and self-awareness
- Practicing forgiveness (Tubesing & Tubesing, 1983; Seaward, 2004)

Discussion Questions

1. What are the pros and cons of the time and stress management strategies discussed in this chapter? Do you have others to add that have been successful for you?
2. If you completed a time management log, what were your findings and what strategies will you adapt to improve your time management skills?
3. Review the information regarding stress management. Realistically, how much stress are you experiencing? What strategies will you try to help you cope with stress?

References

Barker, A. M. (1992). *Transformational nursing leadership: A vision for the future.* New York: National League for Nursing.

Davenport, R. (1982). *Making time, making money: A step by step process for setting your goals and achieving success.* New York: St. Martin's Press.

Lazarus, R. (1999). *Stress and emotion: A new synthesis.* New York: Springer Publishing Company.

Seaward, B. L. (1994). *National Safety Council's stress management.* Sudbury, MA: Jones and Bartlett Publishers.

Seaward, B. L. (2004). *Managing stress: Principles and strategies for health and well-being* (4th ed.). Sudbury, MA: Jones and Bartlett Publishers.

Tubesing, N., & Tubesing, D. (1983). *Structured exercises in stress management.* Duluth, MN: Whole Person Press.

Wetmore, D. E. (1999). *The big hole in your day.* Retrieved February 15, 2005, from http://www.balancetime.com/articles/hole_in_your_day.htm

The Health Care Delivery System and Health Care Policy

Introduction

As an advanced practice nurse, understanding the system in which one works is an essential foundation for successful practice. As an advocate for the consumer and provider and/or manager of care, nurses in advanced practice need basic knowledge of:

- the structure, operations, scope, and characteristics of the healthcare delivery system.
- how the healthcare delivery system is financed, including national healthcare expenditures and sources of payment.
- the trends that will influence the future of the system.
- how nurses can influence healthcare policy and how policy influences practice.

The information provided in this part can help the reader move beyond the perspective of the nursing profession to a broader understanding of the organization in which one works, relationships with others on the multidisciplinary team, and the forces that impact current and future practices. The ultimate goal is to prepare the reader as an advanced practice nurse to provide quality, cost-effective care, participate in the design and implementation of programs in a variety of systems, and to assume leadership roles.

As the reader thinks about the information provided in this part it is helpful to think of the issues as a triad of cost, quality, and access. Any change to correct the issue in one will have a significant and possibly negative effect on the other two. For instance, if the nation implemented policies and practices so that every citizen would be insured, there would be a dramatic increase in costs. This could, in turn, have a negative

effect on quality if this new policy were not funded correctly.

The chapters selected for Part II were selected from two books. Chapters 6, 7, and 8 are the first three chapters in the book, *Delivering Health Care in America: A Systems Approach,* by Shi and Singh. These chapters provide a foundation for understanding the healthcare delivery system. In Chapter 6, Shi and Singh paint a realistic—albeit gloomy—portrait of a complex, massive healthcare "system" in the United States. Because of the diversity of stakeholders including multiple providers, multiple payers, and the government, they suggest revolutionary changes in health care will be difficult, if not impossible, to achieve. In Chapter 7, the authors discuss issues of beliefs, values, and health. Although much of the content is not new to nursing—whose theorists and writers have focused on health as a metaparadigm for the profession for over 60 years (see Part IV)—this chapter explores the concept of holistic health and values in depth from the perspective of policy and leadership. Chapter 8 goes back in time and discusses the historical developments that have shaped the American healthcare delivery system. This knowledge provides the advanced practice nurse with an understanding of the current and future trends in health care and nursing.

Chapters 9 and 10, from the book, *Health Care USA,* by Sultz and Young, were selected to provide greater depth of information about healthcare financing and managed care. In Chapter 9, the information about the nation's healthcare expenditures and sources of payment presents data from the Center for Medicaid and Medicare, which collects, analyzes and disseminates this information annually. Updated information can be accessed from their Web site at http://www.cms.hhs.gov/

nationalhealthexpenddata/01_overview.asp?. Besides the statistical data presented in multiple tables, there is summary information analyzing the current data and projections for the future. Additionally, the journal, *Health Affairs,* presents a summary of the data and analysis in the first quarter of each year. Both should be valuable resources for the present and future. Chapter 10 provides a practical foundational knowledge for managing financial resources. The goal of these two chapters is to provide a basic understanding and foundation of healthcare finance. It is, however, important for nurses in advanced practice to seek help and consultation from the financial experts in their organization and to form close collaborative relationships with them.

Chapter 11 provides an in-depth look at managed care, its historical development, and its impact on clinical practice. In Chapter 12, a discussion of the future of the healthcare delivery system provides the reader with thought-provoking information about trends and issues that will affect the role of the advanced practice nurse.

Using knowledge about the healthcare delivery system, the two concluding chapters apply this understanding to healthcare policy and the role of the advanced practice nurse. In Chapter 13, Milstead provides a comprehensive definition of and stages of healthcare policy formation and the role that nursing should play in this arena. Of importance in this chapter is to gain an appreciation of how policy impacts on research, practice, and education. In Chapter 14, Dodd provides practical advice about strategies to employ in influencing national, state, and local politics.

Part II

The Health Care Delivery System and Health Care Policy

CHAPTER 6   A Distinctive System of
             Health Care Delivery

CHAPTER 7   Beliefs, Values, and
             Health

CHAPTER 8   The Evolution of Health
             Services in the United
             States

CHAPTER 9   Financing Health Care

CHAPTER 10   Managing Financial
             Resources

CHAPTER 11   Managed Care

CHAPTER 12   The Future of Health
             Services Delivery

CHAPTER 13   Advanced Practice
             Nurses and Public
             Policy, Naturally

CHAPTER 14   Making the Political
             Process Work

Chapter 6

A Distinctive System of Health Care Delivery

Leiyu Shi and
Douglas A. Singh

CHAPTER OBJECTIVES

1. Understand how the healthcare delivery system is organized in the United States.
2. Outline the four key functional components of a healthcare delivery system.
3. Discuss the primary characteristics of the U.S. healthcare system.
4. Emphasize why it is important for advanced nurse practitioners to understand the intricacies of the healthcare delivery system.

Introduction

The United States has a unique system of healthcare delivery. It is unlike any other healthcare system in the world. Most developed countries have national health insurance programs run by the government and financed through general taxes. Almost all citizens in such countries are entitled to receive healthcare services. Such is not the case in the United States, where not all citizens are automatically covered by health insurance. The U.S. healthcare delivery system is not a system in the true sense, even though it is called a system when reference is made to its various features, components, and services. Hence, it may be somewhat misleading to talk about the American healthcare delivery "system" because a real system does not exist (Wolinsky, 1988). The U.S. healthcare system is unnecessarily fragmented, which is perhaps its central feature (Shortell, Gillies, Anderson, Erickson, & Mitchell, 1996). The delivery system has continued to undergo periodic changes, mainly in response to concerns with cost, access, and quality. In spite of these efforts, providing at least a basic package of health care at an affordable cost to every man, woman, and child in America remains an unrealized goal. It is highly unlikely that this goal will materialize anytime soon, mainly because expanding access to health care, while containing overall costs and maintaining expected levels of quality, is a daunting challenge.

An Overview of the Scope and Size of the System

Table 6–1 illustrates the complexity of healthcare delivery in the United States. Many organizations and individuals are involved in health care. These range from educational and research institutions, medical suppliers, insurers, payers, and claims processors to healthcare providers. Multitudes of providers are involved in the provision of preventive, primary, subacute, acute, auxiliary, rehabilitative, and continuing care. An increasing number of managed care organizations (MCOs) and integrated networks now provide a continuum of care covering many of the service components.

The U.S. healthcare delivery system is massive. Total employment in various health delivery settings is approximately 10 million, including approximately 744,000 professionally active doctors of medicine (MDs), 2.2 million active nurses, 168,000 dentists, 226,000 pharmacists, and more than 700,000 administrators in medical and healthcare settings. Approximately 325,000 physical, occupational, and speech therapists provide rehabilitation services. The vast array of healthcare institutions includes 5,760 hospitals, 16,100 nursing homes, and 4,300 inpatient mental health facilities. Nearly 1,000 federally qualified health center grantees, with over 5,700 clinical sites, provide preventive and primary care services to approximately 16 million people living in medically underserved rural and urban areas yearly. Various types of healthcare profession-

als are trained in 150 medical and osteopathic schools, 56 dental schools, 91 schools of pharmacy, and more than 1,500 nursing programs located throughout the country. There are 174.5 million Americans with private health insurance coverage, 41.7 million Medicare beneficiaries, and 42.5 million Medicaid recipients. Health insurance can be purchased from over 1,300 health insurance companies and 64 Blue Cross/Blue Shield plans. Multitudes of government agencies are involved with the financing of health care, medical and health services research, and regulatory oversight of the various aspects of the healthcare delivery system (American Association of Colleges of Osteopathic Medicine, 2007; American Association of Colleges of Pharmacy, 2007; American Association of Medical Colleges, 2007; American Dental Education Association, 2007; America's Health Insurance Plans, 2004; Blue Cross/Blue Shield Association, 2007; Kaiser Family Foundation Commission on Medicaid and the Uninsured, 2005; Kaiser Family Foundation Medicare Policy Project, 2005; National Association of Community Health Centers, 2006; National Center for Health Statistics, 2006).

A Broad Description of the System

U.S. health care does not consist of a network of interrelated components designed to work together coherently, which one would expect to find in a veritable system. To the contrary, it is a kaleidoscope of financing, insurance, delivery, and payment mechanisms that remain unstandardized and loosely coordinated. Each of these basic functional components—

Table 6-1 THE COMPLEXITY OF HEALTHCARE DELIVERY

Education/ Research	Suppliers	Insurers	Providers	Payers	Government
Medical schools	Pharmaceutical companies	Managed care plans	Preventive Care	Blue Cross/Blue Shield plans	Public insurance financing
Dental schools	Multipurpose suppliers	Blue Cross/ Blue Shield plans	Health departments	Commercial insurers	Health regulations
Nursing programs	Biotechnology companies	Commercial insurers	Primary Care	Employers	Health policy
Physician assistant programs		Self-insured employers	Physician offices	Third-party administrators	Research funding
Nurse practitioner programs		Medicare	Community health centers	State agencies	Public health
Physical therapy, occupational therapy, speech therapy programs		Medicaid	Dentists		
Research organizations		VA	Nonphysician providers		
Private foundations		Tricare	Subacute Care		
US Public Health Service (AHRQ, ATSDR, CDC, FDA, HRSA, IHS, NIH, SAMHSA)			Subacute care facilities		
Professional associations			Ambulatory surgery centers		
Trade associations			Acute Care		
			Hospitals		
			Auxiliary Services		
			Pharmacists		
			Diagnostic clinics		
			X-ray units		
			Suppliers of medical equipment		
			Rehabilitative Services		
			Home health agencies		
			Rehabilitation centers		
			Skilled nursing facilities		
			Continuing Care		
			Nursing homes		
			End-of-Life Care		
			Hospices		
			Integrated		
			Managed care organizations		
			Integrated networks		

financing, insurance, delivery, and payment—represents an amalgam of public (government) and private sources. Thus, government-run programs finance and insure health care for select groups of people who meet each program's prescribed criteria for eligibility. To a lesser degree, government programs also engage in delivering certain health services directly to the recipients of care, such as veterans, military personnel, and the uninsured who may depend on city and county hospitals or limited services offered by public health clinics. However, the financing, insurance, payment, and delivery functions are largely in private hands.

The market-oriented economy in the United States attracts a variety of private entrepreneurs driven by the pursuit of profits in carrying out the key functions of healthcare delivery. Employers purchase health insurance for their employees through private sources, and people receive healthcare services delivered by the private sector. The government finances public insurance through Medicare, Medicaid, and the State Children's Health Insurance Program (SCHIP) for a significant portion of the very low-income, elderly, disabled, and pediatric populations. But insurance arrangements for many publicly insured people are made through private entities, such as HMOs, and healthcare services are rendered by private physicians and hospitals. The blend of public and private involvement in the delivery of health care has resulted in:

- a multiplicity of financial arrangements that enable individuals to pay for healthcare services.
- numerous insurance agencies employing varied mechanisms for insuring against risk.
- multiple payers that make their own determinations regarding how much to pay for each type of service.
- a large array of settings where medical services are delivered.
- numerous consulting firms offering their expertise in planning, cost containment, quality, and restructuring of resources.

There is little standardization in a system that is functionally fragmented. The various system components fit together only loosely. Such a system is not subject to overall planning, direction, and coordination from a central agency, such as the government. Due to the missing dimension of system-wide planning, direction, and coordination, there is duplication, overlap, inadequacy, inconsistency, and waste leading to complexity and inefficiency. The system does not lend itself to standard budgetary methods of cost control. Each individual and corporate entity within a predominantly private entrepreneurial system seeks to manipulate financial incentives to its own advantage without regard to its impact on the system as a whole. Hence, cost containment remains an elusive goal. In short, the U.S. healthcare delivery system is a behemoth that is almost impossible for any single entity to manage and control. It is also an economic megalith. The U.S. economy is the largest in the world, and, compared to other nations, consumption of healthcare services in the United States represents a greater proportion of the country's total economic output. While crediting the system with delivering some of the best medical care in the world, at least according to some standards, it falls short of delivering equitable services to every American.

An acceptable healthcare delivery system should have two primary objectives: (1) it must enable all citizens to access healthcare services, and (2) the services must be cost effective and meet certain established standards of quality. In many ways, the U.S. healthcare delivery system falls short of these ideals. On the other hand, certain features of U.S. health care are the envy of the world. The United States leads the world in the latest and the best in medical technology, medical training, and research. It offers some of the most sophisticated institutions, products, and processes of healthcare delivery. These achievements are indeed admirable, but a lot more remains unaccomplished.

Basic Components of a Health Services Delivery System

As illustrated in Figure 6–1, a healthcare delivery system incorporates four functional components—financing, insurance, delivery, and payment—that are necessary for the delivery of health services. The four functional components make up the quad-function model. Healthcare delivery systems differ depending on the arrangement of the four components. The four functions generally overlap, but the degree of overlapping varies between a private and a government-run system and between a traditional health insurance and managed care-based system. In a government-run system, the functions are more closely integrated and may even be indistinguishable. Managed care arrangements also integrate the four functions to varying degrees.

Financing

Health care often requires costly diagnostic tests and procedures and lengthy hospital stays. Financing is necessary to obtain health insurance or to pay for healthcare services. For most privately insured Americans, health insurance is employer based; that is, health care is financed by their employers as a fringe benefit. An employee's dependent spouse or children may also be covered by the employer. Most employers, except for the very large ones, purchase health insurance for their employees through an insurance company selected by the employer. In recent years, employers have shifted their purchases from traditional insurance companies to MCOs.

Insurance

Insurance protects the insured against catastrophic risks when they need expensive healthcare services. The insurance function also determines the package of health services the insured individual is entitled to receive. It specifies how and where healthcare services will be received. The insurance company or MCO also functions as a claims processor and manages the disbursement of funds to the providers of care.

Delivery

The term *delivery* refers to the provision of healthcare services and the receipt of insurance payments directly for those services. Common examples of providers who deliver care and services include physicians, dentists, optometrists, and therapists in private practices, hospitals, diagnostic and imaging clinics, and suppliers of medical equipment (e.g., wheelchairs, walkers, ostomy supplies,

Figure 6–1 The Complexity of Healthcare Delivery

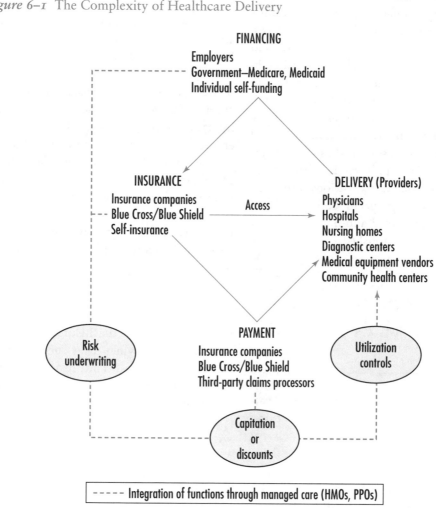

and oxygen). With few exceptions, most providers render services to people who have health insurance.

Payment

The payment function deals with reimbursement to providers for services delivered. Reimbursement is the determination of how much to pay for a certain service. Funds for actual disbursement come from the premiums paid to the insurance company or MCO. In the case of an insurance company, when a covered individual receives healthcare services, the provider of services either requires payment up front or agrees to bill the insurance company on behalf of the patient. In the former case, the patient files a claim with the insurance company to be reimbursed for a portion of the fees and charges paid to the provider. The most common practice, however, is for the insurance company to pay its portion to the provider directly. When receiving services under a managed care plan, the patient is usually required to pay only a small out-of-pocket amount, such as $15 or $20, to see a physician. The remainder is covered by the managed care plan.

A Disenfranchised Segment

Since the United States has an employer-based financing system, it is not difficult to see why the unemployed generally have no health insurance. However, even some employed individuals may not have health insurance coverage for two main reasons: (1) In most states, employers are not mandated to offer health insurance to their employees; therefore, some employers, due to economic constraints, do not offer it. Some small businesses simply cannot get group insurance at affordable rates and therefore are not able to offer health insurance as a benefit to their employees. (2) In many work settings, participation in health insurance programs is voluntary and does not require employees to join when an employer offers health insurance. Some employees choose not to sign up mainly because they cannot afford the cost of health insurance premiums. Employers rarely pay 100% of the insurance premium; most require their employees to pay a portion of the cost, called premium cost sharing. Others require their employees to pay the full cost, in which case health insurance becomes even more unaffordable. Even when the employee has to pay 100% of the premium, the benefit is that employees get group rates through their employer that are generally lower than what the rates would be if the employees were to purchase health insurance on their own. Employees who do not have health insurance offered by their employers and those who are self-employed have to obtain health insurance on their own. Individual rates are typically higher than group rates, and, in some instances, health insurance is unavailable when adverse health conditions are present.

In the United States working people earning low wages are the most disenfranchised because most of them are not eligible for public benefits and they cannot afford premium cost sharing. The United States has a significant number of uninsured—those without private or public health insurance coverage. In 2004, the proportion of Americans under age 65 without health insurance was estimated at 41.6 million, or 16–17% of the total population (National Center for Health Statistics, 2006). The U.S. government finances health benefits for certain special populations, including government employees, the elderly (age 65 and over), people with disabilities, some people with very low incomes, and children from low-income families. The program for the elderly and certain disabled individuals is called Medicare. The program for the indigent, jointly administered by the federal government and state governments, is named Medicaid. The program for children from low-income families, another federal/state partnership, is called the State Children's Health Insurance Program (SCHIP). For such public programs, the government may function as both financier and insurer, or the insurance function may be carved out to an HMO. Private providers, with a few exceptions, render services to these special categories of people. The government pays for the services, generally by establishing contractual arrangements with selected intermediaries for the actual disbursement of payments to the providers. Thus, even in government-financed programs, the four functions of financing, insurance, delivery, and payment may be quite distinct.

Transition from Traditional Insurance to Managed Care

Under traditional insurance, the four basic health delivery functions have been fragmented; that is, the financiers, insurers, providers, and payers have often been different entities, with a few exceptions. For example, self-insured employers, Medicaid in some states, and most participants in Medicare have integrated the functions of financing and insurance. Commercial insurers have integrated the functions of insurance and payment. During the 1990s, however, healthcare delivery in the United States underwent a fundamental change involving a tighter integration of the basic functions of financing, insurance, payment, and delivery through managed care.

Previously, fragmentation of the functions meant a lack of control over utilization and payments. The quantity of health care consumed refers to utilization of health services. Traditionally, determination of the utilization of health services and the price charged for each service were left up to the insured individuals and their physicians. Due to rising healthcare costs, current delivery mechanisms have instituted some controls over both utilization and price.

Managed care is a system of healthcare delivery that (1) seeks to achieve efficiencies by integrating the basic functions of healthcare delivery, (2) employs mechanisms to control (manage) utilization of medical services, and (3) determines the price at which the services are purchased and, consequently, how much the providers get paid. The primary financier is still the employer or the government, as the case may be. Instead of purchasing health insurance through a traditional insurance company, the employer contracts with an MCO, such as an HMO or a PPO, to offer a selected health plan to its employees. In this case, the MCO functions like an insurance company and promises to provide healthcare services contracted under the health plan to the enrollees of the plan. The term enrollee (member) refers to the individual covered under the plan. The contractual arrangement between the MCO and the enrollee—including the collective array of covered health services that the enrollee is entitled to—is referred to as the health plan (or plan, for short). The health plan uses selected providers from whom the enrollees can choose to receive routine services. This primary care provider—often a physician in general practice—is customarily charged with the responsibility to determine the appropriateness of higher level or specialty services. The primary care provider refers the patient to receive specialty services if deemed appropriate.

Managed care integrates the four basic functions of healthcare delivery. Even though financing is primarily through the employers, health plans set up negotiated fee arrangements through contracts with the providers. The negotiated fee arrangements are based on either capitation or discounts. Capitation is a payment mechanism in which all healthcare services are included under one set fee per covered individual. In other words, it is a predetermined fixed payment per member per month (PMPM). As an alternative to capitation, some MCOs negotiate discounts against the providers' customary fees. Generally, HMOs use capitation, whereas PPOs use discounts. Managed care topics are discussed in greater detail in Chapter 11.

Costs are also managed indirectly through control over utilization. The plan underwrites risk; that is, in setting the premiums, the plan relies on the expected cost of healthcare utilization. There is a risk that expenditures for providing healthcare services may exceed the premiums collected. The plan thus assumes the role of insurance. The plan pays the providers (through capitation or discounted fees) for services rendered to the enrollees and thus assumes the payment function. Delivery of services may be partially through the plan's own hired physicians, but most services deliver through contracts with external providers, such as physicians, hospitals, and diagnostic clinics.

Primary Characteristics of the U.S. Healthcare System

In any country, certain external influences shape the basic character of its health services delivery system. These forces consist of the political climate of a nation, economic development, technological progress, social and cultural values, physical environment, population characteristics, such as demographic and health trends, and global influences (Figure 6–2). The combined interaction of these environmental forces influences the course of healthcare delivery.

Ten basic characteristics differentiate the U.S. healthcare delivery system from that of other countries:

1. No central agency governs the system.
2. Access to healthcare services is selectively based on insurance coverage.
3. Health care is delivered under imperfect market conditions.
4. Third-party insurers act as intermediaries between the financing and delivery functions.
5. Existence of multiple payers makes the system cumbersome.
6. Balance of power among various players prevents any single entity from dominating the system.
7. Legal risks influence practice behavior.
8. Development of new technology creates an automatic demand for its use.
9. New service settings have evolved along a continuum.
10. Quality is no longer accepted as an unachievable goal in the delivery of health care.

No Central Agency

The U.S. healthcare system is not administratively controlled by a department or an agency of the government. Most other developed nations have national healthcare programs in which every citizen is entitled to receive a defined set of healthcare services. Availability of free services can break a system financially. To control costs, these systems use global budgets to determine total healthcare expenditures on the national scale and to allocate resources within the budgetary limits. Availability of services as well as payments to providers is subject

Figure 6–2 External Forces Affecting Healthcare Delivery

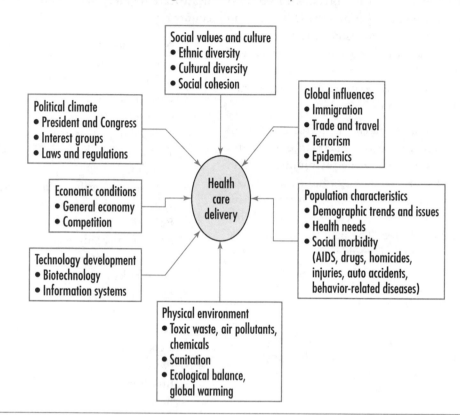

to such budgetary constraints. The government also controls the proliferation of healthcare services, especially costly medical technology. System-wide controls over the allocation of resources determine to what extent government-sponsored healthcare services are available to the citizenry. For instance, the availability of specialized services is restricted.

By contrast, the United States has mainly a private system of financing as well as delivery. Private financing, predominantly through employers, accounts for approximately 55% of total healthcare expenditures; the government finances the remaining 45% (National Center for Health Statistics, 2006). Private delivery of health care means that the majority of hospitals and physician clinics are private businesses, independent of the government. No central agency monitors total expenditures through global budgets and controls the availability and utilization of services. Nevertheless, the federal and state governments in the United States play an important role in healthcare delivery. They determine public-sector expenditures and reimbursement rates for services provided to Medicaid, SCHIP, and Medicare beneficiaries. The government also formulates standards of participation through health policy and regulation, meaning that providers must comply with the standards established by the government to be certified to provide services to Medicaid, SCHIP, and Medicare beneficiaries. Certification standards are also regarded as minimum standards of quality in most sectors of the healthcare industry.

Partial Access

Countries with national healthcare programs provide universal access; that is, health care is available to all citizens. Such is not the case in the United States. Access means the ability of an individual to obtain healthcare services when needed. In the United States, access is restricted to (1) those who have health insurance through their employers, (2) those covered under a government healthcare program, (3) those who can afford to buy insurance out of their own private funds, and (4) those who are able to pay for services privately. Health insurance is the primary means for ensuring access. Even though the United States offers the best medical care in the world, such care is generally available primarily to those who are adequately covered under a health insurance plan or who have adequate means to pay for it privately.

As stated previously, a relatively large segment of the U.S. population is uninsured. For continuous basic and routine care—commonly referred to as primary care—the uninsured are often unable to see a physician unless they can pay the physician's fees or unless they have access to a federally qualified health center (FQHC). FQHCs provide primary care and enabling services in medically underserved urban and rural areas, regardless of patients' ability to pay. Uninsured patients who cannot afford to pay for private physicians and do not have access to free care at a health center often wait until health

problems develop to seek care. At that point, they may be able to receive services in a hospital emergency department, for which the hospital does not receive any direct payments (unless the patient is able to pay). Uninsured Americans, therefore, are able to obtain medical care for acute illness. Hence, one can say that the United States does have a form of universal catastrophic health insurance even for the uninsured (Altman & Reinhardt, 1996). It is well acknowledged that the absence of insurance inhibits the patient's ability to receive well-directed, coordinated, and continuous health care through access to primary care services and, when needed, referral to specialty services. Experts generally believe that the inadequate access to basic and routine primary care services is one of the main reasons why the United States, in spite of being the most economically advanced country, lags behind other developed nations in measures of population health, such as infant mortality and overall life expectancy.

Imperfect Market

Under national healthcare programs, patients have varying degrees of choice in selecting their providers; however, true economic market forces are virtually nonexistent. In the United States, even though the delivery of services is largely in private hands, health care is only partially governed by free market forces. The delivery and consumption of health care in the United States do not quite meet the basic tests of a free market, as described in the following paragraph. Hence, the system is best described as a quasi-market or an imperfect market. Following are some key features characterizing free markets.

In a free market, multiple patients (buyers) and providers (sellers) act independently. In other words, in a free market, patients can choose to receive services from any provider. Providers neither collude to fix prices, nor are prices fixed by an external agency. Rather, prices are governed by the free and unencumbered interaction of the forces of supply and demand (Figure 6–3). Demand, in turn, is driven by the prices prevailing in the free market. Under free market conditions, the quantity demanded will increase as the price is lowered for a given product or service. Conversely, the quantity demanded will decrease as the price increases.

At casual observation, it may appear that multiple patients and providers do exist. Most patients, however, are now enrolled either in a private health plan or in government-sponsored Medicare, Medicaid, or SCHIP programs if they meet the eligibility criteria. These plans act as intermediaries for the patients. Also, the consolidation of patients into health plans has the effect of shifting the power from the patients to the administrators of the plans. The result is that, in many respects, the health plans, not the patients, are the real buyers in the healthcare services market. Private health plans, in many instances, offer their enrollees a limited choice of providers rather than an open choice.

Theoretically, prices are negotiated between the payers and providers. In practice, however, prices are determined by the payers, such as managed care, Medicare, and Medicaid. Because

Figure 6–3 Relationship between Price, Supply, and Demand under Free-Market Conditions

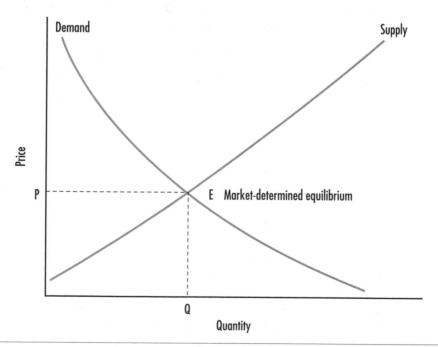

prices are set by agencies external to the market, they are not governed by the unencumbered forces of supply and demand.

For the healthcare market to be free, unrestrained competition must occur among providers based on price and quality. Generally speaking, free competition exists among healthcare providers in the United States. The consolidation of buying power in the hands of private health plans, however, is forcing providers to form alliances and integrated delivery systems on the supply side. Integrated delivery systems are networks of health services organizations. In certain geographic sectors of the country, a single giant medical system has taken over as the sole provider of major healthcare services, restricting competition. As the healthcare system continues to move in this direction, it appears that only in large metropolitan areas will there be more than one large integrated system competing to get the business of the health plans.

A free market requires that patients have information about the availability of various services. In reality, patients do not always have adequate information about services. Technology-driven medical care has become highly sophisticated. New diagnostic methods, intervention techniques, and drugs that are more effective fall in the domain of the professional physician. Also, medical interventions are commonly required in a state of urgency. Hence, patients have neither the skills nor the time and other resources to obtain necessary information when needed. Channeling all healthcare needs through a primary care provider is likely to reduce this information gap when the primary provider acts as the patient's advocate or agent. On the other hand, the Internet is becoming a prominent source of medical information. Pharmaceutical advertising is also having an impact on consumer expectations.

In a free market, patients have information on price and quality for each provider. The current system has other drawbacks that obstruct information-seeking efforts. Item-based pricing instead of package pricing is one such hurdle. Surgery is a good example to illustrate item-based pricing. Patients can generally obtain the fees the surgeon would charge for a particular operation. But the final bill, after the surgery has been performed, is likely to include charges for supplies, use of the hospital's facilities, and services performed by providers, such as anesthesiologists, nurse anesthetists, and pathologists. These providers, sometimes referred to as phantom providers functioning in an adjunct capacity, bill for their services separately. Item billing for such additional services, which sometimes cannot be anticipated in advance, makes it extremely difficult to ascertain the total price before services have actually been received. Package pricing and capitated fees can help overcome these drawbacks, but they have made relatively little headway for pricing medical procedures. Package pricing refers to a bundled fee for a package of related services. In the surgery example, this would mean one all-inclusive price for the surgeon's fees, hospital facilities, supplies, diagnostics, pathology, anesthesia, and postsurgical follow-up. As discussed earlier, with capitation all healthcare services are included under one set fee per covered individual. Capitation is more encompassing than package pricing. Whereas package pricing covers services bundled together for one episode, capitation covers all services an enrollee may need during an entire year.

In recent years, quality of health care has received much emphasis. Performance rating of health plans has met some success. However, apart from some sporadic news stories and selectively published health plan, provider, and hospital "report cards," the public still has scant information on the quality of healthcare providers.

In a free market, patients must directly bear the cost of services received. The purpose of insurance is to protect against the risk of unforeseen catastrophic events. Since the fundamental purpose of insurance is to meet major expenses when unlikely events occur, having insurance for basic and routine health care undermines the principle of insurance. When people buy home insurance to protect their property against the unlikely event of a fire, they generally do not anticipate the occurrence of a loss. The probability that they will suffer a loss by fire is very small. Also, if a fire occurs and causes major damage, insurance will cover the loss, but the policy does not cover routine wear and tear on the house such as chipped paint or a leaking faucet. Health insurance, however, generally covers basic and routine services that are predictable. Health insurance coverage for minor services, such as colds and coughs, earaches, and so forth amounts to prepayment for such services. Health insurance has the effect of insulating patients from the full cost of health care. There is a moral hazard that once enrollees have purchased health insurance, they will use healthcare services to a greater extent than if they were without health insurance. Even certain referrals to higher-level services may be forgone if the patient has to bear the full cost of these services.

In a free market for health care, patients as consumers make decisions about the purchase of healthcare services. The main factors that severely limit the patient's ability to make healthcare purchasing decisions have already been discussed. Even with the best intentions, the circumstances surrounding sickness and injury generally prohibit comparative shopping based on price and quality. Further, such information is not easily available. At least two additional factors limit the ability of patients to make decisions. First, decisions about the utilization of health care are often determined by need rather than price-based demand. Need has generally been defined as the amount of medical care that medical experts believe a person should have to remain or become healthy (Feldstein, 1993). Needs can also be based on self-evaluation of one's own health status. Second, the delivery of health care can result in demand creation. This follows from self-assessed need, which, coupled with moral hazard, leads to greater utilization. This creates an artificial demand because prices are not taken into consideration. Practitioners who have a financial interest in additional treatments also create artificial demand (Hemenway & Fallon, 1985), commonly referred to as supplier-induced demand or provider-induced demand. Functioning as the patients' agents, physicians exert enormous influence on the demand for healthcare services (Altman & Wallack, 1996). Research studies have pointed to physicians' behavior of creating demand for their own financial benefit (see, for instance, the work of McGuire & Pauly, 1991). Demand creation occurs when physicians prescribe medical care beyond what is clinically necessary. It can include practices such as making more frequent follow-up appointments than necessary, prescribing excessive medical tests, and performing unnecessary surgery (Santerre & Neun, 1996).

Third-Party Insurers and Payers

Insurance often functions as the intermediary among those who finance, deliver, and receive health care. As discussed earlier, health care is primarily financed by employers in the private sector and by the government in the public sector. Because the government is a large economic machine, it can self-insure against risk. Even though the government assumes the insurance function, payments to providers are generally handled through insurance intermediaries. Some large employers may also be able to self-insure; however, most private employers purchase health insurance from an insurance company or MCO. The employer's role is essentially relegated to selecting health plans and assisting employees with the enrollment process. The insurance company takes over most other administrative functions associated with the plan. The providers as well as the enrollees must comply with the policies set forth by the insurance company in matters associated with the provision of and payment for health services. Delivery of health care is often viewed as a transaction between the patient and the provider. But insurance and payment functions introduce a third party into the transaction (Griffith, 1995), the patient being the first party and the provider the second party.

The intermediary role of insurance creates a wall of separation between the financing and delivery functions so that quality of care often remains a secondary concern. In normal economic markets, the consumer is armed with the power to influence demand based on the price and quality of goods and services. Another way to illustrate this concept is to say that, in a free market, consumers vote with their dollar bills for the best candidate among competing prod-

ucts, based on the price and quality of each product. The insurance intermediary generally does not have the incentive to be the patient's advocate on either price or quality. At best, employees can air their dissatisfactions with the plan to their employer, who has the power to discontinue the current plan and choose another company. In reality, however, employers may be reluctant to change plans if the current plan offers lower premiums compared to a new plan. National healthcare programs have even fewer incentives for promoting quality, although they can contain costs by artificially fixing prices.

Multiple Payers

A national healthcare system is also sometimes referred to as a single-payer system because there is generally one primary payer, the government. When delivering services, providers send the bill to an agency of the government that subsequently sends payment to each provider.

By contrast, the United States has a multiplicity of health plans and insurance companies because each employer is free to determine the type of health plan it offers. Each plan spells out the type of services the enrollee can receive. Some plans make an arbitrary determination of how much they will pay for a certain type of service. For Medicare and Medicaid recipients, the government has its own set of regulations and payment schedules.

Multiple payers often represent a billing and collection nightmare for the providers of services. Multiple payers make the system more cumbersome in several ways, including the following:

- It is extremely difficult for providers to keep tabs on the numerous health plans. For example, it is difficult to keep up with which services are covered under each plan and how much each plan will pay for those services.

- Providers must hire a battery of claims processors to bill for services and monitor receipt of payments. Billing practices are not always standardized. Each payer establishes its own format.

- Payments can be denied for not following exactly the requirements set by each payer.

- Denied claims necessitate rebilling.

- When only partial payment is received, some health plans may allow the provider to bill the patient for the amount the health plan will not pay, called balance billing. Other plans prohibit balance billing. Even when the balance billing option is available to the provider, it triggers a new cycle of billings and collection efforts.

- Providers must sometimes engage in lengthy collection efforts including writing collection letters, turning delinquent accounts over to collection agencies, and finally writing off as bad debt the amounts that cannot be collected.

- Government programs have complex regulations for determining that payment is made for services actually delivered. Medicare, for example, requires each provider to maintain lengthy documentation on services provided.

When all the costs of billing, collections, bad debts, and maintaining medical records are aggregated for the entire system, the United States ends up spending far more in administrative costs than the national healthcare system of any country in the world.

Power Balancing

The U.S. health services system involves multiple players (not just multiple payers). The key players in the system have been physicians, administrators of health service institutions, insurance companies, large employers, and the government. Big business, labor, insurance companies, physicians, and hospitals make up the powerful and politically active special interest groups represented before lawmakers by high-priced lobbyists. Each player has its own economic interests to protect. Physicians, for instance, want to maximize their incomes and have minimum interference with the way they practice medicine; institutional administrators seek to maximize payment (commonly referred to as reimbursement) from private and public insurers. Insurance companies and MCOs are interested in maintaining their share of the healthcare insurance market; large employers want to minimize the costs they incur for providing health insurance as a benefit to their employees. The government tries to maintain or enhance existing benefits for select population groups and simultaneously reduce the cost of providing these benefits. The problem is that the self-interests of different players are often at odds. For example, providers seek to maximize government reimbursement for services delivered to Medicare, Medicaid, and SCHIP beneficiaries, but the government wants to contain cost increases. Employers dislike rising health insurance premiums. Health plans, under pressure from the employers, may constrain fees for the providers, who resent any cuts in their incomes.

The fragmented self-interests of the various players produce countervailing forces within the system. One positive effect of these opposing forces is that they prevent any single entity from dominating the system. On the other hand, each player has a large stake in health policy reforms. In an environment that is rife with motivations to protect conflicting self-interests, achieving comprehensive system-wide reforms is next to impossible, and cost containment remains a major challenge. Consequently, the approach to healthcare reform in the United States is often characterized as incremental or piecemeal.

Legal Risks

America's society is a litigious one. Motivated by the prospects of enormous jury awards, Americans are quick to drag the alleged offender into the courtroom at the slightest perception of incurred harm. Private healthcare providers have become increasingly more susceptible to litigation. By contrast, in national healthcare programs, the governments are immune from lawsuits. Hence, in the United States, the risk of malpractice lawsuits is a real consideration in the practice of medicine. To protect themselves against the possibility of litigation, some practitioners engage in what is referred to as defensive medicine by prescribing additional diagnostic tests, scheduling return checkup visits, and maintaining copious documentation. Many of these additional efforts may be unnecessary; hence, they are costly and inefficient.

High Technology

The United States has been the hotbed of research and innovation in new medical technology. Growth in science and technology often creates demand for new services despite shrinking resources to finance sophisticated care. People generally want the latest and the best, especially when health insurance would pay for new treatments. Physicians and technicians want to try the latest gadgets. Hospitals compete on the basis of having the most modern equipment and facilities. Once capital investments are made, their costs must be recouped through utilization. Legal risks for providers and health plans alike may also play a role in discouraging denial of new technology. Thus, several factors promote the use of costly new technology once it is developed.

Continuum of Services

Medical care services are generally classified into three broad categories: curative (e.g., drugs, treatments, and surgeries), restorative (e.g., physical, occupational, and speech therapies), and preventive (e.g., prenatal care, mammograms, and immunizations). Health care service settings are no longer confined to the hospital and the physician's office, where many of the aforementioned services were once delivered. Several new settings, such as home health, subacute care units, and outpatient surgery centers, have emerged in response to the changing configuration of economic incentives. Table 6–2 depicts the continuum of healthcare services.

Quest for Quality

Even though the definition and measurement of quality in health care are not as clear cut as they are in other industries, the delivery sector of health care has come under increased pressure to develop quality standards and to demonstrate compliance with those standards. There are higher expectations for improved health outcomes at the individual and the broader community levels. The concept of continuous quality improvement has also received much emphasis in managing healthcare institutions.

Table 6–2 The Continuum of Healthcare Services

Types of Health Services	Delivery Settings
Preventive care	Public health programs Community programs Personal lifestyles
Primary care	Physician's office or clinic Self-care Alternative medicine
Specialized care	Specialist provider clinics
Chronic care	Primary care settings Specialist provider clinics Home health Long-term care facilities Self-care Alternative medicine
Long-term care	Long-term care facilities Home health
Subacute care	Special subacute units (hospitals, long-term care facilities) Home health Outpatient surgical centers
Acute care	Hospitals
Rehabilitative care	Rehabilitation depart- ments (hospitals, long- term care facilities) Home health Outpatient rehabilitation centers
End-of-life care	Hospice services provided in a variety of settings

Figure 6–4 Trends and Directions in Healthcare Delivery

◊ Illness ⟶ Wellness
◊ Acute care ⟶ Primary care
◊ Inpatient ⟶ Outpatient
◊ Individual health ⟶ Community well-being
◊ Fragmented care ⟶ Managed care
◊ Independent institutions ⟶ Integrated systems
◊ Service duplication ⟶ Continuum of services

Trends and Directions

Since the final 2 decades of the 20th century, the U.S. healthcare delivery system has continued to undergo certain fundamental shifts in emphasis summarized in Figure 6–4. Later chapters discuss these transformations in greater detail and focus on the factors driving them.

Promotion of health at lesser cost has been the driving force behind these trends. An example of a shift in emphasis is the concept of health itself; the focus is changing from illness to wellness. Such a change requires new methods and settings for wellness promotion, although the treatment of illness continues to be the primary goal of the health services delivery system. Many of these changes are interrelated. A change in one area requires a modification in other areas. For example, the system of managed care has been necessary for shifting the emphasis from illness to wellness, from acute care to primary care, and from inpatient to outpatient settings. These fundamental moves will shape the future of the healthcare system.

Significance for Healthcare Practitioners and Policy Makers

An understanding of the healthcare delivery system is essential for managers and policy makers. In fact, an understanding of the intricacies within the health services system would be beneficial to all those who come in contact with the system. In their respective training programs, health professionals, such as physicians, nurses, technicians, therapists, dietitians, pharmacists, and others, may understand their own individual roles but remain ignorant of the forces outside their profession that could significantly impact current and future practices. An understanding of the healthcare delivery system can attune health professionals to their relationship with the rest of the healthcare environment. It can help them better understand changes and their potential impact on their own practice. Adaptation and relearning are strategies that can prepare health professionals to cope with an environment that will see ongoing change long into the future.

Policy decisions to address specific problems must also be made within the broader macro context because policies designed to bring about change in one healthcare sector can have wider repercussions, both desirable and undesirable, in other areas of the system. Policy decisions and their implementation are often critical to the future direction of the healthcare delivery system. However, in a multifaceted system, future issues will be best addressed by a joint undertaking that involves a balanced representation of the key players in health services delivery—physicians, insurance companies, managed care organizations, employers, institutional representatives, and the government.

Conclusion

The United States has a unique system of healthcare delivery. The basic features that characterize this system, or patchwork of subsystems, include the absence of a central agency to govern the system, unequal access to healthcare services due to lack of health insurance for all Americans, healthcare delivery under imperfect market conditions, existence of multiple payers, third-party insurers functioning as intermediaries between the financing and delivery aspects of health care, balancing of power among various players, legal risks influencing practice behavior, new and expensive medical technology, a continuum of service settings, and a focus on quality improvement. No country in the world has a perfect system. Most nations with a national healthcare program also have a private sector that varies in size. The developing countries of the world face serious challenges due to scarce resources and strong underlying needs for services.

Healthcare administrators must understand how the healthcare delivery system works and evolves. Such an understanding improves their awareness of the position their organization occupies within the macro environment of the system. It also facilitates strategic planning and compliance with health regulations, enabling them to deal proactively with both opportunities and threats and enabling them to effectively manage healthcare organizations. The systems framework provides an organized approach to an understanding of the various components of the U.S. healthcare delivery system.

Under free-market conditions, there is an inverse relationship between the quantity of medical services demanded and the price of medical services. That is, quantity demanded goes up when the prices go down and vice versa.

On the other hand, there is a direct relationship between price and the quantity supplied by the providers of care. In other words, providers are willing to supply higher quantities at higher prices, and vice versa. In a free market, the quantity of medical care that patients are willing to purchase, the quantity of medical care that providers are willing to supply, and the price reach a state of equilibrium. The equilibrium is achieved without the interference of any nonmarket forces. It is important to keep in mind that these conditions exist only under free-market conditions, which are not characteristic of the healthcare market.

Discussion Questions

1. Why do cost containment, quality, and access remain elusive goals in U.S. health services delivery?
2. Name the four basic functional components of the U.S. healthcare delivery system. What role does each play in the delivery of health care?
3. Discuss the intermediary role of insurance in the delivery of health care and its effect on the practice of the advanced nurse practitioner.
4. Who are the major players in the U.S. health services system? What are the positive and negative effects of the often-conflicting self-interests of these players?
5. Why is it important for nurses in advanced practice to understand the intricacies of the healthcare delivery system?
6. What kind of an approach do you recommend for charting the future course of the healthcare delivery system?
7. What is the healthcare continuum, and how does it impact on advanced nursing practice?

References

Altman, S. H., & Reinhardt, U. E. (1996). Introduction: Where does healthcare reform go from here? An uncharted odyssey. In S. H. Altman & U. E. Reinhardt (Eds.), *Strategic choices for a changing healthcare system* (pp. xxi–xxxii). Chicago: Health Administration Press.

Altman, S. H., & Wallack, S. S. (1996). Healthcare spending: Can the United States control it? In S. H. Altman & U. E. Reinhardt (Eds.), *Strategic choices for a changing healthcare system* (pp. 1–32). Chicago: Health Administration Press.

American Association of Colleges of Osteopathic Medicine. (2007). Retrieved October 10, 2007, from http://aacom.org/colleges

American Association of Colleges of Pharmacy. (2007). Retrieved October 10, 2007, from http://aacp.org/issi/membership/schools.asp?VID=6&CID=593&DID=4224&TrackID=

American Association of Medical Colleges. (2007). Retrieved October 10, 2007, from http://aamc.org/medicalschools.htm

American Dental Education Association. (2007). Retrieved October 10, 2007, from http://adea.org/DMS/instlinks/default.htm

America's Health Insurance Plans. (2004). *2002 AHIP survey of health insurance plans: Chart book of findings.* Washington, DC: America's Health Insurance Plans.

Blue Cross/Blue Shield Association. (2007). *Find your local Blue Cross/Blue Shield company.* Retrieved October 10, 2007, from http://www.bcbs.com/coverage/find/plan

Feldstein, P. J. (1993). *Health care economics.* (4th ed.). New York: Delmar Publishing.

Griffith, J. R. (1995). *The well-managed health care organization.* Ann Arbor, MI: AUPHA Press/Health Administration Press.

Hemenway, D., & Fallon, D. (1985). Testing for physician-induced demand with hypothetical cases. *Medical Care, 23*(4), 344–349.

The Kaiser Family Foundation Commission on Medicaid and the Uninsured. (2005). *Medicaid enrollment in 50 states: June 2005 data update.* Retrieved October 10, 2007, from http://kff.org/medicaid/7606.cfm

The Kaiser Family Foundation Medicare Policy Project. (2005). *Medicare chart book, 2005.* Available at http://kff.org/medicare/7284.cfm

McGuire, T. G., & Pauly, M. V. (1991). Physician response to fee changes with multiple payers. *Journal of Health Economics, 10*(4), 385–410.

National Association of Community Health Centers (NACHC). (2006). *A sketch of community health centers: Chart book, 2006.* Washington, DC: NACHC.

National Center for Health Statistics. (2006). *Health, United States, 2006: With chartbook on trends in the health of Americans.* Hyattsville, MD: Department of Health and Human Services.

Santerre, R. E., & Neun, S. P. (1996). *Health economics: Theories, insights, and industry studies.* Chicago: Irwin.

Shortell, S. M., Gillies, R. R., Anderson, D. A., Erickson, K. M., & Mitchell, J. B. (1996). *Remaking health care in America: Building organized delivery systems.* San Francisco: Jossey-Bass Publishers.

Wolinsky, F. D. (1988). *The sociology of health: Principles, practitioners, and issues* (2nd ed.). Belmont, CA: Wadsworth Publishing Company.

Chapter 7

Beliefs, Values, and Health

Leiyu Shi and
Douglas A. Singh

CHAPTER OBJECTIVES

1. Examine the determinants of health.
2. Explore the American beliefs and values governing the delivery of health care.
3. Appreciate the implications of the concepts for advanced practice nursing and for the promotion of health and prevention of disease.
4. Discuss the implications of the goals and initiatives of *Healthy People 2010* on advanced nursing practice.

Introduction

From an economic perspective, curative medicine seems to produce decreasing returns in health improvement with increased healthcare expenditures (Saward & Sorensen, 1980), and there is increased recognition of the benefits to society from the promotion of health and prevention of disease, disability, and premature death. Although the financing of health care has mainly focused on curative medicine, some strides are being made toward an emphasis on health promotion and disease prevention. Progress in this direction has been slow because

of the social values and beliefs that emphasize disease rather than health. The common definitions of health, as well as measures for evaluating health status, reflect similar inclinations. This chapter proposes a holistic approach to health, although such an ideal would be very difficult to fully achieve. For example, it is not easy for a system to enact a change in self-imposed risk behaviors among the population. Regardless, the healthcare delivery system must allocate resources and take other measures to set a change in course. The 10-year *Healthy People* initiatives, undertaken by the U.S. Department of Health and Human Services since 1980, illustrate steps taken in this direction, even though these initiatives generally have been strong in rhetoric but weak in strategy.

Beliefs and values ingrained in the American culture have also been influential in laying the foundations of a system that has remained predominantly private, as opposed to a tax-financed national healthcare program. Social norms also help explain how society views illness and the expectations it has of those who are sick.

This chapter further explores the issue of equity in the distribution of health services using the contrasting theories of market justice and social justice. The conflict between market and social justice is reflected throughout U.S. healthcare delivery. For the most part, strong market justice values prevail, particularly during economic recessions. However, some components of healthcare delivery in the United States do reflect strong social justice values.

Significance for Managers and Policy Makers

Materials covered in this chapter have several implications for health services managers, policy makers, and advanced practice nurses. The health status of a population has a tremendous bearing on the utilization of health services, assuming that the services are readily available. Planning of health services must be governed by demographic and health trends and initiatives toward reducing disease and disability. The concepts of health, its determinants, and health risk appraisal should be used to design appropriate educational, preventive, and therapeutic initiatives. There is a growing emphasis on evaluating the effectiveness of healthcare organizations

based on the contributions they make to community and population health. The concepts discussed in this chapter can guide administrators in implementing programs of most value to their communities. The exercise of justice and equity in making health care available to all Americans remains a lingering concern. This monumental problem will require a joint undertaking from providers, administrators, policy makers, and other key stakeholders. Quantified measures of health status and utilization can be used by managers and policy makers to evaluate the adequacy and effectiveness of existing programs, plan new strategies, measure progress, and discontinue ineffective services.

Basic Concepts

Health

In the United States, the concepts of health and health care have largely been governed by the medical model, or more specifically, the biomedical model. The medical model presupposes the existence of illness or disease. It therefore emphasizes clinical diagnosis and medical interventions to treat disease or symptoms of disease. The medical model defines health as the absence of illness or disease. The implication is that optimum health exists when a person is free of symptoms and does not require medical treatment. However, it is not a definition of health in the true sense, but a definition of what ill health is not (Wolinsky, 1988). Accordingly, prevention of disease and health promotion is relegated to a secondary status. Therefore, when the term *healthcare delivery* is used, in reality, it refers to medical care delivery.

Medical sociologists have gone a step further in defining health as the state of optimum capacity of an individual to perform his or her expected social roles and tasks, such as work, school, and doing household chores (Parsons, 1972). A person who is unable (as opposed to unwilling) to perform his or her social roles in society is considered sick. However, this concept also tends to view health negatively because many people continue to engage in their social obligations despite suffering from pain, cough, colds, and other types of temporary disabilities, including mental distress. In other words, a person's engagement in social roles does not necessarily signify that the individual is in optimal health.

An emphasis on both physical and mental dimensions of health is found in the definition of health proposed by the Society for Academic Emergency Medicine, according to which health is "a state of physical and mental well-being that facilitates the achievement of individual and societal goals" (Ethics Committee, Society for Academic Emergency Medicine, 1992). This view of health recognizes the importance of achieving harmony between the physiological and emotional dimensions.

Currently, the World Health Organization's (WHO) definition of health is most often cited as the ideal for healthcare delivery systems. WHO defines health as "a complete state of physical, mental, and social well-being, and not merely the absence of disease or infirmity" (WHO, 1948). WHO's definition specifically identifies social well-being as a third dimension of health. In doing so, it emphasizes the importance of positive social relationships. Having a social support network is positively associated with life stresses, self-esteem, and social relations. The social aspects of health also extend beyond the individual level to include responsibility for the health of entire communities and populations. WHO's definition recognizes that optimal health is more than a mere absence of disease or infirmity. Since it includes the physical, mental, and social dimensions, WHO's model can be referred to as the biopsychosocial model of health. WHO has also defined a healthcare system as all the activities whose primary purpose is to promote, restore, or maintain health (McKee, 2001). As this chapter points out, health care should include much more than medical care. Thus, health care would include a variety of services believed to improve a person's health and well-being.

In recent years, a growing interest has emerged in holistic health, which emphasizes the well-being of every aspect of what makes a person whole and complete. Thus, holistic medicine seeks to treat the individual as a whole person (Ward, 1995). Holistic health incorporates the spiritual dimension as a fourth element—in addition to the physical, mental, and social aspects—as necessary for optimal health (Figure 7–1). A growing volume of

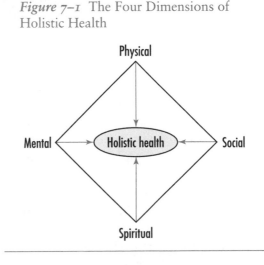

Figure 7–1 The Four Dimensions of Holistic Health

medical literature points to the healing effects of a person's religion and spirituality on morbidity and mortality (Levin, 1994). Numerous studies point to an inverse association between religious involvement and all-cause mortality (McCullough, Hoyt, Larson, Koenig, & Thoresen, 2000). Religious and spiritual beliefs and practices have shown a positive impact on a person's physical, mental, and social well-being. They may affect the incidences, experiences, and outcomes of several common medical problems (Maugans, 1996). For instance, people with high levels of general religious involvement are likely to suffer less from depressive symptoms and disorders (McCullough & Larson, 1999). Spiritual well-being has been recognized as an important internal resource for helping people cope with illness. For instance, a study conducted at the University of Michigan found that 93% of the women undergoing cancer treatment indicated that their religious lives helped them sustain their hopes (Roberts, Brown, Elkins, & Larson, 1997). Studies have found that a large percentage of patients want their physicians to consider their spiritual needs, and almost half expressed a desire that the physicians pray with them if they could (see Post, Puchalski, & Larson, 2000). However, many physicians feel that spiritual matters fall outside their expertise, or that they would be intruding into patients' private lives. Also, caution about ethical issues and religious coercion are valid concerns. Referral to a chaplain or pastoral leader is often a more appropriate alternative (Post et al., 2000).

The spiritual dimension is frequently tied to one's religious beliefs, values, morals, and practices. More broadly, it is described as meaning, purpose, and fulfillment in life; hope and will to live; faith; and a person's relationship with God (Marwick, 1995; Ross, 1995; Swanson, 1995). A clinically tested scale to measure spiritual well-being includes categories such as belief in a power greater than oneself, purpose in life, faith, trust in providence, prayer, meditation, group worship, ability to forgive, and gratitude for life (Hatch, Burg, Naberhaus, & Hellmich, 1998).

Some of the nation's leading medical schools now offer courses that explore spiritual issues in health care and how to address such issues in patient care delivery (American Physical Therapy Association, 1997). Spiritual assessment instruments have been developed to assist physicians and other clinicians in spiritual history taking (Maugans, 1996; Puchalski & Romer, 2000). The Committee on Religion and Psychiatry of the American Psychological Association has issued a position statement to emphasize the importance of maintaining respect for a patient's religious/spiritual beliefs. For the first time, "religious or spiritual problem" has been included as a diagnostic category in DSM-IV. The holistic approach to health also alludes to the need for incorporating alternative therapies into the predominant medical model.

Tamm (1993) observed that different groups in society—including physicians, nurses, and patients—look at health and disease from partly different vantage points, those that are holistic and those that emphasize illness and disease. Such tensions can have significant implications for the delivery of health services, especially in a pluralistic society such as the United States. Although the medical model plays a key role in the delivery of health care, integration of the concepts of holistic health can optimize well-being and promote early recovery from sickness.

Illness and Disease

Once the existence of illness and/or disease is recognized, it triggers care seeking and care utilization behaviors. Health services professionals diagnose illness and prescribe treatment mainly to ease symptoms. In most cases, once relief is obtained, the individual is declared well, regardless of whether or not the underlying cause of disease is cured.

The terms *illness* and *disease* are not synonymous, although they are often used interchangeably as they will be throughout this book. Illness is recognized by means of a person's own perceptions and evaluation of how he or she feels. For example, an individual may feel pain, discomfort, weakness, depression, or anxiety, but a disease may or may not be present. From a sociocultural standpoint, people consider themselves ill when they feel they are not quite able to perform the tasks or roles that society expects from them (Wolinsky, 1988). For example, due to a severe headache, a person may feel unable to go to work or attend school. The person may take pain medication and rest. If symptoms persist, the person may seek professional medical help. During an initial visit, a primary care physician may find nothing wrong physically. The person may still suffer from pain and discomfort and may forgo engagement in social roles, but the person is not declared diseased. He or she may subsequently be referred to a neurologist—a specialist in diseases of the nervous system—who may discover some nervous disorder and prescribe treatment. At this point, the person is declared diseased. Thus, the determination that disease is present is based on professional evaluation, rather than the patient's. It reflects the highest state of professional knowledge, particularly that of the physician, and it

requires therapeutic intervention (May, 1993). In this example, both illness and disease were found to be present, but that is not always the case. Certain diseases, such as hypertension (high blood pressure), are asymptomatic and not always manifested through illness. A hypertensive person has a disease but may not know it. Thus, it is possible to be diseased without feeling ill. Likewise, one may feel ill and yet not have a disease.

Diseases are often caused by more than a single factor. For example, the mere presence of tubercle bacillus does not mean that the infected person will develop tuberculosis. Other factors, such as poverty, overcrowding, and malnutrition, may be essential for the disease to develop (Friedman, 1980). One useful explanation of disease occurrence (for communicable diseases in particular) is provided by the tripartite model sometimes referred to as the epidemiology triangle (Figure 7–2). Of the three elements in the model, the host is the organism—generally, a human—that becomes sick. However, for the

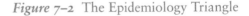

Figure 7-2 The Epidemiology Triangle

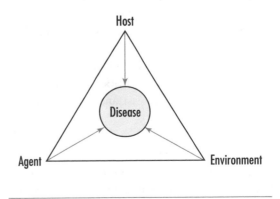

host to become sick, at least one factor, an agent, must be present, although presence of an agent does not ensure that disease will occur. In the tuberculosis example, tubercle bacillus is the agent for tuberculosis. Other examples are chemical agents, radiation, tobacco smoke, dietary indiscretions, and nutritional deficiencies. Factors associated with the host include genetic makeup, level of immunity, fitness, and personal habits and behaviors. Such factors are associated with the contracting of an agent or making the agent active. The third factor, environment, is external to the host. The environment is a moderating factor that can either enhance or reduce susceptibility to disease. It includes the physical, social, cultural, and economic aspects of the environment. Sanitation, air pollution, cultural beliefs, social equity, social norms, and economic status are examples. Because the three factors commonly interact to produce disease, the model has important implications for disease prevention. Risk factors— attributes that increase the likelihood of developing a particular disease or negative health condition at some time in the future— can be traced to the agent, the host, and/or the environment. A risk factor can be associated with any of the factors listed earlier, such as tobacco smoke or poor diet (associated with the agent), genetic makeup or levels of fitness (associated with the host), and poor sanitation or low socioeconomic status (associated with the environment). Preventive interventions to eliminate risk factors constitute an important strategy to reduce occurrence of disease and to promote better health.

Behavioral Risk Factors

Certain individual behaviors and personal lifestyle choices represent important risk factors

for illness and disease. For example, smoking has been identified as the leading cause of preventable disease and death in the United States because it significantly increases the risk of heart disease, stroke, lung cancer, and chronic lung disease (Centers for Disease Control and Prevention, 1999b). Substance abuse, inadequate physical exercise, a high-fat diet, irresponsible use of motor vehicles, and unsafe sex are additional examples of behavioral risk factors. (Table 7–1 presents the percentage of the U.S. population with selected behavioral risks.)

Acute, Subacute, and Chronic Conditions

Disease can be classified as acute, subacute, or chronic. An acute condition is relatively severe, episodic (of short duration), and often treatable (Timmreck, 1994). It is subject to recovery. Treatments are generally provided in a hospital. Examples of acute conditions are a sudden interruption of kidney function or a myocardial infarction (heart attack). A subacute condition is between acute and chronic but has some acute features (Thomas, 1985). It can be a postacute condition requiring treatment after discharge from a hospital. Examples include ventilator and head trauma care. A chronic condition is less severe but of long and continuous duration (Timmreck, 1994). The patient may not fully recover. The disease may be kept under control through appropriate medical treatment, but if left untreated, the condition may lead to severe and life-threatening health problems. Examples are asthma, diabetes, and hypertension. Contributors to chronic disease include ethnical, cultural, and behavioral factors and the social and physical environment, discussed later in this chapter.

Table 7–1 PERCENTAGE OF POPULATION WITH BEHAVIORAL RISKS

Behavioral Risks	Percentage of Population	Year
Alcohol (12 years and over)	50.3	2004
Marijuana (12 years and over)	6.1	2004
Cocaine use (12th graders)	2.3	2005
Cocaine use (10th graders)	1.5	2005
Cocaine use (8th graders)	1.0	2005
Cigarette smoking (18 years and over)	20.8	2004
Hypertension (20–74 years)	25.3	2001–04
Overweight (20–74 years)	66.0	2001–04
Serum cholesterol (20–74 years)	16.0	2001–04

Note: Data are based on household interviews of a sample of the civilian noninstitutionalized population 12 years of age and over in the coterminous United States.

Source: Data from National Center for Health Statistics. *Health, United States, 2006.* Hyattsville, MD: Department of Health and Human Services, 2006, pp. 266, 271, 273, 279, 287.

Health Promotion and Disease Prevention

As discussed earlier, the medical model of health and health care emphasizes clinical interventions once disease has been diagnosed. The wellness model, on the other hand, emphasizes efforts and programs geared toward prevention of disease and maintenance of an optimum state of well-being. It is well recognized that medical care alone cannot promote health. To promote optimum health, a healthcare delivery system must provide medical treatment but also use disease prevention and health promotion strategies. The two should complement each other.

The concept of health promotion and disease prevention is built on three factors: (1) An under-standing of risk factors associated with host, agent, and/or environment. Risk factors and their health consequences are evaluated through a process called health risk appraisal. Only when the risk factors and their health consequences are known can interventions be developed to help individuals adopt healthier lifestyles. (2) Interventions for counteracting the key risk factors include two main interventions: (a) behavior modification geared toward the goal of adopting healthier lifestyles and (b) therapeutic interventions. Both are discussed in the next paragraph. (3) Adequate public health and social services, as discussed later in this chapter, includes all health-related services designed to minimize risk factors and their negative effects in order to prevent disease, control disease outbreaks, and contain the spread of infectious agents. The goal is to maximize the health of a population.

Various avenues can be used for motivating individuals to alter behaviors that may contribute to disease, disability, or death. Behavior can be modified through educational programs and incentives directed at specific high-risk populations. In the case of cigarette smoking, for example, health promotion aims at building people's knowledge, attitudes, and skills to avoid or quit smoking. It also involves reducing advertisements and other environmental inducements that promote nicotine addiction. Financial incentives, such as a higher cigarette tax, are used to discourage purchase of cigarettes.

Therapeutic interventions generally fall into three areas of preventive effort: primary prevention, secondary prevention, and tertiary prevention.

Primary prevention refers to activities undertaken to reduce the probability that a disease will develop at some point in the future (Kane, 1988). Its objective is to restrain the development of a disease or negative health condition before it occurs. Therapeutic intervention would include physicians' efforts to assist their patients in smoking cessation (Breslow, 1989). Smoking cessation can prevent lung cancer; an increase in physical activity can prevent heart disease; teen driver education can prevent disability and death from auto accidents; and safety practices can reduce serious injuries in the workplace. Prenatal care is associated with lower infant mortality rates. Immunization has had a greater impact on prevention against childhood diseases and mortality reduction than any other public health intervention besides clean water (Plotkin & Plotkin, 1999). Hand washing, refrigeration of foods, garbage collection, and protection of the water supply are other examples of primary prevention (Timmreck, 1994). There have been numerous incidents where emphasis on food safety and proper cooking could have prevented outbreaks of potentially deadly episodes, such as those caused by *E. coli*.

Secondary prevention refers to early detection and treatment of disease. Health screenings and periodic health examinations are examples. The main objective of secondary prevention is to block the progression of disease or an injury from developing into an impairment or disability (Timmreck, 1994). Screening tests, such as hypertension screening, Pap smears, and mammograms, have been instrumental in prescribing early treatment.

Tertiary prevention refers to rehabilitative therapies and the monitoring of health care processes to prevent complications or to prevent further illness, injury, or disability. For example, regular turning of bed-bound patients prevents pressure sores; infection control practices in hospitals and nursing homes are designed to prevent iatrogenic illnesses; that is, illnesses or injuries caused by the process of health care. Tertiary prevention may also involve patient education and behavior change to prevent recurrence of disease (Timmreck, 1994). Examples include nutrition counseling and smoking cessation to keep disease in check.

As shown in Table 7–2, prevention, early detection, and treatment efforts helped reduce cancer mortality quite significantly between 1991 and 1995. This decrease was the first sustained decline since record keeping was instituted in the 1930s. The decline in breast cancer has been credited to early detection and treatment advances. The drop in cervical cancer has been attributed to the widespread use of Pap screening. Later data, however, show that the declines in cancer death rates are moderating, most likely due to other factors, such as aging.

Table 7-2 ANNUAL PERCENT DECLINE IN
CANCER MORTALITY 1991–2003

Type of Cancer	1991–95	1994–2003
All cancers	3.0	1.1
Breast cancer	6.3	2.5
Cervical cancer	9.7	3.6
Ovarian cancer	4.8	0.5
Prostate cancer	6.3	3.5

Source: Data from National Center for Health Statistics of the Centers for Disease Control and Prevention, National Cancer Institute, SEER Cancer Statistics Review, 1975–2003 (Table I–7).

Developmental Health

Development refers to growth in skill and capacity to function normally (Hancock & Mandle, 1994). Early childhood development influences a person's health in later years. The foundations laid in the early years often determine the individual's future adjustments to life (Berger, 1988) and shape individual behaviors. Children who fail to acquire certain skills in childhood often have real difficulties as adults (Wynder & Orlandi, 1984). The importance of early childhood development has important implications for health services delivery in two main areas: (1) Expectant mothers need adequate prenatal care. The health promotional needs of the expectant mother and the fetus are so closely intertwined that they must be considered a unit (Hancock & Mandle, 1994). (2) Adequate child care is needed, especially during the first few years of growth. Immunization, nutrition, family and social interaction, and health care are key developmental elements until a child reaches adulthood. Preventable developmental disabilities impose an undue burden on the healthcare delivery system.

Public Health

Almost all Americans consider public health important. However, public health remains poorly understood by its prime beneficiaries, the public, as well as by many of its dedicated practitioners. For some people, public health evokes images of a massive social enterprise or welfare system. To others, the term describes the professionals and workforce responsible for dealing with important health problems that confront the population. Still another image of public health is that of a body of knowledge and techniques that can be applied to health-related problems (Turnock, 1997). None of these ideas adequately reflects what public health is.

Two definitions have been found to be particularly helpful in characterizing public health. The first, by the Institute of Medicine (IOM), proposes that the mission of public health is to fulfill "society's interest in assuring conditions in which people can be healthy" (IOM, 1988). Public health deals with broad societal concerns about ensuring conditions that promote optimum health for society as a whole.

The practices of medicine and public health have followed divergent paths, mainly due to a lack of an infrastructure to support collaboration between the two sectors (Lasker, Abramson, & Freedman, 1998). As a point of distinction, it can be said that medicine focuses on the individual patient—diagnosing symptoms, treating and preventing disease, relieving pain and suffering, and maintaining or restoring normal function. Public health, on the other hand, focuses on populations (Lasker, 1997). The emphases in modern medicine are on the biological causes of disease and developing treatments and therapies. Public health focuses on identifying the environmental, social, and behavioral risk factors that cause disease and on developing and implementing population-based interventions to minimize the risk factors (Peters, Drabant, Elster, Tierney, & Hatcher, 2001). While medicine focuses on the treatment of disease and recovery of health, public health deals with various efforts to prevent disease and promote health.

To promote and protect society's interest in health and well-being, public health must influence the social, economic, political, and medical care factors that affect health and illness. Public health activities can range from providing education on nutrition to passing laws that enhance automobile safety. Public health includes dissemination to the public and to health professionals of timely and appropriate information about important health issues. Another distinguishing characteristic of public health is the broader range of professionals involved, compared to the delivery of medical services. The medical sector encompasses physicians, nurses, dentists, therapists, social workers, psychologists, nutritionists, health educators, pharmacists, laboratory technicians, health services administrators, and so forth. In addition to these professionals, public health also involves professionals such as sanitarians, epidemiologists, statisticians, industrial hygienists, environmental health specialists, food and drug inspectors, toxicologists, and economists (Lasker, 1997).

The second definition, given more than 8 decades ago, characterizes public health as the science and art of preventing disease, prolonging life, and promoting health and efficiency through organized community effort (Winslow,

1920). Accordingly, public health is a broad social enterprise that seeks to apply the current knowledge pertaining to health and disease in ways that will have the maximum impact on the health status of a population (Turnock, 1997).

Health Protection

Environmental health has been an integral component of public health ever since John Snow, in the 1850s, successfully traced the risk of cholera outbreaks in London to the Broad Street water pump (Rosen, 1993). Since then, environmental health has specifically dealt with preventing the spread of disease through water, air, and food (Schneider, 2000). Environmental health science, along with other public health measures, was instrumental in reducing the risk of infectious diseases during the last century. For example, in 1900, pneumonia, tuberculosis, and diarrhea along with enteritis were the top three killers in the United States (Centers for Disease Control and Prevention, 1999a); that is no longer the case today (see Table 7–3). With the rapid industrialization during the 20th century, environmental health faced new challenges due to serious health hazards from chemicals, industrial waste, infectious waste, radiation, asbestos, and other toxic substances. Due to actual and potential industrial accidents, a third major role of public health emerged—that of health protection (in addition to prevention and health promotion). However, due to the complexity of dealing with numerous toxins, many environmental responsibilities were specifically assigned to newly created agencies, such as the Environmental Protection Agency (EPA) and the Occupational Safety and Health Administration (OSHA). Rapid cleanup, evacuation of the affected population, and transfer of victims to

Table 7–3 LEADING CAUSES OF DEATH, 2003

Cause of Death	Deaths	Percentage
All causes	2,448,288	100.0
Diseases of the heart	685,089	28.0
Malignant neoplasms	556,902	22.7
Cerebrovascular diseases	157,689	6.4
Chronic lower respiratory diseases	126,382	5.2
Unintentional injuries	109,277	4.5
Diabetes mellitus	74,219	3.0
Influenza and pneumonia	65,163	2.7
Alzheimer's disease	63,457	2.6
Nephritis, nephrotic syndrome, and nephrosis	42,453	1.7
Septicemia	34,069	1.4

Source: Data from National Center for Health Statistics. *Health, United States, 2006.* Hyattsville, MD: Department of Health and Human Services, 2006, p. 187.

medical care facilities have been the main types of response when accidents occur. Firefighters, police, paramedics, and other civil defense agencies cooperate in such efforts and coordinate functions with local medical centers and public health agencies.

Since the horrific events of what is now commonly referred to as 9/11 (September 11, 2001), the United States has opened a new chapter in health protection. As the nation was still recovering from the shock of the attacks on New York's World Trade Center, attempts to disseminate anthrax through the U.S. Postal Service were discovered. In June 2002, President George W. Bush signed into law the Public Health Security and Bioterrorism Response Act of 2002. The term *bioterrorism* encompasses the use of chemical, biological, and nuclear agents to cause harm to relatively large civilian populations. Dealing with such a threat requires large-scale preparations, which include appropriate tools and training for workers in medical care, public health, emergency care, and civil defense agencies at the federal, state, and local levels. It requires national initiatives to develop countermeasures, such as new vaccines, a robust public health infrastructure, and coordination between numerous agencies. It requires an infrastructure to handle large numbers of casualties and isolation facilities for contagious patients. Hospitals, public health agencies, and civil defense need to be linked together through information systems. Containment of infectious agents, such as smallpox, would require quick detection, treatment, isolation, and organized efforts to protect the unaffected population. To address these issues, President Bush has proposed substantial increases in funding for bioterrorism.

Even broader provisions are contained in the Homeland Security Act of 2002, signed into law in November 2002. The legislation calls for a major restructuring of the nation's resources with the primary mission of helping prevent, protect against, and respond to any acts of terrorism in America. The legislation is also designed to enhance the nation's ability to prevent and detect bioterrorist attacks. For example, it calls for improved inspections of food products entering the United States. It provides for better tools to contain attacks on the food and water supplies, protect the nation's vital infrastructures, such as nuclear facilities, and track biological materials anywhere in the United States. Chapter 12 discusses future trends and the changing role of public health to address such potential threats.

To prevent the introduction, transmission, and spread of severe acute respiratory syndrome (SARS), a contagious disease that is accompanied by fever and symptoms of pneumonia or other respiratory illness, President Bush signed an executive order on April 4, 2003, to designate SARS as a communicable disease and for the apprehension, detention, or conditional release of individuals with SARS. The order also covers other suspected communicable diseases that include cholera, diphtheria, infectious tuberculosis, plague, smallpox, yellow fever, and viral hemorrhagic fevers such as Ebola.

The global threat of avian influenza has also solicited a public health and government response. The Centers for Disease Control and Prevention launched a Web site dedicated to educating the public about avian influenza, how it is spread, and past and current outbreaks. The Web site contains specific information for health professionals, travelers, the poultry industry, state departments of health, and people with possible exposures to avian influenza (Centers for Disease Control and Prevention, 2007). In

January 2006, President Bush pledged $334 million to support the global campaign against avian influenza through improved surveillance and response systems, assistance to countries threatened by the virus, and public awareness campaigns (White House, 2006).

Quality of Life

The term *quality of life* is used in a denotative sense to capture the essence of overall satisfaction with life during and following a person's encounter with the healthcare delivery system. Thus, the term is employed in two different ways. First, it is an indicator of how satisfied a person was with the experiences while receiving health care. Specific life domains, such as comfort factors, respect, privacy, security, degree of independence, decision-making autonomy, and attention to personal preferences are significant to most people. These factors are now regarded as rights that patients can demand during any type of healthcare encounter. Second, quality of life can refer to a person's overall satisfaction with life and with self-perceptions of health, particularly after some medical intervention. The implication is that desirable processes during medical treatment and successful outcomes would subsequently have a positive effect on an individual's ability to function, carry out social roles and obligations, and have a sense of fulfillment and self-worth.

Determinants of Health

The determinants of health—factors that influence individual and population health status—are well established. Starfield (1973) suggested that health status is determined by a confluence of factors that can be classified into four major categories: (1) a person's individual behaviors,

(2) genetic makeup, (3) medical practice, and (4) the environment. The Centers for Disease Control and Prevention (CDC) (1979) estimated that 50% of premature deaths in the U.S. population was directly related to individual lifestyle and behaviors, 20% was attributed to an individual's inherited genetic profile, and only 10% could be ascribed to inadequate access to medical care. The remaining 20% of premature mortality could be attributed to social and environmental factors (Figure 7–3).

In 1974, Blum (1981) proposed an environment of health model later called the force field and well-being paradigms of health (Figure 7–4). Blum proposed four major inputs that contributed to health and well-being. These main influences (called force fields) are the environment, lifestyle, heredity, and medical care, all of which must be considered simultaneously when addressing the health status of an individual or a population. The four wedges in Figure 7–4 represent the four major force fields. The size of each wedge signifies its relative importance. Thus, the most important force field according to this model is the environment, followed by lifestyles and heredity. Medical care has the least impact on health and well-being. Although both the CDC and Blum models point to the same four factors, they are slightly different. The CDC model emphasizes causes leading to premature death and points to individual lifestyle behaviors as the main contributor. Blum's model emphasizes overall well-being, including health, and points to environmental factors as the main contributors.

The determinants of health have made a major contribution to the understanding that a singular focus on medical care delivery is unlikely to improve the health status of any given population. Instead, a more balanced approach to public policy addresses broad social and economic concerns in society. The following discussion and examples show that, regardless of the type of healthcare system a nation may have, social policies must address a multiple of factors for improving the health and well-being of a

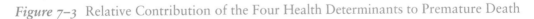

Figure 7–3 Relative Contribution of the Four Health Determinants to Premature Death

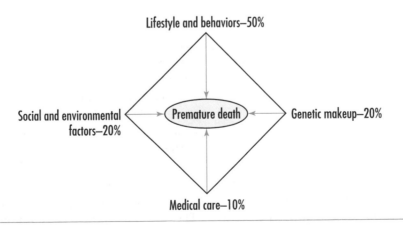

Figure 7–4 The Force Field and Well-Being Paradigms of Health

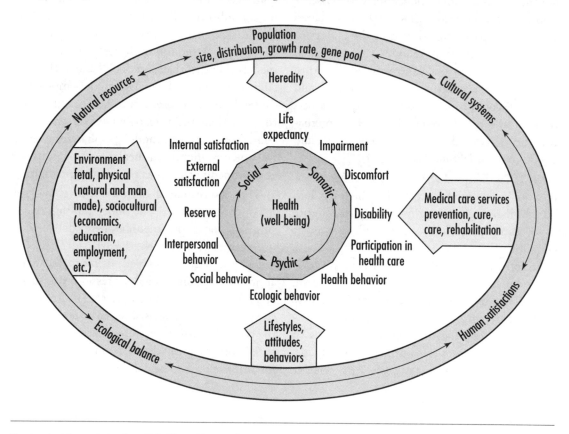

Reprinted with permission from H.L. Blum, Planning for Health, © 1981, Human Sciences Press.

population. From a healthcare delivery perspective, the goal of providing adequate primary care to everyone may be more important than providing access to the latest technology.

Environment

Environmental factors encompass the physical, socioeconomic, sociopolitical, and sociocultural dimensions. Among physical environmental factors are air pollution, food and water contaminants, radiation, toxic chemicals, wastes, disease vectors, safety hazards, and habitat alterations. The relationship of socioeconomic status (SES) to health and well-being may be explained by the general likelihood that people who have better education also have higher incomes. They live in better homes and locations where they are less exposed to environmental risks, have better access to health care, and are more likely to avoid risk behaviors, such as smoking and drug abuse. The relationship between education and health status has been well established. Less educated Americans die younger compared to their better educated counterparts. Diseases mainly responsible for this disparity in mortality are ischemic heart disease, lung cancer, stroke, pneumonia, congestive heart failure, and lung disease, which are, incidentally, all smoking-related diseases (Tanne, 2002). Unemployment may affect social health because of reduced social functioning, mental health because of increased levels of stress, and physical health due to various stress-related illnesses.

A significant body of literature in recent years has demonstrated the association of income inequality with a variety of health indicators, such as life expectancy, age-adjusted mortality rates, and leading causes of death (Kaplan, Pamuk, Lynch, Cohen, & Balfour, 1996; Kawachi, Kennedy, Lochner, & Prothrow-Stith, 1997; Kennedy, Kawachi, & Prothrow-Stith, 1996; Mackenbach, Kunst, Cavelaars, Groenhof, & Geurts, 1997). The greater the economic gap between the rich and the poor in a given geographic area, the worse the health status of the population in that area will be. It has been suggested that wide income gaps produce less social cohesion and greater psychosocial stress and, consequently, poorer health (Wilkinson, 1997). For example, social cohesion, characterized by a hospitable social environment in which people trust each other and participate in communal activities, is linked to lower overall mortality and better self-rated health (Kawachi et al., 1997; Kawachi, Kennedy, & Glass, 1999). Researchers have postulated that the political and policy context that creates income inequality is a precursor to health inequalities (Dye, 1991). Political traditions more committed to redistributive policies, such as those followed by social democratic governments, are generally more success-

ful in improving the health of populations, such as reducing infant mortality (Navarro & Shi, 2001). However, even countries with national health insurance programs, such as England, Australia, Denmark, and Sweden, experience persistent and widening disparities in health according to socioeconomic status (Pincus, Esther, DeWalt, & Callahan, 1998). Pincus and colleagues proposed that poor health in socio logically disadvantaged populations results more from unfavorable social conditions and ineffective self-management than from limitations in access to medical care.

The availability of primary care may serve as one alternative pathway through which income inequality influences population-level health outcomes. Shi and colleagues (Shi, Starfield, Kennedy, & Kawachi, 1999; Shi & Starfield, 2001) examined the joint relationships among income inequality, availability of primary care, and certain health indicators. The results indicate that the availability of primary care physicians, in addition to income inequality, significantly correlates with reduced mortality, increased life expectancy, and improved birth outcome. In another study using the 1996 Robert Wood Johnson Community Tracking Study household survey, they also examined whether income inequality and primary care, measured at the state level, predict individual morbidity, as measured by self-rated health status while adjusting for potentially confounding individual variables (Shi, Starfield, Politzer, & Regan, 2002). The results of the study indicate that the distributions of income and primary care in states were significantly associated with individuals' self-rated health. There was a gradient effect of income inequality on self-rated health, and individuals living in states with a higher primary care physician-to-population ratio were more likely to report good health than those living in states with a lower ratio. These studies made the authors conclude that from a policy perspective, improvement in individuals' health is likely to require a multi-pronged approach that addresses individual socioeconomic determinants of health, social, and economic policies that affect income distribution and strengthens primary care aspects of health services.

The environment can also have a significant influence on developmental health. It has been shown, for example, that children who are isolated and do not socialize much with their peers tend to be overrepresented in groups of delinquents and adults with mental health problems (Wynder & Orlandi, 1984). Current research points out that the experiences that children receive and the way adults interact with them in the early years have a major impact on children's mental and emotional development. Neuroscientists have found that good nurturing and stimulation in the first 3 years of life—a prime time for brain development—activate neural pathways in the brain that might otherwise atrophy, and may even permanently increase the number of brain cells. Hence, the importance of quality of child care provided in the first 3 years of life is monumental (Shellenbarger, 1997).

Lifestyle

Lifestyle or behavioral risk factors were discussed earlier. This section provides some illustrations of how lifestyle factors are related to health. Studies have shown that diet and foods, for example, play a major role in most of the significant health problems of today. Heart disease, diabetes, stroke, and cancer are but some of the diseases with direct links to dietary choices. Throughout the world, incidence and mortality rates for many forms of cancer are rising. Yet research has clearly indicated that a significant portion of cancer is preventable. The role of diet and nutrition in cancer prevention has been one of the most exciting and promising research areas over the past few years. Researchers now estimate that 40–60% of all cancers, and as many as 35% of cancer deaths, are linked to diet (American Institute for Cancer Research, 1996). Current research also shows that a diet rich in fruits, vegetables, and low-fat dairy foods and with reduced saturated and total fat can substantially lower blood pressure. Thus, a nutritional approach can be effective in both preventing and treating hypertension (Appel et al., 1997). The role of exercise and physical activity as a potentially useful, effective, and acceptable method for reducing the risk of colon cancer is also significant (Macfarlane & Lowenfels, 1994). Research findings have also confirmed the association between recreational and/or occupational physical activity and a reduced risk of colon cancer (White, Jacobs, & Daling, 1996).

Heredity

Heredity is a key determinant of health because genetic factors predispose individuals to certain diseases. For example, cancer occurs when the body's healthy genes lose their ability to suppress malignant growth or when other genetic processes stop working properly, although this does not mean that cancer is entirely a disease of the genes (Davis & Webster, 2002).

A person can do little about the genetic makeup he or she has inherited. However, lifestyles and behaviors that a person may currently engage in can have significant influences on future progeny. Advances in gene therapy hold the promise of treating a variety of inherited or acquired diseases.

Medical Care

Even though the other three factors (environment, lifestyle, and heredity) are more important in the determination of health, well-being, and susceptibility to premature death, medical care is nevertheless a key determinant of health. Both individual and population health are closely related to having access to adequate preventive and curative healthcare services. Despite the fact that medical care, compared to the other three force fields, has the least impact on health and well-being, the American public's attitudes toward improving health are based on more medical research, development of new medical technology, and spending more on high-tech medical care. Yet, significant declines in mortality rates were achieved well before the modernization of Western medicine and the escalation in medical care expenditures.

Overarching Factors and Implications for Healthcare Delivery

The force fields illustrated in Blum's model (Figure 7–4) are affected by broad national and international factors, such as a nation's population characteristics, natural resources, ecological balance, human satisfactions, and cultural systems. The type of healthcare delivery system can be included among these factors. Historically, public health and environmental interventions, such as improved nutrition, san-

itation, and immunization, have contributed to significant declines in mortality. Currently, tobacco use, diet and activity patterns, microbial and toxic agents, alcohol and drug abuse, firearms, sexual behavior, and motor vehicle accidents continue to impose a substantial public health burden. Yet the preponderance of healthcare expenditures is devoted to the treatment of medical conditions (e.g., heart disease, cancer, and stroke) rather than to the prevention and control of factors that produce those medical conditions in the first place. This misdirection can be traced to the conflicts that often result from the beliefs and values ingrained in the American culture.

Cultural Beliefs and Values

Cultural beliefs and values are among the overarching factors that influence the key determinants of health, according to Blum's model. A value system orients the members of a society toward defining what is desirable for that society. It has been observed that even a society as complex and highly differentiated as the United States can be said to have a relatively well-integrated system of institutionalized common values at the societal level (Parsons, 1972). Although such a view may still prevail, the American society now has several different subcultures that have grown in size due to a steady influx of immigrants from different parts of the world. There are sociocultural variations in how people view their health and, more important, how such differences influence people's attitudes and behaviors concerning health, illness, and death (Wolinsky, 1988).

Societal values and cultural beliefs are among the external forces that influence how health care is delivered. Decisions about who will receive what type of services can often be culture based. For example, cross-cultural perspectives show wide variations among countries in the way people prioritize who should receive scarce medical resources. In traditional Indian and Chinese cultures, boys are valued more than girls are. Girls are more likely to suffer from poor nutrition and lack of health care. Other culture-based differences exist among some African tribes in how they distribute scarce medical resources among those who may be in equal need of those services (Brown, 1992). Modernization, education, and adoption of Western values are changing some of the cultural orientations toward the use of health care in these countries. On the other hand, certain beliefs and values remain firmly ingrained despite modern influences. In a multicultural society such as the United States, beliefs and values in certain groups that are foreign to the Western culture need to be treated with sensitivity by the providers of health care.

The current system of health services delivery traces its roots to the traditional beliefs and values espoused by the American people. The value and belief system governs the training and general orientation of healthcare providers, type of health delivery settings, financing and allocation of resources, and access to health care. Healthcare systems in other countries also reflect deeply rooted beliefs and values that, largely, make people oppose any major reforms. For example, Canadians are very much opposed to some recent proposals recommending an increased role of private sector companies in the delivery of health services. Canadians also prefer increased spending on health and social programs than receiving a tax cut from the government. Americans, on the other hand, are skeptical of any heavy-handed government involvement in the healthcare system.

Some of the main beliefs and values predominant in the American culture are outlined below:

1. A strong belief in the advancement of science and the application of the scientific method to medicine were instrumental in creating the medical model that primarily governs healthcare delivery in the United States. In turn, the medical model has fueled the tremendous growth in medical science and technological innovation. As a result, the United States has been leading the world in new medical breakthroughs. These developments have had numerous implications for health services delivery, including:

   a. They increase the demand for the latest treatments and raise patients' expectations of finding a cure.

   b. Medical professionals have been preoccupied almost exclusively with clinical interventions, whereas the holistic aspects of health and use of alternative therapies have been deemphasized.

   c. Healthcare professionals have been trained to focus on physical symptoms.

   d. Few attempts have been made to integrate diagnosis and treatment with health education and disease prevention.

   e. The concern with nonhealth has funneled most research efforts away from the pursuit of health into development of sophisticated medical technology. Commitment of resources to the preservation and enhancement of health and well-being has lagged far behind.

f. Medical specialists using the latest technology have been held in higher esteem and have earned higher incomes than general practitioners and health educators.

g. The desirability of healthcare delivery institutions, such as hospitals, is often evaluated by their acquisition of advanced technology.

h. While biomedicine has taken central stage, diagnosis and treatment of mental health have been relegated to a lesser status. Difficulties linking certain behaviors to mental disorders have been at least partially responsible for the secondary status of mental health services in the healthcare delivery system.

i. The biomedical model has also isolated the social and spiritual elements of health.

2. The United States has been a champion of capitalism. Due to a strong belief in capitalism, health care has largely been viewed as an economic good (or service), not as a public resource.

3. A culture of capitalism promotes entrepreneurial spirit and self-determination. Hence, individual capabilities to obtain health services have largely determined the production and consumption of health care—which services will be produced, where, and in what quantity, and who will have access to those services. Some key implications are:

a. Financing of health care through individual health insurance coverage has made access to health care a social privilege.

b. A clear distinction exists between the types of services for poor and affluent communities and between those in rural and urban locations.

c. The culture of individualism emphasizes individual health rather than population health. Medical practice, therefore, has been directed at keeping the individual healthy rather than keeping the entire community healthy.

4. A concern for the most underprivileged classes in society—the poor, the elderly, the disabled, and children—led to the creation of the public programs Medicare, Medicaid, and SCHIP.

5. Principles of free enterprise and a general distrust of big government have kept the delivery of health care largely in private hands. Hence, a separation also exists between public health functions and private practice of medicine.

A Social Model of Health

The social model of health views health and well-being in terms of a person's capacity to function socially and to perform the expected societal roles was discussed earlier. A person unable to perform the social roles is declared sick and is expected to adopt the sick role (Wolinsky, 1988). Parsons (1972) also viewed illness as a socially institutionalized role type that has four specific features: (1) The sick individual is not held responsible for his or her sickness. (2) Being sick is recognized as the legitimate basis for society to exempt the individual from his or her social role obligations. (3) The individual is exempted from social roles on the condition that he or she recognizes that being sick is undesirable and that the individual has the obligation to try to get well. (4) The sick individual must seek competent help and cooperate with medical agencies trying to help the individual get well.

The model has two important implications for healthcare delivery. First, the primary focus is on the individual. Societal roles are mainly passive and consensual—agreeing to release the individual from his or her social obligations and, because illness is only partially and conditionally legitimated (Parsons, 1972), maintaining some sort of surveillance over the individual to ensure that he or she is carrying through with the sick role obligations. More important, society is not required to furnish medical services. The sick individual must seek appropriate medical care and comply with the prescribed regimen. Family members or significant others may assist the individual.

Second, the social model assumes that the sick role obligations are carried out within the context of the medical model of health services delivery. Parsons implied that even though people have an obligation to prevent threatened illness (Parsons, 1972), society does not hold the individual responsible for his or her diseased condition. Even though personal lifestyles and behaviors can substantially increase the risk of high-cost illness, society does not impose any sanctions on the individual for diseases acquired as a direct result of personal indiscretions. The reason, perhaps, is that society also does not assume any responsibility for providing medical care. It is interesting to note that in recent debates and court cases seeking damages for treatment costs for certain groups of smokers who developed lung disease, society has put the entire blame on the tobacco industry while absolving the individual smokers of any personal responsibility.

Equitable Distribution of Health Care

Scarcity of economic resources is a central economic concept. From this perspective, health care can be viewed as an economic good. Two fundamental questions arise with regard to how scarce healthcare resources ought to be used: (1) How much health care should be produced? (2) How should health care be distributed? The first question concerns the appropriate combination in which health services ought to be produced in relation to all other goods and services in the overall economy. If more health care is produced, people will have to forgo some other goods, like food, clothing, and transportation. The second question affects individuals at a more personal level. It deals with who can receive which type of medical services and who will be restricted from accessing services.

The production, distribution, and subsequent consumption of health care must be perceived as equitable. No society has found a perfectly equitable method to distribute limited economic resources. In fact, any method of resource distribution leaves some inequalities. Societies, therefore, try to allocate resources according to some guiding principles acceptable to each society. Such principles are generally ingrained in a society's value and belief system. It is generally recognized that not everyone can receive everything medical science has to offer. The fundamental question that deals with distributive justice or equity is who should receive the medical goods and services that society produces (Santerre & Neun, 1996). By extension, this basic question about equity includes not only who should receive medical care but also which type of services and in what quantity.

A just and fair allocation of health care poses conceptual and practical difficulties; hence, a theory of justice needs to resolve the problem of healthcare allocation (Jonsen, 1986). The principle of justice derives from ethical theories, especially those advanced by John Rawls, who defined justice as fairness (Darr, 1991). Even though various ethical principles can be used to guide decisions pertaining to just and fair allocation of health care in individual circumstances, the broad concern about equitable access to health services is addressed by the theories referred to as market justice and social justice. These two contrasting theories govern the production and distribution of healthcare services.

Market Justice

The principle of market justice ascribes the fair distribution of health care to the market forces in a free economy. Medical care and its benefits are distributed based on people's willingness and ability to pay (Santerre & Neun, 1996). In other words, people are entitled to purchase a share of the available goods and services that they value. They are to purchase these valued goods and services by means of wealth acquired through their own legitimate efforts. This is how most goods and services are distributed in a free market. The free market implies that giving people something they have not earned would be morally and economically wrong.

Chapter 6 discussed several characteristics that describe a pure market. Those market characteristics are a precondition because market justice requires that health care be delivered in a free market. In addition, the principle of market justice is based on the following key assumptions:

- Health care is like any other economic good or service. If health care was considered different from other economic products, it could not be governed by free market forces of supply and demand.
- Individuals are responsible for their own achievements. When individuals pursue their own best interests, the interests of society as a whole are best served (Ferguson & Maurice, 1970).
- People make rational choices in their decisions to purchase healthcare products and services. People demand health care because it can rectify a health problem and restore health, can reduce pain and discomfort and make people feel better, and can reduce anxiety about their health and well-being. Therefore, people are willing to purchase healthcare services. Grossman (1972) proposed that health is also an investment commodity. People consider the purchase of health services as an investment. For example, the investment has a monetary payoff when it reduces the number of sick days, making extra time available for productive activities, such as earning a living. Or it can have a utility payoff—that is, a payoff in terms of satisfaction—when it makes life more enjoyable and fulfilling.
- People, in consultation with their physicians, know what is best for themselves. This assumption implies that people place a certain degree of trust in their physicians and that the physician–patient relationship is ongoing.
- The marketplace works best with minimum interference from the government.

In other words, the market rather than the government can allocate healthcare resources in the most efficient and equitable manner.

The classical ethical theory known as deontology may be applied to market justice. Deontology (from the Greek word *deon*) asserts that it is an individual's duty to do what is right. The results are not important. Deontology emphasizes individual responsibilities as in a physician–patient relationship. A physician is duty-bound to do whatever is necessary to restore a patient's health. The patient is responsible for compensating the physician for his or her services. The destitute and poor may be served by charity, but deontology largely tends to ignore the importance of societal good. It does not address what responsibilities people have toward the society.

Market justice may also be associated with the libertarian view that equity is achieved when resources are distributed according to merits. That is, health care should be distributed according to minimum standards and financed according to willingness to pay. According to this view, equality in health status need not be a central priority (Starfield, 1998).

Under market justice, the production of health care is determined by how much the consumers are willing and able to purchase at the prevailing market prices. It follows that in a pure market system, individuals without sufficient income face a financial barrier to obtaining health care (Santerre & Neun, 1996). Thus, prices and ability to pay ration the quantity and type of healthcare services people would consume. The uninsured and those who lack sufficient income to pay privately generally face barriers to obtaining health care. Such limitations to obtaining health care are referred to as "rationing by ability to pay" (Feldstein, 1994, p. 45), demand-side rationing, or price rationing.

The key characteristics and their implications under the system of market justice are summarized in Table 7–4. Market justice emphasizes individual rather than collective responsibility for health. It proposes private rather than government solutions to social problems of health.

Social Justice

The idea of social justice is at odds with the principles of capitalism and market justice. The term *social justice* was invented in the 19th century by the critics of capitalism to describe the good society (Kristol, 1978). According to the principle of social justice, the equitable distribution of health care is a societal responsibility. This can best be achieved by letting a central agency, generally the government, take over the production and distribution functions. Social justice regards health care as a social good—as opposed to an economic good—that should be collectively financed and available to all citizens regardless of the individual recipient's ability to pay for that care. Canadians and Europeans, for example, long ago reached a broad social consensus that health care was a social good (Reinhardt, 1994). Public health also has a social justice orientation (Turnock, 1997). Under the social justice system, inability to obtain medical services because of a lack of financial resources is considered unjust. A just distribution of benefits must be based on need, not simply on one's ability to purchase in the marketplace (demand). Need for health care is determined either by the patient or by a health professional. The principle of social justice is also based on certain assumptions, which include:

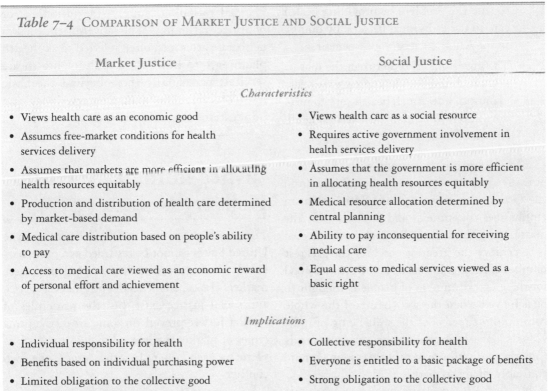

Table 7–4 COMPARISON OF MARKET JUSTICE AND SOCIAL JUSTICE

Market Justice	Social Justice
Characteristics	
• Views health care as an economic good	• Views health care as a social resource
• Assumes free-market conditions for health services delivery	• Requires active government involvement in health services delivery
• Assumes that markets are more efficient in allocating health resources equitably	• Assumes that the government is more efficient in allocating health resources equitably
• Production and distribution of health care determined by market-based demand	• Medical resource allocation determined by central planning
• Medical care distribution based on people's ability to pay	• Ability to pay inconsequential for receiving medical care
• Access to medical care viewed as an economic reward of personal effort and achievement	• Equal access to medical services viewed as a basic right
Implications	
• Individual responsibility for health	• Collective responsibility for health
• Benefits based on individual purchasing power	• Everyone is entitled to a basic package of benefits
• Limited obligation to the collective good	• Strong obligation to the collective good
• Emphasis on individual well-being	• Community well-being supersedes that of the individual
• Private solutions to social problems	• Public solutions to social problems
• Rationing based on ability to pay	• Planned rationing of health care

- Health care is different from most other goods and services. Health-seeking behavior is governed primarily by need rather than by how much it would cost.
- Responsibility for health is shared. Individuals are not held totally responsible for their condition because factors outside their control may have brought on their condition. Society feels responsible for a lack of control of certain envi-

ronmental factors, such as economic inequalities, unemployment, unsanitary conditions, or air pollution.
- Society has an obligation to the collective good. The well-being of the community is superior to that of the individual. An unhealthy individual is a burden on society. A person carrying a deadly infection, for example, is a threat to society. Society, therefore, is obligated

to cure the problem by providing health care to the individual because by doing so the whole society would benefit.

- The government, rather than the market, can better decide, through rational planning, how much health care to produce and how to distribute it among all citizens.

Social justice is consistent with the theory of utilitarianism, a teleological principle (from the Greek *telos*, meaning end). Utilitarianism emphasizes happiness and welfare for the masses; it ignores the individual. Society's goal is to achieve the greatest good for the greatest number of people. In this case, the greatest good for the greatest number of people is thought to be achieved when the well-being of the whole community supersedes the well-being of individuals. By implication, the government is thought to distribute healthcare resources more equitably than the market.

Social justice finds its ethical roots in the egalitarian view that equity is achieved when resources are distributed according to needs. That is, more resources are made available to populations that need more services because of their greater social or health disadvantage (Starfield, 1998).

Under social justice, how much health care to produce is determined by the government; however, no country can afford to provide unlimited amounts of health care to all its citizens (Feldstein, 1994). The government then also finds ways to limit the availability of certain healthcare services by deciding, for instance, how technology will be dispersed and who will be allowed access to certain types of high-tech services, even though basic services may be available to all. This concept refers to planned rationing, supply-side rationing, or nonprice rationing. The government makes deliberate attempts, often referred to as "health planning," to limit the supply of healthcare services, particularly those beyond the basic level of care. The main characteristics and implications of social justice are summarized in Table 7–4.

Justice in the U.S. Health Delivery System

The market for healthcare delivery in the United States cannot be regarded as a pure market. It is characterized as a quasi or imperfect market. Hence, elements of both market justice and social justice exist, but the principles of market justice prevail. In some areas, the principles of market justice and social justice complement each other. In other areas, the two conflict.

Health Insurance

In a society with strong market justice values, individuals paying for their own care would predominantly finance the medical care system. A multitude of private health insurance plans would prevail. In a society with strong social justice principles, the government, through general tax revenues, would finance the medical care system (Long, 1994).

In the United States, the principles of market justice and social justice complement each other with private, employer-based health insurance for mainly middle-income Americans (market justice), publicly financed Medicaid, Medicare, and SCHIP coverage for certain disadvantaged groups, and workers' compensation for those injured at work (social justice). The two principles collide, however, regarding the large number of uninsured who cannot afford to purchase private health insurance and do not meet the eligibility criteria for Medicaid, Medicare, SCHIP, or other public programs. Americans have not been able to resolve the question of who should provide health insurance to the uninsured.

Organization of Healthcare Delivery

In a market justice-dominant society, the number and type of physicians produced by the educational system are determined by the desires of would-be physicians and their assessment of the chances of future success. Physicians themselves decide where they will be located to practice, without necessarily taking into account the needs of the population (Long, 1994). Physicians are compensated mostly on a fee-for-service basis, the fees being established by the physicians themselves. Similarly, hospital location and operations are influenced by financial viability without regard to duplication or shortages of services and technology. In a society with strong social justice values, the number, type, and location of physicians and hospitals, reimbursement to providers, and distribution of medical technology are determined by the government, supposedly based on the health needs of the populations.

In the United States, private and government health insurance programs enable the covered populations to have access to healthcare services delivered by private practitioners and private institutions (market justice). Tax-supported county and city hospitals, public health clinics, and community health centers can be accessed by the uninsured in areas where such services are available (social justice). Publicly run institutions generally operate in large inner cities and certain rural areas. Conflict between the two principles of justice arises in small cities and towns and large rural sections where such services are not available. Medicare and Medicaid make their own determinations on how much to pay for the services. These characteristics do not fully harmonize with the pure market justice principles.

Equity in the U.S. Healthcare Delivery System

Equity advocates argue that health insurance should be universally extended to all Americans (Santerre & Neun, 1996). Major healthcare reform proposals to establish universal access were advanced shortly after Bill Clinton became president in 1992. The first lady, Hillary Rodham Clinton, took the lead in championing the cause. In a speech delivered to the American Medical Association on June 13, 1993, Mrs. Clinton said, "We must guarantee all Americans access to a comprehensive package of [health] benefits, no matter where they work, where they live, or whether they have ever been sick before" (Clinton, 1995). In response to such proposals, a market advocate labeled the Clinton health plan as radical because under such a policy proposal "every person would have the same comprehensive coverage designed by the government, regardless of their health status, health habits, and preferences for insurance coverage. The only individual choice would be to select more or less expensive versions of this same coverage, like the opportunity to choose first class or coach but not the destination of a flight"

(Niskanen, 1995). As discussed earlier, such American ideals reflect strong individualistic values underlying market justice.

The health policy agenda of George W. Bush, the president succeeding Bill Clinton, has adhered to these individualistic values. The major elements of Bush's health platform include: (1) the promotion of health savings accounts (HSAs), which allow people to create tax-free accounts to pay for out-of-pocket medical expenses; (2) efforts to increase transparency (i.e., readily available information) in healthcare pricing and quality, to allow people to make better decisions about their healthcare choices; and (3) the endorsement of health information technology (HIT) to "facilitate the rapid exchange of health information" (White House, 2007). The president has also called for expansion of the community health center program, providing preventive and primary healthcare services to an estimated 16 million people in underserved communities who otherwise would lack access to care. This initiative seems more oriented toward social justice than Bush's other initiatives. However, community health centers derive a significant proportion of their operating revenues from Medicaid reimbursements. During Bush's tenure as president, Medicaid cuts at the federal and state levels, coupled with rising healthcare costs and increasing numbers of uninsured people, have threatened health centers' efforts to provide care to vulnerable populations (National Association of Community Health Centers, 2005).

Americans have a tradition of reliance on individual responsibility and a commitment to the ideal of a limited national government, which are more in accord with the principles of market justice than social justice. In contrast, western Europe, Canada, and most developed countries have adopted a public policy of universal access. Even though they reflect social justice values, such policies were not motivated primarily by concerns about justice and equality but by social objectives—to have a more productive labor force, to have a healthy citizenry for national defense, and to bring stability against social unrest (President's Commission, 1983).

Equality of individuals has always been a prominent American value, but "the traditional emphasis has been on equal civil and political liberties rather than on economic equality" (President's Commission, 1983, p. 14). Social justice represents an effort to stretch the idea of justice to cover economic equality as well (Kristol, 1978). If health care is regarded as a basic right, then an important measure of a just system of healthcare allocation would be equal access to medical services. In the United States, this ideal of equality blurs when it comes to equal access to comprehensive medical care (Brown, 1992).

Distributional Efficiency

Equity requires distributional efficiency, which deals with the amount of resources to allocate and how to distribute them. Since resources are scarce, equity requires that their distribution be efficient, otherwise some people may be denied the benefit of the wasted resources. At a more practical level, resources equate to total expenditures for delivering health care. Market justice assumes that the market would handle the distribution of resources most efficiently, that is, market forces would govern allocation of health dollars. Market justice advocates would also argue that the government is inefficient and resorts to rationing to cover up its inefficiencies. However, in evaluating efficiency, a greater emphasis is being placed on health outcomes. From this perspective, the United States has failed to achieve distributional efficiency, compared to other industrialized nations. The United States tops all other countries in per capita expenditures on health care, but the American population as a whole lags far behind in key indicators of health, such as life expectancy and infant mortality. This largely attributes to significant disparities in health within U.S. subpopulation groups.

Limitations of Market Justice

The principles of market justice work well in the allocation of economic goods when their unequal distribution does not affect the larger society. For example, based on individual success, people live in different sizes and styles of homes, drive different types of automobiles, and spend their money on a variety of things, but the allocation of certain resources has wider repercussions for society. In these areas, market justice has severe limitations, including:

1. Market justice principles generally fail to rectify critical human concerns. Pervasive social problems, such as crime, illiteracy, and homelessness, can significantly weaken the fabric of a society. Indeed, the United States has recognized such issues and instituted programs based on social justice to combat the problems through added police protection, publicly supported education, subsidized housing, and, more recently, national initiatives against terrorism. Health care is an important social issue because it not only affects human productivity and achievement, but it also provides basic human dignity.

2. Market justice does not always protect a society. Individual health issues can have

negative consequences for society because ill health is not always confined to the individual. The acquired immune deficiency syndrome (AIDS) epidemic is an example in which society can be put at serious risk. Initial spread of the SARS epidemic in Beijing was largely due to patients with SARS symptoms being turned away by hospitals since they were not able to pay in advance for the cost of the treatment. Similar to clean air and water, health care is a social concern that, in the long run, protects against the burden of preventable disease and disability, a burden that is ultimately placed on the shoulders of society.

3. Market justice does not work well in healthcare delivery. The decade of the 1990s was characterized by unprecedented economic growth and creation of wealth in the United States. This period of prosperity, however, did not reduce the number of Americans without health insurance. In a nation where the benefits of health care are employment based, this condition is truly a paradox given a low rate of unemployment compared to many other industrialized nations. The experience clearly shows that equitable delivery of health care requires social justice-based solutions.

Integration of Individual and Community Health

In recent years, it has been recognized that the typical emphasis on the treatment of acute illness in hospitals, biomedical research into disease, and high technology has not improved the population's health. The notable concern to contain rising healthcare costs and a paradigm shift toward delivery of health services through managed care have also prompted a reevaluation of the traditional medical model. It has been proposed that the medical model should be replaced with a disease-prevention, health-promotion, or primary care model (Shortell, Gillies, & Devers, 1995). More precisely, this is a call for integration of the two models rather than a total abandonment of the medical model in favor of the other. Society continues to need the benefits of modern science and technology for the treatment of disease. Disease prevention, health promotion, and primary care can prevent certain health problems from occurring, delay the onset of disease, and prevent disability and premature death. An integrated approach will not make disease, disability, and death go away; but it will improve the overall health of the population, enhance people's quality of life, and conserve healthcare resources.

An integrated approach must go beyond a simple merger of the medical and wellness models. The real challenge for the healthcare delivery system is to incorporate these models within the holistic context of health. The Ottawa Charter for Health Promotion, for instance, mentions caring, holism, and ecology as essential issues in developing strategies for health promotion (de Leeuw, 1989). *Holism* and *ecology* refer to the complex relationships that exist among the individual, the healthcare delivery system, and the physical, social, cultural, and economic environmental factors. *Environment*, in this context, could be viewed as an extension of the social dimension of health discussed earlier in this chapter. In addition, as the increasing body of research points out, the spiritual dimension must be incorporated into the integrated model.

Another equally important challenge for the healthcare delivery system is to focus on both individual and population health outcomes. The nature of health is complex, and the interrelationships among the physical, mental, social, and spiritual dimensions are not well understood. How to translate this multidimensional framework of health into specific actions that are efficiently configured to achieve better individual and community health is the greatest challenge any healthcare system could possibly face.

For an integrated approach to become reality, resource limitations would make it necessary to deploy the best U.S. ingenuity toward health-spending reduction, elimination of wasteful care, promotion of individual responsibility and accountability for one's health, and improved access to services. In a broad sense, these services include medical care, preventive services, health promotion, and social policy to improve education, lifestyles, employment, and housing (Figure 7–5). The Ottawa Charter has proposed

Figure 7-5 Integrated Model for Holistic Health

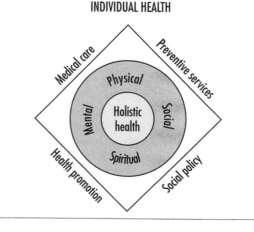

INDIVIDUAL HEALTH

achieving health objectives through social public policy and community action. An integrated approach also necessitates creation of a new model for training healthcare professionals by forming partnerships with the community (Henry, 1993). The following paragraphs describe examples of community partnership reflected in community health assessment and *Healthy People* initiatives.

Community Health Assessment

Community health assessment is a method used to conduct broad assessments of populations at a local or state level. For integrating individual and community health, the assessment is best conducted by collaboration among public health agencies, hospitals, and other healthcare providers. Community hospitals in particular are increasingly held accountable for the health status of the communities in which they are located. To fulfill this mission, hospitals must first conduct a health assessment of their communities. Such an assessment provides a broad perspective of a population's health, and it also points to specific needs that healthcare providers can address. It can help pinpoint interventions that should be given priority to improve the population's health status or to address critical issues pertaining to certain groups within the population. Measures of health status discussed later in this chapter are essential to conduct a community health assessment. An assessment also requires an evaluation of health determinants and utilization of medical care services.

Healthy People Initiatives

Since 1980, the United States has undertaken 10-year plans outlining certain key national health objectives to be accomplished during each of the 10-year periods. These initiatives have been founded on the integration of medical care with preventive services, health promotion, and education; integration of personal and community health care; and increased access to integrated services. Accordingly, the objectives are developed by a consortium of national and state organizations, under the leadership of the U.S. surgeon general. The first of these programs, with objectives for 1990, provided national goals for reducing premature deaths and for preserving the independence of older adults. Next, *Healthy People 2000: National Health Promotion and Disease Prevention Objectives*, released in 1990, identified health improvement goals and objectives to be reached by the year 2000. As part of this process, standardized health status indicators (HSIs) were developed to facilitate the comparison of health status measures at national, state, and local levels over time. According to the final review published by the National Center for Health Statistics (2001), the major accomplishments of *Healthy People 2000* included surpassing the targets for reducing deaths from coronary heart disease and cancer; meeting the targets for incidence rates for AIDS and syphilis, mammography exams, violent deaths, and tobacco-related deaths; nearly meeting the targets for infant mortality and number of children with elevated levels of lead in their blood; and making progress in reducing health disparities among special populations.

Healthy People 2010: Healthy People in Healthy Communities, launched in January 2000, continues in the earlier traditions as an instrument to improve the health of the American people in the first decade of the 21st century. The context developed in national objectives for *Healthy People 2010* differs from the framework of *Healthy People 2000*. Advanced preventive therapies, vaccines, and pharmaceuticals, and improved surveillance and data systems are now available. Demographic changes in the United States reflect an older and more racially diverse population. Global forces, such as food supplies, emerging infectious diseases, and environmental interdependence, present new public health challenges. The objectives also define new relationships between public health departments and healthcare delivery organizations (Department of Health and Human Services, 1998). *Healthy People 2010* specifically emphasizes the role of community partners—such as businesses, local governments, and civic,

professional, and religious organizations—as effective agents for improving health in their local communities. In addition, the objectives for 2010 specifically focus on the determinants of health discussed earlier.

Figure 7–6 presents the graphic framework for *Healthy People 2010*. The two overarching goals designed for achievement by *Healthy People 2010* are (Department of Health and Human Services, 2000):

1. *Increase quality and years of healthy life.*
   The first goal is to help individuals of

Figure 7–6 Healthy People 2010: Healthy People in Healthy Communities

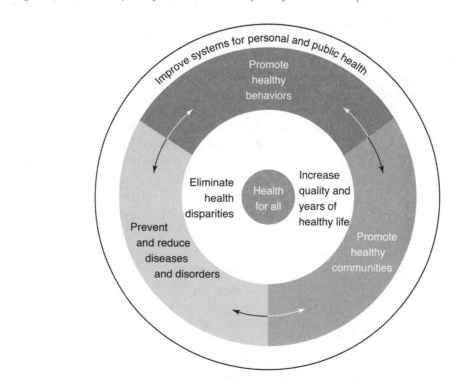

all ages increase life expectancy and improve their quality of life. In particular, differences in life expectancy among populations suggest a substantial need and opportunity for improvement. At least 18 countries with populations of 1 million or more have life expectancies greater than the United States for both men and women. Similar to life expectancy, various population groups show dramatic differences in quality of life. A disproportionate number of Americans in low-income households, women, and those living in rural areas report their health status as fair or poor. These findings lead to the second goal.

2. *Eliminate health disparities.* The second goal of *Healthy People 2010* is to eliminate health disparities among different segments of the population. These include differences that occur by gender, race or ethnicity, education or income, disability, living in rural localities, or sexual orientation. The greatest opportunities for reducing health disparities are in empowering individuals to make

Exhibit 7–1   Healthy People 2010 Focus Areas

1. Access to Quality Health Services	15. Injury and Violence Prevention
2. Arthritis, Osteoporosis, and Chronic Back Conditions	16. Maternal, Infant, and Child Health
3. Cancer	17. Medical Product Safety
4. Chronic Kidney Disease	18. Mental Health and Mental Disorders
5. Diabetes	19. Nutrition and Overweight
6. Disability and Secondary Conditions	20. Occupational Safety and Health
7. Educational and Community-Based Programs	21. Oral Health
8. Environmental Health	22. Physical Activity and Fitness
9. Family Planning	23. Public Health Infrastructure
10. Food Safety	24. Respiratory Diseases
11. Health Communication	25. Sexually Transmitted Diseases
12. Heart Disease and Stroke	26. Substance Abuse
13. HIV	27. Tobacco Use
14. Immunization and Infectious Diseases	28. Vision and Hearing

Source: Department of Health and Human Services. *Healthy People 2010* (Conference Edition, in Two Volumes). Washington, DC: January 2000.

informed healthcare decisions and in promoting community-wide safety, education, and access to health care.

To realize these two broad goals, 28 focus areas were identified as measurable targets by 2010 (see Exhibit 7–1).

Using data gathered through January 2005, the Department of Health and Human Services released a midcourse review of progress toward achieving the *Healthy People 2010* goals. With regard to the initiative's first overarching goal (increase quality and years of healthy life), the midcourse review reported life expectancy continues to increase, but significant gender and racial/ethnic differences remain. In addition, the United States continues to have lower life expectancy than many other developed nations. Two quality of life measures (i.e., expected years in good or better health and expected years free of activity limitations) improved slightly while a third quality of life measure (i.e., expected years free of selected chronic diseases) declined slightly (Department of Health and Human Services, 2006).

With regard to the second overarching goal of *Healthy People 2010* (eliminate health disparities), the midcourse review reported very little progress has been made. While there were reductions in several health areas with disparities, there were increases in disparities in other health areas. The midcourse review noted that the lack of data on education, income, and other socioeconomic factors for many *Healthy People 2010* objectives has limited our capabilities to plan programs that are effective in reducing and eliminating disparities (Department of Health and Human Services, 2006).

Conclusion

The system of healthcare delivery in the United States is predominantly private. Many of the peculiarities of this system trace back to the beliefs and values underlying the American culture. The delivery of health care is primarily driven by the medical model, which emphasizes illness rather than wellness. Even though major efforts and expenditures have been directed toward the delivery of medical care, they have failed to produce a proportionate impact on the improvement of health status. Holistic concepts of health care, along with integration of medical care with preventive and health promotional efforts, need to be adopted to significantly improve the health of Americans. Such an approach would require a fundamental change in how Americans view health. It would also require individual responsibility for one's own health-oriented behaviors as well as community partnerships to improve both personal and community health. An understanding of the determinants of health, health education, community health assessment, and national initiatives, such as *Healthy People 2010*, are essential to accomplishing these goals. The emphasis on market justice in the U.S. healthcare delivery system, however, leaves the critical problem of access unaddressed.

Discussion Questions

1. Discuss the differences between health, illness, and disease. How are these concepts related to the role of the advanced nurse practitioner in the delivery of health care?
2. What is the role of the advanced practice nurse in health promotion and disease prevention? Discuss how this differs for each of the roles.
3. Health promotion and disease prevention may require both behavioral modification and therapeutic intervention. Discuss the role of the advanced practice nurse for both
4. What are the main objectives of public health related to the role of the advanced practice nurse?
5. The Blum model points to four key determinants of health. Discuss their implications for healthcare delivery.
6. Discuss the main cultural beliefs and values in American society that have influenced healthcare delivery and how they have shaped the healthcare delivery system.
7. Briefly describe the concepts of market justice and social justice. In what way do the two principles complement each other, and in what way are they in conflict in the U.S. system of healthcare delivery?
8. To what extent do you think the objectives set forth in *Healthy People* initiatives can achieve the vision of an integrated approach to healthcare delivery in the United States? What is the role of the advanced nurse practitioner in advancing these initiatives?

References

American Institute for Cancer Research. (1996). *Food, nutrition and the prevention of cancer: A global perspective.* Washington, DC: World Cancer Research Fund, American Institute for Cancer Research.

American Physical Therapy Association. (1997, October). Religion called valuable health tool. *PT Bulletin, 7.*

Appel, L. J., Moore, T. J., Obarzanek, E., Vollmer, W. M., Svetkey, L. P., Sacks, F. M., et al. (1997). A clinical trial of the effects of dietary patterns on blood pressure. *New England Journal of Medicine, 336*(16), 1117–1124.

Berger, K. S. (1988). *The developing person through the life-span* (2nd ed.). New York: Worth Publishers.

Blum, H. L. (1981). *Planning for health* (2nd ed.). New York: Human Sciences Press.

Breslow, L. (1972). A quantitative approach to the World Health Organization definition of health: Physical, mental and social well-being. *International Journal of Epidemiology, 1*(4), 347–355.

Breslow, L. (1989). Health status measurement in the evaluation of health promotion. *Medical Care, 27*(3), S205–S216.

Brown, K. (1992). Death and access: Ethics in cross-cultural health care. In E. Friedman (Ed.), *Choices and conflict: Explorations in health care ethics* (pp. 85–93). Chicago: American Hospital Publishing.

Centers for Disease Control and Prevention. (1979). *Healthy people: The surgeon general's report on health promotion and disease prevention.* Washington, DC: U.S. Department of Health and Human Services, Public Health Service.

Centers for Disease Control and Prevention. (1999a). *Morbidity and Mortality Weekly Report, 48*(29).

Centers for Disease Control and Prevention. (1999b). Tobacco use—United States, 1900–1999. *Morbidity and Mortality Weekly Report, 48*(43), 986–993.

Centers for Disease Control and Prevention. (2007). *Avian influenza (bird flu).* Retrieved October 10, 2007, from http://www.cdc.gov/flu/avian/

Clinton, H. R. (1995). Health care: We can make a difference. In E. Mansfield (Ed.), *Leading economic controversies of 1995.* New York: W.W. Norton & Company.

Darr, K. (1991). *Ethics in health services management.* Baltimore: Health Professions Press.

Davis, D. L., & Webster, P. S. (2002, November). The social context of science: cancer and the environment. *The Annals of the American Academy of Political and Social Science, 584,* 13–34.

de Leeuw, E. (1989). Concepts in health promotion: The notion of relativism. *Social Science and Medicine, 29*(11), 1281–1288.

Department of Health and Human Services. (1998). *Healthy People 2010 objectives: Draft for public comment.* Washington, DC: U.S. Government Printing Office.

Department of Health and Human Services. (2000). *Healthy People 2010: Understanding and improving health* (2nd ed.). Washington, DC: U.S. Government Printing Office.

Department of Health and Human Services. (2006). *Healthy People 2010: Midcourse review.* Retrieved October 10, 2007, from http://www.healthy people.gov/data/midcourse/default.htm#pubs

Dye, T. R. (1991). *Politics in states and communities* (7th ed.). Englewood Cliffs, NJ: Prentice-Hall.

Ethics Committee, Society for Academic Emergency Medicine. (1992). An ethical foundation for health care: An emergency medicine perspective. *Annals of Emergency Medicine, 21*(11), 1381–1387.

Feldstein, P. J. (1994). *Health policy issues: An economic perspective on health reform.* Ann Arbor, MI: AUPHA/HAP.

Ferguson, C. E., & Maurice, S. C. (1970). *Economic analysis.* Homewood, IL: Richard D. Irwin.

Friedman, G. D. (1980). *Primer of epidemiology.* New York: McGraw-Hill.

Grossman, M. (1972). On the concept of health capital and the demand for health. *Journal of Political Economy, 80*(2), 223–255.

Hancock, L. A., & Mandle, C. L. (1994). Overview of growth and development framework. In C. L. Edelman & C. L. Mandle (Eds.), *Health promotion through the lifespan.* St. Louis, MO: Mosby–Year Book.

Hatch, R. L., Burg, M. A., Naberhaus, D. S., & Hellmich, L. K. (1998). The spiritual involvement and beliefs scale: Development and testing of a new instrument. *Journal of Family Practice, 46,* 476–486.

Henry, R. C. (1993). Community partnership model for health professions education. *Journal of the American Podiatric Medical Association, 83*(6), 328–331.

Institute of Medicine, National Academy of Sciences. (1988). *The future of public health.* Washington, DC: National Academy Press.

Jonsen, A. R. (1986). Bentham in a box: Technology assessment and health care allocation. *Law, Medicine, and Health Care, 14*(3–4), 172–174.

Kane, R. L. (1988). Empiric approaches to prevention in the elderly: Are we promoting too much? In R. Chernoff & D. A. Lipschitz (Eds.), *Health promotion and disease prevention in the elderly* (pp. 127–141). New York: Raven Press.

Kaplan, G. A., Pamuk, E., Lynch, J. W., Cohen, R. D., & Balfour, J. L. (1996). Income inequality and mortality in the United States. *British Medical Journal, 312*(7037), 999–1003.

Kawachi, I., Kennedy, B. P., Lochner, K., & Prothrow-Stith, D. (1997). Social capital, income inequality, and mortality. *American Journal of Public Health, 87,* 1491–1498.

Kawachi, I., Kennedy, B. P., & Glass, R. (1999). Social capital and self-rated health: A contextual analysis. *American Journal of Public Health, 89,* 1187–1193.

Kennedy, B. P., Kawachi, I., & Prothrow-Stith, D. (1996). Income distribution and mortality: Cross sectional ecological study of the Robin Hood index in the United States. *British Medical Journal, 312*(7037), 1004–1007.

Kristol, I. (1978). A capitalist conception of justice. In R. T. De George & J. A. Pichler (Eds.), *Ethics, free enterprise, and public policy: Original essays on moral issues in business* (pp. 57–69). New York: Oxford University Press.

Lasker, R. D., Abramson, D. M., & Freedman, G. R. (1998). *Pocket guide to cases of medicine and public health collaboration.* New York: The New York Academy of Medicine.

Lasker, R. D. (1997) *Medicine and public health: The power of collaboration.* New York: The New York Academy of Medicine.

Levin, J. S. (1994). Religion and health: Is there an association, is it valid, and is it causal? *Social Science and Medicine, 38*(11), 1475–1482.

Long, M. J. (1994). *The medical care system: A conceptual model.* Ann Arbor, MI: Health Administration Press.

Macfarlane, G. J., & Lowenfels, A. B. (1994). Physical activity and colon cancer. *European Journal of Cancer Prevention, 3*(5), 393–398.

Mackenbach, J. P., Kunst, A. E., Cavelaars, A. E., Groenhof, F., & Geurts, J. J. (1997, June). Socioeconomic inequalities in morbidity and mortality in western Europe. *The Lancet, 349,* 1655–1660.

Marwick, C. (1995). Should physicians prescribe prayer for health? Spiritual aspects of well-being considered. *Journal of the American Medical Association, 273*(20), 1561–1562.

Maugans, T. A. (1996). The SPIRITual history. *Archives of Family Medicine, 5*(1), 11–16.

May, L. A. (1993). The physiologic and psychological bases of health, disease, and care seeking. In S. J. Williams & P. R. Torrens (Eds.), *Introduction to health services* (4th ed., pp. 31–45). New York: Delmar Publishers.

McCullough, M. E., Hoyt, W. T., Larson, D. B., Koenig, H. G., & Thoresen, C. (2000). Religious involvement and mortality: A meta-analytic review. *Health Psychology, 19*(3), 211–222.

McCullough, M. E., & Larson, D. B. (1999). Religion and depression: A review of the literature. *Twin Research, 2,* 126–136.

McKee, M. (2001). Measuring the efficiency of health systems. *British Medical Journal, 323*(7308), 295–296.

National Association of Community Health Centers (NACHC). (2005). *The safety net on the edge.* Washington, DC: NACHC.

National Center for Health Statistics. (2006). *Health, United States, 2006.* Hyattsville, MD: Department of Health and Human Services.

Navarro, V., & Shi, L. (2001). The political context of social inequalities and health. *Social Science and Medicine, 52*(3), 481–491.

Niskanen, W. (1995). Government-managed health care. In E. Mansfield (Ed.), *Leading economic controversies of 1995* (pp. 15–20). New York: W.W. Norton & Co.

Parsons, T. (1972). Definitions of health and illness in the light of American values and social structure. In E. G. Jaco (Ed.), *Patients, physicians and illness: A sourcebook in behavioral science and health* (2nd ed.). New York: Free Press.

Peters, K. E., Drabant, B., Elster, A. B., Tierney, M., & Hatcher, B. (2001). *Cooperative actions for health programs: Lessons learned in medicine and public health collaboration.* Chicago: American Medical Association and Washington, DC: American Public Health Association.

Pincus, T., Esther, R., DeWalt, D. A., & Callahan, L. F. (1998). Social conditions and self-management are more powerful determinants of health than access to care. *Annals of Internal Medicine, 129*(5), 406–411.

Plotkin, S. L., & Plotkin, S. A. (1999). A short history of vaccination. In S. A. Plotkin & W. A. Orenstein (Eds.), *Vaccines* (3rd ed., p. 1). Philadelphia: W.B. Saunders.

Post, S. G., Puchalski, C. M., & Larson, D. B. (2000). Physicians and patient spirituality: Professional boundaries, competency, and ethics. *Annals of Internal Medicine, 132*(7), 578–583.

President's Commission for the Study of Ethical Problems in Medicine and Biomedical and Behavioral Research. (1983). *Securing access to health care: The ethical implications of differences in the availability of health services: Vol. 1.* Washington, DC: U.S. Government Printing Office.

Puchalski, C., & Romer, A. L. (2000). Taking a spiritual history allows clinicians to understand patients more fully. *Journal of Palliative Medicine, 3*(1), 129–137.

Reinhardt, U. E. (1994). Providing access to health care and controlling costs: The universal dilemma. In P. R. Lee & C. L. Estes (Eds.), *The nation's health* (4th ed., pp. 263–278). Sudbury, MA: Jones and Bartlett Publishers.

Roberts, J. A., Brown, D., Elkins, T., & Larson, D. B. (1997). Factors influencing the views of patients with gynecologic cancer about end-of-life decisions. *American Journal of Obstetrics and Gynecology, 176,* 166–172.

Rosen, G. (1993). *A history of public health.* Baltimore, MD: Johns Hopkins University Press.

Ross, L. (1995). The spiritual dimension: Its importance to patients' health, well-being and quality of life and its implications for nursing practice. *International Journal of Nursing Studies, 32*(5), 457–468.

Santerre, R. E., & Neun, S. P. (1996). *Health economics: Theories, insights, and industry studies.* Chicago: Irwin.

Saward, E., & Sorensen, A. (1980). The current emphasis on preventive medicine. In S. J. Williams (Ed.), *Issues in health services* (pp. 17–29). New York: John Wiley & Sons.

Schneider, M. J. (2000). *Introduction to public health.* Gaithersburg, MD: Aspen Publishers, Inc.

Shellenbarger, S. (1997, April 9). Good, early care has a huge impact on kids, studies say. *The Wall Street Journal,* B1.

Shi, L., Starfield, B., Politzer, R., & Regan, J. (2002). Primary care, self-rated health, and reductions in social disparities in health. *Health Services Research, 37*(3), 529–550.

Shi, L., Starfield, B., Kennedy, B., & Kawachi, I. (1999). Income inequality, primary care, and health indicators. *Journal of Family Practice, 48*(4), 275–284.

Shi, L., & Starfield, B. (2001). Primary care physician supply, income inequality, and racial mortality in U.S. metropolitan areas. *American Journal of Public Health, 91*(8), 1246–1250.

Shortell, S. M., Gillies, R. R., & Devers, K. J. (1995). Reinventing the American hospital. *The Milbank Quarterly, 73*(2), 131–160.

Starfield, B. (1973). Health services research: A working model. *New England Journal of Medicine, 289*(2), 132–136.

Starfield, B. (1998). *Primary care and health services.* Oxford: Oxford University Press.

Swanson, C. S. (1995). A spirit-focused conceptual model of nursing for the advanced practice nurse. *Issues in Comprehensive Pediatric Nursing, 18*(4), 267–275.

Tamm, M. E. (1993). Models of health and disease. *British Journal of Medical Psychology, 66*(3), 213–228.

Tanne, J. H. (2002). Cause of death among Americans differs with race and education. *British Medical Journal, 325*(7374), 1192–1196.

Timmreck, T. C. (1994). *An introduction to epidemiology.* Sudbury, MA: Jones and Bartlett Publishers.

Turnock, B. J. (1997). *Public health: What it is and how it works.* Gaithersburg, MD: Aspen Publishers, Inc.

Ward, B. (1995). Holistic medicine. *Australian Family Physician, 24*(5), 761–762, 765.

White, E., Jacobs, E. J., & Daling, J. R. (1996). Physical activity in relation to colon cancer in middle-aged men and women. *American Journal of Epidemiology, 144*(1), 42–50.

White House. (2006). *Statement on U.S. pledge of $334 million in global fight against bird flu.* Retrieved October 10, 2007, from http://www.whitehouse.gov/news/releases/2006/01/20060118-6.html

White House. (2007). *Strengthening health care.* Retrieved October 10, 2007, from http://www.whitehouse.gov/infocus/healthcare/

Wilkinson, R. G. (1997). Comment: Income, inequality, and social cohesion. *American Journal of Public Health, 87,* 1504–1506.

Winslow, C. E. A. (1920). The untilled field of public health. *Modern Medicine, 2*(1), 183–191.

Wolinsky, F. (1988). *The sociology of health: Principles, practitioners, and issues* (2nd ed.). Belmont, CA: Wadsworth Publishing.

World Health Organization. (1948). *Preamble to the constitution.* Geneva, Switzerland: World Health Organization.

Wynder, E. L., & Orlandi, M. A. (1984). *The American Health Foundation guide to lifespan health: A family program for physical and emotional well-being.* New York: Dodd, Mead & Company.

Chapter 8

The Evolution of Health Services in the United States

Leiyu Shi and
Douglas A. Singh

CHAPTER OBJECTIVES

1. Discuss historical developments that have shaped the nature of the U.S. healthcare delivery system.
2. Evaluate why the system has been resistant to national health insurance reforms.
3. Explore some of the recent developments and key forces that are likely to shape the delivery of health services in the future.

Introduction

The healthcare delivery system in the United States evolved quite differently than the systems in Europe. American values and the social, political, and economic antecedents on which the U.S. system is based have led to the formation of a unique system of healthcare delivery, as described in Chapter 6. This chapter discusses how these forces have been instrumental in shaping the current structure of medical services and are likely to shape its future. The evolutionary changes discussed here illustrate the American beliefs and values (discussed in Chapter 7) in action, within the context of broad social, political, and economic exigencies. Because social, political, and economic contexts do not remain static, their shifting influences lend a certain dynamism to the healthcare delivery system. On the other hand, beliefs and values remain relatively stable over time. Consequently, in the American healthcare delivery experience, initiatives toward a national healthcare program have failed to make significant inroads, but social, political, and economic forces have led to certain compromises, as seen in the creation of Medicare and Medicaid and other public programs to extend health insurance to certain defined groups of people. Could major social or economic shifts in the future eventually usher in a national healthcare program? It is anyone's guess. Although there is always a possibility that, given the right set of conditions, a national healthcare program could become a reality in the United States, no one seriously thinks that such a drastic change will take place anytime soon. Cultural beliefs and values are strong forces against attempts to initiate fundamental changes in the financing and delivery of health care. Therefore, enactment of major health system reforms would require consensus among Americans on basic values and ethics (U.S. Surgeon General C. Everett Koop, 1982–1989, cited in Kardos & Allen, 1993).

The growth of medical science and technology has also played a key role in shaping the system of health services delivery. Stevens (1971) points out that the technological revolution has been primarily responsible for bringing medicine into the public domain. Advancement of technology has influenced other factors, such as medical education, growth of institutions, and urban development. Hence, American medicine did not emerge as a professional entity until the beginning of the 20th century with the progress in biomedical science. Since then, the U.S. healthcare delivery system has been a growth enterprise. Debates over issues such as methods of financing health care, quality improvement, and the appropriate role of government have also been rooted in the presumed importance of gaining access to ever-rising levels of scientific medicine (Somers & Somers, 1977).

This chapter traces the evolution of healthcare delivery through three major historical phases, each demarcating a major change in the structure of the delivery system. The first phase is the preindustrial era from the middle of the 18th century to the later part of the 19th century. The second phase is the postindustrial era, beginning in the late 19th century. The third, most recent and current phase is marked by the growth of managed care, organizational inte-gration, the information revolution, and glob-alization. We call it the corporate era.

The practice of medicine is central to the delivery of health care; therefore, a major portion of this chapter is devoted to tracing the transformations in medical practice from a weak and insecure trade to an independent, highly respected, and lucrative profession. The growing power of managed care and the corporatization of physician practices, however, have made a significant impact on the practice styles and have compromised the autonomy that physicians had historically enjoyed. The medical profession, in turn, has consolidated into larger organizational units, away from the solo practice of medicine that had once prevailed. Compromises have also occurred.

Medical Services in Preindustrial America

From colonial times to the beginning of the 20th century, American medicine lagged behind the advances in medical science, experimental research, and medical education that were taking place in Britain, France, and Germany. While London, Paris, and Berlin were flourishing as major research centers, Americans had a tendency to neglect research in basic sciences and place more emphasis on applied science (Shryock, 1966). In addition, American attitudes about medical treatment placed a strong emphasis on natural history and conservative common sense (Stevens, 1971). Consequently, the practice of medicine in the United States had a strong domestic, rather than professional, character. Medical services, when deemed appropriate by the consumer, were purchased out of one's own private funds because there was no health insurance. The healthcare market was characterized by competition among providers. The consumer decided who the provider would be. Thus, the consumer was sovereign in the healthcare market, and health care was delivered under free market conditions.

Five main factors explain why the medical profession remained largely an insignificant trade in preindustrial America:

1. Medical practice was in disarray.
2. Medical procedures were primitive.
3. An institutional core was missing.
4. Demand was unstable.
5. Medical education was substandard.

Medical Practice in Disarray

The early practice of medicine could be regarded more as a trade than a profession. It did not require the rigorous course of study, clinical practice, residency training, board exams, and licensing that make it possible to practice today. At the close of the Civil War (1861–1865), "anyone who had the inclination to set himself up as a physician could do so, the exigencies of the market alone determining who would prove successful in the field and who would not" (Hamowy, 1979). The clergy, for example, often combined medical services and religious duties. The generally well-educated clergyman or government official was more learned in medicine than physicians were (Shryock, 1966). Tradesmen, such as tailors, barbers, commodity merchants, and those engaged in numerous other trades, also practiced the healing arts by selling herbal prescriptions, nostrums, elixirs, and cathartics. Midwives, homeopaths, and naturalists could also practice medicine without any restriction. The red and white striped poles (symbolizing blood and bandages) outside barber shops today are reminders that barbers also functioned as surgeons at one time, using the same blade to cut hair, shave beards, and bleed the sick. This era of medical pluralism has been referred to as a war zone by Kaptchuk and Eisenberg (2001) because it was marked by bitter antagonism among the various practicing sects. Later, in 1847, the American Medical Association (AMA) was founded with the main purpose of erecting a barrier between orthodox practitioners and the irregulars (Rothstein, 1972).

In the absence of minimum standards of medical training, entry into private practice was relatively easy for both trained and untrained practitioners. Free entry into medical practice created intense competition. Medicine as a profession was weak and unorganized. Hence, physicians did not enjoy the prestige, influence, and incomes that they do today. Many physicians found it necessary to engage in a second occupation because income from medical practice alone was inadequate to support a family. It is estimated that most physicians' incomes in the mid-19th century placed them at the lower end of the middle class (Starr, 1982). It is estimated that in 1830, there were 6,800 physicians serving primarily the upper classes (Gabe, Kelleher, & Williams, 1994). It was not until 1870 that medical education was reformed and licensing laws were passed in the United States.

Primitive Medical Procedures

Up until the mid-1800s, medical care was based more on primitive medical traditions than science. In the absence of diagnostic tools, a theory of intake and outgo served as an explanation for all diseases (Rosenberg, 1979). It was believed that diseases needed to be expelled from the body. Hence, bleeding, use of emetics (to induce vomiting) and diuretics (to increase urination), and purging with enemas and purgatives (to clean the bowels) were the popular forms of clinical therapy.

When George Washington became ill with an inflamed throat in 1799, he was bled by physicians. One of the attending physicians argued unsuccessfully in favor of making an incision to open the trachea, which today would be considered a more enlightened procedure. The bleeding most likely weakened Washington's resistance, although historians have debated whether it played a role in his death (Clark, 1998).

Surgeries were limited because anesthesia had not yet been developed, and antiseptic techniques were not known. The stethoscope and X-rays had not been discovered, the clinical thermometer was not in use, and the microscope was not available for medical diagnosis. Physicians relied mainly on their five senses and experience to diagnose and treat medical problems. Hence, in most cases, physicians did not possess technical expertise any greater than mothers and grandparents at home or experienced neighbors in the community.

Missing Institutional Core

In the United States, no widespread development of hospitals occurred before the 1880s. A few isolated hospitals were either built or developed in rented private houses in large cities, such as Philadelphia; New York; Boston; Cincinnati, Ohio; New Orleans, Louisiana; and St. Louis, Missouri. In France and Britain, by contrast, general hospital expansion began much before the 1800s (Stevens, 1971). In Europe, medical professionals were closely associated with hospitals. New advances in medical science, which European hospitals readily adopted, were being pioneered. The

medical profession came to be supremely regarded because of its close association with an establishment that was scientifically advanced. In contrast, American hospitals played only a small part in medical practice because most hospitals served a social welfare function by taking care of the poor, those without families, and those away from home on travel. Similarly, dispensaries were established to provide free care to those who could not afford to pay. Urban workers and their families often depended on such charity (Rosen, 1983). Hence, medical practice in the United States was not legitimized because it lacked organizational affiliation.

Starting with Philadelphia in 1786, dispensaries gradually spread to many other cities. They were private institutions financed by bequests and voluntary subscriptions, and their main function was to provide basic medical care and to dispense drugs to ambulatory patients (Raffel, 1980). Dispensaries were independent of hospitals. Generally, young physicians and medical students desiring clinical experience staffed the dispensaries (as well as hospital wards) on a part-time basis for little or no income (Martensen, 1996), which served a dual purpose. It provided needed services to the poor and enabled both physicians and medical students to gain experience diagnosing and treating a variety of cases. Later, as the practice of specialized medicine, as well as teaching and research, was transferred to hospital settings, dispensaries gradually became part of the institutional setting. Many dispensaries were absorbed into hospitals as outpatient departments. Indeed, outpatient or ambulatory care departments became an important locale for specialty consultation services in large hospitals (Raffel, 1980).

In the United States, the almshouse was the precursor of hospitals, but it was not a hospital in the true sense. Almshouses (also called poor-houses because they served primarily the poor) existed in almost all cities of moderate size and were run by the local governments. These institutions served primarily general welfare functions by providing food and shelter to the destitute. Therefore, their main function was custodial. Caring for the sick was incidental because some of the residents would inevitably become ill and would usually be cared for in an adjoining infirmary. Almshouses were unspecialized institutions that admitted poor and needy persons of all kinds who were mostly homeless or away from home, including the elderly, the orphaned, the insane, the ill, and the disabled. Hence, the early hospital-type institutions emerged mainly to take care of indigent people whose own families could not care for them.

Another type of institution, the pesthouse, was operated by local governments to quarantine people who had contracted a contagious disease such as cholera, smallpox, typhoid, or yellow fever. Located primarily in seaports, the primary function of pesthouses was to isolate people with contagious diseases in order to contain the spread of disease to the inhabitants of the cities where they were first diagnosed. These institutions were the predecessors of contagious-disease and tuberculosis hospitals.

Not until the 1850s were hospitals similar to ones in Europe developed in the United States. These early hospitals generally had deplorable conditions because of a lack of resources. Poor sanitation and inadequate ventilation were their hallmarks. Unhygienic practices prevailed because nurses were generally unskilled and untrained. These early hospitals had an unde-sirable image as houses of death. The mortality rate among hospital patients both in Europe and the United States stood around 74% in the 1870s (Falk, 1999). People went into hospitals only because of dire consequences, not by personal choice. It is not hard to imagine why members of the middle and upper classes, in particular, shunned such establishments.

Unstable Demand

Professional services suffered from low demand in the mainly rural, preindustrial society. Much medical care was provided by people who were not physicians. The most competent physicians were located in more populated communities (Bordley & Harvey, 1976). In the small communities of rural America, a spirit of strong self-reliance prevailed. Families and communities were accustomed to treating the sick, often using folk remedies that were passed on from one generation to the next. It was also common to consult published books and pamphlets on home remedies (Rosen, 1983).

The market for physicians' services was also limited by economic conditions. Many families could not afford to pay for medical services. Two factors contributed to the high cost associated with obtaining professional medical care: (1) The indirect costs of transportation and the opportunity cost of travel (i.e., forgone value of time that could be used for something more productive) could easily outweigh the direct costs of physicians' fees. (2) The costs of travel often doubled because two people, the physician and an emissary, had to make the trip back and forth. For a farmer, a trip of 10 miles into town could mean an entire day's work lost. Physicians passed much of their day traveling along backcountry roads. They had to cover travel costs and the opportunity cost of time spent traveling. Mileage charges typically amounted to four or five times the basic fee for a visit if a physician had to travel 5 to 10 miles. Hence, most families obtained only occasional intervention from physicians, generally for nonroutine and severe conditions (Starr, 1982).

Personal health services had to be purchased without the help of government or private insurance. Private practice and fee for service— the practice of billing separately for each individual type of service performed—had been firmly embedded in American medical care. Similar to physicians, dentists were private entrepreneurs who made their living by private fee-for-service dental practice, but their services were not in great demand because there was little public concern about dental health (Anderson, 1990).

Substandard Medical Education

From about 1800 to 1850, medical training was largely received through individual apprenticeship with a practicing physician, referred to as a preceptor, rather than through university education. Many of the preceptors were themselves poorly trained, especially in the basic medical sciences (Rothstein, 1972). By 1800, only four medical schools were operating in the United States: College of Philadelphia (which was established in 1756 and later became the University of Pennsylvania), King's College (which was established in 1768 and later became Columbia University), Harvard University (opened in 1783), and Dartmouth College (started in 1797). These schools were small, graduating only a handful of students each year (Sultz & Young, 1997).

American physicians later initiated the establishment of medical schools in large numbers. It was partly to enhance one's professional status and prestige and partly to enhance one's income.

Medical schools were inexpensive to operate and often quite profitable. All that was required was a faculty of four or more physicians, a classroom, a back room to conduct dissections, and legal authority to confer degrees. Operating expenses were met totally out of student fees that were paid directly to the physicians (Rothstein, 1972). Physicians would affiliate with a local college for the conferral of degrees and use of classroom facilities. Large numbers of men entered medical practice as education in medicine became readily available, and unrestricted entry into the profession was still possible (Hamowy, 1979). Gradually, as physicians from medical schools began to outnumber those from the apprenticeship system, the doctor of medicine degree became the standard of competence. The number of medical schools tripled between 1800 and 1820 and tripled again between 1820 and 1850, numbering 42 in 1850 (Rothstein, 1972). Academic preparation gradually replaced apprenticeship training.

At this point, medical education in the United States was seriously deficient in science-based training, unlike European medical schools. Medical schools in the United States did not have laboratories, and clinical observation and practice were not part of the curriculum. In contrast, European medical schools, particularly those in Germany, were emphasizing laboratory-based medical research. At the University of Berlin, for example, professors were expected to conduct research as well as teach, and were paid by the state. In American medical schools, students were taught by local practitioners who were ill equipped in education and training. Unlike Europe, where medical education was financed and regulated by the government, proprietary medical schools in the United States could set their own standards

(Numbers & Warner, 1985). A year of medical school in the United States generally lasted only 4 months and required only 2 years for graduation. In addition, American medical students customarily repeated the same courses during their second year that they had taken during their first (Numbers & Warner, 1985; Rosner, 2001). The physicians' desire to keep their schools profitable also contributed to low standards and a lack of rigor. It was feared that higher standards in medical education would drive enrollments down, which could lead the schools into bankruptcy (Starr, 1982).

Medical Services in Postindustrial America

In the postindustrial period, American physicians, unlike other physicians in the world, became enormously successful in retaining private practice of medicine and resisting national health care. Consequently, physicians now belong to a well-organized medical profession and deliver scientifically and technically advanced services to insured patients who do not have to bear the bulk of the expenses themselves. Notably, much of this transformation occurred in the aftermath of the Civil War. Social and scientific changes in the period following the war were accompanied by a transition from a rural agricultural economy to a system of industrial capitalism. Mass production techniques used in the war were applied to peacetime industries. Railroads linked the east and west coasts, and small towns became cities (Stevens, 1971).

The American system for delivering health care took its current shape during this period. Private practice of medicine became firmly entrenched as physicians grew into a cohesive profession and gained power and prestige. Organized efforts of the medical profession have also been instrumental in blocking attempts to create a national healthcare program in the United States. The well-defined role of employers in providing workers' compensation for work-related injuries and illnesses, together with other economic considerations, was instrumental in the growth of private health insurance. Rising costs of health care, however, prompted the U.S. Congress to create the publicly financed Medicare and Medicaid programs for the most vulnerable sectors of the population. Cost considerations also motivated the formation of prototypes for modern managed care organizations (MCOs).

Growth of Professional Sovereignty

The 1920s may well mark the consolidation of physicians' professional power. During and after World War I, physicians' incomes grew sharply, and their prominence as a profession finally emerged, although this prestige and power did not materialize overnight. Through the years, several factors interacted in the gradual transformation of medicine from a weak, insecure, and isolated trade into a profession of power and authority. Seven key factors contributed to this transformation:

1. urbanization
2. science and technology
3. institutionalization
4. dependency
5. cohesiveness and organization
6. licensing
7. educational reform

URBANIZATION

Urbanization created increased reliance on the specialized skills of paid professionals. First, it distanced people from their families and neighborhoods where family-based care was traditionally given. Women entered the workforce and could no longer care for sick members of the family. Second, physicians became less expensive to consult as telephones, automobiles, and paved roads reduced the opportunity cost of time and travel, and medical care became more affordable. Urban development attracted more and more Americans to the growing towns and cities. In 1840, only 11% of the U.S. population lived in urban areas; by 1900, it was up to 40% (Stevens, 1971). The trend away from home visits to office practice also began to develop around this time because of urban growth and shifting residential patterns, which made it more difficult to make house calls (Rosen, 1983). Physicians moved to cities and towns in large numbers to be closer to their growing markets. Better geographic proximity increased physicians' productivity. Whereas physicians in 1850 averaged only about five to seven patients a day, by the early 1940s the average load of general practitioners had risen to 18 to 22 patients a day (Starr, 1982).

SCIENCE AND TECHNOLOGY

Exhibit 8–1 summarizes some of the groundbreaking scientific discoveries in medicine. Advances in bacteriology, antiseptic surgery, anesthesia, immunology, and diagnostic techniques, along with an expanding repertoire of new drugs, gave medicine an aura of legitimacy and complexity. Also, the therapeutic effectiveness of scientific medicine became widely recognized.

When advanced technical knowledge becomes essential to practice a profession, and the benefits of professional services are widely recognized, it simultaneously creates greater acceptance and a legitimate need for the services of that profession. Cultural authority refers to the general acceptance of and reliance on the judgment of the members of a profession (Starr, 1982) because of their superior knowledge and expertise. In a sense, cultural authority legitimizes a profession in the eyes of common people. Advances in medical science and technology bestowed this legitimacy on the medical profession because medical practice could no longer remain within the domain of lay competence.

Scientific and technological change also required improved therapeutic competence of physicians in the diagnosis and treatment of disease. Developing these skills was no longer possible without specialized training. Science-based medicine created an increased demand for the advanced services that were no longer available through family and neighbors.

Physicians' cultural authority was further bolstered when medical decisions became necessary in various aspects of healthcare delivery. For example, physicians decide whether a person should be admitted to a medical care institution and for how long, whether surgical or nonsurgical treatments should be used, and which medications should be prescribed. Physicians' decisions have a profound impact on other providers and nonproviders alike. The judgment and opinions of physicians even affect aspects of a person's life beyond the delivery of health care. For example, physicians often evaluate the fitness of persons for jobs during pre-employment physicals that many employers demand. Physicians assess the disability of the ill and the injured, as in workers' compensation cases. Granting of medical leave for sickness and

Exhibit 8–1 Groundbreaking Medical Discoveries

- The discovery of anesthesia was instrumental in advancing the practice of surgery. Nitrous oxide (laughing gas) was first employed as an anesthetic around 1846 for tooth extraction by Horace Wells, a dentist. Ether anesthesia for surgery was first successfully used in 1846 at the Massachusetts General Hospital. Before anesthesia was discovered, strong doses of alcohol were used to dull the sensations. A surgeon who could do procedures, such as limb amputations, in the shortest length of time was held in high regard.
- Around 1847, Ignaz Semmelweis, a Hungarian physician practicing in a hospital in Vienna, implemented the policy of handwashing. Thus, an aseptic technique was born. Semmelweis was concerned about the high death rate from puerperal fever among women after childbirth. Even though the germ theory of disease was unknown at this time, Semmelweis surmised that there might be a connection between puerperal fever and the common practice by medical students of not washing their hands before delivering babies and right after doing dissections. Semmelweis' hunch was right.
- Louis Pasteur is generally credited with pioneering the germ theory of disease and microbiology around 1860. Pasteur demonstrated sterilization techniques, such as boiling to kill microorganisms and withholding exposure to air to prevent contamination.
- Joseph Lister is often referred to as the father of antiseptic surgery. Around 1865, Lister used carbolic acid to wash wounds, and popularized the chemical inhibition of infection (antisepsis) during surgery.
- Advances in diagnostics and imaging can be traced to the discovery of X-rays in 1895 by Wilhelm Roentgen, a German professor of physics. Radiology became the first machine-based medical specialty. Some of the first training schools in X-ray therapy and radiography in the United States attracted photographers and electricians to become Doctors in Roentgenology (from the inventor's name).
- Alexander Fleming discovered the antibacterial properties of Penicillin in 1929.

release back to work require authorizations from physicians. Payment of medical claims requires physicians' evaluations. Other healthcare professionals, such as nurses, therapists, and dietitians, are expected to follow physicians' orders for treatment. Thus, during disease and disability, and sometimes even in good health, people's lives have become increasingly governed by decisions made by physicians.

INSTITUTIONALIZATION

The evolution of medical technology and the professionalization of medical and nursing staff enabled advanced treatments that necessitated the pooling of resources in a common arena of care (Burns, 2004). Rapid urbanization was another factor that necessitated the institutionalization of medical care. As had already occurred in Europe, in the United States the hospital became the core around which the delivery of medical services was organized. Thus, development of the hospital as the center for the practice of scientific medicine and the professionalization of medical practice became closely intertwined. Indeed, the physician and the hospital developed a symbiotic relationship.

For economic reasons, as hospitals expanded, their survival became increasingly dependent on physicians to keep the beds filled because the physicians decided where to hospitalize their patients. Therefore, hospitals had to make every effort to keep the physicians satisfied, which enhanced physicians' professional dominance even though they generally were not employees of the hospitals. It gave physicians enormous influence over hospital policy. Also, for the first time, hospitals began conforming to both physician practice patterns and public expectations about medicine as a modern scientific enterprise. The expansion of surgery, in particular, had profound implications for hospitals, physicians, and the public. As hospitals added specialized facilities and staff, their regular use became indispensable to physicians and surgeons who earlier had been able to manage their practices with little reference to the hospital (Martensen, 1996). Affiliation with establishments symbolizing the scientific cutting edge of medicine lent power and prestige to the medical profession.

Hospitals in the United States did not expand and become more directly related to medical care until the late 1890s. However, as late as the 1930s, hospitals incurred frequent deaths due to infections that could not be prevented or cured. Nevertheless, hospital use was on the rise because of the great influx of immigrants into large American cities (Falk, 1999). From only a few score in 1875, the number of general hospitals in the United States expanded

to 4,000 by 1900 (Anderson, 1990), and to 5,000 by 1913 (Wright, 1997).

Dependency

Patients depend on the medical profession's judgment and assistance. First, the sick role (discussed in Chapter 7) places the patients in a position of dependency because society expects the sick person to seek medical help and try to get well. The person is expected to comply with medical instructions. Second, dependency is created by the profession's cultural authority because its medical judgments must be relied on to (1) legitimize a person's sickness, (2) exempt the individual from social role obligations, and (3) provide competent medical care so the person can get well and resume his or her social role obligations. Third, in conjunction with the physician's cultural authority, the need for hospital services for critical illness and surgery also creates dependency when patients are transferred from their homes to the hospital or to a surgery center.

Once physicians' cultural authority became legitimized, the sphere of their influence expanded into nearly all aspects of healthcare delivery. For example, laws that prohibited individuals from obtaining certain classes of drugs without a physician's prescription were passed. Health insurance paid for treatments only when they were rendered or prescribed by physicians. Thus, beneficiaries of health insurance became dependent on physicians for reimbursable services. More recently, the referral role (gatekeeping) of primary care physicians in managed care plans has increased patients' dependency on primary care physicians for referral to specialized services.

Cohesiveness and Organization

Toward the end of the 1800s, social and economic changes brought about greater cohesiveness among medical professionals. With the growth of hospitals and specialization, physicians needed support from each other for patient referrals and for access to facilities to admit their patients. Standardization of education also advanced a common core of knowledge among physicians. They no longer remained members of isolated and competing medical sects. Greater cohesiveness, in turn, advanced their professional authority (Starr, 1982)

For a long time, physicians' ability to remain free of control from hospitals and insurance companies remained a prominent feature of American medicine. Hospitals and insurance companies could have hired physicians on salary to provide medical services, but individual physicians who took up practice in a corporate setting were castigated by the medical profession and pressured into abandoning such practices. In some states, courts ruled that corporations could not employ licensed physicians without engaging in the unlicensed practice of medicine, a legal doctrine that became known as the "corporate practice doctrine" (Farmer & Douglas, 2001). Independence from corporate control enhanced private entrepreneurship and put American physicians in an enviable strategic position in relation to organizations such as hospitals and insurance companies. Later, a formally organized medical profession was in a much better position to resist control from outside entities.

The American Medical Association (AMA) was formed in 1847 but had little strength during its first half century of existence. Its membership was small, it had no permanent organization, and it had scant resources. The AMA did not attain real strength until it was organized into county and state medical societies, and state societies were incorporated, delegating

greater control at the local level. As part of the organizational reform, the AMA also began in 1904 to concentrate attention on medical education (Bordley & Harvey, 1976). Since then, it has been the chief proponent for the practitioners of conventional medicine in the United States. Although the AMA often stressed the importance of raising the quality of care for patients and protecting the uninformed consumer from quacks and charlatans, its principal goal—like that of other professional associations—was to advance the professionalization, prestige, and financial well-being of its members. The AMA vigorously pursued its objectives by promoting the establishment of state medical licensing laws and the legal requirement that, to be licensed to practice, a physician must be a graduate of an AMA-approved medical school. The concerted activities of physicians through the AMA are collectively referred to as organized medicine, to distinguish them from the uncoordinated actions of individual physicians competing in the marketplace (Goodman & Musgrave, 1992).

LICENSING

Under the medical practice acts established in the 1870s, medical licensure in the United States became a function of the states (Stevens, 1971). By 1896, 26 states had enacted medical licensure laws to license physicians (Anderson, 1990). Licensing of physicians and upgrading of medical school standards developed hand in hand. At first, licensing required only a medical school diploma. Later, candidates could be rejected if the school they had attended was judged inadequate. Finally, all candidates were required to present an acceptable diploma and to pass an independent state examination (Starr, 1982). Through both licensure and upgrading of medical school standards, physicians obtained a clear monopoly on the practice of medicine (Anderson, 1990). Rothstein (1972) suggested that the irregular practitioners at the time probably did more good—or less harm—to their patients than did the orthodox ones, because during this period, medical practices such as bloodletting and the use of potent emetics and lethal cathartics, such as mercury, were common. Hence, it can be concluded that the early licensing laws did not so much protect consumers as they protected practitioners from the competitive pressures posed by potential new entrants into the medical profession. Physicians generally led the campaign to restrict the practice of medicine. In 1888, in a landmark Supreme Court decision, *Dent v. West Virginia*, Justice Stephen J. Field wrote that no one had the right to practice "without having the necessary qualifications of learning and skill" (Haber, 1974). In the late 1880s and 1890s, many states revised their laws to require all candidates for licensure, including those holding medical degrees, to pass an examination (Kaufman, 1980).

EDUCATIONAL REFORM

Advanced medical training was made necessary by scientific progress. Reform of medical education started around 1870 with the affiliation of medical schools with universities. In 1871, Harvard Medical School, under the leadership of a new university president, Charles Eliot, completely revolutionized the system of medical education. The academic year was extended from 4 months to 9, and the length of medical education was increased from 2 years to 3. Following the European model, laboratory instruction and clinical subjects, such as chemistry, physiology, anatomy, and pathology were added to the curriculum.

Johns Hopkins University took the lead in further reforming medical education when it opened its medical school in 1893 under the leadership of William H. Welch, who trained in Germany. Medical education for the first time became a graduate training course requiring a college degree, not a high school diploma, as an entrance requirement. Johns Hopkins had well-equipped laboratories, a full-time faculty for the basic science courses, and its own teaching hospital (Rothstein, 1972). Standards at Johns Hopkins became the model of medical education in other leading institutions around the country. Raising of standards made it difficult for proprietary schools to survive, and in time they were closed.

The Association of American Medical Colleges (AAMC) was founded in 1876 by 22 medical schools (Coggeshall, 1965). Later, the AAMC set minimum standards for medical education, including a 4-year curriculum, but it was unable to enforce its recommendations. In 1904, the AMA created the Council on Medical Education, which inspected the existing medical schools and found that less than half of them provided acceptable levels of training. The AMA did not publish its own findings, but obtained the help of the Carnegie Foundation for the Advancement of Teaching to provide a rating of medical schools (Goodman & Musgrave, 1992). The foundation appointed Abraham Flexner to investigate medical schools located in both the United States and Canada. The *Flexner Report*, published in 1910, had a profound effect on medical education reform. The report was widely accepted by both the profession and the public. Schools that did not meet the proposed standards were forced to close. State laws were established requiring graduation from a medical school accredited by the AMA as the basis for a license to practice medicine (Haglund & Dowling, 1993).

Once advanced graduate education became an integral part of medical training, it further legitimized the profession's authority and galvanized its sovereignty. Stevens (1971) noted that American medicine moved toward professional maturity between 1890 and 1914 mainly as a direct result of educational reform.

Specialization in Medicine

Specialization has been a key hallmark of American medicine. As a comparison, in 1931, 17% of all physicians in the United States were specialists. Today, the proportion of specialists to generalists is approximately 60:40. The ranks of allied healthcare professionals have also diversified, both in medical specialization—such as laboratory and radiological technologists, nurse anesthetists, and physical therapists—and in new or expanded specialist fields—such as occupational therapists, psychologists, dietitians, and medical social workers (Stevens, 1971).

Lack of a rational coordination of medical care in the United States has been one consequence of the preoccupation with specialization. The characteristics of the medical profession in various countries often shape and define the key attributes of their healthcare delivery systems. The role of the primary care physician (PCP), the relationship between generalists and specialists, the ratio of practicing generalists to specialists, the structure and nature of medical staff appointments in hospitals, and the approach to group practice of medicine have all been molded by the evolving structure and ethos of the medical profession. In Britain, for example, the medical profession has divided itself into general practitioners (GPs) practicing in the community and consultants holding specialist positions in hospitals. This kind of stratification did not develop in American medicine. PCPs in America were not assigned the role that GPs had in Britain, where patients could consult a specialist only by referral from a GP. Unlike Britain, where GPs hold a key intermediary position in relation to the rest of the healthcare delivery system, the United States has traditionally lacked such a gatekeeping role. Only in the last decade or 2, under health maintenance organizations (HMOs), has the gatekeeping model requiring initial contact with a generalist and the generalist's referral to a specialist gained prominence. The distinctive shaping of medical practice in the United States explains why the structure of medicine did not develop around a nucleus of primary care, in which, apart from delivering routine and basic care, the PCP also ensures the continuity, coordination, and appropriateness of medical services received by a patient. Only in some managed care models, such as HMOs, has the primary care model gained prominence.

The Development of Public Health

Public health practices in the United States have largely concentrated on sanitary regulation, the study of epidemics, and vital statistics. The growth of urban centers for the purpose of commerce and industry, unsanitary living conditions in densely populated areas, inadequate methods of sewage and garbage disposal, limited access to clean water, and long work hours in unsafe and exploitative industries led to periodic epidemics of cholera, smallpox, typhoid, tuberculosis, yellow fever, and other diseases. Such outbreaks sometimes led to arduous efforts to protect the public interest. For example, in

1793, the national capital had to be moved out of Philadelphia because of a devastating outbreak of yellow fever. This epidemic prompted the city to develop its first board of health in that same year. In 1850, Lemuel Shattuck outlined the blueprint for the development of a public health system in Massachusetts. Shattuck also called for the establishment of state and local health departments. A threatening outbreak of cholera in 1873 mobilized the New York City Health Department to alleviate the worst sanitary conditions within the city. Previously, cholera epidemics in 1832 and 1848–1849 had swept through American cities and towns within a few weeks, killing thousands (Duffy, 1971).

By 1900, most states had health departments that were responsible for a variety of public health efforts, such as sanitary inspections, communicable disease control, operation of state laboratories, vital statistics, health education, and regulation of food and water (Turnock, 1997; Williams, 1995). Public health functions were later extended to fill gaps in the medical care system. Such functions, however, were limited mainly to child immunizations, care of mothers and infants, health screening in public schools, and family planning. Federal grants were also made available to state and local governments for programs in substance abuse, mental health, and community prevention services. Thus, public health has a strong social justice orientation (Turnock, 1997).

Public health remained separate from the private practice of medicine—as it does even today—because of the skepticism of private physicians that the government could take control of private practice of medicine. Physicians realized that the boards of health could be used to control the supply of physicians and to regulate the practice of medicine (Rothstein, 1972). Fear of government intervention, loss of autonomy, and erosion of personal incomes created a wall of separation between public health and private medical practice. Under this dichotomous relationship, medicine has concentrated on the physical health of the individual, whereas public health has focused on the health of whole populations and communities. The extent of collaboration between the two has been largely confined to the requirement by public health departments that private practitioners report cases of contagious diseases such as sexually transmitted diseases, human immunodeficiency virus (HIV) infection, and acquired immune deficiency syndrome (AIDS), and report any outbreaks of cases such as West Nile virus and other types of infections.

The Rise in Chronic Conditions

Until about 1900, infectious diseases posed the greatest health threat to society. The development of public health played a major role in curtailing the spread of infection among populations. Simultaneously, widespread public health measures and better medical care reduced mortality and increased life expectancy. Around 1920, health statisticians noted that chronic illnesses were replacing infectious diseases as the dominant healthcare challenge (Sydenstricker, 1933). Today, chronic conditions are the leading cause of illness, disability, and death in the United States as well as in other developed and developing nations. Almost one half of all Americans have one or more chronic conditions (Foundation for Accountability, 2001). Chronic conditions account for three of every four deaths (The Robert Wood Johnson Foundation, 1996). It is a paradox that despite a remarkable increase in chronic conditions, the U.S. healthcare delivery system is still largely designed to treat acute illness and often fails to meet the full needs of persons with chronic conditions (Hoffman, Rice, & Sung, 1996).

Health Services for Veterans

Shortly after World War I, the government started to provide hospital services to veterans with service-related disabilities and for nonservice disabilities if the veteran declared an inability to pay for private care. At first, the federal government contracted for services with voluntary hospitals, but over time, the Department of Veterans Affairs (formerly called Veterans Administration) built its own hospitals, outpatient clinics, and nursing homes.

Birth of Workers' Compensation

The first broad-coverage health insurance in the United States emerged in the form of workers' compensation programs initiated in 1914 (Whitted, 1993). Workers' compensation was originally concerned with cash payments to workers for wages lost due to job-related injuries and disease. Compensation for medical expenses and death benefits to the survivors were added later.

Between 1910 and 1915, workers' compensation laws made rapid progress in the United States (Stevens, 1971). Looking at the trend, some reformers believed that since Americans had been persuaded to adopt compulsory insurance against industrial accidents, they could also be persuaded to adopt compulsory insurance against sickness. Workers' compensation served as a trial balloon for the idea of government-sponsored universal health insurance in the United States. However, the growth of private health insurance, along with other key factors that will be discussed later, has prevented any proposals for a national healthcare program from taking hold.

Rise of Private Health Insurance

Private health insurance was commonly referred to as voluntary health insurance in contrast to proposals for a publicly organized compulsory health insurance system. The initial role of private health insurance was income protection during sickness and temporary disability. Some private insurance coverage limited to bodily injuries has been available since about 1850. By 1900, health insurance policies became available, but their primary purpose was to protect against loss of income during sickness (Whitted, 1993). In the early 20th century, coverage was added for surgical fees, but the emphasis remained on replacing earned income lost due to sickness or injury. Thus, the coverage was in reality disability insurance rather than health insurance as we know it today (Mayer & Mayer, 1984).

Technological, social, and economic factors created a general need for health insurance. However, certain economic conditions that prompted private initiatives, self-interests of a well-organized medical profession, and the momentum of a successful health insurance enterprise gave private health insurance a firm footing in the United States. Coverage for hospital and physician services began separately and was later combined under the auspices of Blue Cross and Blue Shield. Later, economic conditions during the World War II period laid the foundations for health insurance to become an employment-based benefit.

Technological, Social, and Economic Factors

The health insurance movement of the early 20th century was the product of three converging developments: the technological, the social, and the economic. From a technological perspective, medicine offered new and better treatments. Because of its well-established healing values, medical care was regarded as socially desirable. The value placed on medical services by individuals and society created a growing demand for medical services. From an economic perspective, people could predict neither their future needs for medical care nor the costs, both of which had been gradually increasing. In short, scientific and technological advances made health care more desirable but less affordable. These developments pointed to the need for some kind of insurance to spread the financial risks over a large number of people.

Early Blanket Insurance Policies

In 1911, insurance companies began to offer blanket policies for large industrial populations, usually covering life insurance, accidents and sickness, and nursing services. A few industrial and railroad companies set up their own medical plans covering specified medical benefits, as did several unions and fraternal orders; however, the total amount of voluntary health insurance was minute (Stevens, 1971). Between 1916 and 1918, 16 state legislatures, including New York and California, attempted to enact legislation compelling employers to provide health insurance, but the efforts were unsuccessful (Davis, 1996).

Economic Necessity and the Baylor Plan

The Great Depression, which started at the end of 1929, forced hospitals to turn from philanthropic donations to patient fees for support. Patients then faced not only loss of income from illness but also increasing debt from medical care costs when they became sick. People needed protection from the economic consequences of

sickness and hospitalization. Hospitals also needed protection from economic instability (Mayer & Mayer, 1984). During the Depression, occupancy rates in hospitals fell, income from endowments and contributions dropped sharply, and the charity load almost quadrupled (Richardson, 1945).

In 1929, the blueprint for modern health insurance was established when J. F. Kimball began a hospital insurance plan for public school teachers at the Baylor University Hospital in Dallas, Texas. Kimball was able to enroll over 1,200 teachers who paid $0.50 a month for a maximum of 21 days of hospital care. Within a few years, it became the model for Blue Cross plans around the country (Raffel, 1980). At first, other independent hospitals copied Baylor and started to offer single-hospital plans. It was not long before community-wide plans offered jointly by more than one hospital became more popular because they provided consumers a choice of hospitals. The underwriting was assumed by the hospitals, which agreed to provide services regardless of the remuneration they would receive. Hence, in essence, these were prepaid plans for hospital services. A prepaid plan is a contractual arrangement under which a provider must provide all needed services to a group of members (or enrollees) in exchange for a fixed monthly fee paid in advance.

Successful Private Enterprise— The Blue Cross Plans

A hospital plan in Minnesota was the first to use the name Blue Cross in 1933 (Davis, 1996). The American Hospital Association (AHA) lent support to the hospital plans and became the coordinating agency to unite these plans into the Blue Cross network (Koch, 1993; Raffel, 1980).

The Blue Cross plans were nonprofit—that is, they had no shareholders who would receive profit distributions—and covered only hospital charges, so as not to infringe on the domain of private physicians (Starr, 1982). Later, control of the plans was transferred to a completely independent body, the Blue Cross Commission, which later became the Blue Cross Association (Raffel, 1980). In 1946, Blue Cross plans in 43 states served 20 million members. Between 1940 and 1950 alone, the proportion of the population covered by hospital insurance increased from 9% to 57% (Anderson, 1990).

Self-Interests of Physicians— Birth of Blue Shield

Voluntary health insurance had received the AMA's endorsement, but the AMA had also made it clear that private health insurance plans should include only hospital care. It is therefore not surprising that the first Blue Shield plan designed to pay for physicians' bills was started by the California Medical Association, which established the California Physicians Service in 1939 (Raffel, 1980). By endorsing hospital insurance and by actively developing medical service plans, the medical profession committed itself to private health insurance as the means to spread the financial risk of sickness and assured that its own interests would not be threatened.

From the medical profession's point of view, voluntary health insurance in conjunction with private fee-for-service practice by physicians was regarded as a desirable feature of the evolving health system (Stevens, 1971). Throughout the Blue Shield movement, physicians dominated the boards of directors not only because they underwrote the plans but also because the plans were, in a very real sense, their response to the

challenge of national health insurance. In addition, the plans met the AMA's stipulation of keeping medical matters in the hands of physicians (Raffel & Raffel, 1994).

Combined Hospital and Physician Coverage

Even though Blue Cross and Blue Shield developed independently and were financially and organizationally distinct, they often worked together to provide hospital and physician coverage (Law, 1974). In 1974, the New York superintendent of insurance approved a merger of the Blue Cross and Blue Shield plans of Greater New York (Somers & Somers, 1977). Since then, similar mergers have occurred in most states. Now, in nearly every state Blue Cross and Blue Shield plans are joint corporations or have close working relationships (Davis, 1996).

The for-profit insurance companies were initially skeptical of the Blue Cross plans and adopted a wait-and-see attitude. Their apprehension was justified because no actuarial information was available to predict losses. But lured by the success of the Blue Cross plans, within a few years commercial insurance companies also started offering health insurance.

Employment-Based Health Insurance

As a result of wage freezes during the World War II period, group health insurance became an important component of collective bargaining between unions and employers. In 1948, the U.S. Supreme Court ruled that employee benefits, including health insurance, were a legitimate part of the union–management bargaining process. Health insurance then became a permanent part of employee benefits in the postwar era

(Health Insurance Association of America, 1991). A 1954 revision to the Internal Revenue code also had a profound influence on the expansion of employer-sponsored health insurance. At that time, employer contributions toward the purchase of employee health insurance became exempt from taxable income for the employee. Employment-based health insurance expanded rapidly. The economy was strong during the postwar years of the 1950s, and employers started offering more extensive benefits. This led to the birth of major medical expense coverage to protect against prolonged or catastrophic illness or injury (Mayer & Mayer, 1984). Thus, private health insurance became the primary vehicle for the delivery of healthcare services in the United States.

Failure of National Healthcare Initiatives

Starting with Germany in 1883, compulsory sickness insurance had spread throughout Europe by about 1912. Health insurance in European countries was viewed as a natural outgrowth of insurance against industrial accidents. Hence, it was considered logical that Americans would also be willing to espouse a national healthcare program to protect themselves from the high cost of sickness and accidents occurring outside employment.

The American Association of Labor Legislation (AALL) was founded in 1906. Although the AALL took no official position on labor unions, its membership included some prominent labor leaders (Starr, 1982), but its relatively small membership was mainly academic, including some leading economists and social scientists, whose all-important agenda was to bring about social reform through gov-

ernment action. The AALL was primarily responsible for leading the successful drive for workers' compensation. It then spearheaded the drive for a government-sponsored health insurance system for the general population (Anderson, 1990). The AALL supported the progressive movement headed by former President Theodore Roosevelt, who was again running for the presidency in 1912 on a platform of social reform. Roosevelt, who might have been a national political sponsor for compulsory health insurance, was defeated by Woodrow Wilson. But the progressive movement for national health insurance did not die.

The AALL continued its efforts toward a model for national health insurance by appealing to both social and economic concerns. The reformers argued that it would relieve poverty because sickness usually brought wage loss and high medical costs to individual families. They also argued that it would contribute to national efficiency by reducing illness, lengthening life, and diminishing the causes of industrial discontent (Starr, 1982). Leadership of the AMA at the time showed outward support for a national plan, and the AALL and the AMA formed a united front to secure legislation. A standard health insurance bill was introduced in 15 states in 1917 (Stevens, 1971).

As long as compulsory health insurance was only under study and discussion, potential opponents paid no heed to it; but once bills were introduced into state legislatures, opponents expressed vehement disapproval. Eventually, it turned out that the AMA's support for social change was only superficial.

Repeated attempts to pass national health insurance legislation in the United States have failed for several reasons, which can be classified under four broad categories: (1) political inexpediency, (2) institutional dissimilarities, (3) ideological differences, and (4) tax aversion.

POLITICAL INEXPEDIENCY

Before embarking on their national health programs, countries in western Europe, notably Germany and England, were experiencing labor unrest that threatened political stability. Social insurance was seen as a means to obtain workers' loyalty and ward off political instability. Political conditions in the United States were quite different. There was no threat to political stability. Unlike countries in Europe, the American government was highly decentralized and engaged in little direct regulation of the economy or social welfare. Although Congress had set up a system of compulsory hospital insurance for merchant seamen as far back as 1798, it was an exceptional measure.* Matters related to health and welfare were typically left to state and local governments, and the general rule at these levels of government was to leave as much as possible to private and voluntary action.

The entry of the United States into World War I in 1917 provided a final political blow to the health insurance movement as anti-German feelings were aroused. The U.S. government denounced German social insurance, and opponents of health insurance called it a Prussian menace inconsistent with American values (Starr, 1982).

After attempts to pass compulsory health insurance laws failed at the state levels in California and New York, by 1920 the AALL itself lost interest in an obviously lost cause. Also in 1920, the AMA's house of delegates approved a resolution condemning compulsory health insurance that would be regulated by any state government or the federal government (Numbers, 1985). This AMA resolution opposing national health insurance solidified the profession against "government interference with the practice of medicine."

INSTITUTIONAL DISSIMILARITIES

The preexisting institutions in Europe and the United States were dissimilar. Germany and England had some mutual benefit funds to provide sickness benefits. These benefits reflected an awareness of the value of insuring against the cost of sickness among a sector of the working population. Voluntary sickness funds were less developed in the United States than in Europe, reflecting less interest in health insurance and less familiarity with it. More important, American hospitals were mainly private, whereas in Europe they were largely government operated (Starr, 1982).

Dominance of private institutions of health-care delivery is generally not consistent with national financing and payment mechanisms. For instance, compulsory health insurance proposals of the AALL were regarded by individual members of the medical profession as a threat to their private practice because it would shift their primary source of income from individual patients to the government (Anderson, 1990). Any efforts that would potentially erode the fee-for-service payment system and let private practice of medicine be controlled by a powerful third party—particularly the government—were opposed.

Other institutional forces also were opposed to government-sponsored universal coverage.

---

*Important seaports, such as Boston, were often confronted with many sick and injured seamen who were away from their homes and families. Congress enacted a law requiring that 20¢ a month be withheld from the wages of each seaman on American ships to support merchant marine hospitals (Raffel & Raffel, 1994).

The insurance industry feared losing the income it derived from disability insurance, some insurance against medical services, and funeral benefits (Anderson, 1990). The pharmaceutical industry feared the government as a monopoly buyer, and retail pharmacists feared that hospitals would establish their own pharmacies under a government-run national healthcare program (Anderson, 1990). Employers also generally saw the proposals as contrary to their interests. Spokespersons for American business rejected the argument that health insurance would add to worker productivity. It may seem ironic, but the labor unions—the American Federation of Labor in particular—also denounced compulsory health insurance at the time. Union leaders were afraid that they would transfer over to the government their own legitimate role of providing social benefits, thus weakening the unions' influence in the workplace. Organized labor was the largest and most powerful interest group at that time. Its lack of support is considered instrumental in the defeat of national health insurance (Anderson, 1990).

IDEOLOGICAL DIFFERENCES

As discussed in Chapter 7, the American value system is based on the principles of market justice. Individualism and self-determination, distrust of government, and reliance on the private sector to address social concerns are typical American ideologies, which seem to stand as a bulwark against anything that is perceived as an onslaught on individual liberties. The cultural and ideological values represent the sentiments of the American middle class, whose support is generally necessary for any broad-based reform. Without such support, a national healthcare program was unable to withstand the attacks of its well-organized opponents (Anderson, 1990).

On the other hand, during times of national distress, such as the Great Depression, pure necessity may have legitimized the advancement of social programs, such as the New Deal programs of the Franklin Roosevelt era (for example, Social Security legislation providing old-age pensions and unemployment compensation).

In the early 1940s, during Roosevelt's presidency, several bills on national health insurance were introduced in Congress, but they all died. Perhaps the most notable bill was the Wagner–Murray–Dingell bill drafted in 1943 and named after the bill's congressional sponsors. However, this time World War II diverted the nation's attention to other issues, and without the president's active support, the bill died quietly (Numbers, 1985).

In 1946, Harry Truman became the first president to make an appeal for a national healthcare program (Anderson, 1990). Unlike the progressives, who had proposed a plan for the working class, Truman proposed a single health insurance plan that would include all classes of society. At the president's behest, the Wagner–Murray–Dingell bill was redrafted and reintroduced. The AMA was vehement in opposing the plan. Other healthcare interest groups, such as the American Hospital Association (AHA), also opposed it. By this time, private health insurance had expanded. Initial public reaction to the Wagner–Murray–Dingell bill was positive; however, when a government-controlled medical plan was compared to private insurance, polls showed that only 12% of the public favored extending Social Security to include health insurance (Numbers, 1985).

During this era of the Cold War, any attempts to introduce national health insurance were met with the stigmatizing label of "socialized medicine." The Republicans took control of Congress in 1946, and any interest in enacting national health insurance was put to rest. However, to the surprise of many, Truman was reelected in 1948, promising national health insurance if the Democrats would be returned to power (Starr, 1982). Fearing the inevitable, the AMA levied a $25 fee on each of its members toward a war chest of $3.5 million (Anderson, 1990). It hired the public relations firm of Whitaker and Baxter and spent $1.5 million in 1949 alone to launch one of the most expensive lobbying efforts in American history. The campaign directly linked national health insurance with communism until the idea of socialized medicine was firmly implanted in the public's minds. Republicans proposed a few compromises, but neither the Democrats nor the AMA were interested in them. By 1952, the election of a Republican president, Dwight Eisenhower, effectively ended any further debate over national health insurance. Failure of government-sponsored universal healthcare coverage is often presented as a classic case of the tremendous influence of interest groups in American politics, especially in major health policy outcomes.

TAX AVERSION

An aversion to increased taxes to pay for social programs is another reason why middle-class Americans, who are already insured, have opposed national initiatives to expand health insurance coverage. According to polls, Americans have been found to generally support the idea that the government ought to help people who are in financial need to pay for their medical care. However, most Americans have not favored an increase in their own taxes to pay for such care.

The most recent unsuccessful attempt to bring about a national healthcare program was initiated by the Clinton administration. While seeking the presidency in 1992, Governor Bill Clinton made health system reform a major campaign issue. Not since Harry Truman's initiatives a few decades earlier had such a bold attempt been made by a presidential candidate. As long as the electorate has remained reasonably satisfied with health care—with the exception of uninsured Americans, who have not been politically strong—elected officials have feared the political clout of big interest groups and have refrained from raising tough reform issues. In the Pennsylvania U.S. Senate election in November 1991, however, the victory of Democrat Harris Wofford over Republican Richard Thornburgh sent a clear signal that the time for a national healthcare program might be ripe. Wofford's call for national health insurance was widely supported by middle-class Pennsylvanians. Election results in other states were not quite as decisive on the health reform issue, but various public polls seemed to confirm that after the economy (the United States was in a brief recession at the time), health care was the second most pressing concern on the minds of the American people. One national survey conducted by Louis Harris and Associates reported some disturbing findings about healthcare delivery. Substantial numbers of insured and relatively affluent people said that they had not received the services they needed. The poll also suggested that the public was looking to the federal government, not the states or private sector, to contain rising healthcare costs (Smith, Altman, Leitman, Moloney, & Taylor, 1992). In other opinion polls, Americans expressed concerns that they might not be adequately insured in the future (Skocpol, 1995). Against this backdrop, both Bill Clinton and the running incumbent, President George (Herbert Walker) Bush, advanced healthcare reform proposals.

After taking office, President Clinton made health system reform one of his top priorities. Policy experts and public opinion leaders have since debated over what went wrong. Some of the fundamental causes for the failure of the Clinton plan were no doubt historical in nature, as discussed earlier in this chapter. One seasoned political observer, James J. Mongan, however, remarked that reform debates in Congress have never been about the expansion of healthcare services but about the financing of the proposed services:

> Thus, the most important cause of health-care reform's demise was that avoiding tax increases and their thinly veiled cousin, employer mandates, took priority over expanding coverage. . . . There undoubtedly would have been pitched legislative battles over other issues—how to pay doctors and hospitals, the role of health insurers, the structure of (regional health) alliances—but these debates never happened in detail. The first and only battle . . . was how to pay for reform. . . . What explains this unwillingness to pay for expanded coverage, on the part of citizens and government alike? Any answer must take into account the economic, social, and political context of the past two decades. . . . The social context is that people tend to take for granted the progress achieved through social insurance programs such as Medicare and Social Security, and they perceive little progress or achievement from welfare expenditures targeted on low-income people. Politically, politicians from the courthouse to the White House have played to an anti-tax sentiment and have convinced Americans and American businesses that they are stag-

> gering under an oppressive burden of taxation that saps most productive effort. Although there is little evidence from other countries to support this belief, it is widely held. This climate fosters a self-centeredness—a focus more on the individual's needs than on the community's needs. Some liberals might use a harsher, more grating word—selfishness—to describe this state of mind. But many conservatives would use the phrase rugged individualism to describe the same phenomenon. . . . Somewhere in here is where health reform died. . . . Until we as a nation make the right diagnosis and begin an honest dialogue about our national values, about the balance between self-interest and community interests, we will not see our nation join almost all others in guaranteeing health coverage to all of its citizens (Mongan, 1995, p. 99–101).

When American polls indicated that a fundamental reform was needed, the people did not have in mind more government regulation or any significant redistribution of income through increased taxes. Most important, they did not wish to have a negative effect on their own access to care or the quality of care they would receive (Altman & Reinhardt, 1996).

For now, employer-based private health insurance is firmly entrenched in the United States. Americans, regardless of gender, race, age, or working status, have indicated that employers would be their preferred source for obtaining health insurance (Duchon, Schoen, Simantov, Davis, & An, 2000). Among both the insured and the uninsured, only a relatively small proportion of adults believe that the government would be the best source for obtaining health coverage (Schoen, Strumpf, & Davis, 2000). The confidence expressed by Americans in their ability to pay for a major illness has also improved over time. The proportion reporting such confidence rose from 50% in 1978 to 67% in 2000 (Blendon & Benson, 2001). But the 2006 Health Confidence Survey conducted by the Employee Benefit Research Institute (EBRI) found that the public was increasingly getting dissatisfied with the U.S. health system primarily because of rising healthcare costs. On the other hand, despite the costs, Americans were satisfied with the quality of health care, and only a minority of Americans identified health care as the country's most critical issue (EBRI, 2006).

Although people's sentiments can change with the ebb and flow of the nation's economic state and other pressing concerns, health care has not been a major political issue in recent years. Health care issues played only a minor role in the 2002 congressional elections and the 2004 presidential election, and concerns about the cost of health care were "not breaking through as a top voting issue in the mid-term election" in 2006 (Blendon & Altman, 2006). Americans are more concerned with other social issues, such as crime, education, the war on terrorism, and homeland security. Cost of health care, however, continues to be a major concern. But, direct government involvement to control rising healthcare expenditures is not the approach with which Americans are most comfortable.

Creation of Medicaid and Medicare

Before 1965, private health insurance was the only widely available source of payment for health care, and it was available primarily to middle-class working people and their families. The elderly, the unemployed, and the poor had to rely on their own resources, on limited public programs, or on charity from hospitals and individual physicians. Often, when charity care was provided, private payers were charged more to make up the difference, a practice referred to as cost shifting or cross-subsidization. In 1965, Congress passed the amendments to the Social Security Act that created the Medicare and Medicaid programs, and the government assumed direct responsibility to pay for some of the health care on behalf of two vulnerable population groups—the elderly and the poor (Potter & Longest, 1994).

Medicaid and Medicare are prime representations of the public sector in the amalgam of private and public approaches for providing access to health care in the United States. Through the debates over how to protect the public from rising costs of health care and the opposition to national health insurance, one thing had become clear: Government intervention was not desired insofar as it pertained to how most Americans would receive health care, with one exception. Less opposition would be encountered if reform initiatives were proposed for the underprivileged classes. In principle, the poor were considered a special class who could be served through a government-sponsored program. The elderly—those 65 years of age and over—were another group that started to receive increased attention in the 1950s. On their own, most of the poor and the elderly could not afford the increasing cost of health care. Also, because the health status of these population groups was significantly worse than that of the general population, they required a higher level of healthcare services. The elderly, particularly, had higher incidence and prevalence of disease compared to younger groups. It was also estimated that less than half of the elderly were covered by private health insurance. By this time, the growing elderly middle class was also becoming a politically active force.

Government assistance for the poor and the elderly was sought once it became clear that the market alone would not ensure access for these vulnerable population groups. A bill introduced in Congress by Aime Forand in 1957 provided the momentum for including necessary hospital and nursing home care as an extension of Social Security benefits (Stevens, 1971). The AMA, however, undertook a massive campaign to portray a government insurance plan as a threat to the physician–patient relationship. The bill was stalled, but public hearings around the country, which were packed by the elderly, produced an intense grassroots support to push the issue onto the national agenda (Starr, 1982). A compromised reform, the Medical Assistance Act (Public Law 86-778), also known as the Kerr–Mills Act, went into effect in 1960. Under the act, federal grants were given to the states to extend health services provided by the state welfare programs to those low-income elderly who previously did not qualify (Anderson, 1990). Since the program was based on a means test that confined eligibility to people below a predetermined income level, it was opposed by liberal congressional representatives as a source of humiliation to the elderly (Starr, 1982). Within 3 years, the program was declared ineffective because many states did not even implement it (Stevens, 1971). In 1964, health insurance for the aged and the poor became top priorities of President Johnson's Great Society programs.

During the debate over Medicare, the AMA developed its own "Eldercare" proposal, which called for a federal–state program to subsidize private insurance policies for hospital and physician services. Representative John W.

Byrnes introduced another proposal, dubbed "Bettercare." It proposed a federal program based on partial premium contributions by the elderly and the remainder subsidized by the government. Other proposals included tax credits and tax deductions for health insurance premiums.

In the end, a three-layered program emerged. The first two layers constituted Part A and Part B of Medicare, or Title XVIII of the Social Security Amendment of 1965 to provide publicly financed health insurance to the elderly. Based on Forand's initial bill, the administration's proposal to finance hospital insurance for the elderly through Social Security to provide hospital care and limited nursing home coverage became Part A of Medicare. The Byrnes proposal to cover physicians' bills through government-subsidized insurance became Part B of Medicare. An extension of the Kerr–Mills program of federal matching funds to the states based on each state's financial needs became Medicaid, or Title XIX of the Social Security Amendment of 1965. The Medicaid program was for the indigent, based on means tests established by each state, but it was expanded to include all age groups, not just the poor elderly (Stevens, 1971).

Although adopted together, Medicare and Medicaid reflected sharply different traditions. Medicare was upheld by broad grassroots support and, being attached to Social Security, had no class distinction. Medicaid, on the other hand, was burdened by the stigma of public welfare. Medicare had uniform national standards for eligibility and benefits; Medicaid varied from state to state in terms of eligibility and benefits. Medicare allowed physicians to balance bill, that is, charge the patient the amount above the program's set fees and recoup the difference. Medicaid prohibited balance billing and, consequently, had limited participation from physicians (Starr, 1982). Medicaid, in essence, has created a two-tier system of medical care delivery because some physicians refuse to accept Medicaid patients because of low fees set by the government.

Not long after Medicare and Medicaid were in operation, national spending for health services began to rise. So did public outlays of funds in relation to private spending for health services (Anderson, 1990).

Regulatory Role of Public Health Agencies

With the expansion of publicly financed Medicare and Medicaid programs, the regulatory powers of government have increasingly encroached upon the private sector. This is because the government provides financing for the two programs, but services are delivered by the private sector. After the federal government developed the standards for participation in the Medicare program, states developed regulations in conjunction with the Medicaid program. The regulations often overlapped, and the federal government delegated authority to the states to carry out the monitoring of compliance with the regulations. As a result, the regulatory powers assigned to state public health agencies increased dramatically. Thus, most institutions of healthcare delivery are subject to annual scrutiny by public health agencies under the authority delegated to them by the federal and state governments.

Prototypes of Managed Care

Even though the early practice of medicine in the United States was mainly characterized by private solo practice, three subsequent developments in medical care delivery are noteworthy. All three required some sort of organizational integration, which was a departure from solo practice. These innovative arrangements can also be regarded as early precursors of managed care and integrated organizations (discussed in Chapter 9). The three developments were contract practice, group practice, and prepaid group practice.

CONTRACT PRACTICE

In 1882, the Northern Pacific Railroad Beneficial Association was one of the first employers to provide medical care expense coverage (Davis, 1996). Between 1850 and 1900, other railroad, mining, and lumber enterprises developed extensive employee medical programs. Such companies conducted operations in isolated areas where physicians were generally unavailable. Inducements, such as a guaranteed salary, were commonly offered to attract physicians. Another common arrangement was to contract with independent physicians and hospitals at a flat rate per worker per month, referred to as capitation. The AMA recognized the necessity of contract practice in remote areas, but elsewhere contract practice was regarded as a form of exploitation because it was assumed that physicians would bid against each other and drive down the price. Offering services at reduced rates was regarded by the AMA as an unethical invasion of private practice. When group health insurance became common in the 1940s through collective bargaining, the medical profession was freed from the threat of direct control by large corporations. Health insurance also enabled workers to go to physicians and hospitals of their choice (Starr, 1982).

Corporate practice of medicine—that is, provision of medical care by for-profit corporations—

was generally prohibited by law. It was labeled as commercialism in medicine. In 1917, however, Oregon passed the Hospital Association Act, which permitted for-profit corporations to provide medical services. Whereas health insurance companies, functioning as insurers and payers, acted as intermediaries between patients and physicians, the hospital associations in Oregon contracted directly with physicians and exercised some control over them. Utilization was managed by requiring second opinions for major surgery and by reviewing the length of hospital stays. The corporations also restricted medical fees, refusing to pay prices they deemed excessive. In short, they acted as a countervailing power in the medical market to limit physicians' professional autonomy. Even though physicians resented controls, they continued to do business with the hospital associations because of guaranteed payments (Starr, 1982).

Early contract practice arrangements and the Oregon hospital associations can be viewed as prototypes of managed care. With the growth of managed care, the traditional fee-for-service payment arrangements have been largely replaced by capitation and discounted fees. Mechanisms to control excessive utilization are another key feature of managed care.

GROUP PRACTICE

Group medicine represented another form of corporate organization for medical care. Group practice changed the relationship among physicians by bringing them together with business managers and technical assistants in a more elaborate division of labor (Starr, 1982). The Mayo Clinic, started in Rochester, Minnesota, in 1887, is generally regarded as a prototype of the consolidation of specialists into group prac-

tice. The concept of a multispecialist group presented a threat to the continuation of general practice. It also presented competition to specialists who remained in solo practice. Hence, the development of group practice met with widespread professional resistance (Stevens, 1971). Although specialist group practice did not become a movement, sharing of expenses and incomes, along with other economic advantages, has caused group practices to continue to grow over the years.

PREPAID GROUP PLANS

In time, the efficiencies of group practice led to the formation of prepaid group plans in which an enrolled population received comprehensive services for a capitated fee. The HIP Health Plan of New York (started in 1947) stands as one of the most successful programs providing comprehensive medical services through organized medical groups of family physicians and specialists (Raffel, 1980). Similarly, Kaiser-Permanente (started in 1942) has grown on the West Coast. Other examples are the Group Health Cooperative of Puget Sound in Seattle, Washington (operating since 1947), a consumer-owned cooperative prepaid group practice (Williams, 1993), and the Labor Health Institute in St. Louis, Missouri (1945), a union-sponsored group practice scheme (Stevens, 1971).

The idea of prepaid group practice had limitations. It required the sponsorship of large organizations. HIP, for example, was created by New York's Mayor Fiorello La Guardia for city employees. Industrialist Henry Kaiser initially set up his prepaid plan to provide comprehensive healthcare services to his own employees. For most employers, it was impractical to have their own health plans; they had to rely on health insurance plans offered by the insurance industry. The Kaiser-Permanente health plan was later extended to other employers.

In 1971, President Nixon singled out pre-paid group practice organizations as the model for a rational reorganization in the delivery of health services. They became the prototype of health maintenance organizations, or HMOs (Somers & Somers, 1977). During the Nixon administration, the use of HMOs in the private sector was encouraged by federal legislation, the Health Maintenance Organization Act (HMO Act) of 1973. The HMO Act required employers to offer an HMO alternative to conventional health insurance (Goodman & Musgrave, 1992). MCOs today attempt to combine the efficiencies of contract and group arrangements with the objective of delivering comprehensive healthcare services at predetermined costs.

Medical Care in the Corporate Era

The later part of the 20th century and start of the 21st have been marked by the growth and consolidation of large business corporations, and tremendous advances in global communications, transportation, and trade. These developments are starting to change the way health care is delivered in the United States, and, indeed, around the world. The rise of multinational corporations, the information revolution, and globalization have been interdependent phenomena. The General Agreement on Trade in Services (GATS), which came into effect in 1995, aims to gradually remove all barriers to international trade in services. In healthcare services, GATS may regulate health insurance, hospital services, telemedicine, and acquisition of medical treatment abroad. GATS negotiations, however, have met with controversy as various countries fear that it may shape their domestic healthcare systems (Belsky, Lie, Mattoo, Emanuel, & Sreenivasan, 2004), although most analysts predict that GATS is likely to produce future market liberalization (Mutchnick, Stern, & Moyer, 2005). No one, however, is certain how the increasing corporatization of medicine and exertion of global forces will eventually shape healthcare delivery.

Corporatization of Healthcare Delivery

Corporatization here refers to the ways in which healthcare delivery in the United States has become the domain of large organizations. These corporations may operate either on a for-profit or nonprofit basis, yet they are driven for the most part by the common goal of maximizing their revenues. At least one benefit of this corporatization has been the ability of these organizations to deliver sophisticated modern health care in comfortable and pleasant surroundings. But, one main expectation of delivering the same quality of health care at lesser cost remains largely unrealized.

On the supply side, until the mid-1980s, physicians and hospitals clearly dominated the medical marketplace. Since then, managed care has emerged as a dominant force by becoming the primary vehicle for insuring and delivering health care to the majority of Americans. The rise of managed care consolidated immense purchasing power on the demand side. It was to counteract this imbalance that providers began to consolidate, and larger, integrated healthcare organizations began forming (see Chapter 11). A second influential factor behind healthcare integration was reimbursement cuts for inpatient acute care hospital services in the mid-1980s. To make up for lost revenues in the inpatient sector, hospitals developed various types of outpatient services such as primary care, outpatient surgery, and home health care, and expanded into other differentiated healthcare services such as long-term care and specialized rehabilitation services. Together, managed care and integrated delivery organizations have in reality corporatized the delivery of health care in the United States.

In a healthcare landscape that has been increasingly dominated by corporations, individual physicians have struggled to preserve their autonomy. As a matter of survival, many physicians had to consolidate into large clinics, form strategic partnerships with hospitals, or start their own specialty hospitals. A growing number of physicians have become employees of large medical corporations. Proliferation of these new models of healthcare delivery has made it increasingly difficult for states to maintain outright bans on the employment of physicians (Farmer & Douglas, 2001).

Both managed care and corporate delivery of medicine have made the healthcare system extremely complex from the consumer's standpoint. Managed care was supposedly a market-based reform, but it has stripped the primary consumer, the patient, of practically all marketplace power. Dominance by any entity, whether organized medicine or integrated health organizations, subverts the sovereignty of the healthcare consumer. In this so-called market-driven integration, the consumer continues to wonder, "Where's the market?"

Information Revolution

The delivery of health care is being transformed in unprecedented and irreversible ways by telecommunication. The use of telemedicine and telehealth is on the rise. In a general sense, the terms *telemedicine* and *telehealth* are used interchangeably, although strictly speaking there is a difference, to refer to the integration of telecommunication systems into the practice of protecting and promoting health in distant caregiving. It may or may not incorporate actual physician–patient interactions. Telemedicine came to the forefront in the 1990s with the technological advances in the distant transmission of image data and the recognition that there was inequitable access to medical care in rural America. Federal dollars were poured into rural telemedicine projects.

Telehealth consultations can occur in real time. Videoconferencing is now replacing telephone consultation as the preferred vehicle for behavioral telehealth or telepsychiatry. E-health has also become an unstoppable force that is driven by consumer demand for healthcare information and services offered over the Internet by professionals and nonprofessionals alike (Maheu, Whitten, & Allen, 2001). The Internet has created a new revolution that is increasingly characterized by patient empowerment. Access to expert information is no longer strictly confined to the physician's domain, which in some ways has led to a dilution of the dependent role of the patient.

Globalization

Although there is no standard definition for globalization, it refers to various forms of cross-border economic activities. Globalization is driven by global exchange of information, production of goods and services more economically in developing countries, and increased interdependence of mature and emerging world economies. It confers many advantages, but it also has its downsides.

From the standpoint of cross-border trade in health services, Mutchnick and colleagues (2005) identified four different modes of economic interrelationships:

1. *Use of advanced telecommunication infrastructures in telemedicine.* For example, teleradiology (the electronic transmission of radiological images over a distance) now enables physicians in the United States to transmit radiological images to Australia, where they are interpreted and reported back the next day (McDonnell, 2006). On the other hand, innovative telemedicine consulting services in pathology and radiology are being delivered to other parts of the world by cutting-edge U.S. medical institutions such as Johns Hopkins.

2. *Consumers travel abroad to receive medical care.* Specialty hospitals, such as the Apollo chain in India, offer state-of-the-art technology to foreigners at a fraction of what it would cost to have the same procedures done in the United States or Europe. Physicians and hospitals outside the United States have clear competitive advantages: reasonable malpractice costs, minimum regulation, and lower costs of labor. As a result of these efficiencies, Indian specialty hospitals can do quality liver transplants for one tenth the cost of U.S. hospitals (Mutchnick et al., 2005).

On the other hand, dignitaries and other wealthy foreigners come to multispecialty centers in the United States, such as the Mayo Clinic, to receive highly specialized services.

3. *Foreign direct investment in health services enterprises.* For example, Chindex International, a U.S. corporation, provides medical equipment, supplies, and clinical care in China. Chindex opened the Beijing United Family Hospital and Clinics in 1997 (Mutchnick et al., 2005).

4. *Health professionals move to other countries that present high demand for their services and better economic opportunities than their native countries.* For example, nurses from other countries are moving to the United States to relieve the existing personnel shortage. Migration of physicians from developing countries helps alleviate at least some of the shortage in underserved locations in the developed world. On the downside, the developing world pays a price when emigration leaves these countries with shortages of trained professionals. The burden of disease in these countries is often greater than it is in the developed world, and emigration only exacerbates the ability of these countries to provide adequate health care to their own populations (Norcini & Mazmanian, 2005).

Globalization produces other negative effects that are indirect. Tobacco use is on the decline in many developed countries, yet economic development and emerging markets provide new targets for the tobacco industry. Today, rapid economic development in China and India offers multinational tobacco companies new markets of potential smokers. In addition, as developing countries become more prosperous, they acquire Western tastes and lifestyles. In some instances, negative health consequences follow. For example, increased use of motorized vehicles results in a lack of physical exercise, which, along with changes in diet, are greatly increasing the prevalence of chronic diseases such as heart disease and diabetes in the developing world. On the other hand, better information about health promotion and disease prevention and access to gyms and swimming pools in developing countries are making a positive impact on the health and well-being of their middle-class citizens.

Globalization has also posed some new threats, for instance, the threat of diseases that were previously unknown in the United States. Infectious diseases appearing in one country can spread rapidly to other countries. HIV/AIDS, hepatitis B, and hepatitis C infections have spread worldwide. New viral infections such as avian flu and SARS (severe acute respiratory syndrome) have at times threatened to create worldwide pandemics.

Another ill effect of globalization, bioterrorism, is the latest threat gripping the nation since the tragic events of September 11, 2001. Vital resources are being deployed to counteract the fear of possible clandestine warfare through deadly agents, such as smallpox, a disease that was eradicated from the planet by 1977.

Other Developments in U.S. Health Care

Healthcare delivery in the United States has been driven primarily by economics, but social and political exigencies do call for incremental change from time to time. Two notable examples that fall in the latter category were expansion of social entitlements. The first was the State Children's Health Insurance Program (SCHIP) enacted in 1997, and the second was creation of Part D of Medicare (implemented in 2006) to assist seniors with their prescription drug costs (both are discussed in Chapter 6).

The United States now has an expanding market of self-care products and alternative therapies (discussed in Chapter 7). In a sense, healthcare delivery to a small degree has reverted to the bygone era of familial medicine and use of products and procedures of questionable scientific validity. This consumer-driven phenomenon has not gone unnoticed by the traditional medical establishment. The private medical establishment and the government have intensified efforts to understand the potential benefits as well as any undesirable consequences of alternative treatments.

Conclusion

Figure 8–1 provides a snapshot of the historical developments in U.S. healthcare delivery. The evolution of healthcare services has been strongly influenced by the advancement of scientific research and technological development. Early scientific discoveries were pioneered in Europe, but they were not readily adopted in the United States; therefore, medicine had a largely domestic, rather than a professional, character in preindustrial America. The absence of standards of practice and licensing requirements allowed the trained and untrained alike to deliver medical care. Hospitals were more akin to places of refuge than centers of medical practice. The demand for professional services was relatively low because they had to be purchased privately, without the help of government or health insurance. Medical

Figure 8–1 Evolution of the Healthcare Delivery System

Development of science and technology

Mid 18th to late 19th century	Late 19th to late 20th century	Late 20th to 21st century
• Open entry into medical practice • Intense competition • Weak and unorganized profession • Apprenticeship training • Undeveloped hospitals • Private payment for services • Low demand for services • Private medical schools providing only general education	• Scientific basis of medicine • Urbanization • Emergence of the modern hospital • Emergence of organized medicine • Emergence of scientific medical training • Licensing • Development of public health • Specialization in medicine • Emergence of workers' compensation • Emergence of private insurance • Failure of national health insurance • Medicaid and Medicare • Prototypes of managed care	• **Corporatization** Managed care Health care integration Diluted physician autonomy Complexity for the patient • **Information revolution** Telemedicine E-health Patient empowerment • **Globalization** Global telemedicine Medical travel Foreign investment in health care Migration of professionals Exportation of lifestyles Challenge of new diseases Bioterrorism
Consumer sovereignty	Professional dominance	Corporate dominance

Beliefs and values/Social, economic, and political constraints

education was seriously deficient in providing technical training based on scientific knowledge. The medical profession faced intense competition; it was weak, unorganized, and insecure.

Scientific and technological advances led to the development of sophisticated institutions where better trained physicians could practice their art. The transformation of the United States from a mainly rural, sparsely populated country to one with growing centers of urban population created increased reliance on the specialized skills that only trained professionals could offer. Simultaneously, medical professionals banded together into a politically strong organization.

The AMA succeeded in controlling the practice of medicine mainly through its influence on medical education, licensing of physicians, and political lobbying.

In Europe, national health insurance has been an outgrowth of generous social programs. In the United States, by contrast, the predominance of private institutions, ideologies founded on the principles of market justice, and an aversion to tax increases have been instrumental in maintaining a healthcare delivery system that is mainly privately financed and operated. The AMA and other interest groups have also wielded enormous influence in opposing efforts to initiate comprehensive reforms based on national health insurance. Access to health services in the United States is achieved primarily through private health insurance; however, two major social programs, Medicaid and Medicare, were expediently enacted to provide affordable health services to vulnerable populations.

Growth in science and technology engenders greater specialization, but a lack of rational coordination of medical care in the United States has created a surplus of specialists and has relegated primary care to a secondary status. Public health and private medicine also function in a dichotomous and sometimes adversarial relationship.

The corporate era in health care dawned in the later part of the 20th century. The rise of multinational corporations, the information revolution, and globalization have marked this current era. Managed care represents corporatization of healthcare delivery on the demand side. On the supply side, providers have integrated into various types of consolidated arrangements. The information revolution is characterized by the growth of telehealth (or telemedicine) and e-health. Globalization has made the mature and the emerging world economies more interdependent, which has both advantages and disadvantages.

Discussion Questions

1. How did the emergence of general hospitals strengthen the professional sovereignty of physicians? What effect did this have on nursing and advanced practice nurses?
2. Discuss the key factors that were instrumental in the growth of voluntary health insurance.
3. Discuss, with particular reference to the roles of (a) organized medicine, (b) the middle class, and (c) American beliefs and values, why reform efforts to bring in national health insurance have been unsuccessful in the United States.
4. Which particular factors that earlier may have been somewhat weak in bringing about national health insurance later led to the passage of Medicare and Medicaid?
5. Discuss the government's role in the delivery and financing of health care with specific reference to the dichotomy between public health and private medicine.
6. Discuss some of the forces that are continuing to shape the healthcare delivery system.

References

Altman, S. H., & Reinhardt, U. E., eds. (1996). *Strategic choices for a changing healthcare system.* Chicago: Health Administration Press.

Anderson, O. W. (1990). *Health services as a growth enterprise in the United States since 1875.* Ann Arbor, MI: Health Administration Press.

Belsky, L., Lie, R., Mattoo, A., Emanuel, E., & Sreenivasan, G. (2004). The general agreement on trade in services: Implications for health policy makers. *Health Affairs, 23*(3), 137–145.

Blendon, R. J., & Altman, D. E. (2006). Voters and health care in the 2006 election. *The New England Journal of Medicine, 355*(18), 1928–1933.

Blendon, R. J., & Benson, J. M. (2001). Americans' views on health policy: A 50-year historical perspective. *Health Affairs, 20*(2), 33–46.

Bordley, J., & Harvey, A. M. (1976). *Two centuries of American medicine 1776–1976.* Philadelphia: W.B. Saunders Company.

Burns, J. (2004). Are nonprofit hospitals really charitable? Taking the question to the state and local level. *Journal of Corporate Law, 29*(3), 665–683.

Clark, C. (1998, October 20). A bloody evolution: Human error in medicine is as old as the practice itself. *The Washington Post,* p. Z10.

Coggeshall, L. T. (1965). *Planning for medical progress through education.* Evanston, IL: Association of American Medical Colleges.

Davis, P. (1996). The fate of Blue Shield and the new Blues. *South Dakota Journal of Medicine, 49*(9), 323–330.

Duchon, L., Schoen, C., Simantov, E., Davis, K., & An, C. (2000). *Listening to workers: Findings from The Commonwealth Fund 1999 national survey of workers' health insurance.* New York: The Commonwealth Fund.

Duffy, J. (1971). Social impact of disease in the late 19th century. *Bulletin of the New York Academy of Medicine, 47,* 797–811.

Employee Benefit Research Institute (EBRI). (2006). *2006 health confidence survey: Dissatisfaction with healthcare system doubles since 1998.* Retrieved October 10, 2007, from http://www.ebri.org/pdf/notespdf/EBRI_Notes_11-20061.pdf

Falk, G. (1999). *Hippocrates assailed: The American health delivery system.* Lanham, MD: University Press of America, Inc.

Farmer, G. O., & Douglas, J. H. (2001). Physician "unionization"—A primer and prescription. *Florida Bar Journal, 75*(7), 37–42.

Foundation for Accountability. (2001). *Portrait of the chronically ill in America, 2001.* Portland, OR: The Foundation for Accountability, and Princeton, NJ: The Robert Wood Johnson Foundation.

Gabe, J., Kelleher, D., & Williams, G. (1994). *Challenging medicine.* New York: Routledge.

Goodman, J. C., & Musgrave, G. L. (1992). *Patient power: Solving America's health care crisis.* Washington, DC: CATO Institute.

Haber, S. (1974). The professions and higher education in America: A historical view. In M. S. Gordon (Ed.), *Higher education and labor markets.* New York: McGraw-Hill Book Co.

Haglund, C. L., & Dowling, W. L. (1993). The hospital. In S. J. Williams & P. R. Torrens (Eds.), *Introduction to health services* (4th ed., pp. 135–176). New York: Delmar Publishers.

Hamowy, R. (1979). The early development of medical licensing laws in the United States, 1875–1900. *Journal of Libertarian Studies, 3*(1), 73–119.

Health Insurance Association of America. (1991). *Source book of health insurance data.* Washington, DC: Health Insurance Association of America.

Hoffman, C., Rice, D., & Sung, H. Y. (1996). Persons with chronic conditions: Their prevalence and costs. *Journal of the American Medical Association, 276*(18), 1473–1479.

Kaptchuk, T. J., & Eisenberg, D. M. (2001). Varieties of healing 1: Medical pluralism in the United States. *Annals of Internal Medicine, 135*(3), 189–195.

Kardos, B. C., & Allen, A. T. (1993). Healthy neighbors: Exploring the healthcare systems of the United States and Canada. *Journal of Post Anesthesia Nursing, 8*(1) 48–51.

Kaufman, M. (1980). American medical education. In R. L. Numbers (Ed.), *The education of American physicians: Historical essays.* Berkeley and Los Angeles: University of California Press.

Koch, A. L. (1993). Financing health services. In S. J. Williams & P. R. Torrens (Eds.), *Introduction to health services* (4th ed., pp. 299–331). New York: Delmar Publishers.

Law, S. A. (1974). *Blue Cross: What went wrong?* New Haven, CT: Yale University Press.

Maheu, M. M., Whitten, P., & Allen, A. (2001). *E-health, telehealth, and telemedicine: A guide to start-up and success.* San Francisco: Jossey-Bass.

Martensen, R. L. (1996). Hospital hotels and the care of the "worthy rich." *Journal of the American Medical Association, 275*(4), 325.

Mayer, T. R., & Mayer, G. G. (1984). *The health insurance alternative: A complete guide to health maintenance organizations.* New York: Putnam Publishing Group.

McDonnell, J. (2006). Is the medical world flattening? *Ophthalmology Times, 31*(19), 4.

Mongan, J. J. (1995). Anatomy and physiology of health reform's failure. *Health Affairs, 14*(1), 99–101.

Mutchnick, I. S., Stern, D. T., & Moyer, C. A. (2005). Trading health services across borders: GATS, markets, and caveats. *Health Affairs Web Exclusives, 24*(suppl. 1), W5-42–W5-51.

Norcini, J. J., & Mazmanian, P. E. (2005). Physician migration, education, and health care. *Journal of Continuing Education in the Health Professions, 25*(1), 4–7.

Numbers, R. L. (1985). The third party: Health insurance in America. In J. W. Leavitt & R. L. Numbers (Eds.), *Sickness and health in America: Readings in the history of medicine and public health.* Madison: The University of Wisconsin Press.

Numbers, R. L., & Warner, J. H. (1985). The maturation of American medical science. In J. W. Leavitt & R. L. Numbers (Eds.), *Sickness and health in America: Readings in the history of medicine and public health.* Madison: The University of Wisconsin Press.

Potter, M. A., & Longest, B. B. (1994). The divergence of federal and state policies on the charitable tax exemption of nonprofit hospitals. *Journal of Health Politics, Policy and Law, 19*(2), 393–419.

Raffel, M. W. (1980). *The U.S. health system: Origins and functions.* New York: John Wiley & Sons.

Raffel, M. W., & Raffel, N. K. (1994). *The U.S. health system: Origins and functions* (4th ed.). Albany, NY: Delmar Publishers.

Richardson, J. T. (1945). *The origin and development of group hospitalization in the United States, 1890–1940: University of Missouri Studies, Vol. XX, No. 3.* Columbia: University of Missouri.

The Robert Wood Johnson Foundation. (1996). *Chronic care in America: A 21st century challenge.* Princeton, New Jersey: The Robert Wood Johnson Foundation.

Rosen, G. (1983). *The structure of American medical practice, 1875–1941.* Philadelphia: University of Pennsylvania Press.

Rosenberg, C. E. (1979). The therapeutic revolution: Medicine, meaning, and social change in 19th-century America. In M. J. Vogel (Ed.), *The therapeutic revolution.* Philadelphia: The University of Pennsylvania Press.

Rosner, L. (2001). The Philadelphia medical marketplace. In J. H. Warner & J. A. Tighe (Eds.), *Major problems in the history of American medicine and public health.* Boston: Houghton Mifflin Company.

Rothstein, W. G. (1972). *American physicians in the nineteenth century: From sect to science.* Baltimore: The Johns Hopkins University Press.

Schoen, C., Strumpf, E., & Davis, K. (2000). *A vote of confidence: Attitudes toward employer-sponsored health insurance* (Issue brief). New York: The Commonwealth Fund.

Shryock, R. H. (1966). *Medicine in America: Historical essays.* Baltimore: The Johns Hopkins Press.

Skocpol, T. (1995). The rise and resounding demise of the Clinton plan. *Health Affairs, 14*(1), 66–85.

Smith, M. D., Altman, D. E., Leitman, R., Moloney, T. W., & Taylor, H. (1992). Taking the public's pulse on health system reform. *Health Affairs, 11*(2), 125–133.

Somers, A. R., & Somers, H. M. (1977). *Health and health care: Policies in perspective.* Germantown, MD: Aspen Systems.

Starr, P. (1982). *The social transformation of American medicine.* Cambridge, MA: Basic Books.

Stevens, R. (1971). *American medicine and the public interest.* New Haven, CT: Yale University Press.

Stevens, R. (1989). *In sickness and in wealth.* New York: Basic Books.

Sultz, H. A., & Young, K. M. (1997). *Health care USA: Understanding its organization and delivery.* Gaithersburg, MD: Aspen Publishers, Inc.

Sydenstricker, E. (1933). *Recent trends in the United States.* New York: McGraw-Hill Co.

Turnock, B. J. (1997). *Public health: What it is and how it works* (pp. 3–38). Gaithersburg, MD: Aspen Publishers, Inc.

Whitted, G. (1993). Private health insurance and employee benefits. In S. J. Williams & P. R. Torrens (Eds.), *Introduction to health services* (4th ed., pp. 332–360). New York: Delmar Publishers.

Williams, S. J. (1993). Ambulatory healthcare services. In S. J. Williams & P. R. Torrens (Eds.), *Introduction to health services* (4th ed.). New York: Delmar Publishers.

Williams, S. J. (1995). *Essentials of health services* (pp. 108–134). Albany, NY: Delmar Publishers.

Wright, J. W. (1997). *The New York Times almanac.* New York: Penguin Putnam, Inc.

Chapter 9

Financing Health Care

Harry A. Sultz and
Kristina M. Young

CHAPTER OBJECTIVES

1. Develop an understanding of how health care is financed.
2. Analyze national healthcare expenditures and sources of payment.
3. Discuss the historical development of the national healthcare reimbursement infrastructure.
4. Identify the major factors that impact healthcare costs and the significant trends in healthcare spending.
5. Discuss the role of government as a payer and provider of services and the associated cost.

Introduction

The financing of the U.S. healthcare system has evolved from a variety of influences, including provider, employer, purchaser, consumer, and political factors. These influences continue to produce major tensions in ongoing debates about the role and responsibility of the government as payer, consumer financial responsibility, the relationships of costs to quality, the impact of payment systems on quality, and the overall effects that managed care has on the healthcare delivery system. A focal point of

the debates is the question of whether market-driven or government-driven strategies should be used to control healthcare expenditures (Weil, 1999). Two core issues include controlling rising costs and the estimated 45 million Americans who remain uninsured or underinsured for health care.

The discussion of healthcare finance includes managed care, which as a system of financing linking both the delivery of and payment for services and impacts consumers, purchasers, and providers. Managed care reshaped how healthcare services are delivered and paid for in the

United States and is discussed in depth in Chapter 11.

Healthcare Expenditures in Perspective

National healthcare expenditures in 2003 totaled $1.7 trillion, or 15.3% of the gross domestic product, or GDP (Smith, Cowan, Sensenig, Catlin, & Health Accounts Team, 2005). The rate of growth in healthcare spending has closely paralleled the growth rate of the GDP since 1994 (Center for Medicare and Medicaid Services, n.d.). The share of GDP devoted to health care has remained relatively stable since 1992 (Center for Medicare and Medicaid Services, n.d.) (see Figure 9–1).

During the years 1992–1996, growth in expenditure rates was successively slower than at any time since tracking of national health expenditures began in 1960 (Levit, Smith, Cowan, Lazenby, & Martin, 2002). In contrast, between 1980 and 1990, average annual growth rates exceeded 10% and were major stimuli for numerous cost-containment efforts that created the momentum for healthcare reform (Levit et al., 1997).

Fundamental changes in the nation's healthcare delivery resulting from the impact of a dramatically evolving healthcare industry marketplace accounted for slowing average growth rates. The impact of managed care, through its focus on controlling utilization, was a major factor in slower spending growth. Throughout the decade of the 1990s, market factors that enabled large purchasers of health insurance to negotiate arrangements aggressively with providers contributed significantly to the impact of expenditure-cutting managed

care initiatives. Beginning in the 1980s and continuing through the 1990s, restrictions imposed on hospital and physician practices through prospective payment and restrictive fee schedules also contributed to the decline in health expenditure growth. In the same period, government's contribution to national healthcare expenditures rose from 40.4% to 46.2% (Levit et al., 2000). The initial impact of the Balanced Budget Act of 1997 (BBA) on Medicare spending and savings from the curtailment of fraud and abuse then resulted in a decrease in government healthcare expenditures (Levit et al., 2000). For the first time in 10 years, in 1998 the component of national healthcare expenditures funded from government sources deviated from its pattern of steady increases and declined to 45.5% (Levit et al., 2000). In 2000, two major pieces of legislation added to Medicare funding: the Balanced Budget Refinement Act and the Medicare, Medicaid, and State Child Health Insurance Program Benefits Improvement and Protection Act (Levit et al., 2002). In 2003, public sector spending again slowed because of the expiration of supplemental funding for Medicare providers and sharply slower growth in Medicaid payments. As a result, government's share of total spending in 2003 remained at 45% of national healthcare expenditures (Smith et al., 2005).

Growth in healthcare expenditures results from a complex array of factors, including the rate of excess inflation associated with medical care costs and the general rise of inflation that affects all sectors of the economy. Historically, major factors that resulted in increased healthcare expenditures include the following:

- Applications of more advanced and more types of technology

Figure 9–1 National Health Expenditures as a Share of the Gross Domestic Product

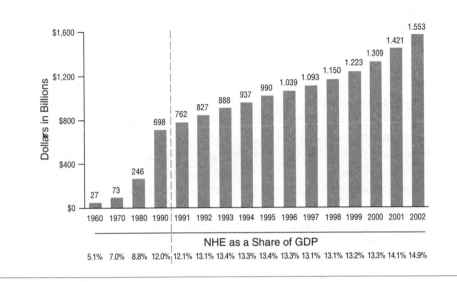

Source: Centers for Medicare and Medicaid Services, Office of the Actuary, National Health Statistics Group.

- Increase in the population of older adults
- Emphasis on specialty medicine
- The uninsured and underinsured
- Labor intensity
- Reimbursement system incentives

An overview of each factor follows.

New Diagnostic and Treatment Technology

The array of medical interventions and diagnostic modalities has increased exponentially in the past 30 years, including a vast expansion of pharmaceuticals to treat acute and chronic conditions. In part, costs rose because of the increase in absolute availability of treatments and diagnostic techniques that did not exist previously. The development of angioplasty as a routine treatment for blocked coronary blood vessels is

one example. The capacity of diagnostic modalities such as magnetic resonance imaging is being continuously upgraded and enhanced through new, computerized technology that is significantly expanding its applications. Many other diagnostic, therapeutic, and surgical techniques are undergoing revolutionary changes resulting from the availability of new equipment and computer-aided technologies. Minimally invasive laparoscopic procedures are just one example of these new techniques. The continued development of innovations can be expected (Coile & Trusko, 1999). Advances of these types have and will continue to come at a significant price. Information technology and computer-aided innovations require expensive software and hardware, new patient care equipment, and highly trained personnel. The large capital investments required create economic and professional imperatives for their use. Historically, the healthcare reimbursement system required neither documentation of the necessity for the use of technologic interventions nor estimates of their benefit. The tendency to favor broad rather than discretionary use grew with the number of interventions available. Managed care organizations, which require preapprovals, procedure authorizations, and physician economic incentives continue the effort to dampen the overuse of technology and avoid unnecessary interventions.

The continuing expansion in the number of new pharmaceutical agents to treat acute and chronic conditions, increased managed care enrollment, providing more access to drug coverage at lower out-of-pocket costs, and direct-to-consumer marketing of prescription drugs via television, radio, and print media combined to make the rise in spending on drugs a focal point of national attention (Levit et al., 2002). Growth in spending for prescription drugs has continued at double-digit levels for several years, and in 2003, prescription drug sales represented $179.2 billion or 11% of the total national health spending (Smith et al., 2005).

Aging Population

Growth in the number of older adults is another major factor in rising healthcare expenditures. The U.S. Administration on Aging reports that in the last century, the number of individuals 65 years of age and older increased by a factor of 11, from 3.1 million in 1900 to 33.2 million in 1994 (U.S. DHHS, 2000) (see Figure 9–2). The age group of 85 years old and older continues to be the fastest growing segment of the older population (Hobbs & Damon, 1999).

Persons over the age of 65 are the major consumers of inpatient hospital care. These individuals account for more than one third of all hospital stays and one half of all days of care in hospitals (Coile & Trusko, 1999). In addition, the aging of the baby-boom population born between 1946 and 1964 is expected to have a profound effect on healthcare services consumption beginning with the second decade of the 21st century. The first wave of the baby-boom population will reach 65 years of age by 2011. From 2011 to 2021, significant growth also will occur within the age bracket of 45 to 64 years, an age group that uses more medical services than do adults in the younger age bracket (Smith, Heffler, Freeland, & National Health Expenditures Team, 1999). These demographic developments embody major implications for future healthcare spending.

The Growth of Specialized Medicine

Growth in specialized medicine occurred in parallel with advancements in medicine's science and technology. Growth in the numbers and types of specialists was accompanied by Americans' high use of specialty care, at least in part driven by specialists' availability. Unlike other industrialized nations, where physician specialists represent half or fewer of physicians in general practice, approximately 65% of practicing physicians in the United States are specialists (U.S. Department of Labor, 2000). In addition to this unbalanced proportion of specialty practitioners, the high value that Americans place on advanced technology has made specialty care synonymous with high-quality care. This perception may be accurate when the most appropriate treatment choice requires a specialist's services, but because specialists' services are generally more costly,

Figure 9-2 Number of Persons 65 or Older (in millions), 1900–2030

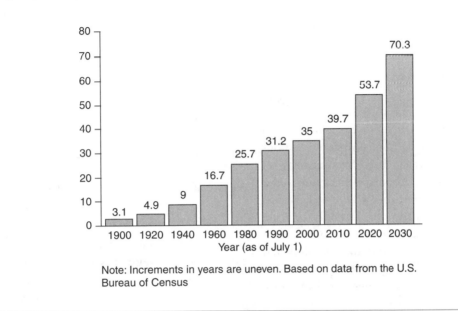

Note: Increments in years are uneven. Based on data from the U.S. Bureau of Census

Sources: Projections of the Total Resident Population by 5 Year Age Groups, Race, and Hispanic Origin with Special Age Categories: Middle Series, 1999 to 2000. U.S. Census Internet release date: January 13, 2000, with Population Projections of the United States by Age, Sex, Race, and Hispanic Origin: 1995–2050, *Current Population Reports*, 25–1130. Data for 2000 are from the 2000 census.

their inappropriate use generates unnecessary expenses. The use of more costly specialists for primary care needs also tends to cause higher use both of diagnostic and therapeutic services than may be necessary for appropriate treatment. Historically, the health insurance models prevalent in the United States carried no prohibitions against self-referrals to specialty care. Patients freely referred themselves to specialists based on their own interpretations of symptoms.

This use of specialists for first-line diagnosis and treatment has been a common and costly practice. Restraining costs associated with inappropriate specialty care continues to challenge managed care organizations, which seek to have patients treated at the lowest cost and most appropriate level of care. The efforts to restrain costs in this manner have raised much public outcry both by physicians and patients concerning the practice of gatekeeping. Numerous legislative initiatives at the state and federal levels pertaining to patients' rights to obtain insurance payment for specialty treatment and physician prerogatives to refer for specialty care without insurance company interference are discussed in the chapter on managed care (see Chapter 11).

The Uninsured and Underinsured

Among all developed countries of the world, the United States has the highest proportion of population with no health insurance coverage (Sloan, Conover, & Hall, 1999). In 2004, the U.S. Bureau of the Census estimated that 45 million Americans, or 15.6% of the population, had no health insurance, an increase of approximately 1.4 million uninsured persons over the prior year (U.S. Department of Commerce, 2004). About 69% of uninsured individuals are in families where at least one person is working full time, and only 19% are in families with no attachment to the work force (The Kaiser Commission on Medicaid and the Uninsured, 2004). Nearly two thirds of the uninsured have incomes less than 200% of the federal poverty level or are from families with low incomes (The Kaiser Commission, 2004). Figure 9–3 provides a snapshot of family income level for the uninsured. In addition, many individuals with health insurance coverage are considered to be underinsured because the extent of their insurance coverage is insufficient to protect them in the event of a major illness or injury.

The lack of health insurance or insufficient coverage carries major consequences by affecting the ability of individuals to receive timely and needed care for prevention, as well as for acute and chronic conditions. The lack of insurance coverage drives individuals to seek care in hospital emergency departments at costs higher than care provided at the physician's office or other ambulatory settings. Furthermore, uninsured or underinsured individuals tend to be low users of preventive services and are known to delay seeking care, even for acute conditions.

These behaviors often result in increased illness severity and more complications, factors that add to diagnostic and treatment costs. Uninsured Americans have been found to be much more likely than insured patients to require avoidable hospitalizations (The Kaiser Commission, 2002). Increased costs are absorbed by providers as free care, passed on to the insured in the form of higher health insurance premiums, or paid by taxpayers in increased taxes levied to support public hospitals or public insurance programs (American College of Physicians—American Society of Internal Medicine, 1999).

A Labor-Intensive Industry

Health care is a labor-intensive industry, with many industry segments operating on a 24-hours-a-day, 7-days-a-week basis. It is one of the largest industries in the United States, employing approximately 12.5 million workers, many of whom represent some of the most highly educated, trained, and compensated individuals in the workforce. The U.S. Department of Labor reports that approximately 16% of all wage and salary jobs created by 2012 will be in health services and that 10 of the 20 occupations expected to grow the fastest will be in health services (U.S. Department of Labor, 2004).

Among the most important factors that continue to produce high employment demands are technologic advances in care and continued growth in the aging population with more intense and diverse healthcare service needs.

Economic Incentives That Fuel Rising Costs

Finally, both private and government healthcare financing mechanisms are recognized as major contributors to rising costs. Until the widespread

Figure 9–3 Characteristics of the Uninsured, 2003

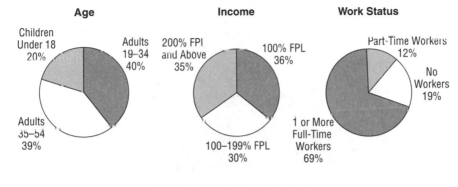

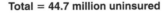

Total = 44.7 million uninsured

Note: The federal poverty level was $18,810 for a family of four in 2003.

Source: Medicare at a Glance—Fact Sheet (No. 1066-06). The Henry J. Kaiser Family Foundation, April 2003. This information was reprinted with permission from the Henry J. Kaiser Family Foundation. The Kaiser Family Foundation, based in Menlo Park, California, is a nonprofit, private operating foundation focusing on the major healthcare issues facing the nation and is not associated with Kaiser Permanente or Kaiser Industries.

introduction of prospective payment and the philosophy and financing mechanisms of managed care began in the 1980s, both government and private third-party payers reimbursed largely on a piecework, fee-for-service, retrospective basis. This system created economic incentives favoring high utilization among both physicians and hospitals. In combination with the other factors fueling increased consumption of healthcare resources, these economic incentives are acknowledged to have played a major role in rising expenditures. The history of failed attempts to change the healthcare financing system is reviewed later in this chapter, providing a foundation for the discussion of managed care's emergence as the predominant form of healthcare financing in the United States.

Components of Healthcare Expenditures

Figure 9–4 depicts the expenditure distribution of the national healthcare dollar. Of the total $1.7 trillion in 2003 healthcare expenditures, the largest portion, $515.9 billion, or 31%, was spent on hospital care. The next largest component of expenditures was physician services, totaling $369.7 billion, or 22% of the healthcare dollar. Prescription drugs consumed a total of $179.2 billion, or 11%. Nursing home care provided in freestanding, nonhospital-based facilities, at $110.8 billion, represented 7% of expenditures. Administration and net costs of private

Figure 9–4   The Nation's Healthcare Dollar 2003: Where It Went

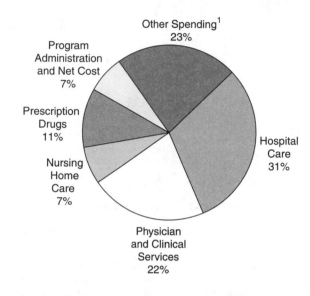

1. "Other Spending" includes dental services, other professional services, home health care, durable medical equipment, over-the-counter medicines, and sundries, public health activities, research and construction.

Source: Centers for Medicare and Medicaid Services, Office of the Actuary, National Health Statistics Group.

health insurance were $119.7 billion, or 7% (Center for Medicare and Medicaid Services, n.d.).

Sources of Healthcare Payment

Figure 9–5 depicts the distribution of national healthcare expenditures by payment source (Center for Medicare and Medicaid Services, n.d.).

Private health insurance currently funds more than one third of total expenditures. In 2003, private health insurance spending totaled $600.6 billion. A slowed rate of growth in private health

insurance expenditures in 2003 suggests that administrative costs and profits are increasing while benefit growth is decreasing (Smith et al., 2005). With benefit costs rising faster than premiums in recent years, insurers have increased their rates to offset higher costs and improve corporate financial performance (Levit et al., 2002).

Public funds contributed a total of 45.6%, or $765.7 billion, to national healthcare expenditures in 2003. Medicare and Medicaid, the federal government's two largest healthcare payment sources, together accounted for 82% of all federal funds expended for health care and 26.3% of total national healthcare expenditures (Center for Medicare and Medicaid Services, n.d.).

Figure 9–5 The Nation's Healthcare Dollar 2003: Where It Came From

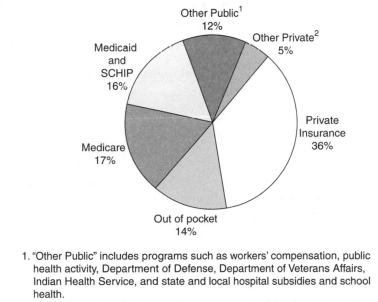

1. "Other Public" includes programs such as workers' compensation, public health activity, Department of Defense, Department of Veterans Affairs, Indian Health Service, and state and local hospital subsidies and school health.
2. "Other Private" includes industrial in-plant, privately funded construction, and nonpatient revenues, including philanthropy.

Source: Centers for Medicare and Medicaid Services, Office of the Actuary, National Health Statistics Group.

Although Medicaid constitutes only 16.8% of payments for hospital care and 7% of physician payments, it is the predominant form of payment for nursing home care. In 2003, federal and state Medicaid sources together provided 46.1%, or $51.1 billion, of nursing home payments. Consumers paid $30.9 billion, 27.9% of the total payments to nursing homes, as out-of-pocket expenditures (Center for Medicare and Medicaid Services, n.d.). Long-term care insurance has been widely available for approximately 20 years. However, premium costs are significant and, as with most insurance products, increase with age. Since 1993, the percentage of nursing home costs covered by private insurance has increased little, from 5.1% to 7.7% in 2003

(Center for Medicare and Medicaid Services, n.d.). State Medicaid programs providing medical assistance to the economically needy continue as a major payment source for individuals who either initially qualified for assistance based on income or subsequently become eligible through depletion of personal assets in paying for long-term institutional care.

Evolution of Health Insurance: Third-Party Payment

Health insurance is the primary source of payment for healthcare costs in the United States.

As a financing mechanism that helps protect individuals from personal monetary devastation when expensive care is required, insurance helps decrease risks of costly delays in seeking treatment for conditions that might otherwise become more serious and more costly. The impact of inadequate or no insurance for over 45 million Americans is repeatedly highlighted in the national debates over the need for healthcare reform that will provide universal coverage.

The U.S. system of health insurance currently includes numerous private entities that provide either indemnity coverage (reimbursement to those insured) or coverage on a prepaid, managed care basis. Government-sponsored and government-administered programs such as Medicare and Medicaid do not provide care directly, but rather contract with providers such as physicians and other health professionals, hospitals, and managed care organizations to deliver healthcare services to their beneficiaries.

The historic definition of insurance by which it is still commonly understood is a mechanism through which individuals pay an advance sum to a pool in which payments from numerous individuals offset the cost of a possible future costly event. Central to this definition is that events insured against are rare or unlikely to befall a particular individual, but can be predicted with a fair level of accuracy in a group. This latter understanding is the basis for payment or premium setting that helps to keep the costs of coverage reasonable for individual participants by pooling risks.

As early as the middle of the 19th century, a movement was started to insure workers against loss of wages resulting from injuries. Later, insurance to cover lost wages resulting from catastrophic illness was added to accident policies. It was not until the 1930s, however, that health insurance as it is known today—that is, insurance that pays all or part of the costs of medical treatment to the provider—was inaugurated. Throughout the 1930s and early 1940s, the voluntary hospital sector and local employers, in part in response to hospitals' difficulty in collecting payment from individuals who lacked financial resources, organized group hospital prepayment plans. This response reflected hospitals' dependence on private payments. In 1935, over 70% of hospital income was derived from private individuals (Stevens, 1989).

In 1930, a group of teachers enacted a contract with Baylor Hospital in Dallas, Texas, to provide coverage for certain hospital expenses (Wilson & Neuhauser, 1982). This initial event created a model for the development of what was to become Blue Cross, a private, not-for-profit insurance empire that grew over the succeeding 4 decades into the dominant form of health insurance in the United States. The Blue Shield plans to provide physician payments began shortly after Blue Cross emerged, and by the early 1940s, numerous Blue Shield plans were operating across the country. In 1946, the American Medical Association financed the Association Medical Care Plans, which later became the National Association of Blue Shield Plans.

These developments, through which health insurance was transformed from a mechanism to reimburse individuals for lost wages resulting from injury or illness to one that reimburses providers for the costs of medical care, carried gigantic implications. The first is antithetical to the central concept of insurance. Whereas insurance originally was designed to guard against the low risk of a rare occurrence, such as premature death, and for unpredictable events such as accidents, today's medical care insurance provides coverage of predictable, routine use of the healthcare system, as well as unforeseen and unpredictable illnesses or injuries. Coverage for routine use of healthcare services added a new dimension to the concept of insurance. Perhaps the term *assurance* more appropriately describes the healthcare payment system that evolved. In Great Britain, *assurance* is used to denote coverage for contingencies that must eventually happen (e.g., life assurance), whereas *insurance* is reserved for coverage of those contingencies (like fire and theft) that may never occur (Kovner, 1995).

The establishment and subsequent proliferation of the "Blues" signaled a new era in U.S. healthcare delivery and financing. They played a significant role in establishing hospitals as the centers of medical care proliferation and technology, and by providing reimbursement for expensive services, they put hospitals within the reach of middle-class working Americans for the first time. The insulation from costs of care provided by the Blues had a major impact on use. By the late 1930s, annual hospital admission rates for Blue Cross enrollees were 50% higher on average than for the nation as a whole, and more than 80% of beneficiaries occupied private or semiprivate rooms (as opposed to wards) (Stevens, 1989). In addition to contributing to increased utilization of hospital services by removing financial barriers, the Blue Cross movement had other major, lasting impacts on national policy making. Rosemary Stevens noted, "In the United States, the brave new world of medicine was specialized, interventionist, mechanistic and expensive—at least as interpreted, through pre-payment, for workers in major organizations" (1989, p. 90). By 1940, the Blue Cross movement represented a major financing alternative, countering forces that had long lobbied politically for a form of national health insurance, a concept opposed

vehemently by private medicine. The plans also stimulated the American Hospital Association and local hospitals to consider providing similar forms of reimbursement for low-income populations, modeled after the Blue Cross divisions of benefits recognizing private, semiprivate, and ward care. This latter movement, which continued for the next 20 years, focused attention on government as a potential source of insurance that was designed for low-income populations, the unemployed, or sporadic seasonal workers and that was modeled along Blue Cross lines (Stevens, 1989).

By 1938, uniform features of all Blue Cross plans were firmly established. These features included not-for-profit status, supervision by state insurance departments, direct payments through contract arrangements with providers, and the use of community rating, in which single premiums were charged to all individuals in a defined group without regard to age, sex, occupation, and health status. Community rating helped ensure nondiscrimination against groups with varying risk characteristics in order to provide coverage at reasonable rates for the community as a whole. However, as commercial insurers entered the healthcare insurance marketplace, using experience rating, basing premiums on historically documented patterns of utilization, Blue Cross plans, to remain competitive, began offering a variety of benefit packages. Ultimately, the Blue Cross plans were compelled to switch to experience-rating schemes to avoid attracting a disproportionate share of high-risk individuals for whom commercial insurance was prohibitively expensive.

Before World War II, commercial insurance companies had little significant involvement with or interest in insuring individuals for healthcare costs. Their portfolios had been limited largely to indemnity payments, considered a much less risky enterprise than insuring for use of the healthcare delivery system. However, post–World War II saw new fringe benefits added to labor contract benefit packages to offset the impact of federal wage and price controls. The financial incentives of these new developments fueled commercial insurers' entry into the healthcare insurance marketplace.

Self-Funded Insurance Programs

Since the late 1970s, self-funding (full or partial) and self-insurance of employee health benefits became increasingly common among large employers. Through the self-funded mechanism, the employer (or other group, such as a union or trade association) collects premiums and pools these into a fund or account from which it pays claims against medical benefits instead of using a commercial carrier. Self-insured plans often use the services of an actuarial firm to set premium rates and a third-party administrator to administer benefits, pay claims, and collect data on utilization. Many third-party administrators also provide case management services for potentially extraordinarily expensive cases to help coordinate care and to control employer risk of catastrophic expenses.

Self-insurance offers significant advantages to employers. Employers can avoid certain additional administrative and other charges made by commercial carriers, such as fees for writing and activating policies. By self-funding benefits, employers also can avoid premium taxes and accrue interest on the cash reserves held in the benefit account. With administrative services-only arrangements, an employer may self-fund

its benefit plan, retain the cash reserve, and use the commercial carrier to process claims and handle related administrative tasks. In another model, the minimum premium plan, the employer shares risk through a contractual agreement with an insurer that assumes liability for certain payments that exceed a predetermined level (Thorpe, 1992). A major stimulus to the development of self-insurance programs has been their exemption from the Employee Retirement and Income Security Act of 1974 (ERISA), which mandates minimum benefits under state law. This exemption has allowed employers much greater flexibility in designing benefit packages and has provided one mechanism to control benefit costs. From 2001 to 2002, premiums for employer-sponsored health plans increased by 12.7%, the highest increase since 1990. In past years, increases in costs for plans in which the employer purchases coverage from an insurer were almost double those for self-insured employers (Gabel et al., 2002). Now, however, significant increases in medical claims expenses and the rise in premium costs are closing the gap between self-insured plans and ones in which the employer purchases coverage from an outside insurer.

Major controversies continue to arise from the ERISA exemption of self-insured employer plans. One controversy is based in states' interpretation of their responsibilities for consumer protection through regulation of the types and scope of required coverage in employer-provided plans. ERISA has historically preempted such regulation. Another major area of dispute centers on the states' losses of premium revenue taxes as they struggle with growing financial burdens of uncompensated care and caring for uninsured populations. An additional area of major national controversy and legal actions surrounding

ERISA is its prohibition against employees suing employer-provided health plans. Under ERISA, organizations that administer employer-based health benefit plans maintain a degree of legal immunity from litigation and liability for withholding coverage or failing to provide necessary care. In 2004, the U.S. Supreme Court upheld a decision that beneficiaries of employment-related managed care plans cannot hold the plans accountable for damages when the beneficiaries are injured as a result of coverage denial decisions (Jost, 2004).

Government as a Source of Payment

The federal, state, and local governments' roles in financing healthcare services have evolved to be of major importance for healthcare services in the United States. Originally focused on specific population groups—most notably providing health care for those in government service, their dependents, and particular population groups such as American Indians—a combination of public programs, chief among them Medicare and Medicaid, now constitutes almost half of the total personal healthcare expenditures (Center for Medicare and Medicaid Services, n.d.).

Government payment for health services includes federal support of U.S. Public Health Service hospitals, the Indian Health Service, state and local inpatient psychiatric and other long-term care facilities, services of the Veterans Affairs hospitals and health services, services provided by the Department of Defense to military personnel and their dependents, workers' compensation, public health activities, and other government-sponsored service grants and initiatives.

In the absence of a comprehensive national health and social services policy, government's role in financing healthcare services can be described as a system only in the loosest interpretation of that term. It may be more accurate to describe government's various roles in healthcare financing as a mosaic of individual programs of reimbursement, direct payments to vendors, grants, matching funds, and subsidies. Some financing programs are interrelated or interdependent, representing tiers, first-pocket, or second-pocket approaches; others are totally independent of each other. Many are overlapping in their intent; some, like the Medicaid program, are conglomerates of federal and state source funds with policy making subject to federal, state, and local administrative and legislative influences.

As a source of healthcare service payments, the system of financing operates primarily in a vendor/purchaser relationship, with government contracting with healthcare services providers rather than providing services itself. An obvious example is the Medicare program, in which the federal government purchases hospital, home health, nursing home, physician, and other medical services under contract with suppliers. The Medicaid system operates similarly. This vendor/purchaser arrangement stands in contrast to other industrialized nations, such as Great Britain, with comprehensive programs of national health insurance in which the government is both the payer and operator of the system. America's history of fierce resistance from the private sector—both organized medicine and, to a lesser degree, the voluntary medicine and hospital system—has served to work against the enactment of a comprehensive national healthcare system. The activity of the private sector lobby can be traced from early attempts to provide some form of national health insurance, beginning in the first decade of the 20th century and continuing through the defeat of the Clinton administration's proposed National Health Security Act. Medicare and Medicaid, the two largest government-funded programs, are discussed later. Attempts at cost containment are discussed relative to each program.

Medicare

If it were not for the successful opposition of the private sector, most notably the American Medical Association, the Social Security Administration would have included a form of national health insurance in 1935. It was not to be for another 30 years, during which time numerous presidential and congressional acts for national health insurance had been proposed and defeated, that Title XVIII of the Social Security Administration, Medicare, was enacted by Congress to take effect in July 1966. Medicare became the second mandated health insurance program in the United States, after workers' compensation.

The enactment of Medicare legislation was a historical benchmark for several reasons. First, it gave every American 65 years old or older covered by the Social Security system entitlement to a range of medical benefits, which signaled a giant step for government's entry into the personal care financing arena. On the federal level, the Medicare program was established under the aegis of the Social Security Administration, and hospital payment was contracted to local intermediaries chosen by hospitals. Over 90% of hospitals chose their local Blue Cross association as the intermediary. As an alternative to government certification required for participation in the Medicare Program, the Social Security Administration agreed that accreditation by the

then-Joint Commission on Accreditation of Hospitals would suffice (Stevens, 1989). The sponsors and advocates of this legislation could not have foreseen its impact on the costs of the delivery system or on the growth of the hospital and healthcare complexes of the United States. Describing the enactment of Medicare as a "watershed," Rosemary Stevens stated:

> Thus with the stroke of a pen, the elderly acquired hospital benefits, the hospitals acquired cost reimbursement for these benefits, the Blue Cross Association was precipitated into prominence as a major national organization (since the national contract was to be with the association, with subcontracting to local plans), and the Joint Commission was given formal government recognition (Stevens, 1989, p. 281).

The act establishing Medicare specifically stated that there should be "prohibition against any federal interference" with the practice of medicine or the way in which medical services were provided (Stevens, 1989, p. 286). However, as could have been predicted, the government's implicit acceptance of responsibility for the care of older adults through the allocation of dollars generated a flood of regulation in the attempt to address both control of expenditures and quality of the medical services and products for which it was now a major payer.

As originally implemented, the Medicare program consisted of two parts, which differed in sources of funding and benefits. Part A provided benefits for care provided in the hospital, outpatient diagnostic services, extended care facilities, and short-term care at home required by an illness for which the patient is hospitalized. This portion of coverage was mandatory and was funded by Social Security payroll taxes. Part B was structured as a voluntary program covering physician services and services ordered by physicians, such as certain diagnostic tests, medical equipment and supplies, and home health services. This portion was funded from beneficiary premium payments, matched by general federal revenues.

Medicare coverage was not fully comprehensive. Beneficiaries were required to share costs through a system of deductibles and coinsurance. A deductible required the beneficiary to reach a set amount in personal outlays each 12-month period before Medicare payment was activated. Coinsurance required that 20% of costs for hospitalization be covered by the patient. The program also set limits on the total days of hospital care that would be paid based on a lifetime pool of days limit. Medicare payments for posthospital stays in extended care facilities were limited to 100 days. These limitations gave rise to a proliferation of supplemental, or "Medi-gap," policies, designed particularly to cover coinsurance requirements for hospital care. Both Blue Cross and commercial insurers wrote these policies.

Almost from its inception, Medicare spending surpassed projections. In the year of enactment, 1965, hospital insurance costs under Medicare were projected at $3.1 billion; in 1970, the figure was revised upward to $5.8 billion (U.S. Senate, Commission of Finance, 1970). Although hospital costs for the growing older adult population increased more rapidly than expected in those 5 years, the rise over projected Medicare expenses could not be explained in major part by that phenomenon. Rosemary Stevens cited a 1976 study by the U.S. Human Resources Administration to help explain the burgeoning Medicare hospital expenses (Stevens, 1989). This study attributed less than 10% of increases to growing utilization and the increasing older adult population. About 23% of the increase over projected hospital costs was attributed to general inflation and the remaining 66% to huge growth in hospital payroll and nonpayroll expenses, including profits.

The reimbursement mechanism for Medicare payment to hospitals mirrored that of the Blue Cross intermediaries. Payment was cost based and retrospective on a per-day-of-stay basis. While facilitating the rapid incorporation of almost 20 million beneficiaries into the new benefit system, the system also fueled use in an era of rapidly advancing medical technology and its introduction of more sophisticated and expensive treatments. Coronary artery bypass grafting and orthopedic prosthetics are just two examples of procedures that were not available on a widespread basis only 10 years earlier, but that rapidly became common treatments of choice, replacing far less costly interventions. Paid on a retrospective basis for costs incurred, hospitals had a strong incentive toward utilization of services and production of charges with no incentives for efficiency.

The 1960s was a period in which aging hospital facilities, many initially constructed or expanded with Hill–Burton funds in the late 1940s and 1950s, were in need of major renovations or modernizations. This was an era in which medical and surgical intensive care services evolved, incurring demand for major capital investments. New technology and treatment advances were rendering hospitals out of date. A 1967 federal conference on medical costs estimated that $10 billion would be needed for modernization of the nation's hospitals (Ball, 1967). The Medicare reimbursement formula, which enabled hospitals to pass a portion of capital costs back to the third-party payer, provided a new opportunity for hospitals to generate additional capital by accumulating operating reserves for capital expansion. This reimbursement feature further promoted maximum use and spending.

In the period of 1966–1978, numerous amendments to the Social Security Act made significant changes both to the Medicare and Medicaid programs. In general, amendments in the first 5 years after passage were largely directed toward increasing the types of covered services and expanding the population of eligible members. During the later period, amendments addressed a rising tide of concerns about the costs and the quality of the programs. Some significant changes to the Medicare program resulting from amendments, and the years they were enacted, include the following (Wilson & Neuhauser, 1982):

1967

- The requirement for physician certification of medical necessity for general hospital admissions and coverage of outpatient hospital services was dropped.
- Full payment of reasonable charges of pathologists and radiologists for inpatient services was authorized, eliminating the deductible and coinsurance requirements.
- Coverage was added for
  —Nonroutine podiatric care under Part B
  —Diagnostic radiographs taken at a patient's home or in a nursing home
  —Durable medical equipment for home use
  —Outpatient physical therapy services under Part B

- A lifetime reserve of 60 days of inpatient coverage for hospital care was added.

1972

- Medicare eligibility was extended to people with disabilities who had received cash benefits under Social Security's disability insurance provisions for at least 24 months.
- Part B premiums were capped at the most recent percentage increase in Social Security cash benefits.
- Coverage was added for
  —Speech–language pathology outpatient services
  —Social Security insureds and their dependents with end-stage renal disease requiring hemodialysis or transplantation
- Requirements were added for
  —Approval of hospital capital expenditures by state or local planning agencies
  —Public disclosures of survey findings in healthcare institutions and agencies with respect to compliance conditions for Medicare participation
  —Professional care review and placement in intermediate care facilities
- Requirements were rescinded for
  —Coinsurance payments for home healthcare services under Part B
  —Medical social services in skilled nursing facilities
- Authorization was granted for
  —Single annual per capita payments to HMOs, provided certain enrollment and other provisions were met, and partial return of cost savings to the HMOs

—Validation of the Joint Commission on the Accreditation of Hospitals survey results through sampling by state Medicare certifying agencies

—Establishment of advance approval of skilled nursing facility and home healthcare benefits and minimum periods of eligibility for posthospitalization services

—Grant and contract funds for experimental and demonstration studies of prospective reimbursement, the 3-day hospital stay requirement for skilled nursing facility admission, ambulatory surgery centers, intermediate care facilities, home health and day care services, reimbursement of nurse practitioner, physician assistant, and clinical psychologist services

—Limited reimbursement for chiropractic services to a specific diagnosis

—Established professional standards review organizations (PSROs)

1977

- Added the following
  —Numerous provisions directed toward control of fraud and abuse
  —Reimbursement for nurse practitioners and physician assistants working in designated rural and urban medically underserved areas, subject to conditions for medical supervisions and other criteria

1978

- Added incentives to the end-stage renal disease program to promote use of less-costly home dialysis and renal transplantation, promote studies of end-stage renal disease, and establish renal disease coordinating activities for program planning and evaluation.

From the mid-1960s through the 1980s, federal initiatives attempted to slow spiraling hospital costs and address quality concerns. Virtually all of these initiatives were unsuccessful. In response to concerns over duplication of services and major capital expenditures for facility expansion, the Comprehensive Health Planning Act was passed in 1966 to provide funds to states to organize local health-planning bodies that would ensure adequate facilities and services on a region-wide basis without unnecessary duplication. Competition for patients and parochial interests of institutions, however, worked against effectiveness in achieving rational regional plans. New York was the first state to adopt certificate-of-need legislation, requiring state permission for major capital expenditures, with permission in part based on appropriateness to a defined regional or area-wide plan. Other states followed rapidly. Again, the intent was to preclude spending for duplicative or unnecessary capital expansion for buildings and technology.

Because interested parties from hospital and other healthcare institutions conducted the initial reviews of planning applications, the processes became relatively meaningless. Similarly, federal legislation was passed in 1974 to form local health systems agencies to replace comprehensive health planning agencies, with the intent to develop plans for local health resources based on quantified population needs. Although the governance structure required participation by consumers, interested parties from the provider groups dominated discussions.

Health systems agencies were fundamentally unsuccessful in materially influencing decisions about service or technology expansion. Their decisions became undeniably political, and attempts to achieve consensus based on real service needs were counterbalanced by community interests in economic and employment expansions. Concurrent with attempts to slow cost increases through a planning approach, a number of other legislative initiatives that were directly related to concerns over Medicare costs and service quality took shape.

The establishment of PSROs in 1972 signaled the first federal attempt to review care provided under Medicare (and Medicaid and certain other federally funded healthcare programs) and to eliminate unnecessary hospital days for federally supported patient care. This program intended to attenuate backlash from the private medical care community by asserting that structured physician review of hospital cases in each locality was the most appropriate means to evaluate the quality and necessity of care. Each local PSRO was a not-for-profit organization composed of a representative group of local physicians. Determinations of the quality and necessity of care were made and passed to the local Medicare intermediary for implementation of payment decisions. Plagued by questionable effectiveness and high administrative costs, PSROs were replaced by peer review organizations (PROs) through a provision of the Tax Equity and Fiscal Responsibility Act of 1982 (TEFRA). The PRO attempted to achieve greater effectiveness in cost control and quality by providing more specific and measurable goals in both areas. Eventually, the PRO's role was extended to include outpatient care, home health care, and care for the military and their dependents. In 1993, the program's mission was

changed again because of high administrative costs and questionable effectiveness. The focus changed from detecting poor clinical quality and overuse to achieving care improvements through measurement and reporting of variation in care quality. Based on standards and outcomes, it was hoped that results shared with hospitals and physicians would provide a basis for working toward quality improvement.

In addition to the expansion of services and facilities occurring in the voluntary hospital sector, investor-owned for-profit hospitals saw the opportunity for expansion offered by Medicare's guarantee of full-cost reimbursement. By 1970, there were 29 investor-owned for-profit hospital chains. Both not-for-profit and for-profit hospital enterprises proliferated without the controlling impact of market competition inherent in providing goods or services directly to consumers. By 1980, over 90% of hospital expenditures were flowing through organized third parties: government, Blue Cross, or commercial insurers.

The Omnibus Budget Reconciliation Acts of 1980 and 1981 added another group of amendments to the Medicare legislation with a strong, continuing cost-containment focus. Many initiatives were directed toward reducing hospitalization and lengths of hospital stay. Representative amendments explicitly advocated the use of home health services as an alternative to hospital care. These included elimination of the limit on the annual number of reimbursable home healthcare visits, elimination of the 3-day hospitalization requirement for home health visit coverage eligibility, and elimination of the need for occupational therapy as a requirement for initial entitlement to home healthcare services. The prior exclusion from Medicare participation of proprietary home healthcare agencies in states that did not require agency licensure also was lifted.

The efforts at cost containment and quality control represented by the legislation of the 1970s and 1980s were followed by an array of initiatives that addressed growing concerns about the value and effectiveness of services being delivered by the rapidly growing outlay of Medicare dollars. Since inception, Medicare legislation required hospitals to conduct utilization review as a safeguard against unnecessary care or poor quality. Compliance was poor, however, because hospitals, unaccustomed to external accountability, did not fully exercise their new obligation to report to outside authorities. This attitude stemmed from strongly held values for autonomy and self-evaluation among hospitals and their medical staff and, in part, from the altruism inherent in the operation of heretofore privately supported institutions. At the same time, the Medicare legislation, seemingly reflecting these altruistic motives, contained no "teeth" to enforce utilization or quality standards or to balance the incentives for service expansion built into the retrospective payment system.

TEFRA, aimed at providing financial incentives to hospitals to contain costs, was followed in 1983 by enactment of a case payment system that radically changed hospital reimbursement under Medicare. In the new scheme, reimbursement for inpatient operating costs shifted from the retrospective to prospective mode. The new reimbursement system was based on preset payments for services rendered to patients with similar diagnoses, rather than on costs incurred. The diagnosis-related group (DRG) payment system based hospital payments on established fees for services required to treat a specific diagnosis rather than on discrete units of services. The

components of each DRG include numerous major diagnostic categories defined by the body's major organ systems. Major diagnostic categories are further subdivided into DRGs based on the patient's diagnosis, demographic characteristics, and relevant clinical data. The payment an individual hospital receives under this system is ultimately calculated using input from a host of other data known to impact costs, such as teaching status and wage data for its geographic area.

The DRG system reversed hospital incentives to consume resources and switched the focus toward efficiency and effectiveness. Instead of financially rewarding hospitals for the high use of services, as was the case under retrospective reimbursement, the DRG system provided incentives for the hospital to spend only what was needed to achieve an optimal patient care outcome. If that outcome could be achieved at a cost lower than the preset payment, the hospital realized an excess payment for the case. If the hospital spent more to treat a particular case than allowed, it had to absorb the excess costs. The DRG system also made financial provisions for cases classified as "outlier" due to complications. The DRG system did not build in allowances to the payment rate for direct medical education expenses for teaching hospitals, hospital outpatient expenses, or capital expenditures. These continued to be reimbursed on a cost basis. The principle of case-based prospective payment was adopted in varying forms by numerous states as a basis for their hospital reimbursement systems, and private third-party payers also adopted the concept.

When the prospective payment system was implemented, many concerns arose from hospitals, healthcare providers, and consumers about its possible effects on the course of healthcare spending, hospital financial viability, physician practice autonomy, and the quality of patient care. The roots of these concerns included questions about

- The new system's effectiveness in controlling cost escalation
- The ability of hospitals to streamline inpatient care delivery sufficiently and quickly enough to avoid major financial losses
- The effects on physician practice patterns of hospitals' pressure to minimize inpatient services and lengths of stay
- The competency and capacity of the home healthcare industry to accommodate service needs of patients discharged in less advanced stages of recovery
- The overall impact on the quality of inpatient outcomes

"Quicker and sicker" was the slogan popularized by the media during the first years of the prospective payment system to characterize the drive to decrease inpatient lengths of stay. The media also popularized the term *patient dumping*. It referred to documented cases of hospitals' inappropriately transferring low-income or uninsured patients at high risk of long, expensive, and potentially unprofitable service needs to other hospitals.

In general, research on the impact of the prospective payment system demonstrated that many early concerns were unfounded and that the system did have a measurable impact on the overall growth of Medicare spending. Also, continuing advancements in medical care and technology were occurring during the early 1980s. These advancements significantly increased the resources available to treat Medicare patients. For example, until 1983, growth rates in

Medicare expenditures for inpatient and outpatient services had increased at comparable rates. Beginning in 1983, the volume of Medicare outpatient services covered under Part B (hospital outpatient services and physician services not included in the prospective payment system) increased dramatically, in part counterbalancing the impact of prospective payment on total Medicare spending (Thorpe, 1992). Medical advancements and changing physician practice patterns also affected costs in the inpatient setting (Thorpe, 1992). The impact of the prospective payment system on the quality of patient care as demonstrated by comparisons of selected quality indicators before and after the system's implementation was the subject of extensive research. The federal Prospective Payment Assessment Commission was established to monitor the effects of the prospective system, and empirical studies reviewed hospital readmission rates as one quality indicator.

On balance, the studies revealed few, if any, effects on Medicare patient readmission rates attributable to the new method of hospital payment (Thorpe, 1992). The RAND Corporation also conducted several studies of another indicator of patient care quality, in-hospital mortality rates. The studies reviewed almost 17,000 records of Medicare patients admitted to hospitals for five common conditions. Findings included a drop of 24% in the average length of hospital stay for these conditions and an overall improvement in mortality rates among the five conditions studied (Thorpe, 1992).

Evidence supports that the prospective payment system slowed hospital cost growth during the early years after implementation, largely through reductions in lengths of stay, hospital personnel, and new medical technologies. However, total Medicare cost growth later reaccelerated, in part because of increased volume in outpatient spending and other factors whose impact have not been clearly determined (Thorpe, 1992). Concerns about the capacity of the home healthcare industry to meet anticipated increases in demand from patients experiencing more rapid hospital discharges dissipated quickly. Both the not-for-profit and proprietary sectors of the industry responded by creating new or expanding existing home healthcare services as components of integrated systems.

Concerns about patient dumping were formally addressed in 1985 by the Consolidated Omnibus Budget Reconciliation Act (COBRA), which included provisions requiring hospitals to provide care to everyone who presented in their emergency departments, regardless of ability to pay. Stiff financial penalties, as well as risk of the loss of Medicare certification by hospitals inappropriately transferring patients, accompanied the Consolidated Omnibus Budget Reconciliation Act provisions.

At least in the early years of the prospective payment system, hospitals did not suffer the negative financial impact predicted by some; they actually posted substantial profits (Thorpe, 1992). In fact, the federal government in part justified later reductions in prospective payment on the basis that early payments were too high relative to costs (Thorpe, 1992). It has even been suggested that the large surpluses generated by not-for-profit hospitals in the early years of prospective payment fueled hospital costs by making new surpluses available for investment (Thorpe, 1992).

From the outset, the prospective payment system's potential cost-containment effectiveness was circumscribed by its limitation to inpatient hospital care only for Medicare recipients. Aggressive shifting of Medicare-covered services

to the outpatient setting and shifting hospital costs onto private pay patients were two major reactions that attenuated the prospective payment system's cost-containment results.

Before the implementation of Medicare DRGs, several states experimented with methods to control rising hospital costs by implementing uniquely designed rate-setting programs known as "all payer" rate systems. These programs enabled states to bring Medicare payments, along with other payers' reimbursement, into a prospective mode. The movement began in Maryland in 1977, when it succeeded in obtaining a Medicare waiver that allowed it to implement its own Medicare payment rules (Kovner, 1995). New York, New Jersey, and Massachusetts followed. The experience of these states was positive in reducing total hospital cost growth, and they succeeded in limiting the difference between private charges and actual costs by capping the differential through statutory limit. This differential previously had been shifted by hospitals to unregulated commercial payers to absorb the amount hospitals were prohibited from charging Medicaid and Blue Cross plans. The differential had provided one method for hospitals to cover costs of uncompensated care. The growth of the uncompensated care volume in the 1980s, along with protests by commercial insurers who felt they were absorbing an unfair portion of that burden through shifting of the differential, led states to implement charity care pools to distribute costs of care more equitably for the uninsured and population groups lacking the means to pay. This was another positive by-product of the all-payer rate system experiments. Ultimately, however, the payment under the new DRG system proved to be more lucrative than under the waivered status of their own systems, and experimenting states dropped their all-payer rate systems; by 1989, all had joined the DRG system.

From the inception of Medicare, physician reimbursement through Medicare Part B was provided on a fee-for-service basis with reimbursement based on prevailing fees for specific services within a specified geographic area. Coupled with a cost-of-living factor designed to provide a payment ceiling specific to a geographic area, a prevailing fee was defined as an amount not to exceed the 75th percentile of charges for a particular service by all physicians within a community. Although physician payments constituted a relatively small portion of total national health expenditures, their rate of increase throughout the 1970s and 1980s in the Medicare program (an average of 18% annually between 1975 and 1987) provoked legislative action (Kovner, 1995).

Medicare first enacted a temporary price freeze for physician services (Thorpe, 1992). Assessments of the effects of the price freeze suggested that the lower fees were offset by an increase in the volume of services (Thorpe, 1992). Several explanations were offered for this phenomenon. One was sheer increases in volume of high-growth services during the 1980s, such as cataract surgery, and the availability of new diagnostic tests. Another was that reductions in out-of-pocket expenses by Medicare recipients drove up the demand for services (Thorpe, 1992). The results of the price freeze highlighted questions about how physicians respond to economic pressures, in particular whether those pressures increase motivation to use more services in order to compensate for lower reimbursement. The concerns over absolute cost increases, undergirded by rising concerns about overuse of costly specialty care, prompted addi-

tional congressional cost-containment action, aimed at physician payments.

The Omnibus Budget Reconciliation Act of 1989 (OBRA) established a new method of Medicare physician reimbursement that became effective in 1992. This new method used a resource-based relative value scale (RBRVS) to replace the fee-for-service reimbursement system based on prevailing fees. Under the old system, payments for services were made at the lower of the physician's usual charge, the actual billed charge, or an average of similar physician charges in a geographic area. Payment increases were capped by the annual amounts of increase in an inflationary factor, the Medicare economic index. The RBRVS system was an attempt to contain costs by instituting the same payments for the same services, whether performed by a generalist or specialist physician. The RBRVS system was structured to include three components in the fee: a measure of total work performed, an allowance for medical practice costs, and an allowance for malpractice insurance expense. The system assigned each service a specified number of relative value units, which are multiplied by a national conversion factor to arrive at the fee. In addition, the relative value units were adjusted for geographic area variations in costs. The hoped-for results were cost containment through reductions in the numbers of expensive procedures and attenuation of the incentive for physicians to specialize.

The OBRA also introduced a cap of 20% above the Medicare-approved amount that could be paid for a specific procedure and created what are known as Medicare volume performance standards, which are another method to cap payment increases on an annual basis.

Altman and Wallack summarized the shortcomings of the RBRVS system:

The fundamental criticism of the RBRVS system is that, while it controls total Medicare spending for physician services in the aggregate, it does so by arbitrarily lowering the prices for all physician services provided under the program and for all physicians. It does not however, provide much of an incentive for the individual physician to question the provision of a given service. On the contrary, by lowering the prices each physician receives per service, the system may be encouraging physicians to offer more services to compensate for lost revenues (1996, p. 18).

The Balanced Budget Act of 1997

Medicare system reforms enacted by the prospective payment system and related regulatory efforts of the 1980s were radical approaches in their times. Indeed, the new fiscal mandates and their accompanying requirements for quality and accountability coupled with the rising influences of managed care, market competition, technology advances, and consumerism produced unprecedented changes in physician practice patterns, hospitals' affinities for technology, and consumer expectations of hospital care. The Medicare prospective payment system even succeeded in demonstrating that in medical care more is not necessarily better, as lengths of stay and service intensity were reduced to accommodate the DRG framework, with no demonstrable negative impact on the overall quality of patient care outcomes.

The first half of the 1990s witnessed one of the most publicly and vigorously debated issues of the century: President Clinton's National Health Security Act. Although the act never reached a congressional vote, many months of debate served to thrust national concerns about health care into the public spotlight. Concerns included increased Medicare spending, lack of access to services, costs to beneficiaries, and provider choice. Popular and political sensitivities to these issues continued to rise against the backdrop of an escalating national dialogue about predictions of the impending insolvency of the Hospital Insurance Trust Fund (Board of Trustees, Hospital Insurance Fund, 1995).

Several trends supported the need for radical changes in the Medicare system. First, the Congressional Budget Office was projecting that Medicare costs would grow at approximately 9% per year, whereas the economy would expand at approximately 5% (Reischauer, 1997). This projection suggested that if costs were not addressed, funding the Medicare program would soon require cuts in other government programs, major increases in taxes, or larger budget deficits, all unsatisfactory alternatives.

Second, the structure of the Medicare program was becoming rapidly outmoded. Medicare remained a largely fee-for-service indemnity program, whereas employer-sponsored plans, Medicaid, and private insurance plans were rapidly embracing managed care principles. Recognition was growing that a program representing 31% of hospital spending and 21% of spending on physician services could not afford to resist current trends in healthcare financing and consumer sensitivity (U.S. DHHS, n.d.).

Third, Medicare coverage left significant gaps requiring co-pays and coinsurance, which many beneficiaries were unable to fill with supplemental "Medi-gap" insurance policies.

Although some Medicare beneficiaries were eligible for Medicaid subsidies of these expenses, subsidies created additional state financial burdens.

After acknowledgment of the president's and Congress's discord on a national health reform program, in 1995, congressional attention was sharply focused on stemming the tide of Medicare cost growth (with federal deficit reduction as a backdrop) and how to achieve broader choices for Medicare beneficiaries, primarily through managed care plans, which were providing models of cost containment and consumer satisfaction (Reischauer, 1997). After 2 decades of experimentation and experience with cost containment and quality improvement measures, a new mandate for reform emerged. Ensuring that the Medicare system could meet the needs of the incoming baby-boom generation with the same benefits afforded to their predecessors formed the challenge (Reischauer, 1997).

During the presidential and congressional campaigns of 1996, public knowledge of the health care issues was brought to light during debate on the National Health Security Act, and emerging consumer concerns about managed care coalesced into the rapid formulation and passage of the Health Insurance Portability and Accountability Act of 1996, also called the Kassenbaum–Kennedy Bill. Important health insurance features of the act included prohibiting insurance companies from denying coverage because of preexisting medical conditions or denying the sale of personal insurance policies to individuals who were previously covered in group plans.

The act required insurance companies to offer group plans to all employers (regardless of size) in markets where they already sold group plans. Furthermore, it prohibited the exclusion of employees or their dependents from group plan participation based on health status. The act ensured that individuals who change jobs would be eligible for coverage immediately, without regard to preexisting medical conditions. It also established a pilot program to enable workers to save tax-free dollars for future medical expenses through medical savings accounts. Another important provision increased the available tax deduction for health insurance premiums of self-employed individuals to 80% by 2006 (The Diabetes Monitor, 1996). Although the act accomplished some beneficial outcomes relative to decreasing the numbers of uninsured, it by no means addressed the serious underlying problems of the healthcare system in general or the Medicare and Medicaid programs.

The 1998 federal budget process reflected pressures to produce a balanced budget and to respond meaningfully to national healthcare issues both from the consumer and cost-containment perspectives. The resulting Balanced Budget Act (BBA) created a major new policy direction for Medicare and Medicaid reforms and took important incremental steps toward universal coverage through an initiative to extend coverage to uninsured children through a $23 billion allocation for new State Children's Health Insurance Programs (SCHIPs) (Balanced Budget Act, 1997).

The act was characterized as containing "some of the most sweeping and significant changes to Medicare and Medicaid since their inception in 1965" (Balanced Budget Act, 1997, p. 1). Overall, the BBA proposed to reduce growth in Medicare and Medicaid spending by a total of $125.2 billion by 2002 (see Figure 9–6).

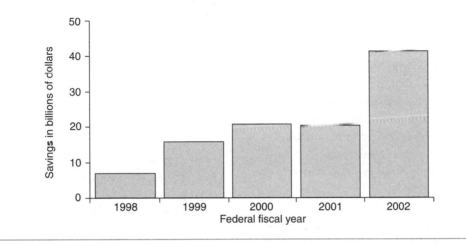

Figure 9-6 Balanced Budget Act of 1997 Projected Savings, 1998–2002

Source: Reprinted from Congressional Budget Office.

Actual Medicare spending for the period 1998–2002 demonstrates the impact of the BBA. After growing at an average annual rate of 11.1% for the 15 years before 1997, the average annual rate of spending growth between 1998 and 2000 dropped to 1.7%, resulting in approximately $68 billion in savings (Medicare Payment Advisory Commission, 2003).

Among the most significant policy shifts intended by the BBA was the departure from the largely fee-for-service model that opened the Medicare program to private insurers through its Medicare+Choice Program. For the first time, this shift allowed sharing of financial risk for the Medicare program with the private sector. The participation of private insurers was intended to increase both the impact of competitive market forces on the program and consumer awareness of alternatives to the fee-for-service system.

In addition to its payment changes, numerous structural and regulatory changes also were contained in the BBA. The Secretary of Health

and Human Services was authorized to carry out a host of initiatives related to the implementation of changes. Federal commissions were constituted to carry out other monitoring and recommendation functions during the BBA implementation. These included a Medicare Payment Advisory Commission and an independent National Bipartisan Commission on the Future of Medicare whose functions entailed

- Reviewing and analyzing of the financial condition of the Medicare program over time
- Formulating recommendations on
  —Ways to ensure the future financial viability of the Hospital Insurance Trust Fund
  —The scope and types of coverage to be included under the Medicare umbrella of approved services
  —The level of premium contribution by beneficiaries

—Age eligibility

—Contributions to medical education

The BBA Medicare savings were to be derived from payment changes to hospitals, physicians, ambulatory care services, post–acute care services (skilled nursing facilities, home healthcare agencies, certain rehabilitation hospitals, hospices, providers of durable medical equipment), and managed care organizations. The balance of targeted savings would result from regulatory changes, decreases in reimbursement of hospitals for medical education expenses, and other changes to both Part A and Part B provisions.

The share of each service's contributions to the total savings is shown in Figure 9–7. Hospitals, the largest Medicare spender, were to contribute more than one third of the total.

In summary, the BBA's major provisions included the following:

1. *Establishing a new Medicare Part C.* Medicare participants were given the choice of remaining in the traditional Medicare fee-for-service program or enrolling in new Medicare+Choice managed care plans with several benefit options.

2. *Changing provider payment methods and amounts.* Increases in direct Medicare payments were reduced for hospitals' inpatient and outpatient services, home health agencies, skilled nursing facilities, physicians, ambulatory surgery centers, clinical laboratories, and durable medical equipment providers.

   Premiums for Part B Medicare beneficiaries were increased. New prospective payment systems were required for hospital outpatient services, skilled nursing facilities, home health agencies, and rehabilitation hospitals. Allowances for

Figure 9–7 Sources, Percent, and Dollar Amount in Billions, of Contributions toward Balanced Budget Act Savings

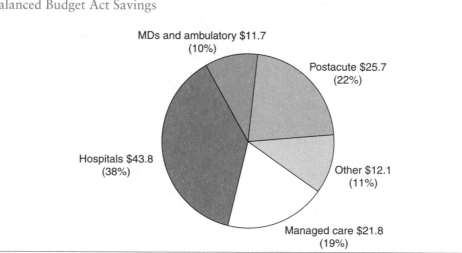

Source: Congressional Budget Office.

indirect medical education expenses of teaching hospitals were reduced. Financial incentives were provided to hospitals for voluntarily reducing the numbers of medical residents.

3. *Conducting demonstration projects.* The BBA required implementation of several demonstration projects encompassing a variety of system changes. One of its most significant mandates changed programs for all-inclusive care for the elderly from demonstration program status to a standard benefit.

4. *Developing prevention initiatives.* Benefits that promoted early disease detection and prevention were added and expanded for services such as mammography, Pap smears, prostate and colorectal cancer screening, diabetes management, osteoporosis screening, and pneumococcal and influenza vaccination.

5. *Providing rural hospital initiatives.* Additional payments were provided to rural hospitals along with enhanced flexibility to maximize Medicare revenue.

6. *Providing antifraud and abuse provisions.* New sanctions were introduced. These sanctions included permanent exclusion from participation in the Medicare program of individuals or entities convicted of three healthcare-related crimes, refusal or termination of Medicare provider agreements with providers convicted of a felony, and civil monetary penalties for accepting kickbacks or contracting or arranging services with excluded providers. Provisions also enabled Medicare to refuse or terminate participation agreements with entities that purposely transfer ownership or

control from an immediate family member in anticipation of a conviction, punitive assessment, or exclusion from a federal healthcare program.

7. *Establishing program integrity provisions.* Provisions addressed nonphysician-provided services and supplies, such as durable medical equipment, nutrition supplies, and home dialysis supplies, and the relationship between the organization or individual ordering and the one providing those services or supplies.

Physicians and others who order laboratory procedures or durable medical supplies were required to provide diagnostic information to support such orders.

Medicare beneficiaries were empowered to request itemized billings and the explanation of benefits included with Medicare statements was required to provide a toll-free number for beneficiaries to obtain further information.

The implementation of the Medicare BBA provisions experienced delays, widespread controversy, and material revisions. Significant changes to the Medicare program structure and the payment methods and amounts for providers all drew fire from industry advocacy groups, professional organizations, and consumers.

In the words of the U.S. comptroller general in testimony before the U.S. Senate Special Committee on Aging in early 1999, "The outcry from providers to undo BBA reforms aimed at savings and efficiency was intense. In response, Congress made refinements" (U.S. Senate Special Committee on Aging, 2000, p. 13). Just before the date when several of the BBA's provisions were to take effect, President Clinton signed the Consolidated Appropriations

Act for Fiscal Year 2000 (CAA). The CAA provided $17 billion in additional allocations for healthcare providers negatively impacted by the BBA and outlined new, later implementation schedules for many of the BBA's original mandates. Examples of some of the CAA's significant provisions were as follows:

- Delay in the implementation of the prospective payment system for hospital outpatient services
- Increases in payments for the care of severely ill skilled nursing facility patients
- Restoration of funding to teaching hospitals
- A moratorium on the imposition of payment limits for certain rehabilitation services
- Adjustments in the prospective payment system for inpatient rehabilitation hospitals

- Postponement of payment rate reductions to home healthcare agencies
- Special payment structure considerations for teaching hospitals and hospitals serving rural communities

The initial impact of BBA reimbursement reductions along with other factors occurring in 1998 appeared to slow the actual rate of Medicare spending growth further than anticipated by the BBA alone (see Figure 9–8). Other factors impacting the rate of Medicare spending growth in 1999 were widespread publication of federal efforts to curtail Medicare fraud and abuse and a dramatic rise in the average time for processing claims as a result of more stringent criteria for claims review (Van de Water, 1999).

Medicare+Choice managed care enrollments after enactment of the BBA totaled approximately 6.5 million by 1999, representing approximately 16% of eligible Medicare beneficiaries. During the initial phases of implementation,

Figure 9–8 Medicare Spending $88.5 Billion Less Than Projected (FYs 1998–2002)

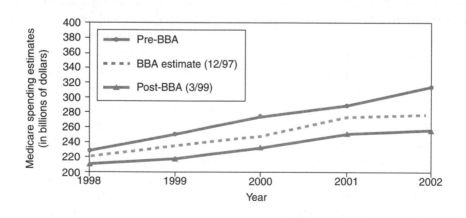

Source: Reprinted from CBO, An Analysis of the President's Budgetary Implications of the BBA of 1997, December 1997, U.S. Congressional Budget Office.

approximately 33 million Medicare beneficiaries chose to remain in the traditional Medicare fee-for-service program (Health Care Financing Administration, 2000).

The BBA Medicare managed care enrollment initiative experienced serious challenges. Managed care organizations, faced with reduced Medicare reimbursement, the costs of working through the federal bureaucracy, and significant market shifts impacting profitability lost their early enthusiasm for participation in the Medicare+Choice Program. Overall, about 2.2 million beneficiaries were affected by plan withdrawals in its first few years of operation (Berenson, 2001). In the effort to stimulate and maintain managed care organization participation in Medicare+Choice, Congress enacted the Balanced Budget Refinement Act of 1999 to slow planned payment reductions, provide bonuses for establishing plans in new geographic areas, and provide exemptions from quality assurance requirements for preferred provider organizations. In addition, the Benefits Protection and Improvement Act of 2000 enacted provisions to increase managed care organization and provider payments (Ross, 2001).

The Medicare Prescription Drug, Improvement, and Modernization Act of 2003

The Medicare Prescription Drug, Improvement, and Modernization Act of 2003 (MMA), renamed the Medicare+Choice managed care option Medicare Advantage, established several new plan options and created a prescription drug program for all Medicare enrollees. Like the Medicare provisions of the BBA, the MMA has been cited as enacting the most far-reaching changes in the Medicare program since its inception (Biles, Dallek, & Nicholas, 2004). The MMA also has been characterized as "one of the most complex pieces of health care legislation to pass Congress" (The Henry J. Kaiser Family Foundation, 2004b, p. 1).

Several factors led to the formulation of the MMA legislation. First, since its inception in 1998, the Medicare+Choice program was plagued by a more than 50% withdrawal rate of health plans, high turnover rates among providers, and sharp premium increases coupled with benefit reductions (Biles et al., 2004). Originally, Medicare+Choice intended to slow the growth of Medicare expenditures and expand consumer choice for health plans. The program failed on both fronts as enrollees' choice was impeded by provider and plan withdrawals and Medicare spent more for Medicare+Choice beneficiaries than those who remained in the traditional fee-for-service Medicare plan (Biles et al., 2004).

The key feature of the MMA is the establishment of a Medicare Part D prescription drug plan to provide financial relief from prescription drug costs to Medicare beneficiaries, especially for low-income individuals. Part D participation is voluntary, but in the effort to promote participation, penalties are built in for failure to enroll during specified open enrollment periods. The MMA also provides financial incentives for employers to continue offering retiree drug benefits with the hope of stabilizing the eroding trend of retiree drug benefits that began in the late 1980s (American Association of Retired Persons, 2005). The prescription drug benefit began with a transitional discount card program in 2004. Beginning in 2006, the MMA provisions began paying for outpatient prescription drugs through private plans that are available both to Medicare

Advantage enrollees and those who chose to remain in the traditional Medicare program. According to the Henry J. Kaiser Family Foundation (2004a), under the standard drug benefit, beneficiaries pay:

- The first $250 in drug costs (deductible)
- 25% of total drug costs between $250 and $2,250
- 100% of drug costs between $2,250 and $5,100 in total drug costs, equivalent to $3,600 out-of-pocket expenses (dubbed "the hole in the doughnut")
- The greater of $2 for generics, $5 for brand drugs, or 5% coinsurance after reaching the $3,600 out-of-pocket limit

Additional payment assistance is available through the MMA for beneficiaries with very low incomes or limited assets.

At the time of passage of the MMA legislation, the cost of the prescription drug benefit was estimated at $400 billion for the 10-year period after inception. In early 2005, the president's federal budget estimates placed the 10-year cost at $720 billion. The discrepancy ignited a storm of responses from Congressional members that awaits further analysis (Pear, 2005).

The MMA provides for several demonstration projects to test potential future improvements in Medicare coverage, expenditures, and quality of care. As outlined by the Center for Medicare and Medicaid Services (2005) summary examples include:

- Competitive bidding for clinical laboratory services
- Recouping Medicare overpayments and identification of underpayments

- Rural hospice care
- Rural community hospitals
- Extended stay clinics in isolated, rural areas
- Case mix adjusted payments for renal dialysis patients
- Prescription of replacement drugs and biologicals
- Patient care quality improvement
- Consumer-directed chronic disease outpatient services
- Physician adoption of health information technology and evidence-based outcome measures
- Chiropractic service coverage
- Homebound services
- Medical adult day care
- Outreach to Medicare beneficiaries

The professional, political, economic, and popular dynamics entailed by the breadth and aggressiveness of the measures contained in the BBA taught important lessons about enacting significant healthcare reform measures. The stakes in maintaining a financially viable system of publicly funded benefits are enormously high for a diverse constituency of providers, payers, and consumers, and they embody major political consequences. As evidenced by reaction to the BBA and resulting congressional and presidential actions, Medicare system financing reform will continue to be a complex and evolving process.

Medicaid

Enacted into law in 1965, Medicaid legislation was passed as Title XIX of the Social Security Act and is administered by the Center for Medicare and Medicaid Services. It is a mandatory joint federal and state program in which federal and state support is shared based on the state's per capita income. Its intent is to provide basic medical care services to the members of the population who qualify by reason of low income or who qualify for welfare or public assistance benefits in the state of their residence. An important distinction exists between benefit programs such as those provided by Medicare, and Medicaid, which represents a type of transfer payment to low-income populations. Medicare, funded from contributions of payroll tax matched by employers, is an entitlement because individuals have contributed to their cost of coverage. On the other hand, Medicaid, which is funded by personal income and corporate and excise taxes, is a transfer payment, representing funds transferred from more economically affluent individuals to those in need (Koch, 1993).

The design, benefit coverage, and joint federal and state reimbursement structure of Medicaid reflects 2 decades of lobbying influence by the hospital industry, state governments, and social welfare reformers to ensure a minimum level of benefits for the economically needy. The Kerr–Mills Act of 1960, an amendment to Title I of the Social Security Act, provided federal aid to states for the voluntary establishment of programs to pay for the medical care of economically needy persons over the age of 65 years. State participation was optional and included specific requirements for the range of medical services covered. The Kerr–Mills program, which was implemented by 25 states, is considered the forerunner of Medicaid (Wilson & Neuhauser, 1982).

Medicaid federal guidelines initially established a mandated core of basic medical services that must be available in each state program. Included were inpatient and outpatient hospital services, physician services, diagnostic services, and nursing home care for adults. Amendments to Title XIX expanded mandated benefits to include home health care, preventive health screening services, family planning services, and assistance to recipients of Supplemental Security Income. State Medicaid programs currently must extend benefits to all pregnant women who meet federal income level guidelines and children whose family incomes fall below specified federal income guidelines. Individual states have broad discretion to include additional services in their Medicaid programs, and many have elected extended benefits well beyond the core of mandated benefits. In doing so, they also may set limitations on the extent of utilization covered for nonmandated benefits. Medicaid also reimburses certain qualified ambulatory care services operated under federal guidelines, notably those serving high-need, underserved population groups, typically in urban centers and rural areas.

Unlike Medicare, which reimburses providers through intermediaries such as Blue Cross, Medicaid reimburses service providers directly. Rate-setting formulas, procedures, and policies vary widely among states. Because of the broad variations in benefits and reimbursement policies, Medicaid has been described as "50 different programs" (Koch, 1993, p. 309).

Along with the rising demand for nursing home care required by older Americans, Medicaid has assumed an increasing share of this costly service burden. The increasing numbers of older adults, coupled with the catastrophic level of expense entailed in long-term institutional and home-based care, have created a rapidly expanding pool of new people who are eligible for Medicaid coverage. Individuals with modest savings and income rapidly deplete personal resources in paying for nursing home or extensive nursing care in the home. The Medicaid program currently funds approximately half of annual expenditures for nursing home care.

Like Medicare, Medicaid spending grew at a rapid pace from 1980 to 1995. Major reasons for the growth in spending included the following:

- Growth in the size of covered populations and expanded coverage and use of services
- Increases in provider payment rates, as compared with general inflation
- The disproportionate share hospital program, which facilitated program expansion and increased federal matching funds
- Growth in the populations of older adults and people with disabilities requiring intensive acute or long-term care and related services
- Advances in medical technology that prolong the lives of extremely low birth weight babies and other severely compromised individuals who require extensive, and often long-term, expensive services

From 1980 to 1990, growth in Medicaid expenditures of almost 300% led to numerous initiatives on the state and federal levels to control spending (Koch, 1993). States tested various prepaid, managed care approaches, and like the Medicare program, some also implemented utilization review requirements and prospective payment systems modeled on DRG reimbursement. In response to the growth in costs, many states obtained waivers from the federal govern-

ment to mandate Medicaid client enrollment in managed care plans. Several states experimented with voluntary Medicaid managed care enrollment, contracting with HMOs on a fully or partially capitated basis to provide some or all of their Medicaid benefits under federally approved demonstration projects.

Since 1993, when federal waivers and demonstration project opportunities were made available to the states, Medicaid managed care enrollment accelerated substantially. Between 1993 and 1996, enrollments increased by over 170% (Center for Medicare and Medicaid Services, 1997). Growth in Medicaid managed care enrollment has continued since 1996, but at a considerably slower pace (see Figure 9–9).

The Balanced Budget Act of 1997

Provisions of the BBA were intended to reduce the growth of federal Medicaid outlays by $10.1 billion by 2002. Savings were expected to result primarily from reductions of disproportionate share payments made to the states, which would be held at 1995 levels for some states and reduced in others. Reductions were expected to have the greatest impact on urban, inner-city hospitals. It was also expected that new state prerogatives to establish their own provider reimbursement rates would result in savings. In 2002, the Center for Medicare and Medicaid Services reported that intended reductions in Medicaid spending growth were attenuated by the Benefits Improvement and Protection Act, which increased limits on states' federal matching funds for disproportionate share payments and by increases in Medicaid enrollment that resulted in sharp increases in the rate of Medicaid spending (Heffler et al., 2002).

The BBA eliminated the requirement for states to obtain federal waivers to mandate

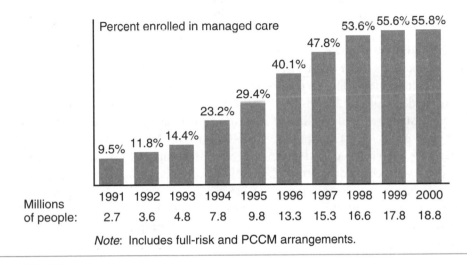

Figure 9–9 Growth in the Share of Medicaid Beneficiaries Enrolled in Managed Care, 1991–2000

Percent enrolled in managed care

Year	1991	1992	1993	1994	1995	1996	1997	1998	1999	2000
	9.5%	11.8%	14.4%	23.2%	29.4%	40.1%	47.8%	53.6%	55.6%	55.8%
Millions of people:	2.7	3.6	4.8	7.8	9.8	13.3	15.3	16.6	17.8	18.8

Note: Includes full-risk and PCCM arrangements.

Source: CMS, 2001.

Medicaid managed care enrollment. It also lifted the requirement for managed care organizations to limit their Medicare and Medicaid enrollment to less than 75% of their total enrollment and introduced administrative structures to encourage marketplace competition.

Additional savings were anticipated from allowing states to reduce their federal cost-sharing requirements for individuals entitled to both Medicare and Medicaid benefits. The BBA also contained new quality improvement standards, beneficiary grievance and resolution processes, and fraud and abuse protections. The issuance of the final rules concerning consumer protection provisions of the BBA was long delayed. First issued by the Clinton administration, the Bush administration delayed its approval three times, ultimately discarding them and issuing its own proposal in 2001. Final adoption occurred in 2002 (Families USA, 2002).

Consumer protections include requirements that enrollees be given the choice of at least two managed care plans, access to adequate provider networks, reasonable access to emergency services, and access to an internal appeals process (Families USA, 2002).

The BBA's child health initiative targeted 10 million children who are eligible for Medicaid but not enrolled or whose family income is too high to qualify for Medicaid but too low to afford private insurance coverage. The BBA granted states federal block grant funds and gave states the authority to use any of three vehicles, singly or in combination, for establishing their programs to provide coverage for uninsured children: increased Medicaid funding, state health insurance programs, or direct payment for services using up to 15% of their block grant funds.

The overarching goal of Medicaid reforms enacted through the BBA was to provide additional flexibility to state Medicaid programs to take creative approaches to reach more individuals with needed services or expand coverage for needed services.

By 1999, all 50 states were receiving federal support from BBA allocations under the SCHIP, and by 2001, 4.6 million children had been enrolled in new or expanded health insurance programs (Center for Medicare and Medicaid Services, 2002). In 2004, the Centers for Medicare and Medicaid Services reported that 5.8 million children were covered under the SCHIP during fiscal year 2003, representing a 9% increase from the prior year (Center for Medicare and Medicaid Services, n.d.). Currently, Medicaid covers approximately one in

five children. Low-income children are more likely to be enrolled in Medicaid or to be uninsured and less likely to have private coverage than children with higher incomes (see Figure 9–10) (The Kaiser Commission on Medicaid and the Uninsured, 2001).

Experience from the first years of Medicaid managed care enrollment demonstrates some evidence of improved access to a regular provider but more difficulties in obtaining care and greater dissatisfaction with care as compared with traditional Medicaid plan enrollees (Richmond & Fein, 1995). In theory, the economic incentives of managed care organizations using full or partial prepaid arrangements with service providers should promote their efforts to ensure timely, appropriate access to preventive services and care. However, with most states

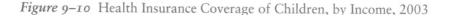

Figure 9–10 Health Insurance Coverage of Children, by Income, 2003

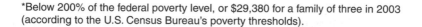

All Children
77.6 million

Low-Income Children*
33.4 million

*Below 200% of the federal poverty level, or $29,380 for a family of three in 2003 (according to the U.S. Census Bureau's poverty thresholds).

Source: Medicare at a Glance—Fact Sheet (No. 1066-06). The Henry J. Kaiser Family Foundation, April 2003. This information was reprinted with permission from the Henry J. Kaiser Family Foundation. The Kaiser Family Foundation, based in Menlo Park, California, is a nonprofit, private operating foundation focusing on the major healthcare issues facing the nation and is not associated with Kaiser Permanente or Kaiser Industries.

paying relatively low provider rates as compared with Medicare and the complex health and social needs of many Medicaid patients, the future success of Medicaid managed care programs to accomplish the goals of improved access and lower costs remains in question.

Other Services Funded by Government

Federal, state, and local governments participate in a broad array of healthcare and health-related programs and services. At the federal level, the Department of Health and Human Services, in addition to encompassing the Centers for Medicare and Medicaid Services, also maintains the other Public Health Service divisions concerned with public health and safety, research, disease prevention, and health promotion. The Veterans Health Administration includes a vast system of hospitals, nursing homes, and outpatient services that serve former members of the armed forces. Administered through the Department of Defense, the Military Health Service program provides healthcare services to all members of the armed forces and their dependents worldwide.

All states bear material responsibility for their Medicaid programs. States also may support medical schools, mental institutions, and departments of health that license and oversee the operation of hospitals and nursing homes. Many states also provide direct care services or support such services at the local level and engage in health education and promotion initiatives.

At the local level, many city and county governments support public hospitals and departments of health. City and county departments of health often provide direct care services for children and adults, monitor and investigate infectious disease cases and implement control measures, and participate in health promotion and education initiatives.

The Future: Continuing Change

The allocation of finite resources in a manner acceptable to political, professional, economic, and consumer constituencies defines the challenge of healthcare financing for the 21st century. Concerns about the resources expended are only one facet of the challenge; patient care results in terms of improved functionality and perceived quality of life are becoming increasingly important considerations.

Concerns about healthcare costs in relationship to the quality of care continue to be at the center of national discussion and debate. The large numbers of uninsured and underinsured individuals, rising health insurance premiums, managed care companies' competitiveness, and continuing impacts of the BBA and future impacts of the MMA are high on consumer, provider, and political agendas. The future integrity of the Medicare program remains a looming concern amid predictions that benefits spending will exceed future revenue.

The control of healthcare services delivery has undergone a shift from the care providers to managed care organizations. With this shift also has come increased consumer influence in response to restrictive managed care reimbursement requirements. New reimbursement arrangements between providers and payers are developing continuously as the system evolves. Market forces in the healthcare delivery industry will continue exerting pervasive and high-impact effects that will drive actions by both public and private policy makers.

The U.S. healthcare delivery system has become the most sophisticated and expensive in the world; however, at the same time, it has been unable to address adequately the issue of universal coverage. Richmond and Fein rationalized this paradox with the thesis that, over the years since World War II, "legislative and regulatory interventions" reflected a "deficit model" in which the expansion of knowledge, services, technology, providers, and facilities was assumed to be able to compensate for any system inadequacies. They suggest that this "expansion ethos" drove system growth and costs with little attention to balancing the allocation of resources to ensure service access for low-income populations and an equitable distribution of services and resources between urban and rural settings (Richmond & Fein, 1995). As pointedly illustrated by the failure of the National Health Security Act, institutional, professional, economic, statutory, and political barriers continue to impede the formulation of a national consensus on appropriate resource allocations and cost controls.

Market forces are reforming healthcare financing and delivery. In the next decade, managed care principles, responding to market forces, will govern the major portion of all U.S. healthcare expenditures, including Medicare and Medicaid. Whether arising from default or initiative, what ultimately emerges as the system of financing and delivery of healthcare services in the United States will likely result from continuing incremental change and system adjustments.

Conclusion

This chapter reviewed the most currently available data on national healthcare expenditures and sources of payment and provided an historical overview of the developments that played major roles in creating the national healthcare reimbursement infrastructure. Major factors that impact healthcare costs were identified and discussed. Significant trends in healthcare spending were reviewed, along with underlying reasons for evolving changes. The roles of government as a payer and provider of services were presented with an overview of the costs associated with government administration of payments and services.

Discussion Questions

1. Update the data in the chapter by using the Center for Medicare and Medicaid Web site to analyze national healthcare expenditures and sources of payment.
2. Using the site, discuss the future projections for healthcare expenditures and sources of payment. What are the implications for advanced practice nursing?
3. Discuss the policy role that advanced practice nurses may assume to influence the government as a payer and provider of services.

References

Altman, S. H., & Wallack, S. S. (1996). Healthcare spending: Can the United States control it? In S. H. Altman & U. E. Reinhardt (Eds.), *Strategic choices for a changing healthcare system* (p. 18). Chicago: Health Administration Press.

American Association of Retired Persons. (2005, February). Will the new Medicare law encourage employers to drop or keep their retiree drug plans? *AARP Bulletin, 46*(2),14. Available from http://www.aarp.org/bulletin

American College of Physicians–American Society of Internal Medicine. (1999, November). *No health insurance: It's enough to make you sick.* Retrieved July 22, 2000, from http://www.acponline.org/uninsured/lack-contents.htm

The Balanced Budget Act of 1997. (1997). Public Law 105-33, Medicare and Medicaid Changes. Washington, DC: Deloitte & Touche LLP and Deloitte & Touche Consulting Group LLC.

Ball, R. M. (1967). Problems of cost—As experienced in Medicare. In *Report of the National Conference on Medical Costs* (p. 65). Washington, DC: U.S. Department of Health, Education and Welfare, Government Printing Office.

Berenson, R. A. (2001, November). Medicare+Choice: Doubling or disappearing? *Health Affairs Web Exclusives,* W66. Retrieved October 10, 2007, from http://content.healthaffairs.org/cgi/reprint/hlthaff.w1.65v1.pdf

Biles, B., Dallek, G., & Nicholas, L. H. (2004, December). Medicare advantage: Déjà vu all over again? *Health Affairs Web Exclusives.* Retrieved October 10, 2007, from http://content.health affairs.org/cgi/reprint/hlthaff.w4.586v1.pdf

Board of Trustees, Federal Hospital Insurance Trust Fund. (1995). *1995 annual report of the board of trustees of the hospital insurance trust fund.* Washington, DC: U.S. Government Printing Office.

Center for Medicare and Medicaid Services. *The nation's healthcare dollar 2003: Where it went.* Retrieved January 6, 2005, from http://www.cms.hhs.gov/statistics/nhe/historical/chart.asp

Center for Medicare and Medicaid Services. *National Health Expenditures aggregate and per capita amounts,% distribution, and average annual % growth by source of funds: Selected calendar years 1980–2003.* Retrieved February 2, 2005, from http://www.cms.hhs.gov/statistics/nhe/historical/t1.asp

Center for Medicare and Medicaid Services. *Nursing home care expenditures aggregate and per capita amounts and % distribution, by source of funds: selected calendar years 1980–2003.* Retrieved February 11, 2005, from http://www.cms.hhs.gov/statistics/nhe/historical/t7.asp

Center for Medicare and Medicaid Services. *Personal healthcare expenditures by type of expenditure and source of funds: Calendar years 1993–2000.* Retrieved February 6, 2005, from http://cms.hhs.gov/statistics/nhe/historical/t9.asp

Center for Medicare and Medicaid Services. (2004, February 12). SCHIP provided health coverage to 5.8 million children in 2003. *HHS News.* Retrieved October 10, 2007, from http://www.hhs.gov/news/press/2004pres/20040212.html

Center for Medicare and Medicaid Services. (1997, January 28). *Managed care in Medicare and Medicaid fact sheet.* HCFA, Washington, DC.

Center for Medicare and Medicaid Services. (2002, February 6). *SCHIP covers 4.6 million children in 2001* [press release]. Available from http://www.hhs.gov/news/press/2002pres/20020206.html

Center for Medicare and Medicaid Services. (2005, January). *CMS demonstration projects under the Medicare Modernization Act (MMA).* Retrieved February 12, 2005, from http://www.cms.hhs.gov/DemoProjectsEvalRpts/downloads/MMAdemolist.pdf

Coile, R. C., Jr., & Trusko, B. E. (1999, August). Healthcare 2020: Challenges of the millennium. *Health Care Management Technology, 20*(7), 37.

The Diabetes Monitor. (1996, August). *Kasselbaum–Kennedy Healthcare reform Act.* Retrieved October 10, 2007, from http://www.diabetesmonitor.com/adv1028.htm

Families USA. (2002, September). *Medicaid managed care final regulations issued.* Retrieved October 10, 2007, from http://www.familiesUSA.org/assets/pdfs/MMCSept2002.pdf

Gabel, J., Levitt, L., Holve, E., Pickreign, J., Whitmore, H., & Dhont, K. (2002). Job-based health benefits in 2002: Some important trends. *Health Affairs, 21*(5), 144.

Healthcare Financing Administration. (2000, August). First Medicare+Choice private fee-for-service plan approved. *Medicare News.* Retrieved July 13, 2000, from http://www.hcfa.gov

Heffler, S., Smith, S., Won, G., Kent Clemens, M., Keehan, S., & Zezza, M. (2002, March/April). Health spending projections for 2001–2011: The latest outlook. *Health Affairs, 21*(2), 211.

The Henry J. Kaiser Family Foundation. (2004a, March). *The Medicare prescription drug law fact sheet.* Retrieved February 1, 2005, from http://www.kff.org/medicare/loader.cfm?url1= commonspot/security/getfile&pageID=33325

The Henry J. Kaiser Family Foundation. (2004b, July). *Consumer protection issues raised by the Medicare Prescription Drug, Improvement and Modernization Act of 2003.* Retrieved February 8, 2005, from http://www.kff.org/medicare/7130.cfm

Hobbs, F. S., & Damon, B. L. (1999, April). 65+ in the United States. *P23-190 current population reports: Special studies,* 2–8. Retrieved June 15, 2000, from http://www.census.gov/prod/1/pop/p23-190/p23-190.html

Jost, T. S. (2004, August). The Supreme Court limits lawsuits against managed care organizations. *Health Affairs Web Exclusives,* W4-417. Retrieved October 10, 2007, from http://content.health affairs.org/cgi/reprint/hlthaff.w4.417v1.pdf

The Kaiser Commission on Medicaid and the Uninsured. (2001, December). *Medicaid and managed care.* Washington, DC: The Henry J. Kaiser Family Foundation. Available from http://www.kff.org

The Kaiser Commission on Medicaid and the Uninsured. (2002, March). *The uninsured: A primer.* Washington, DC: The Henry J. Kaiser Family Foundation.

The Kaiser Commission on Medicaid and the Uninsured. (2004, November). *The uninsured: A primer.* Washington, DC: The Henry J. Kaiser Family Foundation. Retrieved February 10, 2005, from http://www.kff.org/uninsured/7216.cfm

Koch, A. L. (1993). Financing healthcare services. In S. J. Williams & P. K. Torrens (Eds.), *Introduction to healthcare services* (4th ed., p. 309). Albany, NY: Delmar Publishers.

Kovner, A. (1995). *Jonas' healthcare delivery in the United States* (5th ed.). New York: Springer Publishing.

Levit, K., Lazenby, H., Braden, B., Cowan, C., Sensenig, A., McDonnell, P., et al. (1997). National health expenditures, 1996. *Healthcare Financing Review, 19*(1), 162.

Levit, K., Cowan, C., Lazenby, H., Sensenig, A., McDonnell, P., Stiller, J., et al. (2000). Health spending in 1998: Signals of change. *Health Affairs, 19*(1), 124–172, 176, 179.

Levit, K., Smith, C., Cowan, C., Lazenby, H., & Martin, A. (2002, January/February). Inflation spurs health spending in 2000. *Health Affairs, 21*(1), 172.

Medicare Payment Advisory Commission. (2003, March). Context for Medicare spending. In *Report to the Congress: Medicare payment policy* (Chapter 1). Retrieved April 16, 2003, from http://www.medpac.gov/publications/congressional_reports/Mar03_ch1.pdf

Pear, R. (2005, February 9). New White House estimate lifts drug benefit cost to $720 billion. *New York Times.* Retrieved February 12, 2005, from http://www.nytimes.com/2005/02/09/national/09medicare.html

Reischauer, R. D. (1997). Medicare: Beyond 2002, preparing for the baby-boomers. *The Brookings Review, 15*(3), 24, 318.

Richmond, J. B., & Fein, R. (1995). The health care mess: A bit of history. *Journal of the American Medical Association, 273*(1), 69–71.

Ross, M. N. (2001, April). *Improving the Medicare+Choice program: Recommendations of the Medicare Payment Advisory Commission. Statement before the Committee on Finance, U.S. Senate,* pp. 7–8. Retrieved September 4, 2002, from http://www.medpac.gov/publications/congressional_testimony/tst040301Finance_M%20C.pdf

Sloan, F. A., Conover, C. J., & Hall, M. A. (1999). State strategies to reduce the growing numbers of people without health insurance. *Regulation 22*(3), 24.

Smith, C., Cowan, C., Sensenig, A., Catlin, A., Health Accounts Team. (2005, January/February). Health spending growth slows in 2003. *Health Affairs, 24*(1), 185–186, 188, 191.

Smith, S., Heffler, S., Freeland, M., & National Health Expenditures Projection Team. (1999, July/August). The next decade of health spending: A new outlook. *Health Affairs, 18*(4), 89–90.

Stevens, R. (1989). *In sickness and in wealth: American hospitals in the twentieth century.* New York: Basic Books.

Thorpe, K. E. (1992). Health care cost containment: Results and lessons from the past 20 years. In S. M. Shortell & U. E. Reinhardt (Eds.), *Improving health policy and management*. Ann Arbor, MI: Health Administration Press.

U.S. Department of Commerce, U.S. Census Bureau. (2004). *Income stable, poverty up, numbers of Americans with and without health insurance rise, Census Bureau reports*. Retrieved October 10, 2007, from http://www.census.gov/Press-Release/www/releases/archives/income_wealth/002484.html

U.S. Department of Health and Human Services, Administration on the Aging. (2000). *Profile of older Americans: 1999*. Retrieved October 10, 2007, from http://www.aoa.gov/PROF/statistics/profile/1999/profile1999.pdf

U.S. Department of Health and Human Services, Center for Medicare and Medicaid Services, Office of the Actuary, National Health Statistics Group. *Personal healthcare expenditures by type of expenditure and source of funds: Calendar years 1993–2000*. Retrieved October 13, 2002, from http://cms.hhs.gov/statistics/nhe/historical/t9.asp

U.S. Department of Labor, Bureau of Labor Statistics. (2000, April 19). *Occupational outlook handbook* (2001–2002 ed.). Retrieved July 22, 2000, from http://www.stats.bls.gov/oco/ocos074.htm

U.S. Department of Labor, Bureau of Labor Statistics. (2004, September). *Career guide to industries, 2004–2005*. Retrieved February 10, 2005, from http://www.bls.gov/oco/cg/cgs035.htm#outlook

U.S. Senate, Commission of Finance. (1970, February). *Medicare and Medicaid: Problems, issues and alternatives*. Washington, DC: U.S. Senate, Commission of Finance.

U.S. Senate Special Committee on Aging. (2000, February). *Medicare: Program reform and modernization are needed but entail considerable challenges*. 106th Cong., 1st session, 13.

Van de Water, P. N., for the U.S. Congressional Budget Office, U.S. Senate Committee on Finance. (1999, June). *The impact of the Balanced Budget Act on the Medicare fee-for-service program*. Retrieved October 10, 2007, from http://www.cbo.gov/ftpdocs/13xx/doc1322/061099.pdf

Weil, T. P. (1999, Spring). Let's merge competitive and regulatory strategies to achieve cost containment. *Journal of Health Care Finance, 25*(3), 65.

Wilson, F., & Neuhauser, D. (1982). *Health services in the United States* (2nd ed.). Cambridge, MA: Ballinger Publishing.

Chapter 10

Managing Financial Resources

Dori Taylor Sullivan

CHAPTER OBJECTIVES

1. Appreciate how the current healthcare financial environment influences practice as an advanced nurse practitioner.
2. List financial management tools and techniques essential for success as an advanced practice nurse.
3. Discuss the roles and responsibilities that advanced practice nurses have for fiscal accountability.
4. Evaluate the relationship of financial outcomes to the quality of care and service.

Introduction

The responsibilities for financial accountability will differ with each of the roles of advanced practice. Most notably, nurse managers and executives will need advanced competency to lead a department in delivering high quality care and services within the context of the costs of delivering those services in comparison to the established resource allocation (or budget) as well as standards for best practice from others performing similar work (benchmarking). However, nurses in other roles cannot ignore or abandon responsibility for delivering and eval-

uating cost-effective care. This may occur in individual interactions with clients and in developing and evaluating programs, clinical practice guidelines, and/or evidence for costs and quality patient outcomes.

This chapter will start with a brief overview of how changes in the healthcare system and environment have and will continue to influence the advanced practice nurse's financial responsibilities. The second section will review the essential financial management tools and techniques that will position the reader for success in dealing with the money side of an operation. Once we have discussed these tools, we will discuss the major roles and responsibilities advanced practice nurses have for their areas of responsibility. Lastly, we will discuss how financial outcomes relate to and must be considered in tandem with quality indicators for a realistic assessment of goal achievement.

Many nurses become anxious about accountability for running the money side of their practice. Through this chapter, readers will recognize that a fundamental principle of leadership impact relates to the ability to direct resources to priority activities and personnel to achieve the organizational mission and goals. So, increasing knowledge and skills with financial issues and resource allocation will assist the nurse in enacting all of the model leadership competencies. With that said, the advanced practice nurse cannot be expected to have expertise equal to those in the financial management departments. Thus seeking out experts for assistance in developing both operational and program budgets, and for analyzing variances and evaluating outcomes will be essential. But the advanced practice nurse needs to understand foundation principles and financial language in order to communicate needs and understand the advice he or she is given.

The Healthcare Environment: Deciding Whether Health Care Is a Right or a Privilege

As reviewed in the previous chapters, the United States does not have a health system but rather a fragmented approach to dealing with various illnesses. There is a general perception that interest groups representing the most powerful constituencies (often defined as business, the insurance industry, and the medical profession) within the healthcare field have been successful in preventing real change in the healthcare system, despite overwhelming evidence that it isn't working well for many people.

Harrington and Estes (2004) reported that during the 1900s, five major initiatives were undertaken to obtain national health insurance, the most recent being the Clinton health plan in the mid-1990s. However, as the cost of health care in the United States continues to increase more rapidly than the cost of living index and concern is mounting over the dramatic increase in the number of uninsured citizens, a true reworking of the healthcare system may be on the horizon.

Geyman (2003) described six myths that he believes strongly contribute to the inability to create momentum for dramatic healthcare reform. Each of these myths is listed next, and in subsequent sections a brief explanation of the facts disputing their veracity will be provided.

- Everyone gets care anyhow.
- We don't ration care in the United States.
- The free market can resolve our problems in health care.
- The U.S. healthcare system is basically healthy, so incremental change will address its problems.
- The United States has the best healthcare system in the world.
- National health insurance is so unfeasible for political reasons that it should not be given serious consideration as a policy alternative.

Until these myths are widely recognized as untrue, there may not be sufficient momentum to fundamentally redesign and improve the current healthcare system.

Evolution of the Healthcare System in the United States

The expanding knowledge base of medicine, advancing technology, and increasing use of hospitals and other healthcare services have combined with other factors to continue the upward spiraling increases in healthcare costs. A number of changes in the financing or payment systems for health care have been introduced to try to mitigate these effects. We will provide a brief overview of the prior systems and describe newer arrangements to provide the context for why managing financial outcomes is such a critical part of the clinical leader role.

THE FEE-FOR-SERVICE PAYMENT ERA

The fee-for-service payment era is described as the indemnity insurance and cost-plus reimbursement environment. Hospitals worked to attract physicians who would admit their patients and provide necessary diagnostic and treatment services. Expansion in insurance coverage in the 1950s and 1960s generally paid for these services for most employed workers, while Medicare reimbursements significantly covered care for those over 65. Medicaid patients were a minority of patients for many institutions, and the reimbursement rates, although lower than private payers, were closer to actual costs. Little attention was devoted to care access issues by the mainstream populace, most of whom felt they could receive care whenever and wherever they required it. As late as the 1970s, relatively little attention was paid to healthcare costs by either physicians or nurses despite the urgings of administrators. Hospitals and other health-care organizations billed charges that were reimbursed either at face value or at some percentage of the amount, referred to as a discounted fee for service.

During the 1980s, interest in traditional health maintenance organizations (HMOs) like Kaiser Permanente grew, and there was great anticipation of the ability to provide good care while reining in healthcare costs using this model. Looking back, it is clear that not enough focus on the demographics of the early HMO enrollees (mostly healthy young families) may have led to overzealous expectations. Nonetheless, a variety of strategies to manage health care was introduced, and these concepts continue to significantly influence care and reimbursement systems.

In the late 1970s and early 1980s, concerns regarding the cost of health care were growing. Healthcare organizations and especially hospitals began embracing more traditional business approaches in considering their revenues and expenses, the efficiency of their operations, and their organizational structures. Responsibility or cost centers were seen as the location for reducing costs, leading to charging clinical leaders with understanding and managing their budgets, an often unfamiliar task.

THE ADVENT OF PROSPECTIVE PAYMENT AND DIAGNOSTIC RELATED GROUPS

In 1983, a major change in reimbursement called prospective payment was adopted using diagnostic related groups or DRGs. Prospective payment means that the reimbursement for a specified set of services is established before the care is provided. Diagnostic related groups (DRGs) were originally designed as a health services research tool at Yale University; however, policy makers and regulators jumped on this opportunity to drive accountability for costs into healthcare organizations, starting with hospitals. Under the new prospective payment system, hospitals would be allotted a certain amount of reimbursement for their patients according to rates established by patients' diagnoses as categorized through DRGs. Although first applied for Medicare patients only, the use of DRGs and prospective payments was quickly embraced by private insurance companies, who also increased their use of managed care plan techniques for controlling healthcare services and costs.

Devers, Brewster, and Casalino (2004) identified an additional major market and policy response in addition to DRGs that increased price competition from the mid-1980s to the mid-1990s. Managed care companies started selective contracting with hospitals and other healthcare organizations to achieve the best pricing and assurance of the quality of care provided. Due to their size, managed care companies had more negotiating power than individual physicians, and this era also brought new payment arrangements related to sharing risk for high-cost patient stays that exceeded stated norms, also called outliers.

These changes fueled intense scrutiny of the various services and treatments and the costs associated with them in acute care settings; and, since length of stay (LOS) in the hospital is a good predictor of the amount of resources that a patient will consume, LOS became the gold standard for managing care under DRGs.

One of the interesting dialogues that also intensified under the prospective payment system was the issue of costs versus charges. Unlike many other businesses, healthcare organizations had little accurate knowledge of the costs of providing elements of care, and they certainly didn't have good information about the costs of a typical DRG. While in some hospitals charges

for care were defined as a percentage above the costs, in most cases the costs weren't really known and the charges were established through a muddy process that included how much the market would bear. This is important because without knowing the costs of delivery of a certain service or caring for a specific patient DRG, the charges or allocated payment might be insufficient to even cover costs—which means the more a given service is provided, the faster money will be lost! Not surprisingly, hospitals became very interested in managing LOSs, thus an intensified focus on discharge planning and utilization review occurred and evolved toward the current views of case management. Extensive databases (public and proprietary) have been created to provide comparative data for LOS and costs/charges for DRGs so performance could be assessed by each institution. Hospitals struggled to discharge patients within the suggested LOS time frames while they also worked to more accurately estimate the costs of providing care. Prospective payment systems have now migrated to long-term care and home care settings, touching off the same types of issues and reactions as happened in acute care.

One of the most important impacts of that change was the significant increase in patient acuity within the acute care setting and similarly, seeing patients who were sicker with more care needs within community settings like home care due to the earlier discharging. This phenomenon continues today and, coupled with more stringent admission criteria and migration of care services to outpatient settings, is a major factor in the dissatisfaction of many health professional groups whose workload and intensity has also increased.

A second impact was realizing that little was known about the true costs of care for a given diagnosis, since each phase of care (triage, acute care, skilled nursing or long-term care, home care) was considered separately. Thus questions were raised as to whether costs of care increased or decreased or were just shifted to other settings when considering an episode of care rather than just hospital costs.

This recognition and the desire to better coordinate care and control costs led to forming of integrated delivery systems including vertical and horizontal integration strategies. An integrated delivery system (IDS) of a network may be defined as an entity that "provides or arranges to provide a coordinated continuum of services to a defined population and is willing to be held clinically and fiscally accountable for the outcomes and the health status of the population served (Shortell, Gillies, Anderson, Erickson, & Mitchell, 1996, p. 7). Vertical integration refers to formalized relationships (ranging from agreements to ownership by a parent organization) of healthcare agencies that represent the continuum of care. For example, a hospital may have purchased or created a primary care practice, home care agency, and skilled nursing facility so that clients could receive all or most of their care with that IDS. Horizontal integration saw hospitals merge and/or be purchased with the goal of gaining efficiencies of scale as well as market clout and enhanced name recognition to promote growth and profitability. Research (Kitchener, 2004) has suggested that mergers have not been as effective a strategy as is touted and this activity has slowed some in the 2000s.

REENGINEERING AND REDESIGN OF HEALTHCARE SYSTEMS

The 1990s were also characterized by intense reengineering or redesign of patient care delivery systems and models. Major initiatives in cost accounting were launched in many healthcare organizations to better understand the drivers of costs and the actual costs of care for various DRGs. Knowing that in the vast majority of healthcare delivery settings the largest percentage of the budget is personnel, many of the reengineering efforts sought to decrease the overall number of professional staff by redistributing work tasks thought not to require professional knowledge to lesser skilled and lower paid workers. Another hallmark of this period was the decrease in management layers or levels and an increase in the span of control through loss of management positions. While processes of care delivery and support services were included and some successes achieved, the greater share of the changes were in professional roles. Norrish and Rundall (2001) noted that hospital restructuring affects the work of registered nurses in many ways. Their summary of those impacts included:

- nurses spending more time on administration and paperwork with less time in direct patient care—a dissatisfier for many nurses
- contradictory findings as to whether nursing workload increased or decreased depending upon the changes made
- less control over nursing work with managers acquiring additional units to lead and undermining shared governance activities and structures

Nursing was perhaps the major but not the only discipline affected by the redesign trend. Virtually all health professions either added or increased the number of paraprofessional or support staff with the goals of better matching staff skill levels to actual workloads and, of course, to try to reduce costs. Examples in other areas include pharmacy technicians, physical and occupational therapy assistants, social work assistants, and many others.

The early 21st century finds health care still embracing a free market approach with the expectation that competition, with some regulation, will drive down the costs of care. Private insurers and government payers have adopted stringent procedures for preapproving and managing care in most settings, with virtually constant communication and oversight. However, under severe criticism from the general public, steps have been taken to soften the approaches to managing care through legislative actions. While the majority of hospitals and healthcare agencies are not-for-profit entities, an increasing number of for-profit organizations are entering the market.

The operating margin (operating profit divided by revenue as a percentage) for most hospitals has rebounded somewhat from the very low or negative margins of the 1990s, but remained very modest at 1.39% as reported by Moody's for fiscal year 2003. Physician practices, especially primary care, and home care agencies face similar situations. Nursing homes or skilled facilities in a number of states are in a true crisis. So the pressure related to reducing costs of care and delivering high quality care efficiently still dominates most healthcare settings.

How Is Health Care Financed?

Today's healthcare industry consists of private for-profit insurance companies, HMOs, hospitals, physician groups, pharmaceutical companies, medical supply companies, and other health-related businesses (clinics, home care agencies, skilled nursing facilities, etc.). Most of the country has experienced significant consolidation of healthcare entities through the vertical and horizontal integration activities described earlier, resulting in a few larger entities. There is widespread concern that healthcare dollars have been redirected into for-profit entities of the industry, leaving those (organizations and individual professions) who provide care with fewer and fewer resources.

The major payer categories for health care in the United States remain the government, private insurers, and self pay (often referred to as no pay since uninsured people comprise much of this category). The term *payer mix* refers to the percentage of patients in a given healthcare organization that fall into each of these categories. With an aging population and an increasing number of uninsured people, the government (through federal and state programs) is a significant—if not the largest—payer for many healthcare organizations.

Coddington, Keen, Moore, and Clark (1990) predicted the outcomes of continuing with our market-based healthcare system, *all of which have come true in the early years of the 21st century:*

- More than 40 million uninsured
- Continued gaps in safety net coverage
- Double-digit health plan rate increases
- Small employers cutting coverage or even dropping health plans
- Increased co-payments and deductibles for employees
- Large rate increases for private insurers in shrinking markets
- Numerous failures of HMOs and withdrawal from the market by larger insurance companies
- Continued cost shifting in an increasingly fragmented market
- Continued inflation of healthcare costs.

In 2002, $1.5 trillion was spent on health care in the United States. This amount is expected to dramatically increase to $2.5 trillion by 2011 (Heffler et al., 2004), consuming more and more of our gross national product each year.

Comparison of World Health System Outcomes: Do People Get What They Pay for?

It has been estimated that 95% of the nation's trillion-plus dollar budget is spent on medical services with only 5% spent on health promotion and prevention (McGinnis, Williams-Russo, & Knickman, 2002). So it seems clear we still have an illness-oriented system.

The United States is the only country among those classified as Western industrialized nations that does not have some form of national health insurance (Geyman, 2003). While some claim that Americans do not want national health insurance, dissatisfaction with the healthcare system and the aging of the population are two major factors supporting a rise in general support for this concept. More and more often, people have direct knowledge of family or acquaintances who experienced difficulty in accessing or receiving necessary care. There are an estimated 44 million uninsured people in the United States, comprised mainly of the poor and the working poor but with increasing numbers of workers losing or unable to afford health benefits.

It is still often proclaimed that the U.S. healthcare system is the best in the world; however, virtually every health status metric—including how expensive care is—belies that claim. Starfield (2000) detailed the U.S. ranking in health status indicators from a variety of sources and concluded that the United States isn't even close to being the best in the world. Some examples of health indicators showing the worst U.S. performance were: low birth weight babies and child survival at various ages; life expectancy and age-adjusted mortality; disparities in care and outcomes across social groups; and equality of family out-of-pocket expenditures for health care. The facts demonstrate that U.S. citizens pay more for less desirable health status outcomes with difficulties related to access and coordination of care.

Implications for Advanced Practice Nurses

There will continue to be significant pressure to reduce overall healthcare expenditures due to rising healthcare costs as compared to normal inflation. Combined with expectations for continuous improvement and demonstration of quality outcomes, nurses can expect they will need to find ways to manage or reduce costs while maintaining or enhancing the quality of care and services.

Financial Management for Advanced Practice Nurses

In this section, we will present an overview of financial management terms and activities. While there is no expectation that readers will be financial experts, advanced practice nurses must be confident in their ability to manage the fiscal resources associated with their areas of responsibility and understand the terminology and concepts so they can talk to the finance department staff.

The Elements of Financial Management

There are four major elements to financial management: planning, controlling, organizing and directing, and decision making (Baker & Baker, 2004). **Planning** requires establishing goals and developing strategies for achieving those goals; developing a budget is the major activity in this element. **Controlling** involves assuring that the established plans or strategies are being followed, usually consisting of comparing reports of actual performance to targets. **Organizing and directing** relate to using resources to the best advantage. This may be staff, space, supply, and equipment, for example. Finally, **decision making** for each element involves analysis and evaluation to select the best alternatives for action.

ACCOUNTING CONCEPTS

The field of accounting is a critical part of financial management since it organizes information for use according to generally accepted accounting principles. Financial accounting methods are used for external reporting to third parties so that organizations may be compared across similar metrics using generally accepted accounting principles. Financial reporting is a retrospective look at what an organization has done. Managerial accounting is for use within the organization to provide usable information for planning, controlling, organizing and directing, and decision making. Industry performance metrics as well as organization-specific indicators are provided to managers as a guide for assessment and improvement of fiscal matters. In acute care hospitals, we look at metrics such as cost per equivalent discharge and hours of nursing care per patient day translated into

labor dollars. In specific areas, the indicators may relate to number of patient visits or number of procedures, calculating the revenue for those services as compared to the expenses required to provide them.

Financial management occurs within an organizational context based to some extent on the **type of organization,** whether **for profit** or **not for profit.** Nonprofit organizations consist of private or government entities, neither of which pays income taxes. A common misunderstanding is that nonprofits are not allowed to make any money, when in fact they must generate more revenue than expenses to stay in business. What differs is that any margin or profit is invested back into the organization and its mission, whereas in a for-profit company, profits are distributed among owners and/or investors. Most healthcare organizations are nonprofit; however, there is a growing segment of for-profit businesses that own hospitals and most other types of health service delivery organizations.

Two major types of **organizing structures** are most frequently seen in healthcare organizations today. **Traditional bureaucratic structures** divide functions by type and group similar types into larger reporting structures. Each functional area or department is called a responsibility center so that financial assessments of the area may be made. The terms *profit* or *cost center* may also be used. For example, in a health clinic there might be a primary care unit, specialty unit, pediatric unit, dental unit, and administration, human resources, and finance departments. The second structure is organizing by **service lines** or major customer groupings, e.g., cancer, cardiology, and women's health. In the service line model, all of the services required by that client type are grouped so that care is coordinated and customized. Advanced practice nurses will need to understand the managerial structure as well as the financial structure and reporting for their areas, as in some cases they are not the same model.

Managerial Accounting and Financial Analysis

BASIC FINANCIAL TERMS

Revenue is defined as the value of services rendered, expressed at the facility's full established rates. The full rate for a chest X-ray might be $175, with one insurance company plan reimbursing $125 and another company only $110. Payments may be made after services are provided (fee for service or discounted fee for service) or before service is delivered, according to agreements for care. These agreements tend to establish either a predetermined, per person payment or a negotiated amount for specified services based on the characteristics of the group to be served (Baker & Baker, 2004).

Gross revenue is the full value of services provided. Contractual allowances are the deductions for discounts according to the agreements in place. A deduction is also made for bad debt, or the amount of money owed that is not likely to be paid or collected. An advanced practice nurse might work with volume of activity targets such as visits or procedures or patient days rather than actual revenue figures, but obviously these are directly related.

The term *revenue stream* refers to how money flows into the organization or its sources of business. In the most straightforward arrangement, the expenses associated with generating that revenue are considered together to get a sense of the margin or revenue to expense ratio. The margin is the positive (in the black) or negative (in the red) yield after expenses are deducted from revenues.

Expenses are the costs of generating revenue, and, in complex organizations like health care, they are grouped into categories. A major distinction in expenses or costs is whether they are direct or indirect. **Direct costs** can be directly attributed to a responsibility center and tracked. For example, the radiology technologist and the supplies used to perform an X-ray are direct costs. **Indirect costs** reflect costs that are apportioned across responsibility centers to create a complete financial picture of an organization. For example, the patient billing department expenses must be supported across multiple departments as an indirect cost, but they are a necessary cost of doing business. An advanced practice nurse will be more aware of budgeted direct expenses than of indirect costs. Asking about and understanding indirect costs, however, can enhance his or her ability to plan and evaluate the costs of new programs and daily operations. Table 10–1 shows the relationship among some of these financial terms.

Another way that costs are described is whether they are fixed or variable. **Fixed costs** do not change when volume of activity goes up. Rent and minimum staffing requirements are two examples of fixed costs. **Variable costs** go up or down in direct relationship to changes in activity levels. Supply costs may be an example of a variable cost when each procedure uses a prepackaged tray of instruments and supplies. A **semivariable cost** changes with activity but not in direct proportion. Staffing additions are a good example of this category since there might be a one-staff-member increase for three additional patients in a given setting but no further additions until there are five more patients.

Table 10–1 RELATIONSHIP AMONG SELECTED FINANCIAL TERMS

Gross revenue from operations	$1,000,000
– Contractual allowances of discounts	$100,000
– Expenses (direct and indirect)	$850,000
= Net revenue	$50,000

Net revenue/gross revenue = Margin (positive or negative)
Shown as dollar value plus as a percentage of revenue
In this case there is a positive margin of
50,000/1,000,000 = .05 or 5%

FINANCIAL ANALYSIS STATEMENTS

The financial status of an organization is expressed in four standard reports: the balance sheet, statement of revenue and expense, changes in fund balance/net worth, and statement of cash flows (Table 10–2). The **balance sheet** records what an organization owns, what it owes, and basically what it is worth (stated as fund balance for nonprofit organizations). The assets of the organization (what it owns) is equal to its liabilities (what it owes) plus its net worth/fund balance. The balance sheet is described as a snapshot at a point in time (Baker & Baker, 2004). The **statement of revenue and expense** covers a period of time, e.g., a year, and summarizes how much revenue was generated minus the expenses used to generate the revenue, with the balance equaling the operating income. Ideally, revenues exceed expenses,

leading to a positive balance or **margin**, often expressed as a percent of the total operating budget. However, in health care, we sometimes see operating expenses exceeding operating revenues, leading to a negative margin. Some organizations offset this difference with investment income or transfers from other corporation entities like a foundation.

Changes in fund balance/net worth reflect whether an organization is moving in a positive direction by increasing its value or a negative direction by decreasing. An analogy would be whether one's personal savings account combined with the value of one's home is a higher number this year than it was last year. If one had to withdraw $15,000 to repair his or her home, the number may have decreased. The excess of revenues minus expenses from operations plus any gains from investment or nonoperations

Table 10–2 STANDARD FINANCIAL ANALYSIS STATEMENTS

1. Balance sheet
2. Statement of revenue and expense
3. Changes in fund balance/net worth
4. Statement of cash flows

sources are added to the fund balance or net worth of an organization. Last, the **statement of cash flows** translates a variety of accounting elements where the cash has not yet been received along with depreciation of appropriate assets and converts them into cash flow for a designated period. While all four reports are interrelated and important, most clinical managers would focus on the first two to get a sense of the organization's overall financial condition.

The Budget Cycle

All organizations establish a fiscal year (FY), with many using calendar years. In some states, hospitals and sometimes other healthcare organizations are on standardized fiscal years for purposes of regulatory reporting and comparison. At year end, the appropriate financial and accounting procedures are carried out to develop the final financial reports, which are usually audited by an external public accounting firm and certified as accurate in terms of meeting required standards for this type of reporting.

The budget cycle is a series of timed activities planned to arrive at an approved budget prior to the start of the next fiscal year. Depending on the size, complexity, and culture of an organization, planning for the next year's budget might start at the beginning of each fiscal year.

A critical early component of budget planning relates to forecasting and projecting the revenues and expenses for the next fiscal year. Forecasting and projecting may be led by finance executives, strategic planning directors, or other designated personnel. Environmental assessments, contractual changes, and trends in care needs or reimbursement must be analyzed and their relative impact estimated. These conclusions are then translated into what are called budget assumptions, the context for budget development. In addition, the identification of strategic priorities or organizational goals, along with the resources that will be required to accomplish them, must also be factored in, whether they are organization-wide or unit-based initiatives.

Budget Development

The development of a budget requires several steps in addition to forecasting and projections already described. First, an approach to budget development must be selected. A zero-based budget means that each year, those involved with creating the budget assume that there is a clean slate and they start building a budget without regard to the resources allocated for the current fiscal year. Zero-based budgeting can be a useful tool for realigning expenses with changing activity priorities, but it is a difficult and labor intensive process. Most healthcare organizations use some variation of a historical budget that assumes most responsibility centers within the organization will continue to provide similar services, with adjustments made for volumes, new programs, and special projects.

In many organizations, the budget is built by each responsibility center reviewing the general budget assumptions and perhaps collaborating to develop unit-specific assumptions, if appropriate. The role of a clinical leader may involve predicting changes that would affect the unit, including volume of various services, staffing (costs and availability), equipment (needs and costs including replacement), and supplies.

In growing markets (e.g., where the population is increasing) this approach would be used more frequently since volumes and revenues are likely increasing. Using this method, the rolled up budget (adding together all responsibility center requests) may still exceed projected revenue by millions of dollars. The budget review process usually means a process for reducing the requested allocation to try to create a balanced budget. From the perspective of the advanced practice nurse, this approach can be frustrating, as the nurse perceives he or she never gets what he or she needs or requests. It also leads to game playing and padding the budget because people know they will not get what they request, so they request more than what is needed.

More recently, some healthcare organizations in static or highly competitive markets have moved to an approach that we believe is more realistic. Similar to most household budgets, a projection of what the income is likely to be is made first, and then necessary expenses are factored in, followed by funding for whatever discretionary expenditures can be supported. Using this approach, there is little to be gained by having each responsibility center develop a new budget; rather, appropriate changes (adding or subtracting resources) are proposed based on projections and organizational goals. Adjustments are also made for salary increases, inflation of equipment costs, etc., usually by the finance department, after which managers may or may not review the proposed budget. While this can be frustrating, it does reflect the reality of limited resources.

An organization may also use a flexible budgeting approach that indexes or adjusts selected budget categories based on volume or other factors during the budget year. These midyear adjustments may or may not be reflected in budget reports, depending upon the budget software system capability and on the magnitude of the adjustments.

TYPES OF BUDGETS

Typical budgets are organized into operating budgets and capital budgets. **Operating budg-** ets have two major categories, personnel and supplies/equipment. Each type of expense is named and listed on a line in the budget, thus the term *line item*. In most healthcare organizations, personnel costs are by far the largest portion of the budget, so as previously noted much effort goes into determining the necessary staffing mix, pattern, and organization. **Capital budgets** are separately created for expenditures that exceed an established dollar limit that varies across organizations. Similarly, the size of the capital budget is often determined based on what the organization believes it can afford, followed by a process for reviewing and approving capital purchases. One's ability to write a compelling justification for proposed regular and capital budget items is an important skill to acquire. Describing how a new piece of equipment will improve quality of care and decrease the professional time a service requires (and translating this information into financial terms if possible, e.g., a projected savings of 8 hours of professional time per week at $38 per hour for a savings of over $15,000 per year) will be more positively received than citing that two other facilities in the area have the new equipment.

MONITORING BUDGET VARIANCES

The budget variance report, as its name suggests, is a listing of each budget line item and category with the budgeted amount for the month/period and year to date, the actual amount spent for the month/period and year to date, and the difference between the two figures, or variance. The variance is often expressed as the dollar difference and the percentage the variance represents from budget. Table 10–3 shows a budget variance report for a clinical area.

The advanced practice nurse who has direct budget responsibility will be asked regularly to analyze each line item and category, determining which are tracking according to plan and which are outliers, either too high or too low. The next step is to gather the necessary information to understand why an item is over or under budget, and whether this is a good or bad thing. If things are going better than expected, there is an opportunity to learn why and maybe extend that positive impact. More often, the nurse will discover that lines are over budget, and he or she must investigate the causes. Those in a role without direct budget responsibility should recognize that this oversight occurs periodically and that each organization has different review periods.

There are three causes of budget variance for nursing. These are volume, efficiency, and rate variance from the budgeted amount. Volume variances are due to more or fewer patient days or visits; efficiency variance relates to more or fewer hours per patient day, and rate variance relates to salaries (generally the use of overtime). An explanation of the mathematics to complete this easy and very helpful analysis can be found in Finkler and Kovner (2000, p. 300).

FINANCIAL ROLES AND RESPONSIBILITIES OF ADVANCED PRACTICE NURSES

An expert in one's area of specialization, whether with direct responsibility for managing money or with input into budgets and program development, will need the following knowledge and skills:

Table 10–3 SAMPLE BUDGET VARIANCE REPORT FOR A CLINICAL AREA

Description	Dec 05 Budget	Dec 05 Actual	YTD Budget	YTD Actual	Variance	Percentage
Revenue						
Gross	30,000	34,000	90,000	115,000	(25,000)	(27.7%)
Allowance	10,000	14,000	30,000	45,000	(15,000)	(50.0%)
Expenses						
Salaries	21,000	23,000	63,000	65,000	(2,000)	(0.3%)
Fringe	8,400	9,200	25,200	26,000	(800)	(0.3%)
Temporary	1,000	1,200	3,000	2,200	800	26.6%
Med supp	5,000	4,800	15,000	12,000	3,000	20.0%
Office supp	800	800	2,400	2,400	0	0
Telephone	400	500	1,200	1,400	(200)	(16.7%)
Copying	100	140	300	360	(60)	(20.0%)
Travel	75	65	225	210	15	.07%

Year to date (YTD) budget amounts reflect 3 months with fiscal year of October 1–September 30.

- awareness of the region and the discipline's current healthcare environment, especially related to the demand for services, reimbursement mechanisms, workforce supply, and cost pressures
- development of projected revenues and expenses for new and existing programs
- monitoring and responding to budget variances
- participating in benchmarking, either internal or external

It has been said that healthcare issues may be global but the delivery of care and solutions to those issues must be driven locally. Therefore, advanced nurse practitioners must become familiar with the dynamics within their region related to which types of services for care are in demand, what the reimbursement picture is from the major payers, what the pricing range for these services is, and with determination of the quality indicators and outcomes expected. While the literature may provide some general direction, the most current information will come from local sources like the hospital association and its related meeting groups, through professional networking, and from consultants.

The advanced practice nurse's role in projecting revenue and volume for preparation of an annual budget is a critical one, for it is during this process that the decisions that will affect the nurse and his or her patients for at least the next year are made. Once he or she has a sense of the resources likely to be allocated, he or she can begin detailed planning for any changes or improvements that he or she has decided to pursue. Again local networking along with regional or national specialty groups will likely provide the best information for program planning.

One of the most important roles a nurse manager has related to fiscal responsibility is the regular review of budget variance reports. However, whether one is a direct care provider, a manager, or in other roles, understanding the need to analyze and take action in response to budget variance reports is helpful to one's participation in the mission and vision of the organization.

Financial Results and Quality Outcomes

Several authors have proposed methods for assessing overall unit or organizational performance. One of the most popular is the balanced scorecard used in general business and applied to health care (Kaplan & Norton, 1996). The balanced scorecard helps us get a true sense of how an organization or its units are performing by simultaneously considering several performance domains. The original balanced scorecard includes performance measures of finance, internal business processes, learning and growth, and the customer. Many organizations have adapted these categories that are often displayed as quadrants of a table or circle. Table 10–4 shows a sample balanced scorecard for a healthcare organization. The point is that it won't matter much if your financial indicators are excellent if the quality outcomes and satisfaction levels of clients are poor. Similarly, if your quality is wonderful but is costing more than can be supported, the organization cannot sustain success. Benchmarking can provide valuable comparison information when high quality

Table 10–4 EXAMPLE OF A HEALTHCARE ORGANIZATION'S BALANCED SCORECARD

Clinical outcomes and functional status of clients	Operational performance indicators
Customer satisfaction (clients, staff, physicians, payers, community)	Financial performance indicators

information with comparable organizations can be accessed (see Chapter 15).

Conclusion

Often understanding and managing financial resources is one of the more intimidating and challenging skills for nurses in advanced practice. Responsibilities for this will vary according to one's role and the organizational policies and practices in the setting in which one works. However, a basic understanding of the language, processes, and justifications for cost consciousness will make the role transition to advanced practice easier.

Discussion Questions

1. Identify the top two services or activities in the area in which you currently work. If you provide direct services to clients, what types of reimbursement arrangements or contracts are in place? Who are the major payers by percentage of revenue? If your area is considered an area of indirect costs, how is the support for your operation apportioned across the institution?
2. Locate the most recent balance sheet, statement of revenue and expense, and changes in fund value/net worth for your organization. Review these with a manager in nursing or finance to gain an understanding of how to read these.
3. Determine what the operating margin was for the last fiscal year—was it positive or negative, and what does this mean?
4. Review a recent budget variance printout for your department. What were the largest variances, and do you feel confident that you understand why these variances occurred?
5. Review a balanced scorecard for the unit in which you are currently employed. Which aspects of this assessment are meeting targets, and which need improvement?

References

Baker, J. J., & Baker, R. W. (2004). *Health care finance: Basic tools for nonfinancial managers.* Sudbury, MA: Jones and Bartlett Publishers.

Coddington, D. C., Keen, D. J., Moore, K. D., & Clark, R. L. (1990). *The crisis in health care: Costs, choices, and strategies.* San Francisco: Jossey-Bass.

Devers, K. J., Brewster, L. R., & Casalino, L. P. (2004). Changes in hospital competitive strategy: A new medical arms race? In C. Harrington & C. L. Estes (Eds.), *Health policy: Crisis and reform in the U.S. health care delivery system* (4th ed., pp. 174–183). Sudbury, MA: Jones and Bartlett Publishers.

Finkler, S. A., & Kovner, C. T. (2000). *Financial management for nurse executives and managers.* Philadelphia: W. B. Saunders.

Geyman, J. P. (2003). Myths as barriers to health care reform in the United States. *International Journal of Health Services, 33*(2), 315–329.

Harrington, C., & Estes, C. L. (2004). *Health policy: Crisis and reform in the U.S. health care delivery system* (4th ed.). Sudbury, MA: Jones and Bartlett Publishers.

Heffler, S., Smith, S., Won, G., Clemens, M. K., Keehan, S., & Zezza, M. (2004). Health spending projections for 2001–2011: The latest outlook. In C. Harrington & C. L. Estes (Eds.), *Health policy: Crisis and reform in the U.S. health care delivery system* (4th ed., pp. 250–259). Sudbury, MA: Jones and Bartlett Publishers.

Kaplan, R. S., & Norton, D. P. (1996). *Translating strategy into action: The balanced scorecard.* Boston: Harvard Business School Press.

Kitchener, M. (2004). Exploding the merger myth in U.S. health care. In C. Harrington & C. L. Estes (Eds.), *Health policy: Crisis and reform in the U.S. health care delivery system* (4th ed., pp. 162–167). Sudbury, MA: Jones and Bartlett Publishers.

McGinnis, J. M., Williams-Russo, P., & Knickman, J. R. (2002). The case for more active policy attention to health promotion. *Health Affairs, 21*(2), 78–93.

Norrish, B., & Rundall, T. (2001). Hospital restructuring and the work of registered nurses. *The Milbank Quarterly, 79*(1), 55–79.

Shortell, S. M., Gillies, R. R., Anderson, D. A., Erickson, K. M., & Mitchell, J. B. (1996). *Remaking health care in America: Building organized delivery systems.* San Francisco: Jossey-Bass.

Starfield, B. (2000). Is U.S. health really the best in the world? *Journal of the American Medical Association, 284*(4), 483–485.

Chapter 11

Managed Care

Harry A. Sultz and
Kristina M. Young

CHAPTER OBJECTIVES

1. Discuss the historical development of managed care in the United States.
2. Identify the fundamental principles of managed care organizations and practices.
3. Apply current developments in the managed care industry and their impact on advanced nurse practitioners, other providers, and consumers.
4. Identify the role of government in managed care.

Introduction

The national movement to reform the way U.S. health care is financed and delivered emerged in the 1970s. Since 1900, the U.S. government had participated in relatively minor ways in providing and insuring medical care (e.g., workers' compensation benefits, welfare programs of the Social Security Administration). In 1965, the federal government committed to a role as a major payer with the passage of Medicare and Medicaid amendments to the Social Security Act.

Beginning in the 1950s, healthcare technology began developing and expanding at a rapid pace. Hospitals became high-technology centers, consuming upward spiraling volumes of resources in care delivery and billions of dollars in capital to expand, renovate, and update facil-

ities. Physician expenditures also spiraled upward, and costly specialty care burgeoned. By 1970, the U.S. healthcare delivery system had emerged as the world's undisputed leader in high-technology and sophisticated medicine, but not without high costs. In 1960, national hospital care expenditures totaled $9.3 billion; in 1970, $28.0 billion; and in 1980, $102.7 billion. In the decade 1980–1990, national hospital expenditures more than doubled again to $256.4 billion (Health Care Financing Administration, 2000a). Physician service expenditures saw parallel growth. In 1960, they totaled $5.3 billion. In 1970, they reached $13.6 billion, and by 1980, had more than tripled, totaling $45.2 billion. Between 1980 and 1990, physician service expenditures more than tripled again to a total of $146.3 billion

(Health Care Financing Administration, 2000b). In 2000, physician service expenditures stood at $286.4 billion (DHHS, 2002; see Figure 11–1). These increases could not be explained by national economic factors because the rate of growth vastly outstripped inflation and growth in the gross domestic product.

Distanced from the sting of rising healthcare costs by 30 years of employer-funded indemnity health insurance, working Americans used the delivery system without restrictions and very little, if any, cost consciousness. They grew to expect and demand what was perceived as the best care. For most, affordability or costs did not enter into the decision-making equation. Similarly, many physicians were untethered in their treatment decisions by economic considerations among their well-insured patients. The length of hospital stay and the use of consultant specialists and tests were at the physicians' sole medical and economic discretion, without financial implications for the patient.

In the period after Medicare and Medicaid enactment, the hospital industry flourished. In only 4 years after Medicare and Medicaid implementation, net voluntary hospital income increased from $227 million to $400 million (Stevens, 1989). The total assets of not-for-profit voluntary hospitals rose from $16.4 billion to $26.7 billion in the same period (Stevens, 1989). Concerns about rising costs and quality of services began only 1 year after Medicare and Medicaid were enacted and have sustained to the present. Congress and state governments tried with marginal success to reduce or slow the growth of absolute costs. It seemed, however, that no matter how cleverly structured or exquisitely sensitive the control effort, the system was equal to the challenge. The system responded with cost shifting, utilization volume increases,

Figure 11–1 Trend in National Healthcare Expenditures, Hospital Care and Physician Services, Selected Years

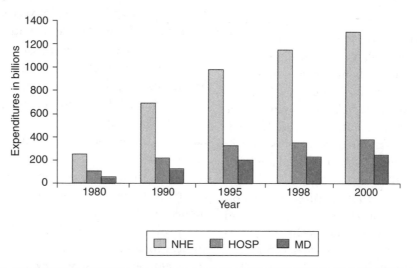

Source: Centers for Medicare and Medicaid Services, Office of the Actuary, National Health Statistics Group.

and justification for added technology and personnel. In addition, emerging environmental factors not within the system's control, such as growing poverty, the AIDS epidemic, inflation, and increasing societal ills, such as substance abuse and violence, added to healthcare costs.

Despite over 60 years of failed political attempts to address the need for national health insurance, it was the growing perception that the United States was losing its competitive base in world manufacturing markets because of escalating costs, in part attributable to employer health insurance expenditures that brought the need for broad reform to the forefront of the U.S. political scene. As Rosemary Stevens stated, "The driving force was cash" (1989, p. 287). In 1982, Chrysler found that it was paying more than $300 million a year for health care, but "didn't know what it was buying or from whom" (Stevens, 1989, p. 309). Lee Iacocca, then chairman of the Chrysler Corporation, went on record as saying that the cost of the company's health insurance premiums was adding an incremental cost to the price of their cars that, if unabated, soon would render the company unable to compete in the marketplace. This statement epitomized the by then ubiquitous signs that serious, major reform measures were necessary.

Throughout the 1980s and early 1990s, the federal administration made reform attempts through legislation introducing Medicare prospective payments, the resource-based relative value scale, and other incremental measures. However, none of these efforts could be characterized as anything other than specific cost-control measures, far from the sweeping reforms clearly needed—reforms that would not only control costs, but would also provide universal access to care for the growing numbers of medically uninsured or underinsured Americans. In 1992, President Bush proposed a type of reform based on a voucher system that would address access for the low-income working population by providing a tax credit to qualifying families. However, it was widely criticized and rapidly defeated as creating another federal financial burden and being ineffective in ensuring the universal access sought by more liberal forces.

The election of President Bill Clinton in 1992 began the first earnest effort to move comprehensive healthcare reform to the front of the political agenda; it became the subject of one of this nation's most widely publicized social reform movements in history. With universal access, a minimum level of benefits to every U.S. citizen, nationwide applications of cost-control strategies based in a competitive marketplace model, and mandated employer participation, Clinton's National Health Security Act attempted to address the concerns about the costs, quality, and access of the U.S. healthcare system of the past 50 years. By the fall of 1994, opposition precluded the bill from reaching the congressional floor. The momentum it created, however, by raising public and corporate awareness continued to fuel a reshaping of the U.S. system of healthcare financing and delivery that began in the mid-1970s. The influence of managed care, the rise of healthcare consumerism, and the impact of market forces joined to create a new healthcare marketplace.

Managed Care Fundamentals

Managed care embodies a direct relationship and interdependence between the provision of and payment for health care. Central to understanding managed care are the population orientation and the organization of care-providing groups or networks who take responsibility and usually share financial risk with the insurer for a population's medical care and health maintenance. The population basis enables the insurer to determine, from actuarial data, the projected use of services related to age, gender, and other factors. Levels of service utilization are estimated as a basis for expected costs over a defined time period. These estimates enable the insurer to establish premiums or charges for benefit coverage. Miller and Luft described the other characteristic of managed care plans—the provider network—as "the single most important feature distinguishing a managed care plan from an indemnity (fee-for-service) plan" (Miller, 1994, p. 439). That feature is key to enabling the insurer to exert influence over the delivery, use, and costs of services.

By linking the insurance of and delivery of services, managed care, in effect, reverses the financial incentives of providers in the fee-for-service model. Fee for service is essentially a piecework, pay-as-you-go system in which the care provider is financially rewarded for high use. The more services are provided, the greater is the reimbursement. Managed care, however, uses the concept of prepayment, in which care providers are paid in advance a preset amount for all of the services their insured population is projected to need in a given time period. Capitation, a method by which providers are paid for services on a per-member-per-month basis, is a common form of prepayment. The provider receives payment whether or not services are used. If a physician exceeds the predetermined payment level, he or she may suffer a financial loss. Similarly, if the physician uses fewer resources than predicted, the excess may be retained as profit.

Fee-for-service payments that withhold a portion of the customary fee (usually 15–20%) are another form of payment that seeks to provide positive financial incentives for efficient resource management. In the withhold scheme, physicians are provided a target amount of resources, usually on an annual basis, to provide a preestablished array of services to a defined population. If the target is met, the withheld amount is returned to the physician. If targets are exceeded, a financial penalty in the form of retention of all or a percentage of the withheld fees is incurred. The intent of these methods is to reverse the provider's financial incentives. Financial benefit derives from controlling, rather than promoting, utilization. Capitation and fee-for-service payments with withholding can be used with all types of individual and institutional providers.

Many other forms of physician payment in managed care systems that address the direction of financial incentives relative to achieving a more efficient use of resources exist. The key element of all such physician prepayment arrangements is to encourage cost-conscious, efficient, and effective care.

The concept of prepayment has been used for decades among certain employer groups that contracted with physician groups and hospitals to serve their employees on a prepaid basis. It was not until the 1970s, however, when increasing concerns over the rising costs of employee health benefits to businesses prompted passage of the Health Maintenance Organization (HMO) Act of 1973, that managed care and the concept of prepayment were thrust into the national forefront.

It is important to distinguish the definition of HMO from the broader definition of managed care. HMOs are organizations or legally organized entities that share the common characteristic of responsibility for both financing and delivering comprehensive healthcare services to a defined group of beneficiaries or members for a prepaid, fixed fee. The HMO's responsibility both for financing and providing healthcare services distinguishes it from the fee-for-service system, in which insurance companies are responsible for reimbursing either the provider or the member for the costs of care but carry no responsibility for providing care or arranging it.

Managed care, although the term implies organization of care, does not in itself refer to any particular type of organizational entity. Managed care rather refers to a body of principles and concepts that govern a variety of insurer and provider relationships. Implicit in the body of principles and concepts is that provision of services is dependent upon provision of payment. Also implicit in the definition of managed care is a requirement of oversight of the enrolled population's use of medical resources as a function of providers' behaviors. The principles and concepts of managed care operate on the assumption that the linkages of service provision and its reimbursement are based on a defined population group for whose insurance a set premium is charged and for whom service costs are reimbursed on a prepaid basis. From its earliest roots, which can be traced back more than 70 years to prepaid health plans, the goal of managed care has been to control costs by controlling healthcare utilization.

With this definition in mind, it becomes clear that HMOs represent a form of managed care but that a virtually infinite number of other provider/insurer relationships are possible using managed care principles. Although managed care and HMOs are not technically synonymous, all HMOs use the concepts and principles of managed care with the goal of controlling costs by controlling utilization. The achievement of this goal is largely based on the transfer of some measure of financial risk from the insurer to the care providers. To a lesser extent, use and, therefore, cost control are also attempted by some managed care plans that transfer some financial risk from the insurer to the managed care member. Transfers of financial risk most commonly take the form of co-payments and deductibles. Co-payments require the member to pay a set fee each time a covered service is received, such as a co-payment for each physician office visit. A deductible requires the member to meet a predetermined, out-of-pocket expenditure level before the managed care organization (MCO) assumes payment responsibility for the balance of charges. Typically, deductible requirements are set for a specific time period and do not carry forward into succeeding periods.

HMO Act of 1973

The HMO Act of 1973 provided both loans and grants for the planning, development, and implementation of combined insurance and healthcare delivery organizations and required that a minimum prescribed array of services be included in the HMO arrangement. These mandated services included

- Physician care
- Outpatient services
- Short-term mental health services
- Specified substance abuse treatment
- Laboratory and radiology services
- Home health care
- Family planning services
- Specified social services

- Immunizations and other preventive health services
- Health education
- Emergency care arrangements
- Arrangements for out-of-area coverage

This legislation also mandated that employers with 25 or more employees offer an HMO option if one was available in their area. The legislation required that employers contribute to employees' HMO premiums in an amount equal to what they contributed to an indemnity plan premium. Initially, this employer mandate helped stimulate growth of HMO membership in regions where federally funded and qualified plans were first established.

As authorized by the 1973 legislation, HMOs were organizations that combined providers and insurers into one organizational entity. As originally established, members of HMOs usually were required to obtain all of their medical care within the organization.

Initially, there were two major types of HMOs. The first was a group, or staff, model and was the type most commonly established from the initial HMO legislation. It employed groups of physicians to provide the majority of ambulatory care needs of its members. Some specialty services were often provided within the HMO and by community physicians under a contracted arrangement with the HMO. In the staff model, the HMO also operated the facilities in which its physicians practiced, providing onsite ancillary support services, such as radiology, laboratory, and pharmacy services. The HMO usually purchased hospital care and other services for its members through fee-for-service or prepaid, contracted arrangements. Established in 1938, the Kaiser-Permanente Health Care System, an early forerunner of the HMO movement, became among the best known staff model HMOs. Staff model HMOs were referred to as "closed panel" because they employed the physicians who provided the majority of their members' care, and those physicians did not provide services outside of the HMO membership. Similarly, community-based physicians could not participate in HMO member care without prearrangement or authorization by the HMO.

The second type of HMO stimulated by the 1973 legislation was the individual practice association (IPA). IPAs are physician organizations comprised of community-based independent physicians, in solo or group practices, who provide services to HMO members. An IPA HMO, therefore, did not operate facilities in which members receive care, but rather provided its members services through private physician office practices. Like the staff model HMO, hospital care and specialty services not available through IPA-participating physicians could be purchased by the HMO from other area providers, either on a prepaid or fee-for-service basis. IPA physicians were allowed to have a nonexclusive relationship with their HMO that permitted them to treat nonmembers as well as members. However, HMO relationships with an IPA could also be established on an exclusive basis. In this scenario, an HMO took the initiative in recruiting and organizing community physicians into an IPA for the purpose of serving its members. Because the HMO was the organizing force in such an arrangement, it was common for the HMO to require exclusivity by the IPA, limiting its services only to that HMO's membership (Kongstvedt, 1989).

The staff model and IPA-type organizations illustrate two major types of HMOs, but each type spawned several hybrids since the 1973 HMO Act. Other major forms of MCOs emerged throughout the 1980s in response to national cost and quality concerns, notably on the part of the federal government and industry as the major health insurance purchasers. Peter Kongstvedt identified three additional HMO models as the most common: group practice, network, and direct contract (Kongstvedt, 1989). In a group practice model, an HMO typically contracts with a multispecialty group practice to provide all of the physician services required by the HMO's enrollees. The physicians remain independent—employed by their group rather than the HMO. Such an arrangement may or may not be exclusive. Depending on the terms of their HMO contract, these physicians may be allowed to see patients insured by other entities or restricted in their practice to see only members of a particular HMO. In the network model HMO, the HMO contracts with more than one group practice and may maintain contracts with several physician groups representing both primary care and specialty practices. The direct contract model HMOs maintain contractual relationships with individual physicians, in contrast to the physician groups as in the IPA and network models. The direct contract approach, although more cumbersome to administer than the other models, gives the HMO the advantages of maintaining a higher level of control over fee arrangements by reducing physician negotiating power to an individual basis and avoiding the risk of lost services to its members by contractual termination of a large group of providers.

The Evolution of Managed Care

Between 1992 and 2000, nationwide managed care enrollment doubled to over 80 million members (The Henry J. Kaiser Family Foundation, 2002; see Figure 11–2). As enrollment accelerated, concerns emerged about MCO restrictions on consumer choice of providers and services. In response, the MCOs spawned what have become known as point-of-service (POS) plans that allow members to use providers outside the MCOs' approved provider networks. To exercise this choice, POS members are charged co-payments and deductibles higher than those charged for in-network services. As managed care enrollment increased and the market became increasingly competitive, MCOs developed more flexible plan offerings that, although more costly to consumers, allowed for more choice in providers. In 2004, POS plans represented 15% of total managed care enrollment (The Henry J. Kaiser Family Foundation and Health Research and Educational Trust, 2004).

Concurrent with the growth of the HMO and managed care movement throughout the 1980s, another organizational entity arose, not technically defined as an HMO, but encompassing important managed care characteristics. Preferred provider organizations (PPOs) were formed by physicians and hospitals to serve the needs of private, third-party payer, and self-insured firms. Through these arrangements, PPOs guarantee a certain volume of business to hospitals and physicians in return for a negotiated discount in fees. PPOs offer attractive features to both physicians and hospitals. Physicians are not required to share in any financial risk as a condition of participation, and PPOs reimburse physicians on the fee-for-service basis to which they are accustomed. By providing predictable admission volume, PPOs helped hospitals to shore up declining occupancy rates and attenuate the competition for

Figure 11–2 Number of Managed Care Enrollees, Selected Years, 1988–2000.

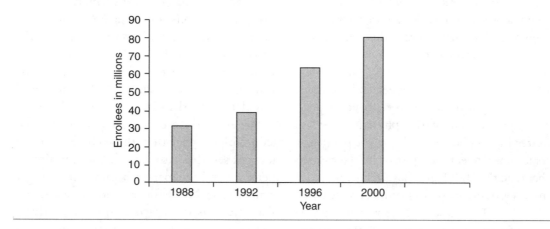

Source: Adapted from The Henry J. Kaiser Family Foundation, "Trends and Indicators in the Changing Healthcare Marketplace," *2002 Chartbook.*

admissions with other hospitals. To control costs, PPOs used negotiated discount fees, requirements that members receive care exclusively from contracted providers (or incur financial penalty), requirements for preauthorization of hospital admission, and second opinions for major procedures, such as surgery. PPOs maintain systems of utilization review and review of hospital lengths of stay as both a prospective and retrospective means to control costs and advocate for more efficient service utilization by hospitals and physicians. As of 2004, PPOs were the most popular managed care plans, with a 55% market share (The Henry J. Kaiser Family Foundation and Health Research and Educational Trust, 2004; see Figure 11–3).

As MCOs continued growing in size and numbers, their organizational forms became significantly more diversified to respond to marketplace demands and to manage operational costs and maximize profits. In 1988, staff models constituted about 42% of MCO member-

ship. By 1999, they represented less than 1% (Interstudy Publications, 1999). This change occurred because of several factors. Staff model MCOs, confronted by the need to expand, were faced with the large capital outlay requirements of constructing or purchasing additional facilities. Increased competition from expanding IPA models, often in the position to offer enrollment without requiring new members to switch physicians for themselves or their dependents, was another factor. Staff model MCOs needed the flexibility of their IPA counterparts to remain competitive in an expanding marketplace. In response, both staff model and group MCOs have increasingly transformed into mixed models that operate both the traditional staff model and an IPA model through contracts with community physicians and practice groups. In 1990, approximately one third of staff models were mixed models. By 1994, 57% of staff models were operating as mixed-model MCOs (Gabel, 1997).

Figure 11–3 Health Plan Enrollment for Covered Workers, by Plan Type, 1988–2004.

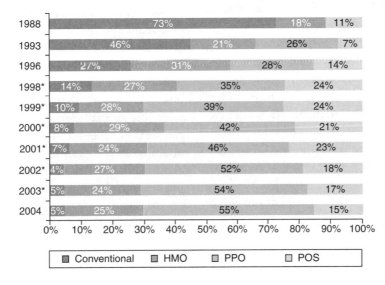

*Distribution is statistically different from the previous year shown at p < 0.5

Source: The Henry J. Kaiser Family Foundation and Health Research and Educational Trust: "Health Employer Benefits 2004 Annual Survey."

MCOs continue offering increasingly diversified products and services to maintain the highest appeal to employer purchasers seeking the cost savings that result from employees' transfer from indemnity plans to MCOs. The ability of an MCO to offer what has become known as the triple option, which includes HMO, PPO, and POS plans, is believed to increase purchaser appeal and competitiveness.

Other trends that emerged in MCOs included increased shifting of financial risk from MCOs to physicians, primarily through increased use of capitation. MCOs also increased patient cost-sharing requirements in the form of co-payments and deductibles as an effort to hold down premiums. Increased patient cost sharing also has been shown to decrease the use of services.

Researchers at Group Health Cooperative of Puget Sound found that adding a $5 co-payment resulted in an 11% reduction in primary care visits, a 3% reduction in specialists visits, and a 14% decrease in physical examinations (Cherkin, Grothaus, & Wagner, 1989). Another trend has been MCOs' increased use of clinical practice guidelines that provide uniform protocols for the treatment of specified medical conditions. Guidelines are advocated by MCOs as one means to promote consistency in clinical practice and thereby reduce costs. Guidelines are assumed by many to promote the quality of clinical outcomes by helping to decrease variability in provider practices. However, because of inadequate data and tracking systems, the process of medical care and its outcomes in MCOs continue to pose important questions about guidelines and their contributions to controlling costs or improving quality (Timmermans & Mauck, 2005).

Whatever the form of organization providing managed care, the inherent operating principles of these organizations recognize that the cost drivers are the forms of payment to providers and incentives implicit to them. There is a massive body of literature spanning 40 years of research suggesting that higher healthcare expenditures do not in all cases contribute to and, in fact, may detract from the quality of care rendered through medical interventions. More recent research data also suggest that major cost savings could be realized by a higher level of scrutiny of the appropriateness of the interventions used (Kovner, 1995). Both directly (by changing reimbursement incentives) and indirectly (by instituting quality control measures that seek to standardize care practices and decrease variation in resource use for the treatment of common illnesses), managed care principles resulted in major shifts in the patient, provider, and payer relationships.

The effects of physician prepayment and the accompanying share of financial risk have a direct impact on the healthcare delivery system far beyond the impact of individual practitioners. Physicians are the predominant influence over the use of virtually all patient care resources. They largely control all hospital admissions, prescription pharmaceuticals consumptions, and laboratory, imaging, and other diagnostic service use. They also control the extent of use of specialty services, surgical services, home health care, and rehabilitation care. Because of the central role of physicians in controlling healthcare resource consumption, MCOs of all types continue to place heavy emphasis on the physician behavior aspect of their systems.

One additional feature common to physician performance in managed care is the emphasis placed on the role of the primary care physician. In recognition of and response to rising concerns about the overuse of specialists and its attendant costs, primary care physicians were assigned the major role in managed care systems. Dubbed "gatekeepers," they are viewed as the most influential resource in ensuring appropriate, timely, and coordinated patient care. By requiring passage through the primary care gate, MCOs seek to avoid unnecessary use of high-cost services for complaints that can be treated effectively at the primary level. Authorization of specialty referrals by the primary physician is used to help ensure coordination and avoid duplication of these services.

Emerging Developments in Managed Care

Today, over 159 million Americans, more than 90% of all privately insured individuals, receive their health insurance through their employer (Fronstin, 2004). In 2004, 95% of all workers covered by employer health benefits were enrolled in some type of managed care plan; only 5% were enrolled in conventional type plans (The Henry J. Kaiser Family Foundation and Health Research and Educational Trust, 2004). The surge in employee enrollment in managed care throughout the 1990s, with accompanying decreases in premium costs, is acknowledged as a significant contributor to the decline witnessed in the average annual growth of national healthcare expenditures throughout this period (U.S. Congressional Budget Office, 1998).

After 4 years of declining costs, health insurance premiums began increasing again in 1998. In that year, premiums rose 8.2%, more than double the increase of the 3 prior years (Levit et al., 2000). Many reasons were offered for the rise in premiums, including the insurance underwriting cycle, in which insurers underprice during periods of market growth and then increase premiums later to restore profitability. Managed care plans realized high profitability in the early 1990s, when large-scale migration occurred from traditional health insurance to managed care plans. After this period of major growth, in 1996 and 1997 nearly two thirds of managed care plans and health insurers suffered losses (National Coalition on Health Care, 2000). Other reasons cited for increasing premiums included investor pressure on insurers to increase profits, rapidly escalating prescription drug costs and use, consumer demands for more choice and access to services, and increasingly difficult negotiations with providers seeking higher reimbursement (National Coalition on Health Care, 2000).

The year 2004 was the fourth consecutive year of health insurance premium increases, although growth slowed from the record pace of 2003. Between 2001 and 2002, premiums rose 12.7%, the largest increase in health insurance costs since 1990 (see Figure 11–4). Unlike earlier increases attributed to the insurance underwriting cycle, current increases reflect insurers' anticipation of higher claims expense, including prescription drug costs (Centers for Medicare and Medicaid Services, 2004b).

The rise in premiums carries significant implications. Increased premium costs, coupled with requirements for larger employee contributions, cause workers to drop coverage. This effect increases in severity as the annual earnings of employees decrease, meaning that lower wage workers who can least afford the risk of high healthcare costs are the most likely to become uninsured. Increased premiums cause employers to pass along higher shares of premium expenses to workers, resulting in significant increases in out-of-pocket employee expenditures. Through what are termed *benefit buy-downs*, employers may shift costs to employees by reducing benefits, requiring more premium cost sharing, higher co-payments, and/or coinsurance and higher co-pays for prescription drugs (Centers for Medicare and Medicaid Services, 2004a). Some experts estimate that for every 1% increase in premiums, 300,000 individuals lose their health insurance coverage (National Coalition on Health Care, 2000). Since 2002, PPO deductibles and employee contributions for all firms have risen 50% (Gabel, Whitmore, Rice, & Lo Sasso, 2004). Cost shifting trends have clear implications for increasing the number of uninsured Americans.

In what is termed the managed care backlash that began in the late 1990s, organized medicine, other healthcare providers, and consumers railed against MCO policies on choice of providers, referrals, and other practices that were viewed as unduly restrictive. A presidential commission was established to review the need for guidelines in the managed care industry (Blendon et al., 1998). In 1998, the president imposed patient protection requirements on private insurance companies providing health coverage to federal workers (Havemann, 1999). Public dissatisfaction with constraints over the right to receive care deemed necessary and the freedom of physicians to refer patients to specialists received wide publicity. Public concerns driving sentiments toward more government regulation of the managed care industry included the belief that managed care

Figure 11-4 Increases in Health Insurance Premiums Compared to Other Indicators, 1988–2004.

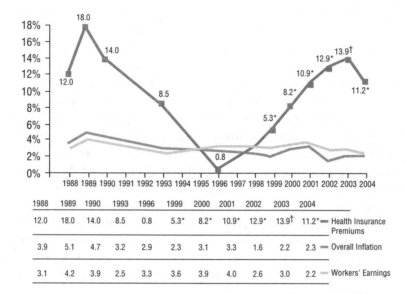

1988	1989	1990	1993	1996	1999	2000	2001	2002	2003	2004	
12.0	18.0	14.0	8.5	0.8	5.3*	8.2*	10.9*	12.9*	13.9†	11.2*■	Health Insurance Premiums
3.9	5.1	4.7	3.2	2.9	2.3	3.1	3.3	1.6	2.2	2.3	■ Overall Inflation
3.1	4.2	3.9	2.5	3.3	3.6	3.9	4.0	2.6	3.0	2.2	▬ Workers' Earnings

*Estimate is statistically different from the previous year shown at $p < 0.05$.
†Estimate is statistically different from the previous year shown at $p < 0.10$.
Note: Data on premium increases reflect the cost of health insurance premiums for a family of four. Historical estimates of workers' earnings have been updated to reflect new industry classifications (NAICS).

Source: The Henry J. Kaiser Family Foundation and Health Research and Educational Trust: "Health Employer Benefits 2004 Annual Survey."

was hurting the quality of patient care and that the managed care industry was not doing as good a job for patients as other sectors of the healthcare industry. Compiled results from a series of public opinion polls shed light on Americans' sentiments about managed care, other healthcare institutions, and the services of other industries. Results demonstrate that in terms of service to consumers, other industries rate well above MCOs. Between 1997 and 2000, the proportion of people who said that managed care companies are doing a good job for consumers declined by 21 percentage points, and managed care con-

sumer satisfaction ranks only slightly above tobacco and oil companies (The Henry J. Kaiser Family Foundation, 2004a; see Table 11–1). First introduced in 1998, a federal patient bill of rights failed to pass. The Bipartisan Patient Protection Act of 2001, introduced by Senators Kennedy and McCain, passed both houses of Congress, but remains in limbo. The states have taken the lead in this arena. By 1999, more than 1,000 managed care laws were enacted by state legislatures (Rogal & Stenger, 2001).

In another response to the managed care backlash, increasing numbers of employers

Table 11-1 CONSUMER VIEWS OF CUSTOMER SERVICE ACROSS VARIOUS INDUSTRIES, 2004

Companies	Percent of Consumers Saying "Good Job"
Tobacco	30
Oil	32
Managed care	38
Pharmaceutical	44
Life insurance	55
Hospitals	78
Airlines	74
Supermarkets	87

Source: Adapted from The Henry J. Kaiser Family Foundation, Health Poll Report, July/August 2004 edition.

began allowing employees to make personal decisions about their coverage, retreating from the standard practice of the employer making benefit decisions on employees' behalf. This movement, dubbed "consumer-driven" health plans, attempts to make patients more knowledgeable about their healthcare choices and associated costs through the provision of comparative information, both in Web-based and traditional formats. Three types of plans are offered. The first uses an account against which the employee may draw to purchase care. When the account is exhausted, employees pay out-of-pocket until an annual deductible is satisfied, after which a major medical plan is activated. The second type allows employees to design their own provider networks and benefits based on anticipated needs and costs. The third uses Web-based information to enable employees to choose from established groupings of provider networks and benefits to customize coverage. It is estimated that about 1% of the employer coverage market, or 1.5 million employees, are enrolled in consumer-driven plans (Gabel, Lo

Sasso, & Rice, 2002). Predictions vary widely regarding the future of such arrangements in the health insurance marketplace. Experts are calling for additional research on the impacts of such plans on care quality, consumer satisfaction, access, and costs (Gabel et al., 2002).

MCOs have undergone many changes in their operating policies, mergers, and consolidations. The most prominent changes have come as responses to consumer demands reflected by state patient protection legislation, a loosening of early restrictions on patient choice of provider, provider specialty referrals, and patient access to information about operating policies, especially regarding denials of payment. A literature analysis of MCO performance between 1997 and 2001 indicates that overall, MCOs have not accomplished their early promises to change clinical practice and improve quality while lowering costs. Analysis findings suggest that a systematic revamping of information systems, coupled with appropriate incentives and revised clinical processes, will be required to produce the desired changes (Miller & Luft, 2002). Recent information indicates that employers are reintroducing previously applied restrictions in their managed care plans in the effort to contain rising costs (Mays, Claxton, & White, 2004).

Medicare and Medicaid Managed Care

The creation of the Medicare+Choice program through the Balanced Budget Act of 1997 (BBA) signaled a new effort to reform the Medicare program. The BBA intended to expand Medicare managed care enrollments by offering a large number of new plan options that include HMOs, preferred provider plans, provider-sponsored organizations, and other insurance plans operated with medical savings accounts. The major models included Medicare risk plans and cost plans. In risk plans, Medicare pays a per-member premium, established on a county-of-residence basis. Risk plans initially required members to receive all of their services within the plan's provider service networks, but were later modified to allow out-of-network options. Typically, risk plans provide coverage for all Medicare-required services and offer additional coverage for added benefits such as pharmacy and vision care. Medicare cost plans reimburse HMOs a predetermined monthly amount per beneficiary based on a total projected budget. Adjustments for variations are made at year end. Unlike in the risk plans, cost plan members were free to obtain services outside of the managed care provider network. Medicare would pay its standard reimbursement, with the member responsible for coinsurance and deductibles.

In 2004, Medicare managed care enrollment stood at 4.6 million, representing 11% of total Medicare beneficiaries and a decline of 1.7 million managed care participants since 2000 (The Henry J. Kaiser Family Foundation, 2004b). Medicare payment reductions, complex administration, market competition, and other factors took a toll on the Medicare+Choice program. After rapid growth in the number of Medicare HMOs available during the 1990s, participation declined (see Figure 11–5). In 1998, there were 346 Medicare HMOs available; by 2004, there were only 145 (The Henry J. Kaiser Family Foundation, 2004b).

The Medicare Prescription and Drug Improvement and Modernization Act of 2003 (MMA), renamed the Medicare+Choice program to Medicare Advantage and added regional PPOs as another plan option (The Henry J. Kaiser Family Foundation, 2004c). Significant changes from prior plan options include new lock-in periods for disenrollment and plan changes, new discounts for drugs beginning in 2004, and payment for drugs beginning in 2006 that will base co-payments and deductibles on income. Drawing on prior negative experiences with provider withdrawals from participation in Medicare+Choice, the Centers for Medicare and Medicaid Services has incorporated features into Medicare Advantage to attract and retain MCO participation. Features include reducing administrative requirements, reducing report duplication, providing start-up funding, sharing financial risk, and providing bonuses (Centers for Medicare and Medicaid Services, 2005). The Medicare managed care option was initially created to improve efficiency and to improve access and coordination of care for beneficiaries. Its history in producing these results has been mixed. Results of the MMA in terms of cost, quality, and provider and beneficiary satisfaction await future assessment (The Henry J. Kaiser Family Foundation, 2004b).

Figure 11-5 Medicare+Choice/Medicare Advantage Plans, 1990–2004.

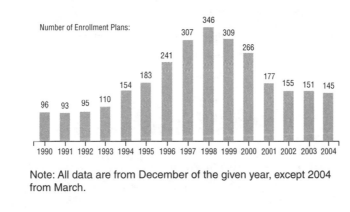

Note: All data are from December of the given year, except 2004 from March.

Source: The Henry J. Kaiser Family Foundation, "Medicare Advantage Fact Sheet," March 2004. The Kaiser Foundation is an independent healthcare philanthropy and is not associated with Kaiser Permanente or Kaiser Industries.

Medicaid managed care enrollment reached 25.2 million by 2003, 59% of the total national Medicaid enrollment (Centers for Medicare and Medicaid Services, 2004; see Table 11–2). All 50 states currently offer some type of Medicaid managed care plans. Managed care for Medicaid recipients is intended to improve access through the establishment of contracted provider networks and promote greater accountability for quality and costs. Enrollment can be either voluntary or mandatory, depending on a particular state's decision. Before the BBA, states wishing to enact mandatory enrollment were required to obtain a federal waiver. Provisions of the BBA lifted this requirement. Where managed care enrollment is mandatory, states are required to offer a choice of managed care plans and make efforts to inform beneficiaries about their choices and how to access enrollment sites.

In general, Medicaid managed care plans use three plan models: primary care case manage-

ment, full-risk HMOs, and prepaid health plans (Holahan, Zuckerman, Evans, & Rangarajan, 1998). Historically, states had difficulty obtaining arrangements with commercial HMOs for Medicaid clients. As a result, several states created Medicaid-only plans. However, with more states mandating HMO enrollment and private sector competition for payments increasing, plans are more amenable to enrolling Medicaid clients.

Carve-outs is a term frequently associated with Medicaid managed care plans. A carve-out refers to one or more services for which a managed care plan is not obligated to provide coverage under its contract with Medicaid. Coverage for services is carved out because a managed care plan is either unable (because of unavailability of services) or unwilling (because of potentially high costs, questionable medical necessity, or both) to include selected services in its Medicaid managed care contract (Holahan et

Table 11-2 MEDICAID POPULATION AND NUMBERS AND PERCENT OF MEDICAID
MANAGED CARE ENROLLMENT, 1996–2003

Year	Total Medicaid Population	Managed Care Population	Other Population	% Managed Care Enrollment
2003	42,740,719	25,262,873	17,477,846	59.11%
2002	40,147,539	23,117,668	17,029,871	57.58%
2001	36,562,567	20,773,813	15,788,754	56.82%
2000	33,690,364	18,786,137	14,904,227	55.76%
1999	31,940,188	17,756,603	14,183,585	55.59%
1998	30,896,635	16,573,996	14,322,639	53.64%
1997	32,092,380	15,345,502	16,746,878	47.82%
1996	33,241,147	13,330,119	19,911,028	40.10%

Source: Centers for Medicare and Medicaid Services.

al., 1998). Mental health and substance abuse treatment services are those most commonly carved out. By retaining the risk for carved-out services, states have been able to increase the involvement of more commercial HMOs in the care of Medicaid recipients. Medicaid has not been immune to rising costs seen in Medicare and the private sector. Medicaid cost growth has outpaced both Medicare and private spending growth trends since 1998, becoming the second largest cost outlay in most state expenditures after education (Centers for Medicare and Medicaid Services, 2004b).

Managed Care Organizations and Quality

As managed care became the predominant mode of healthcare financing, concerns about the quality of care and the criteria and processes used to monitor and report it received increased scrutiny by physicians, other health professionals, the professional literature, the popular media, purchasers, and consumers. Also, with the growth of Medicare and Medicaid managed care enrollment, government and public policy makers became increasingly involved in quality issues. The intensity of scrutiny increased in part because of concerns that as MCOs become more competitive they would reduce services or more tightly restrict their use in the effort to hold down premiums.

Nationally, the most influential MCO quality assurance body is the National Committee on Quality Assurance (NCQA). The NCQA was formed in 1979 in a joint effort of two managed care trade organizations, the American Managed Care and Review Association and Group Health Association of America. The two organizations first merged to become the American Association of Health Plans and then created the NCQA when it appeared that the federal government was considering establishing an entity to monitor health plans. In 1990, the NCQA became an independent, not-for-profit organization, with its primary source of revenue generated from fees for accreditation services (Iglehart, 1996).

Managed care plan organization accreditation by a nationally recognized, independent organization rose in significance among employers, other purchasers, the professional community, and the public. This trend has resulted in increased demands for the NCQA's accreditation services and a doubling of its operations budget since 1993 (Iglehart, 1996). The NCQA evaluates participating organizations on a voluntary request basis, through three primary means. It conducts detailed, on-site reviews of key clinical and administrative processes, uses the Health Plan Employer Data and Information Set to collect data on key health care indicators, and conducts comprehensive managed care subscriber satisfaction surveys (National Committee on Quality Assurance, n.d.). The accreditation process includes advance collection and review of organizational information, and a 3- or 4-day visit by an NCQA team of physicians (often medical directors of other plans) and support staff. The review focuses on six major areas: management, physician credentials, member rights and responsibilities, preventive health services, utilization, and medical records. Samples of actual medical records are reviewed for diagnostic accuracy, appropriateness of care, diagnosis follow-through, and the use of preventive services. MCOs may be granted accreditation for 3 years, 1 year, or on a provisional basis. Beginning in 1999, the NCQA began including outcomes of care and measures of clinical processes in its accreditation reviews, increasing the likelihood that accreditation status will accurately reflect the quality of care delivered (Pawlson & O'Kane, 2002).

The Health Plan Employer Data and Information Set (HEDIS) evolved from a partnership among health plans, employers, and the NCQA in 1989 (Altman & Reinhardt, 1996). It provides a standardized method for MCOs to collect, calculate, and report information about their performance to allow employers, other purchasers, and consumers to compare different plans. HEDIS has evolved through several stages of development and refinements and continues to do so, particularly as it is adapted for use in the Medicare and Medicaid managed care programs. A general version contains 71 measures of MCO performance, divided into the following eight categories:

1. Effectiveness of care—members' receipt of services within specific time frames and the use of preventive services
2. Accessibility and availability of care—timeliness of care, without undue inconvenience
3. Satisfaction with care—summaries of member opinions about the managed care organization and its services
4. Costs of care—premiums, deductibles, and coinsurance
5. Health plan stability—status of the provider network, membership and enrollment trends, organizational structure, and financial status
6. Informed choices—patient education and other efforts to involve members in decisions about their health care
7. Utilization—the rates at which members use services and procedures

8. Descriptive information—factors that define and characterize the MCO and quality improvement activities (Grimaldi, 1997)

Each category also contains its own specific performance measures.

The HEDIS reports are published by the NCQA and often are referred to as MCO report cards. They are available to purchasers and to the public on a Web site (Pawlson & O'Kane, 2002).

A special adaptation of HEDIS was released to the states in 1996 for use in monitoring the performance of contractors providing Medicaid managed care services. The reports are intended to assist MCOs with quality improvement efforts, support states in informing Medicaid recipients about MCO performance, and promote standardization of managed care reporting across the public and private sectors (Grimaldi, 1997). Beginning in 1997, MCOs with Medicare risk contracts were required to provide the Health Care Financing Administration with reports on certain HEDIS measures for their Medicare members.

HEDIS has several significant limitations, which include

- The accuracy of the data is not independently verified.
- Compliance with NCQA reporting guidelines is not independently verified.
- Aggregation precludes analytic flexibility.
- The absence of risk adjustment can produce misleading conclusions.

There is also an overriding concern that report card indicators may be incorporated without adequate scientific proof that they are related to the quality of care (Altman et al., 1996). Nonetheless, the NCQA/HEDIS data provide an important means of accountability to the purchasers and consumers of health care and feedback to its providers that is critical in efforts to achieve improvement. In 2004, 563 commercial Medicare and Medicaid managed health plans with enrollment of over 69 million members representing about one fourth of all Americans reported results to the NCQA. Benchmarked against the performance of the top 10% of all participating health plans, these data disclose quality disparities and gaps that inform purchasers, plan administrators, and policy makers. Comparisons allow the calculation of numbers of avoidable illnesses and deaths for several of the most common costly and deadly health conditions (National Committee on Quality Assurance, 2004). The overarching goal is to showcase excellent performance and create incentives for poorer performers to improve. The NCQA has pay-for-performance initiatives under way that advocate recognition and financial reward for physicians and hospitals that demonstrate outstanding preventive and caregiving practices (National Committee on Quality Assurance, 2004).

MCOs also apply numerous internal techniques to manage quality, many of which directly or indirectly relate to physician performance. Much attention also is focused on the quality of the institutional providers, especially on the hospitals with which they contract for services. Database systems are used to track use of services on both a prospective and retrospective basis to control resource use and monitor quality. Some MCOs employ nurses or other clinically trained professionals to follow potentially expensive cases to ensure care coordination and avoid misuse or duplication of services. The methods being used by MCOs to maintain control of costs and promote quality are numerous, diverse, and growing in sophistication.

The Future of Managed Care

MCOs were at the forefront of reforming the healthcare system's administration and financing. A slowing growth rate of national healthcare expenditures was attributed in significant measure to the growth in MCO enrollment (Levit, Lazenby, Braden, & the National Health Accounts Team, 1998). However, analysts' earlier predictions that managed care premiums would rise materially in 1998 and beyond have proven true. Regulations created in response to the managed care backlash, coupled with new developments in expensive technology, economic and business conditions, and consumer demands, have resulted in significant increases in health insurance costs. Regulation, in addition to a trend that has seen the costs of benefits rising faster than premiums, is resulting in increased costs to employers as well as to consumers through premium increases.

Cost-control initiatives continue to develop as the system evolves. One such initiative is disease management, through which insurers attempt to improve communication, follow-up, and management of patients with chronic conditions with the hope of avoiding costly, unnecessary hospitalizations and emergency treatment. Early research findings on cost savings are equivocal and await further studies to demonstrate whether disease management will actually result in real cost savings (Fireman, Bartlett, & Selby, 2004).

Another development that is likely to bear significant impact on managed care's future is the continuing evolution of the tangled history of the Employee Retirement Income Security Act (ERISA). This act preempts all state laws that relate to employee benefits plans and has been the subject of many years of disputes regarding consumer challenges of managed care regulations under state laws. In 2004, the U.S. Supreme Court upheld the decision that beneficiaries of employment-related managed care plans cannot hold the plans accountable for damages when injured as a result of coverage denial decisions. This decision effectively insulates employment-related health plans from liability for consequences of their treatment decisions until the Congress acts on a managed care bill of rights that establishes national policy for the redress of MCO decisions (Stoltzfus Jost, 2004).

One observation likely to hold true for the foreseeable future is that the market forces in the managed healthcare industry will continue to exert a more fast-paced, pervasive, and high-impact series of effects than initiatives forthcoming from state or federal legislatures. It is likely that states will continue efforts to regulate managed care plans in response to consumer and provider pressures and that interest groups will advocate for an increasing array of mandated benefits and protections. Consolidations and mergers among MCOs are predicted to continue as the market evolves, though at a slower pace than witnessed during the earlier stages of market competition.

Discussion Questions

1. Discuss the historical development of managed care and how it influences the practice of nursing and advanced practice nursing currently.
2. Identify the fundamental principles of managed care organizations and practices. What are the implications for the practice of advanced nursing?
3. How will the current developments and projected trends in the managed care industry impact advanced nurse practitioners, relationships with other providers, and consumers?

References

Altman, S. H., & Reinhardt, U. E. (1996). *Strategic choices for a changing health care system.* Chicago: Health Administration Press.

Blendon, R. J., Brodie, M., Benson, J. M., Altman, D. E., Levitt, L., Hoff, T., et al. (1998). Understanding the managed care backlash. *Health Affairs, 17*(4), 80.

Centers for Medicare and Medicaid Services. (2004a, September 16). *2003 Medicaid managed care enrollment report: National penetration rates from 1996–2003.* Retrieved January 12, 2005, from http://www.cms.hhs.gov/medicaid/managedcare/mmcss03.asp

Centers for Medicare and Medicaid Services. (2004b, March). *Health care industry market update, managed care.* Retrieved October 12, 2007, from http://www.cms.hhs.gov/CapMarketUpdates/Downloads/hcimu32403.pdf

Centers for Medicare and Medicaid Services. (2005, January 21). *Ensuring the success of the new Medicare Advantage program.* Issue Paper no. 28. Retrieved February 4, 2005, from http://www.cms.hhs.gov/medicarereform/issuespapers/title1and2/files/issue_paper_28_-_ensuring_success_for_ma_program.pdf

Cherkin, D., Grothaus, L., & Wagner, E. H. (1989, July). The effect of office visit co-payments on utilization in a health maintenance organization. *Medical Care,* 669–678.

Department of Health and Human Services, Center for Medicare and Medicaid Services, Office of the Actuary: National Health Statistics Group. (2002,

July 17). *National health expenditures aggregate amounts and average annual percent change, by type of expenditure: Selected calendar years, 1980–2000,* 1–5. Retrieved November 29, 2002, from http://cms.hhs.gov./statistics/nhe/historical/t2.asp

Fireman, B., Bartlett, J., & Selby, J. (2004). Can disease management reduce health care costs by improving quality? *Health Affairs, 23*(6), 71–74.

Fronstin, P. (2004, December). *Sources of health insurance and characteristics of the uninsured: Analysis of the March 2004 current population survey.* Issue Brief no. 276. Washington: Employee Benefit Research Institute. Retrieved October 12, 2007, from http://www.ebri.org/pdf/briefspdf/1204ib1.pdf

Gabel, J. (1997). Ten ways HMOs have changed during the 1990s. *Health Affairs, 16*(3), 136.

Gabel, J., Lo Sasso, A. T., & Rice, T. (2002, November 20). Consumer-driven health plans: Are they more than talk now? *Health Affairs Web Exclusives,* W403. Retrieved October 12, 2007, from http://content.healthaffairs.org/cgi/content/full/hlthaff.w2.395v1/DC1

Gabel, J. R., Whitmore, H., Rice, T., & Lo Sasso, A. T. (2004, April 21). Employers' contradictory views about consumer-driven health care: Results of a national survey. *Health Affairs Web Exclusives.* Retrieved February 2, 2005, from http://content.healthaffairs.org/cgi/content/full/hlthaff.w4.210v1

Grimaldi, P. L. (1997, January). HEDIS is bigger and better. *Nursing Management, 28*(1), 18.

Havemann, J. (1999, April 9). Citing success, White House plans to widen patient rights initiative. *The Washington Post*, p. A18. Retrieved June 4, 2000, from http://www.washingtonpost.com

Health Care Financing Administration, Office of the Actuary: National Health Statistics Group. (2000a, January). *Hospital care expenditures aggregate and per capita amounts and percent distribution, by source of funds, selected calendar years, 1960–1998.* Retrieved June 10, 2000, from http://www.hcfa.gov/stats/nhe-oact/tables/t5.htm

Health Care Financing Administration, Office of the Actuary: National Health Statistics Group. (2000b). *Physician service expenditures, aggregate and per capita amounts and percent distribution by source of funds, selected calendar years, 1960–1998.* Retrieved June 10, 2000, from http://www.hcfa.gov/stats/nhe-oact/tables/t.6htm

The Henry J. Kaiser Family Foundation. (2002, May). *Trends and indicators in the changing health care marketplace, 2002 chartbook.* Retrieved October 12, 2007, from http://www.kff.org/insurance/loader.cfm?url=/commonspot/security/getfile.cfm&PageID=14967

The Henry J. Kaiser Family Foundation. (n.d.). *Health poll report: Views of managed care and customer service.* Retrieved January 26, 2005, from http://www.kff.org/health poll report/archive_aug2004/3.cfm

The Henry J. Kaiser Family Foundation. (2004, March). *Medicare Advantage fact sheet.* Retrieved October 12, 2007, from http://www.kff.org/medicare/upload/Medicare-Advantage-Fact-Sheet.pdf

The Henry J. Kaiser Family Foundation. (2004c, March). *The Medicare prescription drug law fact sheet.* Retrieved February 1, 2005, from http://www.kff.org/medicare/loader.cfm?url1=commonspot/security/getfile&pageID=33325

The Henry J. Kaiser Family Foundation and Health Research and Educational Trust. (2004, September). *Employee health benefits 2004 annual survey,* Exhibit 5.1. Retrieved February 4, 2005, from http://www.kff.org/insurance/7148/sections/ehbs04-5-1.cfm

Holahan, J., Zuckerman, S., Evans, A., & Rangarajan, S. (1998). Medicaid managed care in thirteen states. *Health Affairs, 17*(13), 51.

Iglehart, J. K. (1996). The national committee for quality assurance. *New England Journal of Medicine, 335*(13), 995.

Interstudy Publications. (1999, December 10). *Total HMO enrollment continues to increase, though growth rates slow significantly, 3.* Retrieved September 11, 2002, from http://www.hmodata.com/pdf/ir91pr.pdf

Kongstvedt, P. R. (1989). *The managed health care handbook.* Gaithersburg, MD: Aspen Publishers.

Kovner, A. (1995). *Jonas' health care delivery in the United States* (5th ed.). New York: Springer Publishing.

Levit, K., Cowan, C., Lazenby, H., Sensenig, A., McDonnell, P., Stiller, J., et al. (2000). Health spending in 1998: Signals of change. *Health Affairs, 19*(1), 131.

Levit, K. R., Lazenby, H. C., Braden, B. R., & the National Health Accounts Team (1998, January/February). National health spending trends in 1996. *Health Affairs, 17*(1), 35.

Mays, G. P., Claxton, G., & White, J., et al. (2004, August 11). Managed care rebound? Recent changes in health plans' cost containment strategies. *Health Affairs Web Exclusives.* Retrieved February 4, 2005, from http://content.healthaffairs.org/cgi/reprint/hlthaff.w4.427v1.pdf

Miller, R., & Luft, H. (1994). Managed care plans: Characteristics, growth and premium performance. *Annual Review of Public Health, 15,* 439.

Miller, R. H., & Luft, H. S. (2002). HMO plan performance update: Analysis of the literature, 1997–2001. *Health Affairs, 21*(4), 81.

National Coalition on Health Care. (2000). *Deja vu all over again: The soaring cost of private health insurance and its impact on consumers and employers.* Retrieved June 14, 2000, from http://www.americashealth.org/releases/Pemiums_4-24-00.pdf

National Committee on Quality Assurance. (n.d.). *The state of health care quality 2004.* Retrieved February 2, 2005, from http://www.ncqa.org/communications/somc/sohc2004.pdf

National Committee on Quality Assurance. (n.d.). A letter from NCQA President Margaret E. O'Kane. Retrieved February 6, 2005, from http://www.ncqa.org/about/president.htm

Pawlson, L., & O'Kane, M. (2002, May/June). Professionalism, regulation, and the market: Impact on accountability for quality of care. *Health Affairs, 21*(3), 202.

Rogal, D. L., & Stenger, R. J. (2001, August). The challenge of managed care regulation: Making markets work? *Academy Health*, 1. Retrieved October 12, 2007, from http://www.hcfo.org/pdf/managedcare.pdf

Stevens, R. (1989). *In sickness and in wealth: American hospitals in the twentieth century.* New York: Basic Books.

Stoltzfus Jost, T. (2004, August 11). The Supreme Court limits lawsuits against managed care organizations. *Health Affairs Web Exclusives.* Retrieved February 2, 2005, from http://content.healthaffairs.org/cgi/content/full/hlthaff.w4.417

Timmermans, S., & Mauck, A. (2005). The promises and pitfalls of evidence-based medicine. *Health Affairs, 24*(1), 18–28.

U.S. Congressional Budget Office. (1998, January). *Projections of national health expenditures: 1997–2008, the economic and budget outlook: Fiscal years 1999–2008.* Retrieved June 18, 2000, from http://www.cbo.gov/showdoc.cfm?index=316&sequence=13

Chapter 12

The Future of Health Services Delivery

Leiyu Shi and
Douglas A. Singh

CHAPTER OBJECTIVES

1. Assess the trends in employer-based health insurance and evaluate the challenges faced by managed care.
2. Discuss future financing, insurance, and universal access options.
3. Apply future challenges in wellness and prevention, chronic care, and infectious diseases to the role of the advanced practice nurse.
4. Discuss issues pertaining to the future needs for a well-prepared healthcare workforce and the way in which health work is organized.
5. Understand the emphasis on customer service and potential barriers.
6. Discuss new technology frontiers in the areas of clinical care, information systems, and telehealth.
7. Appreciate the need for large-scale integrated data collection and analysis for outcome monitoring.
8. Value collaborative teamwork and cross-training in the delivery of health services as an advanced nurse practitioner.
9. Assess the trends in evidence-based practice and the implications of advanced practice.

Introduction

Predicting the future direction of healthcare delivery in the United States is predicated upon major current developments and the course they might take in the foreseeable future. Future change also relies on historical precedents and a society's fundamental values. These elements come into play particularly when any kind of a sweeping transformation is proposed. For instance, in 1993, President Bill Clinton proposed his national healthcare initiative in an economic, social, and political environment in which healthcare expenditures were getting out of hand and a significant

241

number of Americans were without health insurance. However, the majority of Americans did not think that nationalized health insurance was the right way to address these issues. Most Americans were opposed to uninvited government intervention. The insured Americans were particularly fearful of losing their existing coverage with which they were reasonably satisfied. Middle-class Americans have also held a widespread belief that they pay more than their reasonable share of taxes to support Medicare and Medicaid programs to help the underprivileged. Besides the American middle class, the Clinton plan was also opposed by most providers, particularly by physicians in private practice.

Rejection of the Clinton plan based on ingrained American values provided the impetus for a widespread shift toward managed care, which at that time had already started to emerge as a growing force. Managed care became the natural choice for injecting competition into the financing, insurance, delivery, and payment functions of health care.

At this point, the foundational values of American society remain intact. Hence, no sweeping changes are expected. However, medical cost escalation and cost of health insurance premiums continue to outpace both general inflation and general economic growth. For example, premiums for family coverage have risen by 87% since 2000 (Claxton, Gil, Finder, & DiJulio, 2006). Faced with such a cost burden, fewer employers are offering health insurance coverage to their workers. The percentage of firms offering health insurance has fallen from 69% in 2000 to 61% in 2006 (Claxton et al., 2006). Also, since the mid-1990s, there has been steady erosion in retiree health benefits. Buchmueller, Johnson, and Lo Sasso (2006) estimated that in 2003 only about 25% of private-

sector employees worked at establishments that offered retiree health benefits, down from 32% in 1997. At the same time, Americans' appetite for new medical breakthroughs remains unabated. Amid these transitions, any major healthcare reform on a national scale has remained a nonissue. But, in April 2006, Massachusetts restructured its own health insurance markets, imposed assessments on employers who did not provide health insurance to their workers, and pooled private and public resources to cover many of the uninsured. If successful, this model may open the way for other states to initiate health insurance reforms.

Any attempts to project the future of health care provoke more questions than answers. Even though precise forecasts cannot be made, certain fundamental features of healthcare delivery in the United States are assured at least for the foreseeable future. The stable features of the U.S. healthcare system essentially recapitulate some of the points made in earlier chapters. In addition, this chapter provides some insights into current directions that might impact the future financing and delivery of health care. Other discussions revolve around what might be achievable, given the right configuration of broader socioeconomic, cultural, and technological forces, particularly in view of some of the major issues that must be addressed.

Trends in Private and Public Health Insurance

Trends in Employment-Based Insurance

During the era marked by the rapid growth of managed care, the proportion of nonelderly who had employment-based health insurance increased from 64.4% in 1994 to 66.8% in 2000. This was also a period of economic expansion and shortage of skilled workers that created stiff competition for labor. Since then, employment-based coverage has been eroding. It went down to 62.4% in 2004, which is below the level in 1994 (Gold, 2006). Between 2000 and 2004, declines in employment-based coverage were the steepest for younger and low-income people (Holahan & Cook, 2005). In addition, as the U.S. workforce continues to age, the composition of enrollees in employment-based insurance will shift toward older adults, which portends an acceleration in the rate of premium growth. Well before we see the effects of baby boomers' enrollment in Medicare, rising premiums in private health plans could place more pressure on an already strained employment-based health insurance system (Keenan, Cutler, & Chernew, 2006).

Public sector employers, particularly state and local governments, also face challenges similar to those in the private sector. As are major private employers, the public sector is experimenting with numerous cost-containment strategies, including disease and case management, aggressive management of pharmacy benefits, and contracting with managed care (McKethan, Gitterman, Feezor, & Enthoven, 2006).

Given the existing conditions, at least some commentators regard employers as ineffective and unenthusiastic managers of the health benefits they sponsor (Galvin, Delbanco, Milstein, & Belden, 2005). It is suggested that, if possible, employers would like to get out of the business of offering health benefits altogether, but it is unlikely to happen (Galvin & Delbanco, 2006). Research suggests that employers, both large and small, hold a positive view of the value of health benefits in attracting and retaining

workers, improving morale, and increasing workers' productivity. The same employers also believe that all employers should share in the cost of health insurance (Whitmore, Collins, Gabel, & Pickreign, 2006). It appears that employers are sensitive to having to carry the cost burden of those employed elsewhere, such as spouses of employees.

High-Deductible Health Plans

Faced with escalating health insurance premiums, employers appear to be embracing increased responsibility and higher cost sharing by the employees as strategies for reducing their healthcare costs (Claxton et al., 2005a). One emerging health plan type, the high-deductible health plan (HDHP), seems to be gaining some initial momentum. For example, in 2006, among firms that offered employment-based health insurance, 7% offered an HDHP. It was estimated that out of 155 million Americans covered under employment-based health insurance, as many as 2.7 million may be covered under an HDHP (Claxton et al., 2006). However, these plans may become more popular in the future because they carry the lowest premium compared to HMO, PPO, and POS plans, they offer tax advantages to workers, and give the insured control over how the money is spent. Hence, these plans are also loosely referred to as consumer-directed health plans.

There are two basic types of HDHPs. The first type, called health reimbursement arrangements (HRAs), grew out of federal regulations made by the Internal Revenue Service in 2002. The second type, health savings accounts (HSAs), were authorized in the Medicare Prescription Drug, Improvement, and Modernization Act (MMA) of 2003.

An HRA is a medical care reimbursement plan sponsored by an employer. HRAs are typically offered in conjunction with a health plan that carries a high deductible. Generally, health plans that carry at least $1,000 deductible for a single plan and $2,000 for a family plan are considered high-deductible health plans. In this arrangement, employers typically commit a predetermined amount of funds that the employee (and eligible dependents) can use to pay for medical expenses and for premium costs for the HDHP. Once the allocated funds are exhausted, the HDHP health insurance kicks in, in which the employee must first meet the deductible requirements out of pocket. Once the deductible is met, the plan becomes similar to a traditional health plan (Claxton et al., 2005b).

An HSA is a savings account created by an individual to pay for health care. To be eligible to create an HSA, a person must be covered by a qualified health plan, which is an HDHP but also meets other legal requirements. Employers can offer qualified health plans, and both employers and employees can contribute to an HSA, but employer contributions are optional. An HSA offers certain tax advantages to the employee. Any contributions made by the employer are nontaxable. Employee contributions are on a pre–income tax basis. Funds in the HSA are invested and the earnings from investments are tax free. Withdrawals from the account to pay for health care are nontaxable; only withdrawals for nonmedical purposes are taxable. The savings account can build up over time, it belongs to the employee, and is portable (Claxton et al., 2005b). HSAs are an improvement over medical savings accounts (MSAs) that were authorized under the Health Insurance Portability and Accountability Act of 1996, but were available only to small businesses, the self-employed, and the uninsured.

The major problem with HDHPs as a reform effort is that they do not achieve universal coverage, and no one knows their impact on the control of healthcare cost growth. Poor families and individuals with limited tax liability are unlikely to benefit from HSAs' tax incentives. Also, people may skimp on care and delay seeking medical treatment for fear of depleting their accounts, thus jeopardizing their health.

Insurance Restructuring in Massachusetts

In April 2006, Massachusetts became the first state to break the gridlock between Democrats and Republicans and passed a bipartisan plan that would achieve nearly universal coverage in the state. The plan was implemented in July 2007. The individual mandate part of the legislation requires all state residents to have health insurance or face legal penalties. The employer mandate part of the legislation requires all employers with more than 10 workers to offer at a minimum a Section 125 cafeteria plan that permits workers to purchase health insurance with pretax dollars (The Henry J. Kaiser Family Foundation, 2007). Large government subsidies would enable low-income individuals to buy insurance. People whose incomes are less than the federal poverty level will have their premiums paid by the state. Those earning up to 300% of the federal poverty level will pay a subsidized premium.

At the core of the plan is the reorganization of a large part of the state's private insurance system into a single-market structure with uniform rules and a central clearinghouse or connector to facilitate the purchase and administration of private health insurance coverage. The connector relieves employers of the burden of obtaining and administering health insurance coverage. Only plans approved by the state's insurance department may be sold through the connector (Haislmaier & Owcharenko, 2006).

The plan is expected to cost $1.2 billion over 3 years. This funding will be derived from redistribution of existing funding that includes federal Medicaid payments that were previously paid to safety net providers under a federal waiver. Actually, the potential loss of this federal funding is what prompted the state to reform its healthcare system. Also noteworthy is the fact that Massachusetts had enacted a play-or-pay (see explanation of this option later in this chapter) mandate in 1988, but it was never implemented.

Unknown at this point are the answers to some key questions regarding the availability of private plans that the state would consider affordable, whether employers will continue to offer current health insurance or switch to the Section 125 plan, which would be cheaper, and whether the plan can be financed over the long term.

The key features of what the program offers are quite appealing. If successful, the plan is likely to be emulated by other states. The plan has three main desirable features, as described by Haislmaier and Owcharenko (2006):

1. Insurance through the connector is available to all residents of the state.
2. Coverage can become portable among employers within the state, and the coverage can be retained during periods of unemployment, part-time employment, or self-employment.
3. The program will provide a choice of plans. Once a year, participants will be allowed to switch coverage on a guaranteed-issue basis at standard prices.

However, the plan faces many challenges and unknowns, and its full effects will not become known for several months.

Trends in Medicare and Medicaid

The Medicare Part D prescription drug benefit requires beneficiaries to receive drug coverage through private plans. The MMA of 2003 also provides new incentives, including sizable payment increases, to expand the role of private managed care plans to provide all Medicare covered services under the Medicare Advantage option (Biles, Dallek, & Nicholas, 2004). The policy is intended to attract more beneficiaries into managed care from the traditional fee-for-service option. Although only 14% of Medicare beneficiaries have chosen to enroll in Medicare Advantage, the Centers for Medicare and Medicaid Services estimates that by 2013, the proportion of beneficiaries in Medicare Advantage will rise to 30%. This estimate is perhaps based on the current levels of increased payments to private plans, but there is no certainty that Congress will maintain the payment increases when faced with future budget constraints. The program will very likely face budget constraints as, by 2015, annual Medicare expenditures are projected to reach $792 billion, which is more than double the amount of spending in 2005 and represents an average annual increase of 9%. In comparison, national health expenditures are expected to grow at an average rate of 7.2% between 2005 and 2015 (Borger et al., 2006).

The MMA has also attached a means-test feature to Medicare for both Part B and Part D premiums. In Part B, for example, single beneficiaries earning less than $80,000 per year ($160,000 per couple) will pay the standard premium, whereas those earning more will pay a higher income-based premium. As originally crafted, Medicare was not to be a means-tested program. Means-tested premiums may have opened the way for future reforms in which the wealthy would be asked to share a greater cost burden for financing the program.

Total enrollment in Medicaid has increased from 33.5 million in 2000 to 44.5 million in 2005 (Sanofi-Aventis U.S., 2006), and expenditures have jumped from $118 billion to $179 billion (Catlin, Cowan, Heffler, Washington, & the National Health Expenditure Accounts Team, 2007), or from $3,522 to $4,022 on a per capita basis, during the same period. Between 2005 and 2015, Medicaid spending is projected to grow at an average annual rate of 7.8%. Spending is projected to reach $384.4 billion in 2015 (Borger et al., 2006), which is more than double the amount spent in 2005. In 2005, 10 states had at least 90% of their Medicaid recipients enrolled in managed care. Nationwide, 62.2% of Medicaid recipients were in managed care, up from 58.4% in 2003 (Sanofi-Aventis U.S., 2006). There is some evidence that Medicaid recipients enrolled in HMOs incur lower overall expenditures (Kirby, Machlin, & Cohen, 2003). Hence, it is expected that more states will mandate HMO enrollment in the future.

Future Options in Financing and Insurance

National health expenditures are projected to reach $4 trillion by 2015, approximately double the total spending in 2005, despite the fact that healthcare expenditures are expected to grow at a moderate rate of 7.2% annually. The amount of spending is projected to consume 20% of the gross domestic product (GDP) in 2015 (Borger et al., 2006), up from 16% in 2005. Although 88% of insured Americans rate their own health insurance coverage as excellent or good, approximately 20% are dissatisfied with the costs. Also, among the insured, 60% are at least somewhat worried about being able to afford the cost of their health insurance over the next few years, mainly if they lose their jobs. People's inability to pay for care when needed is on the rise; one in four Americans indicated they had a problem paying for care sometime during the previous year (The Henry J. Kaiser Family Foundation, 2006).

Some innovative approaches in healthcare financing and insurance have already started to emerge. This section also includes proposals that might reduce the number of uninsured through innovative financing policies. Given that one out of every five dollars would be consumed by health care, Americans will have to forgo some other goods and services. This will likely lower, at least to some degree, the overall standard of living that Americans have become accustomed to. Erosion in the standard of living is perhaps best reflected in the growing number of poor in the United States. This is simply another social ill effect that unrestrained growth in health care will bring.

Defined Contribution Plans

Currently, the majority of employers offer what is referred to as a defined benefit plan. The employer selects a health insurance plan and commits to providing the health benefits package, generally on a cost-sharing basis. Large employers generally offer a choice of plans that vary in cost. Employees can choose from more expensive and less expensive plans. In the defined benefit health insurance arrangement, consumers have no financial incentives to be prudent purchasers, and patients are almost totally removed from the cost of care. But, the consumer of health insurance and health care is likely to bear more responsibility in the future. The defined contribution approach holds this promise. Defined contribution health insurance products that make use of Internet technologies are also getting some attention. Under a defined contribution plan, employers commit to a fixed dollar amount for health benefits rather than to a predetermined package of health benefits.

The model for a defined contribution approach has, for some time, been used for retirement benefits. A shift occurred in the 1980s on the retirement benefits front when employers began moving away from defined benefit (or pension) plans toward defined contribution (or savings) plans (White, 2001). Many employers see adoption of the defined contribution approach for healthcare benefits as compatible with the need to give employees a greater role in purchasing health insurance as well as healthcare services (Christianson, Parente, & Taylor, 2002). Actually, both HRAs and HSAs, discussed earlier, use certain features of defined contribution arrangements. In the future, other variations of defined contribution arrangements are likely to emerge.

A defined contribution plan could take one of two basic forms. On the more conservative side, employees would simply use the defined contribution to choose among several health plans selected by their employer. On the more radical side, employees could take their defined contribution dollars and purchase their own health insurance. In either case, the employer's share of premium costs is capped at a predetermined fixed dollar amount. One way to ensure that the money is actually applied to health care

is to directly deposit the employer's contribution into employees' HSAs, which the employees are responsible for managing (White, 2001).

In the future, the Internet is likely to play a major role in the purchase of health insurance and in the management of HSAs. Internet-based e-health plans will enable consumers to tailor plans according to individual needs, obtain instant quotes, and make online purchases. Managed care organizations are likely to play a major role by adapting their existing structures to meet the new demand. On the other hand, many of the emerging e-health plans have secured partners, such as Merrill Lynch, Chase Capital Partners, Hewitt Associates, Pricewaterhouse Coopers, and even the Mayo Clinic. These developments may indicate the emergence of the next wave of healthcare financing (White, 2001). In any event, *consumer choice*, *affordability*, *cost effectiveness*, and *better value* are going to be tomorrow's buzzwords.

Defined contribution plans also have implications for the health insurance market. With consumers in the driver's seat, aided by the ability to shop on the Web, insurers will have to come up with differentiated plans that would serve a variety of needs and fit different budgets.

Public Entitlement Programs

Care for the future elderly, particularly as the first wave of baby boomers turns 65 in 2011, has serious implications for the Medicare program. Today's elderly account for 13% of the U.S. population, yet they get more than 60% of all federal social spending (Lamm & Blank, 2005). By 2020, the elderly will constitute 16% of the population, which will put unprecedented financial strains on the younger generations.

The RAND Corporation, in collaboration with Stanford University and the V.A. system of

Greater Los Angeles, explored how changes in medical technology, disease, and disability would affect healthcare spending for the elderly population. Their key finding: Medical innovations will result in better health and longer life, but they will likely increase, not decrease, Medicare spending. Even though the health of the population over age 65 has been improving since the early 1980s, cumulative Medicare spending is relatively unaffected by the health status of new beneficiaries because healthier people live longer and have more years in which to accumulate costs. As in the past, new technologies will increase healthcare expenditures even though such technologies may improve health. The reason is that the reduction in spending resulting from better health will be outweighed by the costs of technologies themselves and by health expenditures during the additional years of life that the technologies may make possible. In short, there are no silver bullets for Medicare's fiscal crisis on the foreseeable horizon (RAND, 2005). Given the grim prospects, Medicare will require a major reform effort and political will to carry out the needed reforms. Means testing has already been addressed earlier. Other reforms will most likely be coordinated along with reforms for the Social Security system, which will also face severe financial shortfalls. Since there is no single magic bullet to cure these programs, the main options will likely include a combination of raising eligibility age, increasing premiums and other mechanisms to shift costs from the program to the beneficiaries, reducing reimbursement to providers, and curtailing benefits. Given the expansion of benefits in recent years, the latter option will be the most controversial, but will likely become necessary.

Given the cost projections presented earlier, the Medicaid program will also have to choose various options to curtail spending, similar to the ones just discussed, but for a couple of exceptions. Age limitation does not apply because eligibility is means tested, and there is perhaps little room, if any, to raise income-based eligibility thresholds. Secondly, shifting costs to the beneficiaries will be impractical because the program serves the indigent. Experiences of some states during the 2001–2003 recession might provide some lessons for the future. A study by Coughlin and Zuckerman (2005) concluded that states relied on a range of short-term solutions instead of reassessing their basic tax structures and policies. By resorting to short-term approaches, some states have created structural deficits that will profoundly influence state policy making for many years to come (Coughlin & Zuckerman, 2005). The implication here is that Medicaid reform will require tax hikes at both the federal and state levels.

Tax Credits and Vouchers

McClellan and Baicker (2002) argued that President George Bush's proposal to introduce tax credits for the purchase of health insurance would enable millions of Americans to purchase private health insurance. It would also improve the functioning of private markets, empower patients to make informed decisions, and increase the use of high-value health care while reducing inappropriate use. To this effect, Congress passed the Trade Adjustment Assistance Act of 2002, which includes health insurance tax credits for displaced workers and retirees who have lost their employer coverage. The work of Patel (2002) suggests that affordable individual health insurance is available for most Americans, but one main barrier is the lack of consumer awareness. A variation of this approach is to issue the tax credits in advance in the form of vouchers that enable people, particularly the poor, to purchase insurance.

High-Risk Pools

Tax credits would still leave some people uninsured, particularly those who are considered high risk due to severe illnesses or chronic conditions. High-risk pools target groups that cannot purchase health insurance on their own because of poor health. Over 30 states currently have set up high-risk pools that enable hard-to-insure people to purchase subsidized coverage. In almost all cases, premium rates are capped at 125–150% of the average market rate. Deductibles are generally $1,000 or less, and an 80/20 coinsurance is common. Proposals that the federal government should help states establish these pools are based on the premise that the federal government already is the insurer of last resort in case of major natural catastrophes, and in the housing mortgage market through loan guarantees (Swartz, 2002). Under the Trade Adjustment Assistance Reform Act of 2002, the Centers for Medicare and Medicaid Services (CMS) awarded the entire $80 million dollars that the bill had appropriated. The Deficit Reduction Act of 2005 reauthorized federal funds through fiscal year 2010. Federal grants provide seed money to create new high-risk pools and to cover operational losses.

Future Challenges for Managed Care

The role of managed care, as we know it, is assured in American health care at least for the foreseeable future. For now, status quo has been maintained in employer-sponsored health insurance as employers have been able to pass increased insurance costs to the employees through higher cost sharing in insurance premiums and higher deductibles and co-payments. However, pressures to control healthcare costs are beginning to mount. Once again, managed care will have to adapt and change to remain competitive.

Management of Risk

The greatest challenge in insurance is maintaining a balance between healthy and sick enrollees. However, 30% of persons 21 to 24 years of age are uninsured compared to 13.7% of people 55 to 64 years of age (Serota, 2002). With the shifting demographics of the health insurance pool, managed care in the future will have to focus on managing the risk of an increasing number of people with potentially debilitating chronic illnesses, and also the sickest people in society. As discussed earlier, a growing number of Medicaid and Medicare beneficiaries, most of whom are high risk, are receiving care through managed care plans. Reforms in Medicaid, Medicare, and managed care will be necessary for Managed Care Organizations (MCOs) to do a better job of managing health risk and for keeping costs under control. Future trends point to managed care as a risk-driven healthcare payment system. Instead of diagnosis and treatment as its principal business, the healthcare system will have to predict health risk and try to manage that risk before it turns into illness and cost (Institute of Medicine, 1996). Managing risk will involve population-based efforts to improve overall health status and an increased emphasis on prevention.

Accountability

MCOs in the future will have to be more accountable to both employers and enrollees. Although the choice of health plans by employers is driven primarily by the cost of premiums, accountability measures will be useful for enrollees in making informed decisions about which plan to choose. Such measures would be necessary if e-health programs catch on with the implementation of defined contribution benefits. Clinical practice guidelines to assess and improve the quality of care in MCOs will also become more common.

Comprehensive Reform: If and When It Occurs

At some point, debate over comprehensive reforms leading to universal coverage is likely to arise again. In a system driven by incremental reforms, experimentation with additional ad hoc arrangements is eventually likely to run out of viable options. Comprehensive reform may come up for debate, particularly if employer-based health coverage continues to erode, or if powerful politicians believe Americans are ready for comprehensive reform. The last situation occurred in 1992 when Clinton became president. Past proposals likely to be considered again have included a single-payer system, managed competition, and an employer-based play-or-pay system (see Table 12–1 for summaries of major approaches to finance health care). Assuming that a major reform of the U.S. healthcare system does occur in the future, the single-payer proposal is the least likely to be adopted because this will be the most drastic of the three approaches. Employer mandates enacted in Hawaii in 1974 are also discussed in this section, but are unlikely to be an option today because they will be highly resisted by employers.

Although a universal health insurance program will cover all citizens, access will be restricted to essential care. People wanting access to services beyond what is determined to be essential will have to pay for them (Ginzberg, 1999). Besides, those who currently have good coverage will have to settle for a system that imposes supply-side rationing, and the delivery system will quickly become overburdened with an unanticipated surge in demand for services. Cost-effectiveness criteria will become the gold standard for rationing medicine. There are three major problems with proposals for universal health insurance. (1) To financially sustain such a system Americans will have to "give up a cherished dream: the dream of total, universal care for any ailment freely available on demand" (Lamm & Blank, 2005). (2) Proposed options (discussed in the next section) only deal with insurance financing. They do not address the potential problem with access—how an overburdened system will meet increased demand for services. (3) Americans will have to be willing to pay increased taxes to sustain such a system.

Single-Payer Health Plans

A single-payer health plan would place the responsibility for financing health care with a central agency (most likely the federal government). One major advantage of this system is that all Americans and lawful residents would be entitled to benefits regardless of individual or family income. Private insurance plans and government entitlement programs (Medicaid, Medicare, TriCare, and the Federal Employee Health Benefits program) would no longer be necessary under a single-payer system, although

---

Table 12–1 GENERAL APPROACHES FOR HEALTH CARE FINANCING REORGANIZATION

Option 1: A laissez-faire, free-market approach ("piecemeal")

Pros: • Builds on the current system rather than replacing it.

• Promotes managed care concepts (HMOs, PPOs) that incorporate mechanisms to control costs.

• Gives people an incentive to price-shop for insurance and medical care, improving individual choice and reducing personal costs.

• Maintains private market-based approach.

• Significantly restricts government involvement and regulation compared with the other approaches.

Cons: • Does not mandate coverage for everyone.

• Requires consumers to have a sophisticated knowledge of insurance plans.

• Relies primarily on questionable cost-control strategies already in place.

• Does not address administrative waste.

• Continues a two-tier medical system in which those who can afford it have greater coverage, while low income people receive minimum coverage.

• Lacks coverage for long-term care services.

Option 2: Government-financed public health care system ("single-payer" or "national health insurance")

Pros: • Guarantees access to care for all individuals.

• Ensures coverage regardless of health status, economic status, job loss, or job change.

• Reduces or eliminates many out of pocket costs.

• Controls costs by setting payment rates and global limits on total health care spending.

• Removes employers' responsibility to provide health insurance, though they continue to pay for coverage through taxes.

• Greatly reduces multiple payers, thus lowering administrative costs.

• Spreads risk and cost across entire population.

Cons: • Requires a substantial increase in taxes.

• Puts government in charge of whole system, which could lead to budgetary constraints affecting choice, quality, and use of new technologies.

• May result in waiting lists and shortages due to supply-side rationing.

• Significantly curbs need for private insurance coverage, resulting in thousands of lost jobs throughout the insurance industry.

• Could allow political and ideological biases to influence scientific decisions.

(continues)

Table 12–1   GENERAL APPROACHES FOR HEALTH CARE FINANCING REORGANIZATION
(CONTINUED)

Option 3: Employer-based regulatory approach ("play-or-pay")

Pros: • Provides coverage for everyone.

• Builds on the current system rather than replacing it.

• Eliminates exclusions for preexisting conditions.

• Reduces out of pocket costs substantially for many groups of people.

• Maintains competition among private-market insurance companies.

• Spreads risk and cost across entire population.

Cons: • May offer no real incentive for some employers to "play" because tax route may be cheaper, which could shift millions of employed people into government pool.

• Mandates small businesses to pay, through either health insurance ("play") or higher taxes ("pay").

• Enables many insurance companies to continue to operate, which means some of the administrative costs (e.g., advertising) also continue.

• Increases taxes, although less than for government-based approaches.

---

the market for some private insurance will remain for those desiring coverage beyond what a basic government plan might offer.

According to one proposal, financing would come from an employer excise tax (8.7%) on annual revenues and a payroll tax levied on employees' salaries (2.2%), similar to federal or state income tax (LAPSR, 1996). Additionally, the unemployed, disabled, and elderly would be subsidized through federal and state funds based on their ability to pay (LAPSR, 1996). Healthcare providers would be reimbursed on a fee-for-service scale. Hospitals, nursing homes, and other institutional facilities would be given an annual prospective budget to provide all required care.

A single-payer system could accomplish two major goals of healthcare reform: (1) provide universal coverage and (2) contain costs. By eliminating private health insurance, the single-payer system can lower administrative costs.

But, the bulk of savings will come from supply-side rationing, which is the hallmark of all national health insurance programs.

A single-payer system has other drawbacks. Financing this type of plan primarily with an employer tax would place a financial burden on small businesses. Very likely, an increase in general taxes will also become necessary to support a burgeoning system. In addition, a single-payer system will likely create bureaucratic problems associated with the centralized administrative process. These problems include lack of flexibility and enhanced power and control over providers and businesses. Open rationing of health services will be highly resisted by the American public.

Managed Competition

President Clinton's proposed Health Security Act of 1993 was based largely on the principles of managed competition. The plan proposed to guarantee every citizen the right to receive a comprehensive package of healthcare benefits. Under the proposal, regional alliances would be established to ensure that every citizen was enrolled in a plan. The alliances would function very much like the connector in the Massachusetts health plan discussed earlier; that is, they would act as the fiscal intermediary between the plans and enrollees. Financing for the proposed program was based on cost sharing between employers (80%) and employees (20%).

The advantage of adopting a managed competition arrangement is that the medical infrastructure is already in place, and the private insurance industry, the would-be administrator of care, is well established in the United States. This could facilitate a smooth transition, whereas the single-payer system would require redesigning the entire healthcare delivery system. Also, compared to a single-payer system, managed competition calls for a smaller government bureaucracy.

Unfortunately, managed competition cannot guarantee that everyone would have equal access to care. Inner cities and rural areas in particular would have difficulty attracting enough health plans. A fundamental problem with managed competition is that unless several plans are competing against each other in a given geographic area, the system cannot drive down the cost of health care.

Play-or-Pay Coverage

Employer-based play-or-pay coverage was introduced as a Senate bill in 1989 to achieve universal coverage. Under this system, employers must either provide their employees health insurance (play) or pay into a public health insurance program. The plan requires private or public insurance entities to provide identical benefits to working Americans and their dependents. Medicaid and Medicare would remain to provide care to the elderly, disabled, and poor.

If the employer chooses to pay, financing is through a payroll tax paid by the employer and the employee. The employee is still responsible for co-payments, premiums, and deductibles. Employees could also purchase supplemental health care benefits privately or through their employers.

Because an employer-based system is already in place, this type of plan is less disruptive than a single-payer system. Since many Americans who are uninsured are actually employed, this program could considerably reduce the number of uninsured.

Much like a single-payer system, a play-or-pay system would place an undue economic burden on small businesses because of mandatory employer financing. However, given the choice of "not to play, but pay" many employers, including those who currently provide health insurance to their workers, will choose to pay because, as the recent experience in Massachusetts indicates, it will be cheaper to pay than to play. Consequently, a greater cost burden would fall on the public, who will have to pay higher taxes. This was precisely the reason why Massachusetts did not implement its 1988 enactment of a play-or-pay mandate. California is another state that passed a play-or-pay mandate in 2003, but the law was repealed through a ballot referendum. Another drawback of a play-or-pay system is that it focuses only on the financing of care, and does not address other areas of concern, such as access to care, utilization of services, and quality of care.

Employer Mandates

Employer mandates require employers to help pay for their employees' coverage. Despite the seeming appeal of an employer mandate, only Hawaii has implemented this type of reform. States' ability to adopt employer mandates has been thwarted by the federal Employee Retirement Income Security Act (ERISA), which exempts self-insured businesses from state insurance regulations and taxes. Hawaii is the only state that received a congressional exemption from ERISA for its employer mandate. In spite of employer mandates, almost 10% of the population in Hawaii is uninsured (DHHS, 2006).

Most employers not offering health insurance to their workers would actually like to offer it, but they find it too costly. Other employers do not offer health insurance because most of their employees already have coverage (often from a spouse's employer) or because health insurance is not regarded as necessary to attract or retain the types of employees needed (Friedland, 1996). This is often the case in low-skill jobs.

National and Global Challenges

To restrain the mounting burden of healthcare spending, wellness and disease prevention will have to be incorporated into healthcare delivery. On the other hand, the demands of chronic care and new and resurgent infectious diseases must also be incorporated into medical practice. New healthcare roles are required to coordinate the needs of people with chronic illnesses. Healthcare institutions and private practitioners must coordinate their efforts with public

health agencies to identify emergent diseases and contain the spread of infection.

Future of Wellness, Prevention, and Health Promotion

Because of the changing causes of death, disease patterns, and the economic burden of disease, future healthcare emphasis will shift from acute to preventive care. To keep health benefit costs under control, employers are likely to promote employee health. Coile (2002) proposed that employers might have to take a long-term view instead of depending on short-term solutions. Employers would have to proactively identify employees and dependents with health risk factors and support health promotion strategies to reduce health risks through smoking cessation, weight reduction, and stress management programs (Coile, 2002). Hospitals and managed care plans must continue as the leaders in integrating wellness and health promotion into medical care delivery. The goals and objectives laid out in *Healthy People 2010* (see Chapter 7) are also consistent with this kind of shift in emphasis. However, the epidemic of overweight and obesity threatens to undo much of the progress that has been made in controlling cardiovascular disease, diabetes, and cancer (Satcher, 2006).

Former U.S. Surgeon General David Satcher laid out a three-point plan to increase investment in prevention: At the first level, labeled "downstream," the focus is on the individual and his or her lifestyle and behaviors. For example, regular physical activity, good nutrition, and scheduled immunizations are emphasized here, as well as the importance of avoiding toxins such as tobacco, alcohol, and harmful drugs. At the second level, labeled "midstream," the focus is on the community. For example, investments are needed in public infrastructures that support walking, biking, and physical recreation. Schools should provide physical education. At the third level, labeled "upstream," the focus is on health policy that supports prevention. An example is legislation that promotes physical activity and good nutrition programs in schools (Satcher, 2006). Although putting such a plan into practice will be a challenge, it will require public-private partnership.

Challenges of Chronic Illness Care

In one century, the United States and most other nations have made significant gains in health status and life expectancy—mainly by conquering communicable diseases and developing more affluent lifestyles. However, with a higher life expectancy, such chronic disorders as heart disease and cancer have become the major causes of death. Future trends project an increase in affluence-related diseases, including cardiovascular, oncotic, and degenerative diseases. The more successful health care is at vanquishing disease symptoms and prolonging life, the more people will have to face the inevitable physical deterioration of the aging process.

Changing patterns of diseases are occurring in the shift to more chronic and multifaceted illnesses—a shift that will affect the demand for services and the type of services required. The future healthcare delivery system will have to be configured to meet these impending challenges. At a fundamental level, the shift will be from a reactive approach that responds to illness and its accompanying complications to a proactive approach that focuses on managing the underlying medical conditions.

Approximately one third of Americans with chronic illnesses report that they are in fair to poor health, and too many chronically ill patients are not equipped to deal with their medical problems. According to one report, only 30% of patients with chronic illnesses felt very confident about their ability to decide something as basic as when it is appropriate to see a physician, 20% were not very confident about taking their medications in an appropriate manner, almost 50% had low levels of confidence about eating right, and about 50% could count on a high level of social support. On the other hand, people who suffer from chronic illnesses continue to engage in risky behaviors at rates comparable to the general population, despite the higher risks to their health. The chronically ill also face barriers because of affordability and physical access even though the vast majority has private or public insurance. The frequently expressed need for home care and special transportation services remains unmet for the vast majority of patients (Foundation for Accountability, 2001). On the other hand, expenditures for long-term care are projected to increase at 2.6% annually above inflation to $154 billion in 2010, $195 billion in 2020, and a staggering $270 billion in 2030 (Congressional Budget Office, CBO, 1999). Clearly, the future's healthcare delivery system will need to improve drastically to meet the growing demand for effective chronic care. The system needs to shift decisively from the current acute care model to a chronic care model.

Some of the main initiatives to improve the quality of care and reduce costs of care for the chronically ill have occurred through Medicare policy. For example, Section 721 of the MMA establishes the Chronic Care Improvement Program (CCIP). The CCIP, a new service that is predicated on disease managements being introduced on a pilot basis with the fee-for-service option in Medicare. Other demonstration programs called for by previous legislative action such as the Medicare, Medicaid, and State Children's Health Insurance Program Benefits Improvement and Protection Act of 2000 are in various stages of planning and implementation. However, past demonstration projects have had a less than optimal record of achieving their intended objectives. Hence, more comprehensive, multifaceted innovations that simultaneously address provider practice, patient education, and patient self-management are necessary. Also, given the well-established influence of reimbursement on physician behavior, payment strategies should be restructured to facilitate transition of chronic care principles to the healthcare delivery system (Wolff & Boult, 2005). Reimbursement systems must change in a way that also includes compensation for the services of nonphysician providers, such as nurse practitioners and community health nurses. In addition, healthcare professionals, including physicians, need to receive appropriate training in the management and coordination of the special needs of people suffering from chronic illnesses.

Challenges in Long-Term Care

The financing and delivery of long-term care will remain a major challenge. The good news is that long-term care is typically needed later in life. Even though the first wave of baby boomers will start retiring in 2011, they are not likely to need professional long-term care services until 2025 or later. However, the system must be reformed before that time comes. In their report to the National Commission for Quality Long-Term Care, Miller and Mor

(2006) identified six main areas of concern that must be addressed: financing, resources, infrastructure, workforce, regulation, and information technology.

FINANCING

Currently, most middle-class families are unprepared to meet long-term care expenses. Most people think that Medicare would pay for their long-term care needs. But Medicare covers only short-term postacute care. It is estimated that less than 10% of the elderly have private long-term care (LTC) insurance (Burke, Feder, & Van de Water, 2005). Unless policy initiatives are established to promote long-term care health insurance plans, the public sector will see its expenditures grow rapidly. Purchasing long-term care (LTC) insurance is both expensive and confusing. The Congressional Budget Office (CBO, 2004) recommended improving the way private markets for LTC insurance currently function. For instance, private insurance could be made more attractive to consumers by standardizing insurance policies to allow competing policies to be more easily compared. Currently, state insurance regulations do not require insurance carriers to offer policies that conform to particular design standards. Standardized policies could also stimulate price competition among insurers and help keep premiums lower than they would otherwise be. However, reform is also needed in a public financing system, particularly Medicaid, that pays for the bulk of long-term care costs. The Deficit Reduction Act (DRA) of 2005 tightened Medicaid eligibility rules. The law also extended the time period for asset transfers (called the look-back period) to qualify for Medicaid (Crowley, 2006). In 2004, Medicaid and Medicare financed roughly 60% of all long-term care costs (CBO, 2004).

Without reform, these programs will put enormous financial pressure on the future working population.

RESOURCES

Currently, financing for long-term care in the United States is tilted quite heavily in favor of institutional services rather than community-based services. Costs can be reduced if people who otherwise would be placed in nursing homes can have their needs met using community-based care. However, the Home and Community Based Waiver (HCBW) program has been too restrictive. Some provisions have been made in the DRA to extend community-based care to a larger number of people.

INFRASTRUCTURE

The institutional long-term care sector has been going through a cultural change that has led to the creation of enriched living environments in nursing homes. New architectural designs, living arrangements, and worker and patient empowerment are improving the quality of life in nursing facilities that have adopted innovative models such as Eden Alternative, Green House Project, and Wellspring. Over time, traditional living and care arrangements will be replaced by these and other innovative models.

WORKFORCE

The aging of Americans will shrink the overall pool of workers. Experts think that this will have a particularly drastic effect on the healthcare sector, and long-term care in particular because of low pay and hard work. It is estimated that between 2000 and 2010 alone, when the baby boomers are about to reach retirement age, an additional 1.9 million direct care workers will be needed in long-term care settings

(Department of Health and Human Services, 2003). Another issue that must be addressed is a lack of training in geriatrics among the current workforce (discussed later).

REGULATION

Currently, many experts see fundamental contradictions between the existing regulatory mechanisms that address quality issues in nursing facilities through periodic inspections and sanctioning, and regulations that require the same nursing facilities to implement quality improvement programs. Also, one of the most disconcerting aspects of government regulation of long-term care is its inconsistent application both within and across regions over time (Miller & Mor, 2006). These issues need to be resolved.

INFORMATION TECHNOLOGY

Interoperable IT systems will enable providers to track patients' care across hospitals, nursing homes, home health agencies, and physicians' offices. Such systems are particularly critical in long-term care because the elderly frequently make transitions between long-term care and non–long-term care settings. Currently, such transitions rarely occur smoothly because of high rates of missing or inaccurate information (Miller & Mor, 2006).

Infectious Diseases and Challenges of Globalization

The much-needed shift to combat chronic disease and disability does not mean that infectious disease prevention and control efforts will become unnecessary. In fact, intensified efforts will be required to combat emergent and resurgent infectious diseases. For instance, in the early

1980s, the sudden appearance of a previously unknown disease we now call AIDS challenged the widely held belief that infectious diseases were under control. Since then, other deadly bacterial infections, such as Lyme disease, have appeared. Even though some of the newer infections have not created the panic that AIDS did, the scientific community is baffled by some ordinary bacterial infections that have turned lethal. Another cause of concern is that certain strains of bacteria have become antibiotic resistant from the inadvertent overuse of antibiotics, which presents fresh challenges from infectious diseases, new and old. New forms of influenza virus have periodically raised alarms in the United States. Hantavirus, which is believed to have originated in Korea, has caused some lethal infections in the United States. National public health alerts made headlines in 2002 when encephalitis cases in New York were attributed to the West Nile virus, which then traveled 3,000 miles west to California. This infection had never before been identified in the Western Hemisphere (Novick, 2001), and its emergence in the United States has been attributed to global flow of goods, services, and people. Increase in air travel resulted in the spread of Severe Acute Respiratory Syndrome (SARS) from China to Canada in 2003, and of polio virus from India to northern Minnesota in 2005 (Milstien, Kaddar, & Paule Kieny, 2006).

The aforementioned examples demonstrate that infectious diseases and health care must be viewed from a global perspective. The HIV/AIDS epidemic, for instance, has so far affected Africa the most. The African epidemic received little attention from the United States until very recently when it was recognized that the epidemic posed growing risks to U.S. interests due to increasing globalization. Immigration of people from other countries to the United States, international travel to and from the United States, and shipments coming to the United States from other countries have made it increasingly possible for deadly infections to cross international borders. Data show that the U.S. death rate from infectious diseases has doubled since 1980, and treatment of these diseases uses 15% of total U.S. health spending (Kassalow, 2001). HIV/AIDS, hepatitis C, and other infectious diseases, some currently known and some as yet unknown, will pose growing threats to U.S. interests, particularly as the AIDS crisis is expected to spread rapidly through India, Russia, China, and Latin America, which make up almost 40% of the world's population (Gow, 2002).

The global aspect of infectious diseases emphasizes the need to link together the nation's foreign policy and public health policy. Globalization presents social and economic opportunities from which nations can benefit, but it also holds the potential for a global catastrophe. International cooperation, sharing of information, and technical and financial assistance will be necessary to avert any major health mishaps that could affect millions of people around the world.

Bioterrorism and the Transformation of Public Health

Public health has always been about protecting the population's health. More recently, emphasis on homeland security has lifted public health to a new level of respect and recognition as an instrument to protect the public against new threats to their health and well-being. Actually, the interest in public health in the United States has been like a seesaw, going up during times of danger to people's health and safety, and coming down when no present dangers loom. The importance of public health and deficiencies in the existing public health system received national attention during terrorism-related attempts to bring about an anthrax epidemic in October 2001, soon after the terrorist attacks and destruction of the World Trade Center in New York City on September 11, 2001. Since then, a heightened awareness of potential threats posed by chemical and biological weapons and low-grade nuclear materials has prompted public officials nationwide to review and revamp the system. Most experts believe that the threat of terrorism on American soil will remain with us for the foreseeable future. The nation's central public health agency, the Centers for Disease Control and Prevention (CDC), will continue to play a vital role in recognizing emerging threats and in developing measures to contain any unexpected outbreaks. Public health agencies at local, state, and federal levels have been identifying infrastructure weaknesses and reevaluating plans to protect the American public (Baker & Koplan, 2002). Public health must prepare for threats other than those posed by imported infectious diseases (discussed earlier); possible use of chemical, biological, and nuclear agents; and natural disasters such as Hurricanes Katrina and Rita in the Gulf Coast. Safeguarding the nation's food and water supplies is equally important.

The future effectiveness of public health will involve cooperation among public health agencies at the federal, state, and local levels; other departments of the government, such as the Department of Justice, and the Food and Drug Administration; private and public organizations, such as hospitals, clinics, and nursing homes; private practitioners, such as physicians and nurses; volunteer agencies, such as the American Red Cross and numerous other voluntary organizations; civil defense agencies, such as police and fire departments; businesses; and individuals and groups within communities.

To protect the health and safety of Americans, public health agencies will need to strengthen the 10 core public health functions enumerated by the National Association of County Health Officials (1994) in its *Blueprint for a Healthy Community: A Guide for Local Health Departments.* Those functions are:

1. Conduct a community diagnosis. Collect, manage, and analyze health-related data for information-based decision making.
2. Prevent and control epidemics. Investigate and contain diseases and injuries.
3. Provide a safe and healthy environment. Maintain clean and safe air, water, food, and facilities.
4. Measure performance, effectiveness, and outcomes of health services. Monitor healthcare providers and the healthcare system.
5. Promote healthy lifestyles. Provide health education to individuals and communities.
6. Provide laboratory testing. Identify disease agents.
7. Provide targeted outreach and form partnerships. Assure access to services for all vulnerable populations and the development of culturally appropriate care.
8. Provide personal healthcare services. Treat illness, injury, disabling conditions, and dysfunction (ranging from

primary and preventive care to specialty and tertiary treatment).

9. Promote research and innovation. Discover and apply improved healthcare delivery mechanisms and clinical interventions.

10. Mobilize the community for action. Provide leadership and initiate collaboration.

Effective public health responses will also require revamping the infrastructure and improving skills. Some priorities include workforce development; technical leadership skills for top-level public health professionals; modern information and communication systems; state-of-the-art disease surveillance systems, including early-warning systems; resources to maintain front-line public health response teams in a state of readiness; and rapid deployment of antidotes and vaccines when needed. In addition, periodic readiness assessment, ongoing research, and the upgrading of laboratory capabilities will be needed to ensure readiness for new and yet unknown challenges.

Local and state public health agencies will remain safety-net providers by continuing to deliver certain healthcare services to those in need. Increasingly, however, these governmental agencies will form partnerships with organized healthcare providers to ensure that population-based prevention is available to everyone. To increase efficiencies, consolidation will be effected by regionalizing public health jurisdictions. This would diminish the number of local public health jurisdictions from approximately 3,000 to somewhere between 500 and 1,000 (Mays, Miller, & Halverson, 2000). In some jurisdictions, the privatization of public health services using contractual arrangements with private providers will continue in ways that improve efficiency (Baker & Koplan, 2002).

The Future Outlook for U.S. Hospitals

It appears that a nationwide hospital construction boom is under way to expand capacity, replace aged facilities, or build new full-service or specialty hospitals. Many hospitals are replacing existing semiprivate patient rooms with all private rooms. In many instances, hospitals are also increasing capacity in operating rooms, diagnostic radiology, telemetry observation beds, critical care for newborns and children, and outpatient services. For increasing capacity, the most notable market factor is population growth, particularly in areas where such populations are well insured. At this point, there is little evidence, however, as to how the benefits of increased capacity will balance with the increased costs (Bazzoli et al., 2006). Recent research shows that contrary to popular opinion, the aging of the baby boomers and increased longevity in general will have less of an impact on the future of hospital demand than local population trends and changing practice patterns attributable to advancing medical technology (Strunk et al., 2006). Cost increases in the healthcare system have also been primarily attributed to hospitals. For example, it is estimated that hospitals were responsible for about 28% of the $528 billion increase in healthcare spending between 1998 and 2003 (D'Cruz & Welter, 2005). Hence, hospitals will come under increased scrutiny to contain costs and improve efficiencies.

Hospitals will also be expected to continue to respond to other pressures from their external environments. They will increasingly develop a continuum of medical care services and will continue to engage in providing one-stop shopping for all healthcare needs. Hospitals will also continue to reinvest capital in the development of integrated delivery networks, including joint ventures with other hospitals, physician practices, and managed care organizations.

The hospital of the future will be a health center, not just a medical center. Keeping people healthy will continue to receive a great deal of emphasis, and hospitals will increasingly engage in offering valuable resources to the community on matters of health and well-being and will be held increasingly accountable for the community's health status. Hospitals will work not only to improve community health services but also to develop better programs to measure outcomes.

Other freestanding institutions of healthcare delivery will continue to exert competitive pressures on hospitals. On the other hand, concerns about Medicare's solvency and pickup in cost escalation will impose fiscal pressures. With the growing number of uninsured patients, the workloads of emergency departments are likely to increase, but without any additional reimbursement. This is especially true of public hospitals and those located in urban centers, which will face increasing utilization and financial pressures because these hospitals end up sharing a larger burden of uncompensated care.

Cost pressures are likely to require hospitals to focus on greater labor productivity and reductions in overall staffing. This will require emphasis on multiskilled workers and labor-saving technology.

The Future of the Healthcare Workforce

Healthcare delivery influences and is influenced by the characteristics of the healthcare workforce. Some of the factors influencing the workforce include changes in the utilization of hospital-based and other healthcare services, an increasing elderly population, training and availability of skilled and semiskilled workers, and more women and minorities entering the healthcare workforce. The future healthcare workforce will also be impacted by individual career choices and enrollments in training programs and immigration of trained foreign workers in areas of high labor demand. Shortage of nurses is one of the dominant issues today. However, whether this shortage will continue is debated. Currently, pharmacists, technicians, and therapists are also in short supply (Coile, 2002).

Supply and Demand for Physicians

The Council on Graduate Medical Education (COGME) assessed the likely future supply, demand, and need for physicians in the United States through 2020 for both generalist and specialist physicians. The report concluded that between 2000 and 2020, the number of practicing physicians would rise from approximately 781,000 full-time equivalent (FTE) to 1.02 million FTEs under the most probable aggregate assumptions that take into account physician lifestyle factors such as working fewer hours and increased productivity as a result of new technologies. These figures translate to 283 FTEs per 100,000 population in 2000, and 313 FTEs per 100,000 population in 2020 (Department of Health and Human Services, 2005). On the surface, these figures may indicate a surplus of physicians. However, there are two main factors that suggest that the demand for physicians is likely to grow more rapidly than the supply (Department of Health and Human Services, 2005): (1) A greater proportion of elderly in the population, and (2) the changing age-specific per capita physician utilization rates, with those age 45 and above using more services. When these assumptions are factored in, the demand for physicians in 2020 will be between 1.02 million and 1.24 million. Hence, there could actually be a shortage of physicians by 2020. Also, the problems of specialty maldistribution and geographic maldistribution are likely to continue. By 2010, the number of specialists is expected to reach 152 per 100,000 population (from 140 in 2000), and the number of generalists is expected to remain stable at 67 per 100,000 population (Institute for the Future, 2000). These projections represent a generalist to specialist ratio of 31:69. The COGME forecasted a similar mix for 2020. A shortage of generalists will have serious consequences in a healthcare system that needs to focus more on addressing multiple chronic conditions. Two major forces will negatively affect the supply of generalist physicians in rural America—the number of residency graduates in primary care and the increasing feminization of the physician workforce. During the 1990s, growth of managed care had sparked a renewed interest among medical graduates in pursuing residencies in primary care because a shortage of generalists was widely forecast. Consequently, family practice residencies increased 54% between 1993 and 2000, a trend that would have had a sizable impact on the rural physician workforce (Colwill & Cultice, 2003). However, the new

century has seen a remarkable drop in student interest in primary care. The second factor, feminization of the physician workforce, is also believed to negatively affect the supply of rural practitioners because women have been less likely to select rural practice. The proportion of women in family medicine is expected to double to 40% by 2020 (Colwill & Cultice, 2003).

Supply and Demand for Nurses

The recent shortage of RN-trained nurses in the United States has received much attention. Nurse shortages in the past have been cyclical. The current shortage began in 1998, and in 2006 entered its 9th year, making it the longest shortage in the past 50 years (Auerbach, Buerhaus, & Staiger, 2007). In response, hospitals have used a mix of short-term and long-term strategies to deal with shortages. Among the long-term solutions are investments in training by expanding existing training capacity, opening new schools, and adding fringe benefits focused on education; and improvement of work environments through lengthening or redesigning of orientation programs for new nurses, increasing staffing levels, and work redesign (May, Bazzoli, & Gerland, 2006). Only time will tell if these strategies will produce a lasting effect in alleviating the problem. Other factors, however, seem to suggest that the shortage of nurses will persist in the future. Unlike previous age cohorts of nursing students in the 1970s and 1980s, large numbers of people are entering the profession in their late 20s and early 30s. Based on revised projections taking into account this recent pattern of entry into nursing schools, the total RN workforce size is expected to be 2.45 million in 2012 and 2.47 million in 2020. The authors of these projections, Auerbach and colleagues (2007), used the demand data produced by the Health Resources and Services Administration and estimated a shortfall of 340,000 nurses in 2020. The authors also comment that future changes in the economy, immigration, educational incentives, retirement trends among nurses, wages, delivery of health care, and societal values in general could affect future cohorts' propensities to enter nursing.

Deficits in Geriatric Training

Based on current trends, a shortage of healthcare professionals schooled in geriatrics is a critical challenge. It is estimated that only about 9,000 practicing physicians in the United States (2.5 geriatricians per 10,000 elderly) have formal training in geriatrics. This number is expected to drop down to 6,000 in the near future. Among nurses, less than 0.05% have advanced certification in geriatrics (CDC and Merck Institute of Aging and Health, CDC/Merck, 2004).

The elderly use the majority of home healthcare services and nursing home care, about half of hospital inpatient days, and approximately a quarter of all ambulatory care visits. Growth of the elderly population will impose increased challenges on the healthcare delivery system, which has thus far ignored the need for specialized geriatrics training. Many elderly patients suffer from chronic conditions. Their care is complicated by the presence of comorbidities, use of multiple drug prescriptions, and an increased prevalence of mental conditions and dementia. Evidence shows that care of older adults by healthcare professionals prepared in geriatrics yields better physical and mental outcomes without increasing costs (Cohen et al., 2002). Current trends in the education and training of healthcare professionals shows the

future demand will far outstrip the supply of physicians, nurses, therapists, social workers, and pharmacists with geriatrics training. This problem is compounded due to a shortage of faculty in colleges and universities who are trained in geriatrics. Only 600 medical school faculty out of 100,000 list geriatrics as their primary specialty. Due to this and perhaps other reasons, only 3% of medical students take any elective geriatric courses. In other disciplines, such as nursing, pharmacy, medicine, and dentistry, the majority of educational curricula do not require geriatric training. For example, 60% of nursing schools have no geriatric faculty (CDC/Merck, 2004). A shortage of workforce members prepared in geriatrics affects all settings, but it especially affects nursing facilities that serve large numbers of frail elderly. Geriatrics training is also important in other types of health services, such as oncology, neurology, rehabilitation, and critical care (Kovner, Mezey, & Harrington, 2002). Even though there are some encouraging signs that initiatives are being taken by educational institutions in recognition of a critical deficit in geriatric training, it is not clear how the nation will deal with the impending need.

Workforce Diversity

Women's continual entry into the workforce in large numbers is likely to affect health services delivery. Although further research and time will clarify this impact, health services managers should be prepared to improve the work environment to accommodate the needs of female workers. Examples include day care services and flexible work schedules. MCOs are likely to select women for their staff physicians, nurses, social workers, and case managers. Female physicians are expected to prefer managed care to private practice because MCOs are more likely to provide secure income and regular hours.

The increase in the proportion of non-Whites, particularly in the most populous cities and states, is another change. Already, the states of California, Texas, New York, New Jersey, and Florida have significant minority populations. And estimates say near the middle of this century, more than half of U.S. citizens will be non-White (U.S. Census Bureau, 2001). Consequently, the future healthcare workforce will be much more diverse ethnically and racially. Preparation of a culturally competent healthcare workforce is a growing challenge. The term cultural competence refers to knowledge, skills, attitudes, and behavior required of a practitioner to provide optimal healthcare services to persons from a wide range of cultural and ethnic backgrounds. Development of cultural competence is necessary because most future healthcare professionals will be called upon to deliver services to many patients with backgrounds far different from their own. To do so effectively, healthcare providers need to understand how and why different belief systems, cultural biases, ethnic origins, family structures, and many other culture-based factors influence the manner in which people experience illness, comply with medical advice, and respond to treatment. These variations have implications for outcomes of care (Cohen, Gabriel, & Terrell, 2002).

Changes in the racial/ethnic and gender makeup of the workforce will continue to influence the management of health services organizations. Managers will have to consider cultural backgrounds and attitudes toward work as well as employees' potential language and educational disparities. Having more women in the workforce will require awareness of gender pay

disparities and the need to address family issues, such as child care and maternity leave.

Work Organization

In many healthcare settings, multidisciplinary team approach, collaboration, and cross-training will be used to improve quality and productivity. These approaches improve communication, enable practitioners to address complex clinical cases from different perspectives, and improve productivity by avoiding duplication.

Collaborative Team Approach

Consistent with the concept of total quality management is the use of multidisciplinary teams to provide patient services. The team approach concept is intended to provide comprehensive care and to eliminate duplication of services. For example, diabetes is not only a growing health concern in the United States, but it is also a complex chronic disease. Care for diabetes requires significant daily self-care that includes medication management, proper diet, and physical activity. Insulin dependency creates additional daily tasks such as monitoring of blood glucose levels, administering proper dosages of insulin, and managing hypoglycemic episodes. Further, depression is a common comorbidity accompanying diabetes that can lower physical and mental functioning, which can lead to decreased ability to adhere to the self-care regimens. The result can likely be complications that can eventually lead to serious problems such as blindness, heart disease, and kidney failure. In diabetes management, a collaborative team approach provides numerous benefits to patients and practitioners. Also, a collaborative approach can provide medical students valuable cross-training (Robinson,

Barnacle, Pretorius, & Paulman, 2004). A multidisciplinary team approach is also indispensable in ethical decision making. Most medium- and large-sized hospitals have ethics committees that generally include multiple disciplines, such as physicians, nurses, social workers, administrators, ethicists, and clergy. Development of medical science and new technology create new challenges regarding clinical decisions that defy straightforward answers.

Health services providers and managers are more likely to involve key stakeholders, including patients and the population, in decision making (Issel & Anderson, 1996). By involving the patient in decision making, healthcare organizations hope to improve customer service and control costs. In a wellness-care system, it will become apparent that dictating a treatment regimen that customers do not like and will not comply with will not meet the goals of the organization or the customer (Issel & Anderson, 1996).

Cross-Training

Cross-training of health service workers can include teaching an employee to assume additional clinical or clerical roles or training an employee to work in several different areas (D'Aunno, Alexander, & Laughlin, 1996). The ultimate objectives are to improve staff flexibility, realize greater efficiency, and reduce costs. However, cross-training also benefits the employees by furnishing them with a larger set of skills than they would otherwise have. Although licensure issues can hamper worker cross-training in a number of areas, in other areas licensure conflicts do not arise. For example, one tertiary care setting used a cross-training program to evaluate the feasibility of floating a medical/surgical floor nurse to the

medical intensive care unit, and both units have been jointly managed (Gilbert & Counsell, 2000).

Training workers to become multiskilled health practitioners (MHPs) has several advantages. MHPs are an asset to small rural hospitals that may have difficulty obtaining or maintaining staff in certain specialties. Workers trained in multiple areas can respond to changing needs and demands in the health services industry. Continuity of care may also be enhanced by the use of MHPs because cross-trained nurses can attend to patients throughout their care rather than attending to them in a specific care level setting (D'Aunno et al., 1996).

Enhanced Focus on Customer Service

Market forces have increased competition among healthcare providers and networks of providers. Competition has brought with it more input from payers as well as consumers, increased scrutiny of services, and accountability for outcomes. In response, the healthcare industry is placing more emphasis on patient satisfaction. In a consumer-choice market, an institution's client satisfaction ratings may be the best predictor of future success (Coile, 2002). Healthcare organizations will undoubtedly become more service oriented because those regulations and economic factors that made the industry substantially immune to competition are being dismantled (Eisenberg, 1997).

Health services will not make the transition to service orientation without challenge. Eisenberg (1997) cited four barriers that must be overcome:

1. Healthcare environments are highly regulated on everything from waste disposal to records maintenance. To comply with the extensive regulations requires a great deal of time and resources, which can impede focusing on the consumer.

2. The healthcare industry has a traditional resistance to entrepreneurship. Incentives for efficiency and cost management are uncommon. This is partly because of the large number and various types of payers and the traditional view of health services as a noble and charitable enterprise (Eisenberg, 1997).

3. Health services are typically paternalistic. Because hospitalization generally occurs not by choice but because of necessity, consumers are often in a subordinate role without much decision-making power about what happens to them in the hospital.

4. The traditional medical model tends to depersonalize the patient. Patients are categorized by their condition. Training for health careers predominantly focuses on scientific and technical levels, ignoring customer relations.

To compete in a changing healthcare environment, health services will have to overcome these barriers and make a commitment to customer satisfaction and patient relations. This goal can be accomplished by adopting customer service principles as part of the overall mission and philosophy, empowering staff, improving both internal and external communications, creating feedback systems measuring patient satisfaction, and making service environments more user friendly (Eisenberg, 1997).

New Frontiers in Clinical Technology

Technological progress is behind much of the growth in the health services industry. The Institute for the Future (2000) predicted that eight types of medical technologies would especially affect future delivery of patient care—rational drug design, advances in imaging, minimally invasive surgery, genetic mapping and testing, gene therapy, vaccines, artificial blood, and xenotransplantation.

1. Rational drug design is a step beyond the painstaking and costly random search for new pharmaceuticals that is characterized by trial and error. Now, scientists can study the structure and composition of a receptor or enzyme and actually design new chemicals or molecular entities that bind to the receptors or enzymes. Rational drug design will shorten the drug discovery process. The chief candidates for this process are drugs to treat neurological and mental disorders, and antiretroviral therapies for HIV/AIDS, encephalitis, measles, and influenza.

2. Imaging technologies present an enhanced visual display of tissues, organ systems, and their functions. Current research focuses on four areas: (a) Finding new energy sources and focusing an energy beam to avoid damage to adjacent tissue and to minimize residual damage. (b) Use of microelectronics in digital detectors and advances in the contrast media for a finer detection of abnormalities. (c) Faster and more accurate analysis of images using 3-D technology.

(d) Improvements in display technology to produce higher resolution displays.

3. The latest advances in minimally invasive surgery include image-guided brain surgery, minimal access cardiac procedures, and the endovascular placement of grafts for abdominal aneurysms. The overall impact of minimally invasive procedures on cost efficiency and the patients' quality of life from early recovery assures the growth of this technology and the growth of ambulatory surgi-centers.

4. Genetic mapping has enabled the identification of a wide range of genes that can cause complex diseases, such as diabetes, cancer, heart disease, Huntington's disease, and Alzheimer's disease. The discovery of genetic susceptibility to certain diseases will improve preventive techniques. The term *genometrics* is used for the association of genes with specific disease traits.

5. Gene therapy is a therapeutic technique in which a functioning gene is inserted into targeted cells to correct an inborn defect or to provide the cell with a new function. The future challenge in this area is to develop methods that discriminately deliver enough genetic material to the right cells. Cancer treatment is receiving much attention as a prime candidate for gene therapy since current techniques (surgery, radiation, and chemotherapy) are effective in only half the cases.

6. Vaccines have traditionally been used prophylactically to prevent specific infectious diseases, such as diphtheria, smallpox, and whooping cough.

However, the therapeutic use of vaccines in the treatment of noninfectious diseases, such as cancer, has opened new fronts in medicine. At the same time, development of new vaccines for emerging infectious diseases remains on the research agenda. Making today's vaccines safer for wide-scale preventive use against bioterrorism, in which such agents as smallpox and anthrax may be used, will also be an ongoing challenge.

7. Research will continue on the development of fluids that, in many instances, could be used as substitutes for real blood in transfusions, particularly in war and in natural disasters when supplies may fall short.

8. Transplantation of organs is one of the 20th century's great medical advances. It treats a life-threatening chronic disease by replacing the diseased organ. However, a critical shortage of transplantable tissues remains a major concern. Xenotransplantation, in which animal tissues are used for transplants in humans, is a growing research area. New knowledge and methods in molecular genetics, transplantation biology, and genetic engineering look promising.

The Era of Evidence-Based Health Care

Wide variations in clinical practice have finally caught the attention of mainstream media in the United States, raising public awareness of the quality and cost implications of clinical variations (Schaeffer & McMurtry, 2004). There is little evidence that high-spending providers deliver better outcomes. The goal of evidence-based medicine (EBM) is to increase the value of medicine. Even though consumers, as well as practitioners, often fear that reducing costs translates into lower quality, this is not necessarily true. Quality of care can be improved while reducing costs—thus increasing the value of medical care—by reducing misuse and overuse (Slawson & Shaughnessy, 2001). The tools for the practice of evidence-based medicine have been developed for several years, mainly in the form of clinical practice guidelines. Evidence-based practice guidelines are intended to represent best practices and proven therapies.

Several countries have undertaken some significant initiatives in the research and application of EBM. For example, in the United States, the Agency for Healthcare Research and Quality (http://www.ahrq.gov) leads national efforts in the use of evidence to guide healthcare decisions. The establishment of the National Institute for Health and Clinical Excellence (http://www.nice.org.uk) in England, the Scottish Intercollegiate Guidelines Network (http://www.sign.ac.uk), and the National Institute for Clinical Studies (http://www.nicsl.com.au) in Australia have similar responsibilities for developing evidence-based guidelines and for providing information on the clinical aspects and cost effectiveness of interventions (Gerrish et al., 2007).

There is at least some evidence that practitioners may have begun to incorporate EBM into their clinical decision making. For example, Halm and colleagues (2007) reported a remarkable reduction in the proportion of patients undergoing carotid endarterectomy (a surgical procedure that removes the inner lining of the carotid artery if it has become thickened or damaged by plaque) for inappropriate reasons

subsequent to the publication of several large international randomized controlled trials that rationalized the use of the procedure.

On the other hand, the use of guidelines is not widespread in the medical community. Even though the research community has known about clinical variations since the 1970s, and evidence has mounted since then, relatively little has been done to translate this research into actual practice. Many physicians think that guidelines and protocols are either too simple or too complicated, promote "cookbook care," lack creditable authors or evidence, are biased, decrease flexibility, reduce autonomy, and are not applicable to the practice population (Oeyen, 2007).

Future strategies are needed to improve guidelines and protocols and their adherence. At least six recommendations can be made for the future:

1. The issue of practice variations will require the attention of practitioners, payers, and policy makers.

2. Computer-based models will have to be developed to incorporate EBM into medical decision making. Models that are easily usable and understandable are essential.

3. Conducting ongoing clinical trials will be the backbone of EBM. Adherence to clinical guidelines is higher when the recommendations are supported by evidence from randomized controlled trials (Leape et al., 2003).

4. Guidelines and protocols must be revised and kept current to incorporate subsequent scientific evidence.

5. Future practice guidelines must incorporate economic analysis. Mounting healthcare expenditures will pressure

society to make rational choices about when certain types of services become unwarranted. Treatments with cost-effectiveness ratios greater than a widely agreed upon standard may have to be eliminated from recommended practice. Also, future technological change will be driven by assessments that show clear-cut clinical and economic advantages.

6. Financial incentives, including provider payments and patient cost sharing, must be restructured. Reimbursement methods should focus on paying for best achievable outcomes and the most effective care over the course of treatment instead of paying for units of service (Gauthier, Schoenbaum, & Weinbaum, 2006).

In the future, EBM will also transcend what physicians do. For example, the practice of nursing, pharmacology, and other disciplines allied with the practice of medicine will be governed by EBM. Eventually, EBM will become the standard that will govern the multidisciplinary process of healthcare delivery.

Conclusion

At the dawn of the 21st century, the only certainty facing health care is change. Future directions will be determined mainly by social, cultural, technological, and economic changes. Lack of access for the uninsured and cost inflation will continue to haunt the system. In the short run, greater cost shifting will move more expense from employers to employees. A defined contribution from employers is likely to replace the existing defined benefit program. To what extent this shift will occur and to what extent employers may actually abdicate their responsibility to be directly involved in purchasing health insurance will depend largely on the state of the economy and labor markets. Managed care's vast infrastructure will not be easily dismantled. Instead, it is more reasonable to assume that in a changing environment, managed care itself will have to evolve, since employers once again will be in a position to exert enough influence to bring about certain desired changes. Better management of risk and more accountability for cost and quality will be demanded. Universal health care is once again appearing on the national policy agenda. If a national healthcare system becomes a reality, universal access will be restricted to essential care. Those wanting access to services beyond the essentials will have to pay for them.

Under growing cost pressures, wellness and public health will be more strongly emphasized. In a reformed healthcare system, a major challenge will be to forge partnerships between communities and all levels of government. Coordinating functions and developing needed infrastructures have become even more critical due to increased threats of bioterrorism and outbreaks of new infectious diseases.

A rapidly growing elderly population that requires care for chronic ailments and long-term care will pose increased challenges. Physicians will need training to function more effectively in a chronic care environment.

Composition of the healthcare workforce will undergo changes because of a decline in inpatient hospital care, an increasing elderly population, and more women and minorities entering the healthcare workforce. Despite recent efforts to bring about some parity, the problems associated with specialty maldistribution and geographic maldistribution will continue. Even though currently there is a surplus of physicians in the United States, by 2020, a shortage could exist. A shortage of nurses has also been projected, but factors such as economic conditions, immigration, and educational incentives could change the outlook.

As minority populations continue to increase and the workplace becomes increasingly diverse, healthcare managers face the challenge of preparing a culturally competent healthcare workforce. The healthcare workforce also needs to be schooled to give geriatric care. Additional workforce issues include cross-training and the team approach to addressing complex problems.

Health care is often seen as developing into a consumer-choice market. Client satisfaction and customer services will increasingly determine the success of healthcare organizations in a competitive market. However, industry regulations, lack of incentives, paternalism, and predominance of the medical model pose critical barriers to service orientation.

New frontiers will be opened in the application of clinical, informational, and telehealth technology. Technologies such as new drugs, safer procedures, gene therapy, and therapeutic use of vaccines will strongly affect treatments for cancer, HIV/AIDS, and neurological diseases. Sharing of information among providers, intermediaries, and consumers will be necessary to achieve better efficiency and disease management. However, adoption of costly information technology will be driven by cost-benefit considerations.

Evidence-based medicine will play a growing role in the delivery of medical care that is both effective and cost effective. Higher quality at lower cost can be achieved by reducing misuse and overuse based on clinical evidence. Hence, use of clinical practice guidelines that represent best practices and have been proven through clinical trials will become the standard for clinical care delivery.

Discussion Questions

1. Discuss the future direction of employer-based health insurance in the United States.
2. What are managed care's future challenges? How might MCOs address them?
3. What are some of the incremental changes in financing and insurance that the existing healthcare system might see?
4. What proposals might work in a universal access program in the United States, if and when the time comes to debate such proposals?
5. Discuss how the role of public health will change in the future.
6. What are some of the workforce-related challenges the United States will face in the future?
7. Discuss some of the changes in the areas of work organization in healthcare delivery.
8. Give an overview of what new technology might achieve in the delivery of health care.
9. What are the advantages of collaborative teamwork in managing healthcare delivery?
10. What is evidenced-based medicine, and why is it important to advanced nursing practice?

References

Auerbach, D. I., Buerhaus, P. I., & Staiger, D. O. (2007). Better late than never: Workforce supply implications of later entry into nursing. *Health Affairs, 26*(1), 178–185.

Baker, E. I., & Koplan, J. P. (2002). Strengthening the nation's public health infrastructure: Historic challenge, unprecedented opportunity. *Health Affairs, 21*(6), 15–27.

Biles, B., Dallek, G., & Nicholas, L. H. (2004). Medicare advantage: Deja vu all over again? *Health Affairs Web Exclusives, 23*(Suppl. 2), W4-586–W4-597.

Borger, C., Smith, S., Truffer, C., Keehan, S., Sisko, A., Poisal, J., et al. (2006, January–June). Health spending projections through 2015: Changes on the horizon. *Health Affairs Web Exclusives, W61–W73.*

Buchmueller, T., Johnson, R. W., & Lo Sasso, A. T. (2006). Trends in retiree health insurance, 1997–2003. *Health Affairs, 25*(6), 1507–1516.

Burke, S. P., Feder, J., & Van de Water, P. N. (2005). *Developing a better long-term care policy: A vision and strategy for America's future.* Washington, DC: National Academy of Social Insurance.

Catlin, A., Cowan, C., Heffler, S., Washington, B., & the National Health Expenditure Accounts Team. (2007). National health spending in 2005: The slowdown continues. *Health Affairs, 21*(1), 142–153.

CDC/Merck. (2004). *The state of aging and health in America, 2004.* Centers for Disease Control and Prevention/Merck Institute of Aging & Health. Retrieved October 12, 2007, from http://www.cdc.gov/aging/pdf/State_of_Aging_and_Health_in_America_2004.pdf

Christianson, J. B., Parente, S. T., & Taylor, R. (2002). Defined-contribution health insurance products: Development and prospects. *Health Affairs, 21*(1), 49–64.

Claxton, G., Gil, I., & Finder, B. (2005a). *Employer health benefits: 2005 annual survey.* Washington, DC: The Kaiser Family Foundation and Health Research and Educational Trust.

Claxton, G., Gabel, J., Gil, I., Pickreign, J., Whitmore, H., Finder, B., et al. (2005b). What high-deductible plans look like: Findings from a national survey of employers, 2005. *Health Affairs Web Exclusives, 24*(Suppl. 3), W5-434–W5-441.

Claxton, G., Gil, I., Finder, B., & DiJulio, B. (2006). *Employer health benefits: 2006 annual survey.* Washington, DC: The Kaiser Family Foundation and Health Research and Educational Trust.

Cohen, H. J., Feussner, J. R., Weinberger, M., Carnes, M., Hamdy, R. C., Hsieh, F., et al. (2002). A controlled trial of inpatient and outpatient geriatric evaluation and management. *New England Journal of Medicine, 346*(12), 906–912.

Cohen, J. J., Gabriel, B. A., & Terrell, C. (2002). The case for diversity in the health care workforce. *Health Affairs, 21*(5), 90–102.

Coile, R. C. (2002). *Futurescan 2002: A forecast of healthcare trends.* Chicago: Health Administration Press.

Colwill, J. M., & Cultice, J. M. (2003). The future supply of family physicians: Implications for rural America. *Health Affairs, 22*(1), 190–198.

Congressional Budget Office (CBO). (1999). *CBO Memorandum: Projections of expenditures for long-term care services for the elderly.* Washington, DC: CBO.

Congressional Budget Office (CBO). (2004). *Financing long term care for the elderly.* Washington, DC: CBO.

Coughlin, T. A., & Zuckerman, S. (2005). Three years of state fiscal struggles: How did Medicaid and SCHIP fare? *Health Affairs Web Exclusives, 24*(Suppl. 3), W5-385–W5-398.

Crowley, J. S. (2006). *Medicaid long-term care services reforms in the Deficit Reduction Act.* Washington, DC: The Henry J. Kaiser Family Foundation.

D'Aunno, T., Alexander, J. A., & Laughlin, C. (1996). Business as usual? Changes in health care's workforce and organization of work. *Hospital and Health Services Administration, 41*(1), 3–18.

Department of Health and Human Services. (2003). *The future supply of long-term care workers in relation to the aging baby boom generation, Report to Congress.* Washington, DC: Department of Health and Human Services.

Department of Health and Human Services. (2005). *Physician workforce policy guidelines for the United States, 2000–2020.* Washington, DC: Department of Health and Human Services.

Department of Health and Human Services. (2006). *Health, United States, 2006.* Hyattsville, MD: DHHS.

Eisenberg, B. (1997). Customer service in healthcare: A new era. *Hospital and Health Services Administration, 42*(1), 17–31.

Foundation for Accountability. (2001). *Portrait of the chronically ill in America, 2001.* Portland, OR: The Foundation for Accountability, and Princeton, NJ: The Robert Wood Johnson Foundation.

Friedland, R. (1996). The role of managed care in the future. *Generations, 20*(1), 37–41.

Galvin, R. S., Delbanco, S., Milstein, A., & Belden, G. (2005). Has the Leapfrog Group had an impact on the health care market? *Health Affairs, 24*(1), 228–233.

Galvin, R. S., & Delbanco, S. (2006). Between a rock and a hard place: Understanding the employer mindset. *Health Affairs, 25*(6), 1548–1555.

Gauthier, A., Schoenbaum, S. C., & Weinbaum, I. (2006). *Toward a high performance health system for the United States.* New York: The Commonwealth Fund.

Gerrish, K., Ashworth, P., Lacey, A., Bailey, J., Cooke, J., Kendall, S., et al. (2007). Factors influencing the development of evidence-based practice: A research tool. *Journal of Advanced Nursing, 57*(3), 328–338.

Gilbert, M., & Counsell, C. (2000). Intensive care unit cross training: Saving dollars while retaining staff. *Journal of Nursing Administration, 30*(6), 308, 324.

Ginzberg, E. (1999). U.S. health care: A look ahead to 2025. *Annual Review of Public Health, 20,* 55–66. Retrieved October 12, 2007, from http://arjournals.annualreviews.org/doi/full/10.1146/annurev.publhealth.20.1.55

Gold, M. (2006). Commercial health insurance: Smart or simply lucky? *Health Affairs, 25*(6), 1490–1493.

Gow, J. (2002). The HIV/AIDS epidemic in Africa: Implications for U.S. policy. *Health Affairs, 21*(3), 57–69.

Halm, E. A., Tuhrim, S., Wang, J. J., Rojas, M., Hannan, E. L., & Chassin, M. R. (2007). Has evidence changed practice? Appropriateness of carotid endarterectomy after the clinical trials. *Neurology, 68*(3), 187–194.

The Henry J. Kaiser Family Foundation. (2006, October). *Health care in America 2006 survey.* Retrieved October 12, 2007, from http://www.kff.org/kaiserpolls/upload/7573.pdf

The Henry J. Kaiser Family Foundation. (2007, June). *Massachusetts health care reform plan.* Retrieved October 18, 2007, from http://www.kff.org/uninsured/upload/7494-02.pdf

Haislmaier, E. F., & Owcharenko, N. (2006). The Massachusetts approach: A new way to restructure state health insurance markets and public programs. *Health Affairs, 25*(6), 1580–1590.

Holahan, J., & Cook, A. (2005). Changes in economic conditions and health insurance coverage, 2000–2004. *Health Affairs Web Exclusives, 24,* W498–W508.

Institute for the Future. (2000). *Health and health care 2010: The forecast, the challenge.* San Francisco: Jossey-Bass Publishers.

Institute of Medicine. (1996). *2020 vision: Health in the 21st century.* Washington, DC: National Academy Press.

Issel, M., & Anderson, R. (1996). Take charge: Managing six transformations in health care delivery. *Nursing Economics, 14*(2), 78–85.

Kassalow, J. S. (2001). *Why health is important to U.S. foreign policy.* New York: Council on Foreign Relations and Milbank Memorial Fund.

Keenan, P. S., Cutler, D. M., & Chernew, M. (2006). The "graying" of group health insurance. *Health Affairs, 25*(6), 1497–1506.

Kirby, J. B., Machlin, S. R., & Cohen, J. W. (2003). Has the increase in HMO enrollment within the Medicaid population changed the pattern of health service use and expenditures? *Medical Care, 41*(7, Suppl.), III24–III34.

Kovner, C. T., Mezey, M., & Harrington, C. (2002). Who cares for older adults? Workforce implications of an aging society. *Health Affairs, 21*(5), 78–89.

Lamm, R. D., & Blank, R. H. (2005, July/August). The challenge of an aging society. *The Futurist,* 23–27.

LAPSR (Los Angeles Physicians for Social Responsibility). (1996). *Health care reform: Information and commentary.* Retrieved from http://www.labridge.com/psr.healthreform.html

Leape, L. L., Weissman, J. S., Schneider, E. C., Piana, R. N., Gatsonis, C., & Epstein, A. M. (2003). Adherence to practice guidelines: The role of specialty society guidelines. *American Heart Journal, 145*(1), 19–26.

May, J. H., Bazzoli, G. J., & Gerland, A. M. (2006, January–June). Hospitals' responses to nurse staffing shortages. *Health Affairs Web Exclusives,* W316–W323.

Mays, G. P., Miller, A., & Halverson, P. K. (2000). *Local public health practice: Trends and models.*

Washington, DC: American Public Health Association.

McClellan, M., & Baicker, K. (2002). Reducing uninsurance through the nongroup market: Health insurance credits and purchasing groups. *Health Affairs Web Exclusives*, W363–W366.

McKethan, A., Gitterman, D., Feezor, A., & Enthoven, A. (2006). New directions for public health care purchasers? Responses to looming challenges. *Health Affairs, 25*(6), 1518–1528.

Miller, E. A., & Mor, V. (2006). *Out of the shadows: Envisioning a brighter future for long-term care in America.* Providence, RI: Brown University.

Milstien, J. B., Kaddar, M., & Paule Kieny, M. (2006). The impact of globalization on vaccine development and availability. *Health Affairs, 25*(4), 1061–1069.

National Association of County Health Officials. (1994). *Blueprint for a healthy community: A guide for local health departments.* Washington, DC: NACCHO.

Novick, L. F. (2001). Defining public health: Historical and contemporary developments. In L. F. Novick & G. P. Mays (Eds.), *Public health administration: Principles for population-based management* (pp. 3–33). Gaithersburg, MD: Aspen Publishers, Inc.

Oeyen, S. (2007). About protocols and guidelines: It's time to work in harmony! *Critical Care Medicine, 35*(1), 292–293.

Patel, V. (2002). Raising awareness of consumers' options in the individual health insurance market. *Health Affairs Web Exclusives*, W367–W371.

RAND. (2005). *Future health and medical care spending of the elderly: Implications for Medicare.* Santa Monica, CA: RAND Corporation.

Robinson, W. D., Barnacle, R. E. S., Pretorius, R., & Paulman, A. (2004). An interdisciplinary student-run diabetic clinic: Reflections on the collaborative training process. *Families, Systems, and Health, 22*(4), 490–496.

Sanofi-Aventis U.S. (2006). *Managed care digest series: Government digest.* Bridgewater, NJ: Sanofi-Aventis U.S.

Satcher, D. (2006). The prevention challenge and opportunity. *Health Affairs, 25*(4), 1009–1011.

Schaeffer, L. D., & McMurtry, D. E. (2004). When excuses run dry: Transforming the U.S. health care system. *Health Affairs Web Exclusives*, VAR117–VAR120.

Serota, S. (2002). The individual market: A delicate balance. *Health Affairs Web Exclusives*, W377–W379.

Singh, D. A. (2005). *Effective management of long-term care facilities.* Sudbury, MA: Jones and Bartlett Publishers.

Slawson, D. C., & Shaughnessy, A. F. (2001). Using "medical poetry" to remove the inequities in health care delivery. *Journal of Family Medicine, 50*(1), 51–65.

Swartz, K. (2002). Government as reinsurer for very-high-cost persons in nongroup health insurance markets. *Health Affairs Web Exclusives*, W380–W382.

U.S. Census Bureau. (2001). *Statistical abstract of the United States, 2001.* Washington, DC: U.S. Census Bureau.

White, B. (2001). The future of health care financing. *Family Practice Management, 8*(1), 31–36.

Whitmore, H., Collins, S. R., Gabel, J., & Pickreign, J. (2006). Employers' views on incremental measures to expand health coverage. *Health Affairs, 25*(6), 1668–1678.

Wolff, J. L., & Boult, C. (2005). Moving beyond round pegs and square holes: Restructuring Medicare to improve chronic care. *Annals of Internal Medicine, 143*(6), 439–445.

Advanced Practice Nurses and Public Policy, Naturally

Jeri A. Milstead

CHAPTER OBJECTIVES

1. Discuss the historical and emerging role nursing and nursing organizations have played in public policy.
2. Appreciate the integration of policy, practice, research, and education and its impact on the practice of the advanced practice nurse.
3. Define public policy and its components.
4. List the four stages of the policy processes and understand how to influence this process.
5. Identify future policy issues for the advanced practice nurse role.

Introduction

The advanced practice nurse of the third millennium must be technically competent, use critical thinking and decision models, possess vision that is shared with colleagues and consumers, and function in a vast array of roles. One of these roles is policy expert. In spite of the influence of Florence Nightingale in the 19th century, nurses in the 20th century nearly lost the role of the nurse in the political arena. Only at the end of the 1990s was this aspect of the role becoming integrated into the scope of practice of the advanced practice nurse. Policy and politics is a natural domain for nurses, and the full integra-

tion into practice chronicles nursing's heritage and the evolution of the profession and the healthcare system. Major changes in the profession and society mirror the evolution, including changes in the practice of nursing, the emerging political role of nurses, finding a foundation in theory, and a new organizational paradigm.

Chapter 13

Changes in the Practice of Nursing

The changing paradigm in the delivery of health care of the late 20th century is reflected in changes in the practice of nursing. In the early

1900s when nurses traditionally worked in homes or did home visits through an organized nursing service, nurses focused on personal care of individuals who were sick. As hospitals took on the function of workshops for physicians, nurses were employed to provide care to many individuals in one site. Just as organizational theorists were trying to establish the structure and function of institutional arrangements that developed with the industrial age, nurses were trying to establish the roles and functions of organizational employees in a system that was becoming very complex. Nurses categorized patients as those with primarily medical or primarily surgical problems, which led to the early differentiation of types of floors or areas in which nurses worked and which also differentiated nursing expertise in specific areas. Some nurses became organizational experts as they managed nursing units and whole hospitals.

As early as the 1940s, nurses were creating typographies of areas of nursing. Psychiatric, pediatric, obstetrical, medical, and surgical nursing were considered distinct clinical areas that were required for basic practice and, as such, were tested in early examinations for licensure. By the 1950s, nursing programs long had recognized the teaching of nursing as an area that required knowledge beyond the traditional baccalaureate degree. Bachelor of science degrees in nursing education (BSNE) had been offered at the undergraduate level to prepare nurses to teach in diploma schools of nursing. BSNE programs were phased out as specialization in all areas of nursing education, and clinical practice was ascribed to the master's level.

After World War II, veterans (including nurses) pursued college degrees through the GI bill. With the dearth of advanced nursing education programs, many nurses enrolled as education majors. Students and faculty in many areas were struggling with the impact of an explosion of knowledge and questioned whether their fields were science and whether the discipline fit the definition and expectations of a profession. For example, the discipline of political economy changed its name to political science and many nursing programs became nursing science programs. Practitioners of nursing adopted the scientific process and embraced the scientific theory of assessing, planning, implementing, and evaluating what nurses do. Nursing education programs sought courses in the natural sciences (chemistry and physiology) and social sciences (sociology and psychology) to provide a foundation for the nursing courses that were evolving with theories and models. Research became important to confirm nursing's position as a profession, but many of the studies examined the behavior of the nurse or the system of nursing education rather than clinical practice. The endorsement of the scientific approach as a logical, linear, and sequential process concomitantly rejected any indication of intuition or discernment of knowledge in any way other than what could be calculated by quantitative measures. The wisdom that was transferred through generations of nurses almost was lost by the insistence in academic programs of a focus on hard science.

By the 1960s, special care areas were surfacing in hospitals. As machines were invented for diagnostic testing and monitoring of patients, as early computers were developed, and as statistics evolved into a special branch of mathematics, physicians and nurses were placing patients into geographic and medically focused units where care could be concentrated. The emergence of coronary care units was quickly followed by the creation of intensive care units that soon became differentiated as surgical, trauma, neonatal, and other narrow domains. Nurses and physicians needed more knowledge and clinical skills to understand the medical, nursing, and technological advances that were occurring, and specialization became formalized into programs.

As nurses came to understand more about what constituted the practice of nursing, the boundaries of nursing expanded. Breaking free of the old-fashioned perspective of the nurse as handmaiden to the physician, nurses in the 1970s and 1980s sought autonomy as independent practitioners of nursing. Nurse practitioner programs were created to relieve a shortage of physicians. However, rather than becoming "junior doctors," nurse practitioners pushed out the margins of the discipline of nursing. Physical examinations, formerly limited to the scope of practice of physicians, were incorporated into nursing education programs, and physical examinations became essential to clinical nursing practice. Assertiveness training was taught in schools of nursing, which produced articulate registered nurses who could speak up. The nursing process became the watchword of the profession, and national standards were adopted based on assessment, diagnosis, planning, implementation, and evaluation criteria. Nursing theories were developed and research was conducted to test the theories. Certification in specialty areas acknowledged the clinical competence of nurses in distinct practice areas. Intensive care nurses became certain of and comfortable with their clinical knowledge and used it to provide physicians with indispensable data and to suggest treatment options. The rise in the number of baccalaureate-prepared nurses triggered a move toward graduate education. The number of doctoral programs in nursing

was increasing. Although the improving image of nursing still did not command the respect from physicians, nurses gained respect and trust with the public.

By the 1990s, nurses were found in many settings. In addition to staff nurses, hospitals employed nurses as unit managers, educators in staff-development departments, coordinators of outpatient services, senior administrators, and creators of data-and-information systems. Nurses also served as infection-control officers, materials coordinators, patient-relations officials, and heads of quality improvement. Outside the hospital, nurses provided direct care in hospices and homes, in occupational health departments of business and industry, in prisons and correctional facilities, in schools, in interdisciplinary teams concerned with the health of astronauts, and in a host of military situations. Nonhospital, nondirect care opportunities found nurses directing their own continuing education companies, staffing professional and specialty associations, and combining nursing knowledge and skill with law and business degrees, in marketing and product sales, in pharmaceutical companies (as salespersons, researchers, and lobbyists), and in computer sales. Professional nurses also were contributing their expertise through positions as executive directors or members of boards of directors of social and health-related associations such as Planned Parenthood, Inc. Nurses were appointed to state boards of nursing; a few ran for public office; and some nurses directed or staffed offices of federal and state legislators, legislative committees and commissions, and bureaucratic agencies. The scope of nursing practice had expanded, and most state nurse practice acts reflected the changes in their legal definitions of nursing.

Laws that govern nursing define the practice of nursing and set the scope of practice of professional nurses. Early definitions of practice focused on the provision of direct care; later definitions added functions and roles such as "teaching, counseling, administration, research, consultation, supervision, delegation and evaluation of practice" and "observation, care, and counsel of the ill, injured, infirm, the promotion and maintenance of health" (Laws governing nursing, 1994, p. 3). Clearly, the role of the nurse had been expanded beyond caring for the sick patient. Laws governing advanced practice nursing have emerged to offer title protection and legal guidance. Because all laws are the result of compromise, nurse practice acts reflect what is acceptable at the time, not the ideal.

The Emerging Political Role of Nurses

As early as the 1960s, social scientists from a broad array of disciplines had investigated the concept of occupational and professional roles. Concepts such as role ambiguity, role congruence, role conflict, and role taking were frequently cited in the literature (Argyris, 1962). Haas's (1964) early study of nurses clarified that role had four dimensions: task, authority or power, deference or prestige, and affect or feelings. In spite of Haas's study, however, the term *role* still is synonymous with task in most of the literature, and readers miss, therefore, a full understanding of the concept. There has been a major shift in the roles that nurses assume. In addition to clinical experts, nurses have become entrepreneurs, decision makers, and political activists. Many nurses realized that in order to control practice and move the profession of

nursing forward as a major player in the health-care arena, nursing and nurses had to be involved in the legal decisions about the health and welfare of the public, decisions that often were made in the governmental arena.

For many nurses, political activism meant letting someone else get involved. For some nurses, political activism meant dusting off the page in the high school or college *Problems in Government* textbook that presented an algorithm about how a bill becomes a law. A focus on the legislative process in which bills are drafted and passed by the Senate and the House of Representatives stimulated some grassroots connections between nurses and their legislative members. Nurses began to tune in to bills that affected a specific disease entity (e.g., diabetes), a population (e.g., the elderly), an issue (e.g., drunk driving), or a personal passion. Nurses learned to write letters to congresspersons and to visit them in their offices on occasion.

Organized nursing, especially the American Nurses Association (ANA), realized early that decisions that affected nurses and their patients often were made in Washington, DC. ANA moved its national headquarters to that city in 1992 (Kelly & Joel, 1995) to establish visibility and make a statement about the seriousness of the purpose of the organization. ANA created political action committees (PACs) that developed processes for endorsing public officials through statements or with financial contributions to their campaigns. ANA also created a department of governmental affairs that employed full-time registered lobbyists who developed ongoing relationships with elected and appointed officials and their staffs. The development of staff relationships was especially critical as nurses learned that the way to access governmental decision makers was through their staff. By developing credibility with those active in the political process and demonstrating integrity and moral purpose as client advocates, nurses slowly became players in the complex process of policy making.

The ANA and its state and district levels educated nurses about the political process through continuing education programs, legislation committee structures, and the creation of Senate and congressional district coordinators. The latter were nurses who volunteered to create ongoing relationships with their U.S. senators and representatives in order to serve as liaisons between legislators and organized nursing. The creation of the Nurses Strategic Action Team (N-STAT) and state nurses association legislative liaison programs provided a grassroots network of nurses throughout the country who are informed when immediate action is needed and who respond quickly to their legislative representatives.

Political appointments of nurses were sporadic but strong appointments. Kristine Gebbie, RN, served as the AIDS czar in the 1990s. Sheila Burke, RN, was chief of staff to Senate Majority Leader Bob Dole, and Dr. Mary Wakefield, RN, was chief of staff for Senators Quentin Burdick and Pete Conrad. Carolyne Davis, RN, served as head of the Health Care Financing Administration, the agency responsible for the third-largest federal budget and for shaping Medicare and Medicaid policy. Virginia Trotter Betts, RN, a former president of ANA, was appointed senior health policy advisor of the U.S. Department of Health and Human Services during the Clinton administration. Also during that administration, Dr. Beverly Malone, RN, another former ANA president, served as deputy assistant secretary for Health and Human Services. Dr. Malone went on to become

the general secretary of the Royal College of Nursing in England, Scotland, and Northern Ireland. These prestigious and powerful appointments came after many years of involvement in politics and with policy makers.

Nurses learned that by using nursing knowledge and skill they could gain the confidence of government actors. Communications skills that were learned in basic skills classes or in psychiatric nursing classes are critical in listening to the discussion of larger health issues and in being able to present nursing's agenda. Personal stories gained from professional nurses' experience anchor altruistic conversations with legislators and their staffs in an important emotional link toward policy design. Nurses' vast network of clinical experts produces nurses in direct care who provide persuasive, articulate arguments with people on Capitol Hill during appropriations committee hearings and informal meetings.

Nurses began to participate in formal, short-term internship programs with elected officials and in bureaucratic agencies. Most of the programs were created by nurses' organizations that were convinced of the importance of political involvement. The interns and fellows learned how to handle constituent concerns, how to write legislation, how to argue with opponents and remain colleagues, and how to maneuver through the bureaucracy. They carried the message of the necessity of the political process to the larger profession, although the rank and file still were not active in this role.

As nurses moved into advanced practice and advanced practice demanded master's degree preparation, the role of the nurse in the policy process became clearer. Through the influence of nurses with their legislators, clinical nurse specialists, certified nurse midwives, certified registered nurse anesthetists, and nurse practitioners were named in several pieces of federal legislation as duly authorized providers of health care. The process was slow; however, the deliberate way of including more nurse groups over time demonstrated that to get a foot in the door is an effective method of allowing change within the seemingly slow processes of government. Some groups of nurses did not understand the political implications of incrementalism (the process of making changes gradually) and wanted all nurse groups named as providers at one time. They did not understand that most legislators do not have any idea what registered nurses do. Those nurse lobbyists who worked directly with legislators and their staff bore the brunt of discontent within the profession and worked diligently and purposefully to provide a unified front on Capitol Hill and to expand the definition of provider at every opportunity. The designation of advanced practice nurses as providers was an entry to federal reimbursement for some nursing services, a major move toward improved client and family access and health care. Advanced practice nurses (APNs) became acutely aware of the critical importance of the role of political activist. Not only did APNs need the basic knowledge, they understood the necessity of practicing the role, developing contacts, working with professional organizations, writing fact sheets, testifying at hearings, and maintaining the momentum to move an idea forward.

However, most nurses still focus their political efforts and skills on the legislative process. They do not have an understanding of the comprehensiveness of the policy process, the much broader process that precedes and follows legislation. For APNs to integrate the policy role into the character of expert nurse, they must recognize the many opportunities for action. APNs

cannot afford to do their own thing, that is, just provide direct patient care. They cannot ignore the political aspects of any issue. Nurses who have fought the battles for recognition as professionals, for acknowledgment of autonomy, and for formal acceptance of clinical expertise worthy of payment for services have enabled APNs today to provide reimbursable, quality services to this nation's residents. The American Association of Colleges of Nursing (Essentials of Baccalaureate Education, 1998; Essentials of Masters Education, 1996) underscored the importance of understanding and becoming involved in policy formation and the organization and financing of health care for the APN with its documents on essential components of baccalaureate and master's education in nursing.

Finding a Foundation in Theory and Research

As nurses in the middle of the 20th century sought more education in institutions of higher learning, they found few nursing programs at the master's and doctoral levels. However, potential nurse scholars were exposed to an array of disciplines from which they could study. Many of those disciplines enjoyed an academic history and were respected for having a body of knowledge. Education, psychology, anthropology, and sociology were the most common academic fields entered by early nurse scholars, and the nurses soon adapted concepts, models, and theories to nursing practice. The process of teaching and learning, principles of adult education, and styles of leadership were drawn from the field of education. Psychology and sociology lent nursing a rational approach to studying behavior, helped nurses ascribe determinants of social and asocial conduct, and provided nursing with a theoretical foundation in interpersonal therapeutic communications. Through the study of anthropology, nurses learned about the customs and values of people different from themselves, the commonalities of human behavior, and the rigors of conducting field research. Aspects of these disciplines became integrated into nursing education, research, and practice.

Nurses became interested in the idea and applicability of theory and within a generation had begun considering the philosophical foundations and theories of nursing. Early nurse theorists, such as Peplau (1952), Orem (1971), and Henderson (1966), concentrated on organizing clinical practice as a deliberate, reasoned response by the nurse to sick people. This move toward intentional activity based on astute observations and thoughtful connections served nursing well. Nursing became "as much an intellectual activity as a physical endeavor" (Halloran, 1983, p. 17). Nursing theories were extrapolated from systems theory as Rogers (1970) and King (1971) developed and refined their thinking about the discipline. Watson (1979) and Benner (1984), building on humanistic concepts and examining the essence of the profession, furthered the theoretical foundation of nursing as they challenged others to conceptualize and redefine commonly held assumptions and relationships. Leininger (1978) confronted nursing's ethnocentricity and provided theoretical groundwork for cultural care from a global perspective. Nurse scholars in other countries, such as Grijpdonk in Belgium and Van de Brink Tjebbes in The Netherlands, developed theories that are being tested for applicability in their own and other cultures (R. Martijn, personal communication, November 12, 1997). These early nurse theorists, among

others, changed the direction of nurses from dependent workers to autonomous thinkers.

The link between nursing research and advanced nursing practice became evident as nurses moved into graduate programs. Master's and doctoral education required research courses, practica, theses, and dissertations. The knowledge and skills that nurses developed served as a foundation for study in a wide array of disciplines and in as many areas of nursing as are available. Although much research was completed, not all of it added to the body of knowledge of clinical nursing. Early studies focused on attitudes and behaviors of nurses and nursing students. Inquiry into theories and models of education, instructional methods, and curriculum development and evaluation contributed to improved presentation of nursing in the academic setting and to the teaching/learning processes practiced by nurses in clinical settings.

Clinical nursing research became a focus area in the 1990s when outcome data were needed to defend nurse decisions. Clinical research cited in nursing journals moved from a few published studies to a wave of clinical trials in a variety of patient care areas. Brooten and Naylor (1995) referred to "nurse dose" (the amount and type of nursing needed to produce an effect of nursing care) as critical in determining outcomes. Blank (1997) named nursing case management as the vehicle through which health care will be restructured as the quality of nursing care is measured through clinical outcomes. Clinical pathways were espoused as a successful way to demonstrate the importance of outcomes to healthcare providers and payers (Porter-O'Grady, 1996; Zander, 1990). Hegyvary (1992) expanded the concept and proposed that patient outcomes reflect the economic, organizational, political, and social context within which they are studied. Far beyond local impact, the influence of nurse experts can never be overestimated for their work with the federal Agency for Healthcare Policy and Research (AHCPR) in the development of clinical practice guidelines. As AHCPR evolved into the Agency for Healthcare Research and Quality (AHRQ), health services research took on an important role in further defining what nursing is and the value of nurses.

The initial link between nursing and policy can be viewed as beginning in the 1960s when nurses sought federal funding for research. The explosion of social programs and the raising of social consciousness that occurred in the 1960s and 1970s in the United States alerted nurses to the value of political activity. The professional association provided a structure for the voice of nursing and developed a cadre of nurses who contributed to policy formation and were committed to political activism.

Today's nurses have a much clearer understanding of what constitutes nursing and how nurses must integrate political processes into their practices to further the decisions made by policy makers. Nurses continue to focus on the individual, family, community, and special populations in the provision of care to the sick and infirm and on the activities that surround health promotion and the prevention of disease and disability. Advanced practice nurses have a foundation in expert clinical practice and can translate that knowledge into understandable language for elected and appointed officials as the officials respond to problems that are beyond the scale or impact of individual healthcare providers. As nurses continue to refine the art and science of nursing, forces external to the profession compel the nursing community to consider another

aspect—the business of nursing—that is paradoxical to the long history of altruism.

A New Organizational Paradigm

The whole economic basis of capitalism, i.e., the manufacturing system, had become outdated by the beginning of the new millennium. Traditional organizational structures that were invented in the late 19th century to accommodate the move from a farm-and-feudal system to an urban-industrial system no longer fit a new age. Hierarchical, bureaucratic institutions had been the norm and centralized, top-down administration had been the method of control. Information was the new commodity, and communications systems were needed to create and disseminate the plethora of new material. The computer chip may someday replace the printing press and forced a move to a new organizational model (Porter-O'Grady & Wilson, 1995). Efficiency and cost containment led to downsizing and rightsizing, which often were euphemisms for "smallsizing" that translated into firings and layoffs. Machine workers had been replaced by technologists, who were being replaced by "knowledge workers" (Drucker, 1959, p. 40). Knowledge workers required new structures and processes for doing their work.

The new paradigm for organizations in the 21st century begins with changes within one's head; that is, a move to a perspective that is outside the usual way of thinking. What work is done, where it is done, and how it is done are mundane questions that demand creative answers. Large manufacturing plants no longer are needed if merchandise can be made elsewhere and retailers can rely on just-in-time inventories. The very question of what product should be produced requires evaluation. The where of work has changed. Offices do not have to exist in a skyscraper, because a computer can be located at the beach, in a mountain retreat, or in a kitchen. However, the new worker cannot afford the isolation and detachment noted in the title character of *Bartleby, the Scrivener* (Melville, 1853), who simply preferred not to be a part of the group. Drucker (1995) insisted that knowledge workers have two new requirements: (1) they work in teams, and (2) if they are not employees, they must be affiliated with an organization. He emphasized that organizations are important because they provide a continuity that enables the worker to convert specialized knowledge into performance. Drucker (1999) also noted that productivity is an organization's greatest challenge. This is especially true in a company in which thinking and making decisions are the major processes. Systems thinking, a metaparadigmatic approach, is crucial to the effectiveness of an organization in the 21st century (Flood & Senge, 1999).

An organization must have a mission that is publicized and in which all workers (both traditional employees and managers) can invest their energies. Structures and processes should be constructed to facilitate the work of the institution (Wheatley, 1992). Part of the new paradigm is based on the assumption that prior worker-and-manager practices that evolved from the old bureaucratic model are outdated and must be replaced with collaborative communications that can mobilize and empower all people in the organization (Champy, 1995). People do not expect establishments to remain static or stable; organizations learn new lessons continuously or they fail (Senge, 1990). Peters (1988) addressed the chaotic nature of new companies as being patterned and dynamic—two characteristics of organizations in the new paradigm that provide direction for all levels of workers. Peters (1997) also noted that innovative organizations are inhabited by innovative people who seek affiliation with others in new, productive coalitions.

Partnerships are valued over competition, and the old rules of business that rewarded power and ownership have given way to accountability and shared risk. Reengineering the old systems to the new systems does not mean merely automating processes or restructuring the organizational chart. Reengineering involves a radical, cross-functional, futuristic change in the way people think (Porter-O'Grady & Malloch, 2002), a reframing or "discontinuous thinking" (Blancett & Flarey, 1995, p. 16). Long-term planning is replaced by strategic planning, and vertical work relationships are replaced with networks and webs of people and knowledge. All workers at all levels share a commitment to the organization and an accountability to define and produce quality work (Covey, 1991). All workers share responsibility for self-governance, from which both the organization and the worker benefit (Porter-O'Grady, Hawkins, & Parker, 1997). Control is replaced by leadership. The new leader does not use policing techniques of supervision but enables and empowers colleagues through vision, trust, and respect (Bennis & Nanus, 1985; Kouzes & Posner, 1987; Porter-O'Grady & Wilson, 1999). Encouragement, appreciation, and personal recognition are celebrated together in an effective organization (Kouzes & Posner, 1999). Table 13–1 presents a framework for organizations in this century.

Kennedy and Charles (1997) assert that, rather than the authority or blind obedience of the

Table 13–1 FRAMEWORK FOR EFFECTIVE ORGANIZATIONS IN THE 21ST CENTURY
• Mission: vision, product/outcome
• Structure: network, linkages, distribution of power, risk management
• Processes: production, challenge, correction
• Culture: communication, technology, access, recognition

industrial establishment, the new leader must return to the origin of the word *author* and serve as coach and mentor by helping others learn. Much as Siddhartha learned that knowledge can be transmitted to others but wisdom must be experienced (Hesse, 1951), the worker of the 21st century needs the knowledge that is passed on from those who have learned over time in order to experience the wisdom necessary to be competent and fulfilled in the new organization.

The Changing Paradigm in Health Care

The impact of the enormous changes occurring in business and industry in the late 20th century was reflected in the healthcare delivery system. Hospitals faced a dinosaur-like future due to several changes. The traditional medical model of a complex hospital system of sick care, a profusion of technology, and ethical questions that could not have been anticipated at the beginning of the century were pointing to a serious need for reform in the healthcare system. The United States was spending 13% of its gross national product on health care, a figure that caused great concern to government officials and economists.

Cost containment began with congressional demand for prospective payment for Medicare recipients through diagnosis-related groups (DRGs). Government-funded Medicare, the largest payer of healthcare services to the elderly in the country, replaced the retrospective method of payment for primarily hospital services (i.e., nursing services) with a system that linked medical diagnoses to length of stay (Fuchs, 1993). Private insurance companies followed the government's lead and reinvented their methods of payment, changing to a prospective system.

Hospital administrators, faced with decreasing income, were forced to contain costs. Nursing care long had been considered by financial personnel as an expenditure, and nurses were not usually thought of as income generators. The actual cost of nursing care was unknown, and few nurses knew how to calculate it or even what factors to consider. Financial analysts and business executives who did not understand the value of quality care became focused on costs and profit. Nursing, a profession that had matured over a few short decades into a confident discipline, found itself confronted with assaults from business decisions that affected the type, setting, scope, and quality of nursing care. How nursing services are produced and calculated, how much nursing care is required for each recipient, and how to decide what mix of service providers is needed became very important questions.

A pecking order in which nurses were subservient to physicians, which was especially noticeable in hospitals, had been established.

Rules were valued, and compliance with rules was the measure of success. "Doctor's orders" were considered inviolate commands, and nurses' clinical knowledge and judgment were discounted. This arrangement generated physician–nurse games in which communication from nurses was couched in passive, circuitous language. Separation of disciplines occurred as health workers focused on distinct parts of the person's illness or problems. Compartmentalization served a pyramidal system but did not contribute to a holistic approach to providing comprehensive health care.

Nurses were confronted with a system that was changing around them and that sometimes produced subtle changes whose impact was not recognized immediately. Nurse managers found themselves dealing with budgets, variances, and other business-related activities for which they had not been educated. Nurses without appropriate education in management and community health were forced to seek referrals for patients who were being discharged after brief hospitalization and to ensure continuity of care in homes and other healthcare agencies.

Corporate mergers and acquisitions and other organizational arrangements resulted in a tumultuous hospital-cum-healthcare system in which layoffs, staff reductions, and elimination of positions and departments affected nurses in many ways. Nurse administrators encountered executive decisions to downsize when new systems and processes were not yet in place. For example, the position of nurse manager was eliminated in many hospitals in the 1990s with the expectation that staff nurses would assume responsibility and accountability for managerial activities, but the requisite education and training were not provided. Licensed nurses were replaced in many institutions with unlicensed assistive personnel who were given inadequate training in a short time and expected to provide comprehensive care with little supervision to ill patients with complex conditions. Staff nurses worried that patient and nurse safety was jeopardized.

The Pew Health Professions Commission (1995) studied the training and practice of healthcare professionals and recommended revolutionary changes in how the professions are regulated and educated. From interdisciplinary and multidisciplinary courses and programs to single professional licensure, the recommendations focused on preparing nurses, physicians, dentists, pharmacists, and other healthcare professionals for practice within the new healthcare paradigm. The Pew Commission encouraged cross-training for multiskilled allied health workers. Nurses understood early that the new definition of interdisciplinary means nursing, allied health, medicine, and other health professions. On the other hand, many physicians think interdisciplinary means specialists in orthopedics, cardiology, radiology, and pulmonology who work together, and allied health professionals believe the term means collaboration among occupational therapists, physical therapists, and physicians' assistants. There still is work to be done to convince all healthcare providers of the value of an interdisciplinary team for the patient and the provider.

Nurses who weathered drastic organizational changes were seldom acknowledged as having to face problems. Noer (1993) was one of the few authors who wrote about the guilt and depression felt by those who did not lose their jobs but were expected to carry on in sometimes deprived circumstances. Nurses took the lead in efforts to redesign nursing systems by proposing systems that replaced the industrial-age concept of responsibility that bred paternalism with accountability, in which empowerment, partnerships, and leadership are fostered (Porter-O'Grady & Wilson, 1995). Reengineering the workplace for nurses demanded a transformation to professional practice (Blancett & Flarey, 1995). Some healthcare systems did not integrate information technology into the new order, resulting in restructured old systems rather than new paradigms of health care, according to nursing informatics expert Roy Simpson (personal communication, June 6, 1998).

Health care in the 20th century was delivered most often through hospitals, although there was a major move to the community in the last decades (Aiken, 1990). In the 1990s, new systems of nurse empowerment were created by visionary nurse leaders such as Blancett and Flarey (1995); Porter-O'Grady and Wilson (1995); and Wolf, Boland, and Aukerman (1994a, b). Nursing responses to external forces of managed care centered on a system of case management in which the nurse, preferably an advanced practice nurse, brokered and coordinated care for clients before, during, and after hospitalization (Ethridge & Lamb, 1989; Genna, 1987; Maurin, 1990; Mundinger, 1984; Zander, Etheredge, & Bower, 1987). Models of case management were created for many organizational structures, acute care facilities, hospices, and community health enterprises (Bower, 1992). As case managers, APNs took the lead in including members of other disciplines in decisions about the health care of clients, families, and communities.

Early in the 21st century, hospitals were investing in corporate partnerships with other healthcare and business organizations. Many mergers and acquisitions resulted in staff cuts, and nurses and other healthcare professionals (e.g., pharmacists, physicians, physical therapists) were forced to rethink the way in which care was provided. Collaboration became a necessity, and whole departments have begun to build coalitions with each other to reduce complexity and improve communication. Healthcare report cards provided a mixed response as to their utility in making informed choices about hospitals and physicians (Dranove, Kessler, McClellan, & Satterthwaite, 2003). After the 1999 Institute of Medicine report (Koln, Corrigan, & Donaldson, 1999) noted the large number of medical errors in hospitals, over 90 major industries formed the Leapfrog Group (Milstead, 2003) that recommended urban hospitals adopt computerized physician order entry, evidence-based hospital referrals, and the use of intensivists. Evidence-based nursing practice developed at the same time and provided credibility for nursing interventions.

Venegoni (1996) identified five significant factors that influenced the changes in healthcare systems for the 21st century: (1) place (site of delivery); (2) people (who receives care); (3) preventive model (reward for health, not sickness); (4) paradigm (quality improvement and customer satisfaction); and (5) process (modern technology). The comparison of the old hospital paradigm and the emerging model (Table 13–2), illustrates a practical expression of Venegoni's factors.

Nurses were taking on new positions in all types of healthcare systems and had become sophisticated providers of care. Beyond that, nurses were beginning to integrate the roles of educator, researcher, administrator, and political activist. As client advocates, nurses speak out on issues of prevention of illness and disability, safety and environmental hazards, and informed consent. Nurses have come to realize the critical nature of involvement with legislators who

Table 13-2 COMPARISON OF OLD HEALTH CARE PARADIGM WITH NEW PARADIGM

Old Paradigm	New Health Care Paradigm
Hospital based, acute care	Short-term hospital: same-day surgery, 23-hour stays; prehospital testing and precertification; telehealth/ telemedicine; home health; mobile vans; school and mall clinics
Specialty units	Cross-training (multiskilled workers): LDRP, OR/PACU, CCU/telemetry
Hierarchical management	Decentralization (unit budget, scheduling, variance); shared governance; strategic plan
Physician as captain of ship; others are followers	Inter/multidisciplinary team, collaboration; case management (registered nurse/broker)
Nurse as employee; job focused, "refrigerator nurse"	Nurse as professional: career-focused clinical ladder; continuing credentials; tuition reimbursement, paid certification exam
Medical condition; focus on segment	Holistic person in family/community; pastoral care, parish nurse
"Sick" care; focus on cure	Health care, health promotion, prevention programs; focus on cure, care, and continuity of care; complementary health alternatives
Cost containment; focus on billing	Focus on patient and accountability of caregivers/agency; electronic patient record, patient/continuous quality improvement, care maps
Written medical record	Integrated electronic records: smart card, bedside computers
Fee for service	Managed competition (HMO, PPO, IPA)
Physician as employer	Physician as employee; capitation system
One insurance plan	Variety of insurance options ("covered lives"): basic plan, dental, eye, long-term care, cancer, disability
80–100%	Greater deductible, lower percentage coverage, or co-payment insurance

make policies such as laws, regulations, and programs that affect nurses, patients, and the healthcare system. A more comprehensive understanding of the societal mandate for nursing services requires that nurses assume an active part of a complex system of sociocultural, economic, and political forces. Nurses, especially those in advanced practice, are expanding the scope of nursing in direct care by addressing healthcare issues that are a matter of public interest. Decisions that affect the public interest are made over time in the policy arena.

What Is Public Policy?

In this chapter, policy is an overarching term used to define both an entity and a process. Although there has not been a clear definition of policy in the nursing literature (Rodgers, 1989), scholars in political science have developed definitions and models from which nursing can benefit. The purpose of public policy is to direct problems to government and secure government's response (Jones, 1984). Although there has been much discussion about the boundaries and domain of government and the extent of difference between the public and private sectors, that debate is beyond the scope of this chapter.

The definition of public policy is important because it clarifies common misconceptions about what constitutes policy. The process of creating policy can be focused in many arenas, and most of these are interwoven. For example, environmental policy deals with health issues such as hazardous material, particulate matter in the air or water, and safety standards in the workplace. Education policy, more than tangentially, is related to health—just ask school nurses. Regulations define who can administer medication to students; state laws dictate what type of sex education can be taught. Defense policy definitely is related to health policy when developing, investigating, or testing biological and chemical warfare.

Policy as an Entity

As an entity, policy is seen in many forms as the standing decisions of an organization (Eulau & Prewitt, 1973). As formal documented directives of an organization, official government policies reflect the beliefs of the administration in power and provide direction for the philosophy and mission of government organizations. Specific policies usually serve as the shoulds and thou shalts of agencies. Some policies, known as position statements, report the opinions of organizations about issues that members believe are important. For example, state boards of nursing (government agencies created by legislatures to protect the public through the regulation of nursing practice) publish advisory opinions on what constitutes competent and safe nursing practice.

The term *policy* is used often to refer to goals, programs, and proposals. Although such substitution may be confusing in conceptualizing policy, the term may be seen as a type of verbal shorthand for colleagues who are discussing a specific program or program goal. For example, nurses who talk about the gag-rule policy of the Reagan administration understand that they are discussing programs, such as Title X of the Medicare program related to family planning that forbade health professionals from discussing abortion as an option to clients in agencies that received federal funding. A similar gag rule occurred in the 1990s when many health maintenance organizations forbade physicians to discuss treatment options with patients.

Agency policies can be broad and general, such as those that describe the relationship of an agency to other governmental groups. In the most narrow sense, policies can be specific announcements, such as operational procedures. Procedure manuals in government hospitals that detail steps in performing certain nursing tasks are examples of specific policy activities. Both general and specific policies serve as guidelines for employee behavior within an institution.

Although the terms *policies* and *procedures* often are used interchangeably, policies usually are considered more broad.

Laws are types of policy entities. As legal directives for public and private behavior, laws serve to define action that reflects the will of society—or at least a segment of society. Laws are made at the international, federal, state, and local levels and have the impact of primary place in guiding conduct. Lawmaking usually is the purview of the legislative branch of government in the United States, although presidential vetoes, executive orders, and judicial interpretations of laws have the force of law.

Judicial interpretation is noted in three ways. First, courts may interpret the meaning of laws that are written broadly or with some vagueness. Laws often are written deliberately with language that addresses broad situations. Agencies that implement the laws then write regulations that are more specific and that guide the implementation. However, courts may be asked to determine questions in which the law is unclear or controversial (Williams & Torrens, 1988). For example, the 1973 Rehabilitation Act prohibited discrimination against the handicapped by any program that received federal assistance. Although this may have seemed fair and reasonable at the outset, courts were asked to adjudicate questions of how much accommodation is fair (Wilson, 1989). Second, courts can determine how some laws are applied. Courts are idealized as being above the political activity that surrounds the legislature. Courts also are considered beyond the influence of politically active interest groups. The court system, especially the federal court system, has been called upon to resolve conflicts between levels of government (state and federal) and between laws enacted by the legislature and interpretation by powerful interest groups. For example, courts may determine who is eligible or who is excluded from participation in a program. In this way, special interest groups that sue to be included in a program can receive "durable protection" from favorable court decisions (Feldstein, 1988, p. 32). Third, courts can declare the laws made by Congress or the states unconstitutional, thereby nullifying the statutes entirely (Litman & Robins, 1991). Courts also interpret the Constitution, sometimes by restricting what the government (not private enterprise) may do (Wilson, 1989).

Regulations are another type of policy initiative. Although they often are included in discussions of laws, regulations are different. Once a law is enacted by the legislative branch, the executive branch of government is charged with administrative responsibility for implementing the law. The executive branch consists of the president and all of the bureaucratic agencies, commissions, and departments that carry out the work for the public benefit. Agencies within the government formulate regulations that achieve the intent of the statute. On the whole, laws are written in general terms, and regulations are written more specifically to guide the interpretation, administration, and enforcement of the law. The Administrative Procedures Act (APA) was created to provide opportunity for citizen review and input throughout the process of developing regulations. The APA ensures a structure and process that is published and open, in the spirit of the founding fathers, so that the average constituent can participate in the process of public decision making.

All of these entities evolve over time and are accomplished through the efforts of a variety of actors or players. Although commonly used, the terms *position statement, resolution, goal, objective, program, procedure, law,* and *regulation* really are not interchangeable with the word *policy*. Rather, they are the formal expressions of policy decisions. For the purposes of understanding just what policy is, nurses must grasp policy as a process.

Policy as a Process

In viewing policy as a guide to government action, nurses can study the process of policy making over time. Milio (1989) presents four major stages in which decisions that translate to government policies are made: (1) agenda setting, (2) legislation and regulation, (3) implementation, and (4) evaluation. Agenda setting is concerned with identifying a societal problem and bringing it to the attention of government. Legislation and regulation are formal responses to a problem. Implementation is the execution of policies or programs toward the achievement of goals. Evaluation is the appraisal of policy performance or program outcomes.

Within each stage, formal and informal relationships are developed among actors both within and outside of government. Actors can be individuals, such as a legislator, a bureaucrat, or a citizen. Actors also can be institutions, such as the presidency, the courts, political parties, or special-interest groups. A series of activities that brings a problem to government occurs, which results in direct action by the government to address the problem. Governmental responses are political; that is, the decisions about who gets what and when and how they get it are made within a framework of power and influence, negotiation, and bargaining (Lasswell, 1958).

One must recognize that the policy process is not necessarily sequential or logical. The definition of a problem, which usually occurs in the agenda-setting phase, may change during legislation. Program design may be altered significantly during implementation. Evaluation of a policy or program (often considered the last phase of the process) may propel onto the national agenda (often considered the first phase of the process) a problem that differs from the original. However, for the purpose of organizing one's thoughts and conceptualizing the policy process, the policy process is examined from the linear perspective of stages.

Even before the process itself can be studied, nurses must understand why it is so important to be knowledgeable about the components and the functions of the process and how this public arena has become an integral part of the practice of advanced nursing.

Why Nurses and Public Policy?

Registered professional nurses have studied the basics of how a bill becomes a law in their baccalaureate programs. An extension of the focus on legislation usually is provided in graduate schools. However, most nurses (and most nurse educators) do not have a clear understanding of the total policy process. To focus on legislation misses a whole range of governmental and political activities—activities in which professional nurses should have a central place. In the 1990s, the healthcare delivery system was the subject of a major thrust of reform. Reform is a political process in which priorities are determined and public policy decisions are made. Nurses, as the largest group of healthcare professionals in the country and as the providers of the most direct and continuous care to individuals and groups, were at the table. That is, nursing was included in the short list of groups convened by a presidential mandate that were instrumental in assisting the government in the mid-1990s to make changes that would directly affect the health of citizens and the legal purview of the healthcare professions. The nursing presence was a direct result of the many years of leadership exerted by a few nurses (mostly through the professional associations) who have understood the importance and have worked tirelessly to develop relationships, to identify problems and suggest solutions, and to demonstrate willingness to compromise in the present to secure greater gain in the future. Although the federally directed process of reform did not result in substantial change, all of the issues that nursing brought to the discussion were still being addressed after legislation failed. These issues, such as universal access to health care, a basic services package, an emphasis on health promotion and disease prevention, catastrophic coverage for long-term care, and an initial emphasis on at-risk populations such as women and children (Nursing's Agenda, 1994), fell to the states for discussion.

Nurses and nursing are at the center of issues of tremendous and long-lasting impact, such as access to providers, quality of care, and reasonable cost. In addition, issues crucial to the profession are being decided, such as who is eligible for government reimbursement for services and what is the appropriate scope of practice of registered nurses in advanced practice. If nurses wait until legislation is being voted on before they become involved, it will be too late to affect decisions. Nurses have learned the legislative process. Nurses have written letters and made visits to their legislators. Now nurses must move forward and apply the knowledge of the whole policy process by speaking out to a variety of appropriate governmental actors and institutions so that nursing can move issues onto the national agenda, lobby Congress with alternatives, and provide nursing expertise as policies and programs are being designed. In addition, nurses must be the watchdogs as pro-

grams are implemented so that target groups are served and services are appropriate. Nurses should be experts at program evaluation and continuing feedback to ensure that old problems are being addressed, new problems are being identified, and appropriate solutions are being considered. The opportunities for nursing input throughout the policy process are unlimited and certainly not confined narrowly to the legislative process. Nurses are articulate experts who can address both the rational shaping of policy and the emotional aspects of the process. Nurses cannot afford to limit their actions to monitoring bills; they must seize the initiative and use their considerable collective and individual influence to ensure the health, welfare, and protection of the public and healthcare professionals.

An Overview of the Policy Process

Advanced practice nurses should have an overview of the total process so that they do not get stuck on legislation. Many useful articles and books have been written about policy in general and even about specific policies, but few have addressed the scope of the policy process or defined the components. The elements of agenda setting (including problem definition), government response (legislation, regulation, or programs), and policy and program implementation and evaluation are distinct entities but are connected as parts of a whole tapestry in the process of public decision making.

Agenda Setting

Getting a healthcare problem to the attention of government can be a tremendous first step in getting relief. The actual mechanism of defining a healthcare problem is a major political issue in which APNs can participate, especially in a collective manner as an interest group. Problem definition often is influenced by special-interest groups. When acquired immune deficiency syndrome (AIDS) was first diagnosed in the 1980s, the disease was perceived as a problem of homosexuals and intravenous drug users. Within this definition, assumptions were made by government officials that the disease might be confined to a small population. Federal health agencies were not likely to obtain a large budget for a disease that affected small groups, especially those considered outside the mainstream of American values. Gay rights activist organizations such as the Gay Men's Health Crisis (GMHC) and AIDS Coalition to Unleash Power (ACTUP) were special-interest groups that were instrumental in persuading the government to alter the definition of the AIDS problem by broadening it to include persons other than homosexuals. As AIDS became known in hemophiliacs, infants, and heterosexual men, the problem became redefined as a community health problem. From this perspective, AIDS was perceived as having an impact on a larger segment of the population, including mainstream Americans. Government officials in the administrative and legislative branches were pressured to assume responsibility for addressing an epidemic. Officials were able to identify a variety of departments and agencies beyond the traditional health and human services, such as the Department of Defense and the Bureau of Indian Affairs, that could seek funding for programs of research and treatment. Defining the problem differently increased access to the national agenda.

APNs must come to understand the concepts of windows of opportunity, policy entrepreneurs, and political elites. Sound bites and word bites are tools that were introduced by people who were invested in getting the AIDS crisis onto the national agenda (Milstead, 1993). Gay rights groups used radical political action tactics borrowed from the civil rights movement of the 1960s and 1970s to get their message heard by those in Washington, DC. Activists conducted sit-ins and marches, testified at hearings, ridiculed weak efforts to provide research and treatment, and held press conferences. During the press conferences, self-taught activists learned that although a person may be recorded by microphone or video camera during a speech, only a few seconds would be broadcast on the news. Activists prepared written scripts of selected material from their interviews in advance of the interviews and presented the scripts to the media people. This allowed the speakers to talk at length about their issues and yet focus the media replay to ensure that a specific message was promoted.

Government Response

The government response to public problems often emanates from the legislative branch and comes in three forms: (1) laws, (2) rules and regulations, and (3) programs. Because only senators and representatives can introduce legislation (not even the president can bring a bill to the floor of either house), these elected officials command respect and attention. The work of legislation is not clear cut or linear. Informal communication and influence are the coin of the realm when trying to construct a program or law from the often vague wishes of disparate groups. The committee structure of both houses is a powerful method of accomplishing the work of government.

Conference committees are known as the third house of Congress (How our laws are made, 1990) because of their power to force compromise and bring about new legislation. APNs must appreciate the difference between the authorization and appropriations processes and seek influence in both arenas. Becoming involved directly with legislators and their staffs has been a training ground for many APNs. Supporting or opposing passage of a bill often has served as the first contact with the political process for many nurses. However, this place often has been the stopping point for many nurses because they were unaware of other avenues of involvement, such as the follow-up process of regulations and rule making.

Lowi (1969) noted that administrative rule making often takes place as an effort to bring about order within environments that are unstable and full of conflict. Some regulations codify precedent; others break new ground and address issues not previously explicated. An example of the latter is the Federal Trade Commission's (FTC) trade regulation rules. In 1964, the FTC, whose mission is to protect the consumer and enforce antitrust, wrote regulations requiring health warnings on cigarette packages. The tobacco industry reacted so fiercely that Congress quickly passed a law that nullified the regulations and replaced them with less stringent ones (West, 1982). Other ways to sanction agencies whose rules are viewed as too restrictive are to reduce budget allocations and increase the number of adjudications or trial-like reviews. Advanced practice nurses must become knowledgeable about the regulatory process so that they can spot opportunities to contribute or intervene prior to final rule making (The regulatory process, 1992).

Programs are concrete manifestations of solutions to problems. Program design often is a joint effort of legislative intent, budgetary expediency, and political feasibility (the latter meaning "an interest group arrangement hammered out in Congress" [Skocpol, 1995, p. 283]). There are many opportunities for nurses in advanced practice to become involved in the design phase of a program. Selecting an agency to administer the program, choosing the goals, and selecting the tools that will ensure eligibility and participation are all decisions in which the APN should collaborate.

Policy and Program Implementation

It is important that APNs keep reminding their colleagues that the phases of the policy process are not linear and that policy activities are fluid and move within and among the phases in dynamic processes. The implementation phase includes those activities in which legislative mandates are carried out, most often through programmatic means. The implementation stage also includes a planning ingredient. Problems occur in program planning if technological expertise is not available. This is particularly important to nurses, who are experts in the delivery of health care in the broadest sense.

If government officials do not know qualified, appropriate experts, then decisions about program planning and design often are determined by legislators, bureaucrats, or staff who know little or nothing about the problem or the solutions. As excellent problem solvers, APNs have many opportunities to offer ideas and solutions. One strategy is to employ second-order change to reframe situations and recommend pragmatic alternatives to implementors (de Chesnay, 1983; Watzlawick, Weakland, & Fisch, 1974). Bowen (1982) used probability theory to demonstrate how program success could be improved. She suggested putting several clearance points (instances where major decisions are made) together so that they could be negotiated as a package deal. She also advocated beginning the bargaining process with alternatives that have the greatest chance for success and using that success as a foundation for building more successes, a strategy she referred to as a "bandwagon approach" (p. 10). In the past, nurses have done the opposite: focused on failure and perceived lack of nursing power. APNs have begun to note successes in the political arena and are building a new level of success and esteem. The nurse in advanced practice today uses the strategies of packaging, success begets success, and persistence in a deliberate way so that nurses can increase their effective impact in the implementation of social programs. Although nurses most often work toward positive impact, they have found that opposition to an unsound program can have a paradoxical positive effect. Although not in the public arena, an example of phenomenal success in the judicious use of opposition occurred when the professional body of nursing rose up as one against the American Medical Association's 1986 proposal to create a new type of low-level healthcare worker called a registered care technician. The power emerged as over 40 nursing organizations stood together in opposition to an ill-conceived proposal that would have placed patients in jeopardy and created dead-end jobs.

Policy and Program Evaluation

For nurses who have worked within the nursing process of clinical reasoning (Pesut & Herman,

1999), the process of evaluation seems to be a logical component of the policy process. Evaluation is the systematic application of methods of social research to public policies and programs. Evaluation is conducted "to benefit the human condition to improve profit, to amass influence and power, or to achieve other goals" (Rossi & Freeman, 1995, p. 6). Evaluation research is a powerful tool for defending viable programs, for altering structures and processes in order to strengthen programs, and for providing rationale for program failure. Goggin, Bowman, Lester, and O'Toole (1990) proposed that researchers investigate program implementation within an analytical framework rather than a descriptive one. They argued that a third generation of research established within a sound theory would strengthen the body of knowledge of the policy process. APNs can contribute to both the theory and the method of evaluation.

Evaluation must be started early and continued throughout a program. An unconscionable example of a program that should have been stopped even before it was begun is the Tuskegee experiment. From 1932 to 1972, a group of African Americans was used as a control group and denied antibiotic treatment for syphilis even after treatment was known to be successful (Thomas & Quinn, 1991). Beyond evaluation research, this study clearly points out the moral and ethical concerns that are mandated when researchers work with human beings. Should a study or program be started at all? At what point should it be stopped? What is involved in informed consent? If a program involves experimental therapy, what are the methods for presenting subjects with relevant data so that participation preferences are clear (Bell, Raiffa, & Tversky, 1988)? These kinds of questions should be considered automatically by today's researchers, but it is the responsibility of APNs as consumer agents to ask the questions if they have not been asked or if there is any doubt about the answers.

A Bright Future

The multiple roles of the APN—provider of direct care, researcher, consultant, educator, administrator, consumer advocate, and political activist—reflect the changing and expanding character of the professional nurse. Today is the future; nursing action today sets the direction for what health care becomes for projected generations. As true professionals with a societal mandate and a comprehensive body of knowledge, nurses function as visionaries who are grounded in education, research, and experience. APNs serve as the link between human responses to actual and potential health problems and the solutions that may be addressed in the government arena. Full integration of the policy process becomes evident when professional nurses discern early the social implications of health problems, seize the opportunity to inform public officials with whom the nurses have credible relationships, provide objective data and subjective personal stories that help translate big problems down to a level of understanding, propose alternative solutions that acknowledge reality, and participate in the evaluation process to determine the effectiveness and efficiency of the outcomes.

Educating Our Political Selves

Nurses in advanced practice should be expert in the knowledge and skills of political activity. Basic content in undergraduate nursing programs must be reexamined in light of the needs of the profession. Educators must do more than plant the seeds of interest and excitement in baccalaureate students. Educators must model activism by talking about the bills they are supporting or opposing, by organizing students to assist in election campaigns, and by demanding not only that students write letters to officials but that they mail them and provide follow-up. Educators can develop games in which students maneuver through a virtual bureaucracy to move a health problem onto the agenda. Brainstorming techniques can lead students to discover innovative alternative solutions. Baccalaureate students can analyze policy tools to discover how and when to use them. Teachers of research methods and processes can use political scenarios to point out how to phrase clinical questions so that legislators will pay attention. Program effectiveness can be studied in research and clinical courses. The theoretical components taught in class and followed by practical application through participation in political and legislative committees in professional organizations must serve as basic training for the registered nurse.

Graduate education must demand demonstrated knowledge and application of more extensive and sophisticated political processes. Nursing must increase the total of those with master's degrees and doctoral degrees beyond 9.6% and 0.6%, respectively, of nearly 2.7 million registered nurses (Spratley, Johnson, Sochalski, Fritz, & Spencer, 2000). All graduate program faculty should serve as models for political activism. The atmosphere in master's and doctoral programs should heighten the awareness of students who are potential leaders. Faculty will motivate students by displaying posters that announce political events and by including students in discussions of nursing issues framed in a policy context. Students who spot educators at rallies and other political and policy occasions are learning by example. Faculty should advertise their experiences as delegates to political and professional conventions. A few faculty will serve as mentors for students who need to move from informal to sustained, formal contact with policy makers and for those who have a policy track in their career trajectories. Both faculty and students should consider actual experience in government offices as a means of learning the nitty-gritty of how government functions and of demonstrating their own leadership capabilities. The Nurses' Directory of Capitol Connections (Bull, Sharp, & Wakefield, 2000) is an excellent resource for identifying a wide range of opportunities for participation of nurses who work in the policy arena.

If students hesitate and seem passive about involvement, educators must help these nurses determine where their passions are. This may help students focus on where they might start. Often the novice can be enticed by centering on a clinical problem.

Identifying Problems

Advanced practice nurses, by definition, are "professional nurses who have successfully completed a graduate program in nursing or a related area that provides specialized knowledge and skills that form the foundation for expanded roles in health care" (ANA House of Delegates, 1993, p. 5). According to this definition, APNs function in the provision of direct clinical care; as educators, administrators, and researchers; in consultative and counseling roles; and with a variety of titles. Within this broad interpretation, APNs have the capacity and opportunity to identify and frame problems from multiple sources.

CLINICAL PROBLEMS

The choice of a clinical problem on which to focus one's energy is a major decision. A nurse may be working in a specialized area and may see a need for more research or alternatives to treatment. For example, those who work with patients and families with breast cancer already may have a passion for issues critical to this area. Other current topics receiving attention include diabetes, obesity, AIDS, early detection and treatment of prostate cancer, child and parent abuse, cardiac problems in women, and empowering caregivers (Hash & Cramer, 2003; Pierce & Steiner, 2003). Professional problems that are especially critical to nurses in advanced practice include reducing barriers that prevent practice autonomy and reimbursement for nursing services. Workplace issues include advocacy for workplace safety and management strategies for training and redeploying nurses as work sites change. Related social problems that affect nurses include the increase of street violence and bioterrorism. There is a plethora of problems and irritations that can arouse the passion of a nurse in advanced practice.

FUNDING FOR EDUCATION

Preparing nurses at the graduate level, either with master's or doctoral degrees, has been a problem on several levels. The first concern was with a cyclical shortage of nurses, especially during war time when nurses left hospital employment and entered the armed forces. The Social Security Act of 1935 and, a decade later, the National Mental Health Act of 1946 provided some federal funding for graduate education and research (Lash, 1986). By the 1950s, nurses were seeking graduate degrees, but there were not enough programs in nursing. Part of the problem was that not enough nurses held doctoral degrees and could teach in graduate programs (Aiken, 1986). Organized nursing knew that federal legislators had initiated a GI bill that provided money to attend college for those who served in World War II. Nursing advocates convinced legislators that nurses were a scarce national resource, and funds were appropriated for nursing education through the Nurse Training Acts (NTAs) that began in 1943. Funding encouraged the initiation of new graduate nursing education programs, such as nurse-practitioner programs. By 1966, an amendment created grants for students, and the 1972 bill awarded capitation grants to nursing education programs to expand enrollment and increase graduations. With the infusion of federal dollars, the quantity and quality of educators and education improved (Kelly & Joel, 1995).

Nursing education as a functional area lost ground with the expansion of technology, the explosion of knowledge, and the increase in clinical master's degrees that began in the 1990s. Nursing's heritage of experienced teachers (education majors were acceptable routes for women/nurses who pursued higher education in the first half of the 20th century) was supplanted with clinically competent APNs who often were not schooled in principles of teaching and learning. Funding for nurses who sought baccalaureate and master's degrees focused on clinical nursing. Although this was appropriate in order to accommodate new knowledge about genetics, immunology, pharmacology, ethics, and other important content, teaching was slowly squeezed out. In the first decade of the 21st century, academic institutions face not only a shortage of faculty, but a shortage of faculty who have backgrounds in the principles of education. A few colleges and universities have begun doctoral programs with a focus on teaching, and many master's programs offer an education track. Funding for scholarships and loans in the early 2000s reflects a beginning recognition of the need for adequately prepared nurse-teachers.

SUPPORT FOR NURSING ADMINISTRATION

The only area of nursing education in which federal funding was not provided directly was in nursing administration. Even though NTA criteria for student qualifications clearly eliminated those studying nursing administration by denying their eligibility, potential leaders in that specialty became very important as managed care schemes replaced traditional fee-for-service arrangements. Nurses' need for knowledge about budgets, organizations, change theory, human resource strategies, and other formerly tangential material became critical in the 1990s. Federal money for education in that area had not been a priority, and nurse administrators have had to shoulder the burden of their education alone with the hope of executive and entrepreneurial opportunities through which they could recoup some of their financial investment. Federal nurse traineeships did change the eligibility in the late 1990s to include nurses with administration majors, but the funding competed with that for clinical scholarships.

INVESTMENT IN NURSING RESEARCH

From early nurse scientist programs that encouraged research training in physical and behavioral science programs to later grants that allowed nursing education programs to develop researchers in nursing, federal funds have provided the impetus for scientific inquiry into nursing concerns. Pre- and postdoctoral fellowships for nurse scientists and new investigator awards fostered research activity and the education of future researchers. Faculty development grants and research conferences made it possible to study and disseminate findings. The creation of the National Center for Nursing Research and its later elevation to the National Institute of Nursing Research (NINR) were outgrowths of struggles within the profession and between nursing and federal officials in efforts to secure funding for nursing research, especially clinical research (Brown, 1986). Although funding increased slowly over the years, NINR remains the lowest-funded institute of National Institutes of Health (NIH).

Government responds to social problems that either are too big for the private sector or are particular to the mission of government. The leadership role of government has been pictured by Osborne (1992) as steering rather than rowing in the 1800s with the provision of land grants for colleges and in the 1990s with funding for advanced practice nurses. Nurses must steer the course as healthcare experts by staying involved in the political process and influencing health policy. All registered nurses, especially those in advanced practice, have an extraordinary investment in the new structures and processes that will continue to be negotiated to provide health care to the citizens and residents of the United States.

Expanding the Framework

Nurses were central players in early discussions of a new healthcare delivery system (Backer, Costello-Nikitas, & Mason, 1993). The 1990s' nursing agenda for healthcare reform was a timely and fresh approach that rejected the traditional medical model and instead focused on the consumer as well as the provider. Nurse practitioners, clinical nurse specialists, and those in the new paradigm of the blended role in advanced practice spoke out as agents of patients and families to ensure that critical elements that affect healthcare cost, quality, and access are incorporated into current and future organizational arrangements for the delivery of care. Nurses and nursing were a strong political force in discussions of what healthcare delivery should be.

Practice the Rules of Debate

Nurses absolutely must get their act together and work toward a unified voice on issues that affect the public health and the nursing profession. Whatever their differences in the past— anger from entry-into-practice arguments that have dragged on for over half a century; disparagement and animosity among those with varied levels of education; cerebral and pragmatic concerns about gaps between education and practice, practice and administration, or administration and education—nurses must put these kinds of divisive, emotional issues behind them if they expect to be taken seriously as professionals by elected and appointed public officials and policy makers. Nurses cannot afford to stop arguing critical issues internally, but they must learn how to argue heatedly among themselves—and then go to lunch together. Nurses can learn lessons from television shows such as *Crossfire*, *The McLaughlin Group*, and *The Capital Gang* about how to challenge, contest, dispute, contend, and debate issues passionately and then shake hands and respect the opponent's position. Passionate issues must not polarize the profession any longer and, more important, must not stand in the way of a unified voice to the public.

STRENGTHEN ORGANIZED NURSING

The most productive and efficient way to act together is through a strong professional organization. As organizations in general have restructured and reengineered for more efficient operation, so will the professional associations. APNs have a knowledge base that includes an understanding of how organizations develop and change. This theoretical knowledge must serve as a foundation for leadership in directing new organizational structures that are responsive to members and other important bodies. National leaders must talk with state and local leaders as new configurations are conceived. States must confer among themselves to share innovations and knowledge about what works and what does not.

The Nursing Organizations Alliance (Saver, 2003), composed of the presidents and executive directors of over 50 major nursing organizations, held an inaugural meeting in 2003. The alliance is a loose collection of groups that provides a forum to discuss and debate issues important to a wide range of perspectives. Time will tell how effective this organization will be in serving as an internal medium for airing differences and coming to consensus.

Issues such as the role of collective bargaining units within the total organizational structure, the position of individual membership vis-à-vis state membership, the political role of a specialized interest group (nurses) in creating public policy, and the issue of international influence in nursing and health care require wisdom and leadership that APNs must exert as the American Nurses Association addresses its place as a major voice of this country's nurses. One united voice is necessary to carry nursing's messages to the public. For example, the Tri-Council of Nursing (ANA, American Association of Colleges of Nursing, American Organization of Nurse Executives, and the National League for Nursing) took a single message to Congress to increase funding for NINR and to authorize and appropriate funding for the Nurse Reinvestment Act (to create scholarships for students and faculty).

Issues inherent in multistate licensure are being debated today, and the outcome will reflect the extent to which nurses will use concepts of telehealth in their practices. Because APNs already are eligible for Medicare reimbursement for telehealth services that are provided in specified rural areas (Burtt, 1997), these nurses are rich resources and must be included in reasoned discussions on this issue. State boards of nursing in every state and jurisdiction face issues of appropriate methods of recognizing advanced nursing practice, the role of the government agency in regulating nursing and other professions, and the analysis of educationally sound and legally defensible examinations for candidates.

Nurses who have been reluctant to become political cannot afford to ignore their obligations any longer. Each nurse counts, and, collectively, nursing is a major actor in the effort to ensure the country's healthy future. Nurses have expanded their conception of what nursing is and how it is practiced to include active political participation. A nurse must choose the governmental level on which to focus: federal, regional, state, or local. The process is similar at each level: identify the problem and become part of the solution.

Advanced practice nurses understand the scope of service delivery, continuity of care, appropriate mix of caregivers, and the expertise that can be provided by multidisciplinary teams.

By being at the forefront of understanding, nurses have a moral and ethical mandate to participate in the public-policy process. Dynamic political action is as much a part of the advanced practice of nursing as is expert direct care.

WORK WITH THE POLITICAL SYSTEM

By now, many APNs have developed contacts with legislators and have appointed officials and their staffs. A new group that holds great potential for nurse interaction is the Congressional Nursing Caucus in the U.S. House of Representatives, begun in 2003 by Representatives Lois Capps (D-California) and Ed Whitfield (R-Kentucky). This bipartisan group assembles to educate Congress on all aspects of nursing—education, practice, research, leadership. Members will hold briefings on the nurse shortage, patient and nurse safety issues, preparedness for bioterrorism, and other relevant and pertinent issues and concerns. The caucus will serve as a "clearinghouse for information and a sounding board for ideas brought forth by the nursing community" (Nevada Nurses Association, 2003, p. 1). APNs must stay alert to issues and be assertive in bringing problems to the attention of policy makers. It is important to bring success stories to legislators and officials—they need to hear what good nurses do and how well they practice. Sharing positive information will keep the image of nurses in an affirmative and constructive picture. Legislators must run for office (and U.S. Representatives do this every 2 years), so media coverage with an APN who is pursuing noteworthy accomplishments is usually welcomed eagerly.

Conclusion

Nurses in advanced practice must have expert knowledge and skill in change, conflict resolu-

tion, assertiveness, communication, negotiation, and group process to function appropriately in the policy arena. Professional autonomy and collaborative interdependence are possible within a political system in which consumers can choose access to quality health care that is provided by competent practitioners at a reasonable cost. Nurses in advanced practice have a strong, persistent voice in designing such a healthcare system for today and for the future.

The policy process is much broader and more comprehensive than the legislative process. Although individual components can be identified for analytical study, the policy process is fluid, nonlinear, and dynamic. There are many opportunities for nurses in advanced practice to participate throughout the policy process. The question is not whether nurses should become involved in the political system, but to what extent. In the whole policy arena, nurses must be involved with every aspect. Knowing all of the components and issues that must be addressed within each phase, the nurse in advanced practice finds many opportunities for providing expert advice. APNs can use the policy process, individual components, and models as a framework to analyze issues and participate in alternative solutions.

Nursing has a rich history. The professional nurse's values of altruism, respect, integrity, and accountability to consumers remain strong. In some ways, the evolution of nursing roles has come full circle, from the political influence recognized and exercised by Nightingale to the influence of current nurse leaders with elected and appointed public officials. The APN of the 21st century practices with a solid political heritage and a mandate for consistent and powerful involvement in the entire policy process.

Discussion Questions

1. Compare the definition of nursing according to Nightingale, Henderson, the ANA, and your own state nurse practice act. What is the difference in a legal definition and a professional definition? What are the similarities? What did the definitions include or not include that reflected the state of nursing at the time? Construct a definition of nursing for today and 10 years from now.

2. How do research and policy interact and inform each other?

3. Identify a current healthcare policy related to poverty or public health. What governmental agency is responsible for developing the policy? For enforcing the policy? How has the policy changed over time? What are the consequences of not complying with the policy?

4. Discuss the major components of the policy process and discuss the fluidity of the process. Point out how players move among the components in a nonlinear way.

5. How can nurses become more knowledgeable about the policy process? Choose at least three activities in which you will participate.

6. Using Table 13–2 as a guide, write in activities and practices that you see or in which you are involved within the new paradigm.

7. Discuss at least five strategies for helping nurses integrate policy skills into their practices.

References

Aiken, L. H. (1986). Nursing education: The public policy debate. In J. C. McCloskey & H. K. Grace (Eds.), *Current Issues in Nursing* (2nd ed., pp. 680–696). Boston: Blackwell Scientific Publications.

Aiken, L. H. (1990). Charting the future of hospital nursing. *Image: Journal of Nursing Scholarship, 22*(2), 72–78.

American Nurses Association. (1994). *Nursing's agenda for health care reform*. Washington, DC: American Nurses Publishing, Inc.

ANA House of Delegates. (1993). *Regulation of advanced nursing practice* (action report). Washington, DC: American Nurses Publishing Co.

Argyris, C. (1962). *Interpersonal competence and organizational effectiveness*. Homewood, IL: Dorsey Press.

Backer, B. A., Costello-Nikitas, D., & Mason, D. J. (1993). Power at the policy table—when women and nurses are involved. *Revolution, 3*(2), 68–71, 74–76.

Bell, D. E., Raiffa, H., & Tversky, A. (1988). *Decision making*. Cambridge, MA: Cambridge University Press.

Benner, P. G. (1984). *From novice to expert: Excellence and power in clinical nursing practice*. Menlo Park, CA: Addison-Wesley.

Bennis, W., & Nanus, B. (1985). *Leaders*. New York: Harper and Row.

Blancett, S. S., & Flarey, D. L. (1995). *Reengineering nursing and health care: The handbook for organizational transformation*. Gaithersburg, MD: Aspen Publishers, Inc.

Blank, A. E. (1997). Linking the restructuring of nursing care with outcomes. In E. L. Cohen & T. G. Cesta (Eds.), *Nursing case management* (2nd ed., pp. 261–273). St. Louis, MO: C. V. Mosby.

Bowen, E. (1982). The Pressman–Wildavsky paradox: Four addenda on why models based on probability theory can predict implementation success and suggest useful tactical advice for implementers. *Journal of Public Policy, 2*(1), 1–22.

Bower, K. A. (1992). *Case management by nurses.* Washington, DC: American Nurses Publishing.

Brooten, D., & Naylor, M. D. (1995). Nurses' effect on changing patient outcomes. *Image: Journal of Nursing Scholarship, 27*(2), 95–99.

Brown, B. J. (1986). Past and current status of nursing's role in influencing governmental policy for research and training in nursing. In J. C. McCloskey & H. K. Grace (Eds.), *Current issues in nursing* (2nd ed., pp. 697–712). Boston: Blackwell Scientific Publications.

Bull, J., Sharp, N., & Wakefield, M. (2000). *Nurses' directory of capitol connections* (5th ed.). Fairfax, VA: George Mason University Center for Health Policy, Research and Ethics.

Burtt, K. (1997, November/December). Nurses use telehealth to address rural health care needs, prevent hospitalizations. *The American Nurse, 29*(6), 21.

Champy, J. (1995). *Reengineering management.* New York: Harper Business.

Covey, S. R. (1991). *Principle-centered leadership.* New York: Summit Books.

de Chesnay, M. (1983). The creation and dissolution of paradoxes in nursing practice. *Topics in Clinical Nursing, 5*(3), 71–80.

Dranove, D., Kessler, D., McClellan, M., & Satterthwaite, M. (2003). Is more information better? The effects of "report cards" on health care providers. *Journal of Political Economy, 3*(11), 555–585.

Drucker, P. F. (1959). *Landmarks of tomorrow.* New York: Harper.

Drucker, P. F. (1995, February). The age of social transformation. *Quality Digest,* 36–39.

Drucker, P. F. (1999). Knowledge worker productivity: The biggest challenge. *California Management Review, 4*(21), 79–94.

Essentials of baccalaureate education for professional nursing practice, The. (1998). New York: American Association of Colleges of Nursing.

Essentials of master's education for advanced practice nursing, The. (1996). New York: American Association of Colleges of Nursing.

Ethridge, P., & Lamb, G. (1989). Professional nursing case management improves quality, access, and cost. *Nursing Management, 20*(3), 30–35.

Eulau, H., & Prewitt, K. (1973). *Labyrinths of democracy.* Indianapolis, IN: Bobbs-Merrill.

Feldstein, P. J. (1988). *The politics of health legislation.* Ann Arbor, MI: Health Administration Press.

Flood, R. L., & Senge, P. M. (1999). *Rethinking the fifth discipline: Learning within the unknowable.* London: Routledge.

Fuchs, V. R. (1993). *The future of health policy.* Cambridge, MA: Harvard University Press.

Genna, J. (1987, November/December). AIDS management. *Healthcare Forum Journal,* 18–48.

Goggin, M. L., Bowman, A. O'M., Lester, J. P., & O'Toole, L. J., Jr. (1990). *Implementation theory and practice: Toward a third generation.* New York: HarperCollins Publishers.

Haas, J. E. (1964). *Role conception and group consensus.* (Research monograph No. 17). Columbus, OH: The Ohio State University, Bureau of Business Research.

Halloran, E. J. (1983). Staffing assignment: By task or by patient. *Nursing Management, 14*(8), 17.

Hash, K. M., & Cramer, E. P. (2003). Empowering gay and lesbian caregivers and uncovering their unique experiences through the use of qualitative methods. *Journal of Gay and Lesbian Social Services. Issues in Practice, Policy and Research, 15*(1/2), 47–64.

Hegyvary, S. (1992). *Outcomes research: Integrating nursing practice into the world view: National Institutes of Health, patient outcomes research: Examining the effectiveness of nursing practice* (17–24). (DHHS publication No. 93-3411).

Henderson, V. (1966). *The nature of nursing: A definition and its implications for practice, research, and education.* New York: Macmillan.

Hesse, H. (1951). *Siddhartha.* New York: Bantam Books.

How our laws are made. (1990). Washington, DC: United States Government Printing Office, House document 101–139, 4.

Jones, C. O. (1984). *An introduction to the study of public policy* (2nd ed.). Monterey, CA: Brooks/Cole.

Kelly, L. Y., & Joel, L. A. (1995). *Dimensions of professional nursing* (7th ed.). New York: McGraw-Hill, Inc.

Kennedy, E., & Charles, S. C. (1997). *Authority.* New York: Simon & Schuster.

King, I. M. (1971). *Toward a theory for nursing.* New York: John Wiley and Sons, Inc.

Koln, L. T., Corrigan, J. M., & Donaldon, M. S. (Eds.). (1999). *To err is human: Building a safer health system. A report from the Committee on Quality of Healthcare in America, Institute of Medicine, National Academy of Sciences.* Washington, DC: National Academy Press.

Kouzes, J., & Posner, B. (1987). *The leadership challenge.* San Francisco: Jossey-Bass.

Kouzes, J., & Posner, B. (1999). *Encouraging the heart: A leader's guide to rewarding and recognizing others.* San Francisco: Jossey-Bass.

Lash, A. A. (1986). Federal financing and its effect on higher nursing education. In J. C. McCloskey & H. K. Grace (Eds.), *Current issues in nursing* (2nd ed., pp. 663–679). Boston: Blackwell Scientific Publications.

Lasswell, H. D. (1958). *Politics: Who gets what, when, how.* New York: Meridian Books.

Laws governing nursing in South Carolina. (1994). Columbia, SC: South Carolina Department of Labor, Licensing, and Regulation.

Leininger, M. (Ed.). (1978). *Transcultural nursing: Concepts, theories and practices.* New York: John Wiley & Sons.

Litman, T. J., & Robins, L. S. (1991). *Health politics and policy* (2nd ed.). Albany, NY: Delmar Publishers, Inc.

Lowi, T. (1969). *The end of liberalism.* New York: Norton.

Maurin, J. (1990). Case management: Caring for psychiatric clients. *Journal of Psychosocial Nursing, 28*(7), 8–12.

Melville, H. (1853). Bartleby, the scrivener: A story of Wall Street. *Putnam's Monthly Magazine, 2*(911), 546–577.

Milio, N. (1989). Developing nursing leadership in health policy. *Journal of Professional Nursing, 5*(6), 315.

Milstead, J. A. (1993). *The advancement of policy implementation theory: An analysis of three needle exchange programs.* Doctoral dissertation, University of Georgia.

Milstead, J. A. (2003). Leapfrog group: A prince in disguise or just another frog? *Nursing Administration Quarterly, 26*(4), 16–25.

Mundinger, M. (1984). Community-based care: Who will be the case managers? *Nursing Outlook, 32*(6), 294–295.

Nevada Nurses Association. (2005). American Nurses Association commends Reps. Capps, Whitfield for forming congressional nursing caucus. Retrieved October 18, 2007, from http://findarticles.com/p/articles/mi_qa4102/is_200305/ai_n9254257/pg_2

Noer, D. M. (1993). *Healing the wounds.* San Francisco: Jossey-Bass.

Orem, D. E. (1971). *Nursing: Concepts of practice.* Scarborough, Ontario: McGraw-Hill.

Osborne, D. E. (Ed.). (1992). *Reinventing government: How the entrepreneurial spirit is transforming the public sector.* Reading, MA: Addison-Wesley.

Peplau, H. (1952). *Interpersonal relations in nursing.* New York: Springer.

Pesut, D., & Herman, J. (1999). *Clinical reasoning: The art and science of critical and creative thinking* (2nd ed.). Albany, NY: Delmar Learning.

Peters, T. J. (1988). *Thriving on chaos.* New York: Knopf.

Peters, T. J. (1997). *The circle of innovation: You can't shrink your way to greatness.* New York: Knopf.

Pew Health Professions Commission. (1995, November). *Critical challenges: Revitalizing the health professions for the twenty-first century* (3rd report). San Francisco: UCSF Center for the Health Professions.

Pierce, L., & Steiner, V. (2003). The male caregiving experience: Three case studies. *Stroke, 34*(1), 315.

Porter-O'Grady, T. (1996). Accountability and the role of advanced practice. In C. E. Loveridge & S. H. Cummings (Eds.), *Case management in the new paradigm* (pp. 477–480). Gaithersburg, MD: Aspen Publishers, Inc.

Porter-O'Grady, T., Hawkins, M. A., & Parker, M. L. (1997). *Whole-systems shared governance: Architecture for integration.* Gaithersburg, MD: Aspen Publishers, Inc.

Porter-O'Grady, T., & Malloch, K. (2002). *Quantum leadership: A textbook of new leadership.* Gaithersburg, MD: Aspen Publishers, Inc.

Porter-O'Grady, T., & Wilson, C. K. (1995). *The leadership revolution in health care: Altering systems, changing behaviors.* Gaithersburg, MD: Aspen Publishers, Inc.

Porter-O'Grady, T., & Wilson, C. K. (1999). *Leading the revolution in health care: Advancing systems, igniting performance* (2nd ed.). Gaithersburg, MD: Aspen Publishers, Inc.

Rodgers, B. L. (1989). Exploring health policy as a concept. *Western Journal of Nursing Research, 11*(6), 694–702.

Rogers, M. E. (1970). *An introduction to the theoretical basis for nursing.* Philadelphia: F. A. Davis Company.

Rossi, P. H., & Freeman, H. E. (1995). *Evaluation: A systematic approach* (5th ed.). Beverly Hills, CA: Sage Publications.

Saver, C. (2003). Alliance takes another step. *Nursing Spectrum Midwestern Edition, 4*(1), 12.

Senge, P. (1990). *The fifth discipline: The art and practice of the learning organization.* New York: Doubleday.

Skocpol, T. (1995). *Social policy in the United States.* Princeton, NJ: Princeton University Press.

Spratley, E., Johnson, A., Sochalski, J., Fritz, M., & Spencer, W. (2000). *The registered nurse population, March 2000.* U.S. Department of Health and Human Services, Health Resources and Service Administration, Bureau of Health Professions, Division of Nursing. Retrieved October 16, 2007, from http://bhpr.hrsa.gov/healthworkforce/reports/nursing/samplesurvey00/chapter3.htm

The regulatory process. (1992, December 4). *Capitol Update, 10*(23), 1.

Thomas, S. B., & Quinn, S. C. (1991). The Tuskegee syphilis study, 1932 to 1972: Implications for HIV education and AIDS risk reduction education programs in the black community. *American Journal of Public Health, 8*(11), 1498–1505.

Venegoni, S. L. (1996). Changing environment of healthcare. In J. V. Hickey, R. M. Ouimette, & S. L. Venegoni (Eds.), *Advanced practice nursing: Changing roles and clinical applications* (pp. 77–90). Philadelphia: Lippincott.

Watson, J. (1979). *Nursing: The philosophy and science of caring.* Boston: Little, Brown.

Watzlawick, R., Weakland, C. E., & Fisch, R. (1974). *Change.* New York: WW Norton & Co.

West, W. F. (1982, September/October). The politics of administrative rulemaking. *Public Administration Review,* 420–426.

Wheatley, M. (1992). *Leadership and the new science.* San Francisco: Berrett-Koehler.

Williams, S. J., & Torrens, P. R. (Eds.). (1988). *Introduction to health services* (3rd ed.). Albany, NY: Delmar Publishers, Inc.

Wilson, J. Q. (1989). *American government institutions and policies* (4th ed.). Lexington, MA: D.C. Heath and Co.

Wolf, G., Boland, S., & Aukerman, M. (1994a). A transformational model for the practice of professional nursing–Part I: The model. *Journal of Nursing Administration, 24*(4), 51–57.

Wolf, G., Boland, S., & Aukerman, M. (1994b). A transformational model for the practice of professional nursing–Part II: Implementation of the model. *Journal of Nursing Administration, 24*(5), 38–46.

Zander, K. (1990). The 1990s: Core values, core change. *Frontiers in Health Service Management, 2*(1), 39–43.

Zander, K., Etheredge, M., & Bower, K. (Eds.). (1987). *Nursing case management: Blueprints for transformation.* Boston: New England Medical Center.

Chapter 14

Making the Political Process Work

Catherine J. Dodd

CHAPTER OBJECTIVES

1. Develop strategies of political expertise for success in the role of the advanced nurse practitioner.
2. List 10 specific strategies and their rationale.

Introduction

An old politician (Otto von Bismarck) once said, "Those who like sausages and laws should never watch either be made." Legislated health policy rarely resembles its ideological beginnings. However, if pragmatic idealists, both the self-appointed guardians of the public good and elected officials, fail to participate in the political process, the creation of health policy will be designed by and left in the hands of the well-financed interest groups motivated only by profit.

- Politics has been defined as: the art and science of government
- Political affairs has been defined as: competition between competing interest groups of individuals for power and leadership (Webster's Ninth New Collegiate Dictionary, 1984).

The process by which scarce resources are divided is almost without exception a political one characterizing competition among interest groups. It is rarely fair. Political decisions are not made during the hearings in the hallowed halls of the Capitol. Political decisions are made long before the day of the vote; they are based on external influences which may or may not include expert knowledge. Politics determines the outcomes of proposals in the workplace, the neighborhood, and in kindergarten class. Consider these examples: Ms. Gee's kindergarten class has a clown coming to perform. Ms. Gee assigns seats in the class based on which students had put away their art supplies even though some students would not be able to see over tall students seated in the front. Ms. Gee's decision was a political one that granted privileges and rewarded one kind of behavior over another. Similarly, a state legislator may vote to fund a new health center because it will be in a neighborhood within her district even though without continued funding a clinic in another legislative district serving people who have no other healthcare options will close. Political decisions influence many aspects of our daily lives. Those who fail to participate in the political process are allowing the decisions to be made by people who may seek to control resources for their own personal and/or political gain.

Developing and maintaining political power and expertise is like exercising to strengthen your abdominal muscles . . . the personal trainer says, "If you don't use it, you lose it." Following the trainer's instructions can prevent painful injuries. Political expertise is essential for success in organizations, institutions, and local, state, and national government.

Ten Universal Commandments of Politics and Reasons to Obey Them

1. The Personal Is Political. Each of Us Is Just One Personal or Social Injustice Away from Being Involved in Politics. Every Vote Counts.

The more voices that participate in our democracy, the more likely it will be that the weak voices are heard. People who choose not to vote, and/or not to be involved in politics, are stuck with what those who do vote choose. Each person can make

a difference, especially when one illustrates how the outcome of an election may affect the lives of those who do not believe that their voice counts. Many elections throughout the country are decided by one vote per precinct or less.

Entire advocacy organizations have been started because of a single injustice or tragedy. Movements have begun because an individual brought together others of like minds and took action. Elected officials are inspired to introduce legislation because of their own personal experience or that of someone they know. Representative Caroline McCarthy, LPN, ran for Congress and was elected after her husband and child were shot on the New York subway. She promised the voters that she would fight for stricter gun laws.

Mothers Against Drunk Driving (MADD) was founded by a mother whose child was killed by a drunk driver. Today, MADD chapters exist all over the country; their members include relatives and friends of victims of drunk drivers as well as supportive members of the public. MADD has been extremely effective in achieving its objectives, at the local level lobbying for speed bumps and the installation of stoplights, increasing penalties for drunk driving at the state level, and placing restrictions on alcohol advertising at the national level.

Hundreds of AIDS and HIV organizations grew out of personal tragedy. AIDS activists have created an effective lobby. The lobbying techniques used by AIDS-funding activists include traditional lobbying in legislatures and Congress, as well as nontraditional civil disobedience demonstrations.

National Rifle Association (NRA) enthusiasts, who believe their personal freedom will be impinged upon by limiting access to automatic weapons, frequently initiate very successful letter-writing and e-mail campaigns in key congressional districts to protect their constitutional rights. NRA activists also raise money for key candidates from members all over the country.

2. *Friends Come and Go but Enemies Accumulate.*

This old adage can be applied to many relationships. Its application includes two important concepts: Activists should never surprise their friends, and politics makes strange bedfellows. It is imperative to not jeopardize working relationships by publicly opposing someone, not inviting them to a meeting, or by voting against them without talking to them before taking action. Maintaining a relationship does not require disclosing strategy, it means simply showing respect for the right of others to have a different perspective. Trust and respect are commodities in politics that, once lost, are rarely regained. While people may disagree on one issue, there may exist agreement on another and a relationship sustained by respect allows for discussion, compromise, and progress. Handling conflicts respectfully will allow for future collaboration. Maintaining working relationships allows for strange bedfellows. Managing conflicts respectfully allows for future collaboration with partners who may agree with one's position on other issues.

Advocates for women's and children's health frequently testify to protect women's reproductive freedom and argue against the testimony of advocates from conservative religious organizations. However, on issues affecting children's health, the organizations come together as strange bedfellows and make powerful allies.

3. *Politics Is the Art of the Possible. Count Votes in Advance. The Majority Rules.*

In the policy and legislative arena, no one gets everything he or she wants and hence, without both compromise and strategy, no one gets anything. Successful politicians strive for what is possible. In diverse political cultures in which there are many different opinions and philosophies, successful legislators are those with an ability to find compromises acceptable to the majority that do not destroy the intent of the original legislation. Votes are not won during dramatic debate on the floor of the House or Senate. Votes are won one by one by talking to individual legislators, seeking their support, finding out what compromises would be required to gain their support. Sometimes asking others for assistance in lining up additional votes is necessary. In general, people like to help. Once someone commits support, they are unlikely to renege on that commitment because it jeopardizes their credibility. Nurse-midwives quickly learned the meaning of compromise and securing votes one by one.

Nurse-midwives seeking a change in their state practice act had far fewer numbers and much less political clout than the opposing physician lobbies. First, they asked the OB/GYNs with whom they worked for support on the idea. Then, they met with the leadership of the physicians' organizations and gained support from one organization based on compromised language that mirrored the national standards for nurse-midwifery practice. United, the OB/GYNs and nurse-midwives took consumers and business people to meet with each legislator on key committees where the proposed legislation would be heard. One by one, legislators agreed to support the legislation. Some members of the legislative committees were unwilling to vote in favor of the bill until they were certain it would pass. Legislators do not willingly vote for legislation that is opposed by powerful lobbies if they believe the legislation is going to fail anyway (because, as stated in the second commandment of politics, friends come and go but enemies accumulate, and no one wants to alienate powerful lobbies if the bill will fail anyway). In this example, only one more vote was needed. An intense lobbying effort by consumers in one legislator's district and the nurse-midwives' willingness to compromise as requested by that legislator, even though the compromise lessened the value of the legislation, resulted in gaining that vote, giving the bill a majority and passing it out of committee.

If the margin for passage is close, how a legislator votes usually depends on whether the voters in his/her district care about the issue and/or on which side of the issue donors to his/her election are. Advocates need to be certain of those votes they can count on and then ensure that the supporting legislators, board members, and so forth will be in attendance the day the vote is scheduled, especially if the vote will be close.

A Republican RN state legislator who lived in a competitive swing district (one with equal numbers of voters registered as Democrats and Republicans) had been lobbied by many nurse supporters and contributors to support a bill that provided protection from discrimination for lesbians and gays. When the roll was called on the vote, she did not vote. The bill passed by several votes. When asked why she did not vote in favor, she replied that if her vote would have meant the difference, she would have voted in favor of the bill. However, because it was an election year and voters in her district were very conservative, she could not afford to have the more conservative members of her party run someone against her based on this vote.

Many people wonder why so few pieces of legislation are passed and signed into law. The answer is twofold. Since the 1994 elections, Congress and state legislatures have become more partisan and the voters have become disillusioned with incumbent career politicians. For example, in 1993, Congress spent an entire year debating Clinton's healthcare reform proposal. Second, the 1994 elections produced a class of freshmen (new Senators and Representatives) dominated by citizen politicians or businessmen on sabbaticals. For the first time in 40 years, the Republican party gained a majority in both houses of Congress (the Senate and the House of Representatives). The Republicans elected to the 104th Congress were very conservative, and their majority created a more conservative Congress.

All votes cast in the 104th Congress were significantly more conservative on health, education, human services, and environmental issues than previous Congresses. Democrats representing swing districts voted more conservatively than they might have previously in an attempt to appeal to moderate Republicans in their districts during an election year. This same trend was evidenced throughout the country at the state and local level, as conservative (religious anti-women's reproductive choice) campaign strategists successfully ran candidates in primaries rebuffing career politician incumbent (generally) Democrats.

Partisan ideology has taken the place of pragmatic problem solving. The freshman businessmen/owners elected often lacked experience in negotiating with others who have entirely different philosophies or agendas and simply refused to do so, creating legislative gridlock. In the corporate world, business owners who cannot agree on terms merely find other contractors. Elected officials do not have this option; their associates in Congress are elected by constituents, not hired by them. The increased partisanship in halls of government across the country produced very few compromises. Leadership in both parties is necessary for legislators to work together and one by one meet, talk, and identify compromises.

In order for legislation to pass, a majority of members of the legislature need to vote for it. The majority rules in more ways than one. Parties have philosophies and agendas. The majority party determines what issues will be debated and if the debate will allow alternatives or compromise. Many pieces of legislation are introduced and never put on the agenda for consideration if the party in the majority does not want the issue considered.

In 2002, Representative Lois Capps, RN, a Democrat, worked with the American Nurses Association and other nursing organizations to craft the Nurse Reinvestment Act (NRA). The act authorized funds for recruitment into the profession through media and funding for scholarships and grants to schools. Representative Capps went to Republican colleagues she had worked with and talked about the nursing shortage in their respective districts. She was able to gather many Republican cosponsors before introducing the NRA despite a new and growing budget deficit. Rep. Capps easily brought her Democratic colleagues on in support and the NRA was one of a handful of pieces of legislation signed into law by President George W. Bush during a very partisan period in Congress. Representative Capps used her individual relationships with fellow legislators. She had RNs throughout the country lobbying their Congress members, and she was polite, persistent, and persuasive.

4. Be Polite, Be Persistent, Be Persuasive, and Be Polite. Send Thank-You Notes, Write, Write, Write, Ghost Write, and Write.

Letters from voters who live in the elected official's district make a difference. Some elected officials believe their constituency goes beyond their legislative district; for example, an RN legislator may consider and respond to the opinions of RNs regardless of where they live. If a legislator is not on the committee that is scheduled to hear the bill an activist is interested in, he should find out who the staff person is for the committee. He should address his letter to the chair of the committee in care of the staff person, and then send a copy of the letter to his legislator.

Elected officials listen to those who elect them and/or support them financially in their campaigns. Perennial voters (those who vote in every election rain or shine) tend to be more highly educated and are more likely to write a letter or craft an e-mail message. That is why individually written letters (mailed/faxed/or e-mailed, not chain messages) are the most effective lobbying tools, because elected officials know that people who take the time to write letters are voters. Preprinted letters or postcards are effective only in specific mass strategy campaigns. Phone calls are best used to gather information about the legislator's position in advance. When calling, callers should ask to speak to the staff person responsible for the issue to be discussed. They should thank the staff person for their assistance, and if the legislator agrees with the caller's position, activists should write a letter/message so that it acknowledges his or her position and states that they are pleased with it. In general, phone calls urging a vote are used in last-minute attempts and are only considered an effective lobbying tool if they are from constituents who leave their address and ask for a written response explaining how the elected official plans to vote or voted.

Communication with legislators should establish credibility of the sender as a constituent (i.e., a nurse, a mother, etc.) and should be polite, persuasive, and succinct. Communications should state the sender's position early in the communication, offer support for the position with research or personal experience/belief, and ask for a response prior to the vote. This is not a term paper and need not be perfect grammatically, only persuasive. It is likely to be read only by staff (unless the sender has a personal relationship with the elected official). Multiplying the effectiveness of this effort by demonstrating broad support/opposition can be accomplished by assisting, collecting, and mailing similar letters from friends, family, and colleagues. When one letter arrives in a legislator's office it is recorded; when 10 arrive it becomes an issue of constituent concern. When 20 individually written communications arrive, staff alert the elected official. To be effective, letters must arrive before the vote is scheduled. The earlier the better. If the bill fails and is introduced in subsequent years, activists must write again, again, and again as necessary.

If the legislator, organizational board member, or coworker takes the desired action, it is important for everyone to follow their mom's advice: Write a thank-you note. Everyone enjoys being recognized and thanked. Those colorful envelopes in the mail are the first to be opened by each of us and elected officials are no exception. Politicians, like relatives and friends, remember people who send thank-you notes.

Be polite. In talking to legislators, staff, or the press, one should never say or put in writing anything one does not want printed on the front page of the newspaper. Many a career has ended because of an angry quote.

Letters to the editor and op-ed columns in local newspapers are extremely effective lobbying tools. The editorial section of the newspaper is the first section read by political staff each day because the opinions expressed are those of voters. Politicians give extra credence to these letters. It is often believed that people who write them subscribe to the paper and are more likely to be voters. Often letters are not printed unless the paper has received more than one on the subject.

Health professionals have very high credibility. So, a letter to the editor published in a local paper from a professional will have significant public influence recognized by politicians. Letters should be well written (they will be read by thousands of people) but should not exceed 250 words. Many papers have publication policies that can be acquired with a call to the paper. Letters can be faxed or mailed, and must include the address of the sender. The same letter, with a different sender, can be submitted to a paper in another geographic area of the state or country. Op-ed pieces should not exceed 750 words and usually require a 4- to 6-week lead time. Communicating first with the editor of the opinion page will increase the likelihood that an op-ed piece will be printed. Op-ed pieces are published on topics of broad interest. Generating letters to the editor to demonstrate interest in the subject/position prior to submitting an op-ed piece, or following the publication of an op-ed piece, is a sophisticated and very effective strategy for influencing public opinion and hence the opinion of elected officials. The best way to plan an editorial page lobbying effort is to become acquainted with the editorial pages of the newspaper.

Be persuasive. Whether it is voting for a piece of legislation when it comes before the legislature or whether it is voting for a candidate in an election, RNs and health professionals are very persuasive. After all, if a professional can convince someone to drink Metamucil, he or she can surely convince them to vote. Health professionals are effective campaigners—door to door, on phone banks, and raising money on behalf of candidates. The public loves nurses. Everyone has a relative who is a nurse or health professional, or a relative who was just cared for by a nurse or doctor. Nurses poll higher in public trust measurements than any other profession. When nurses' or health professionals' popularity is combined with persuasive abilities, a very powerful political advocate is created.

5. Ignore Your Mother's Rule. Talk to Strangers, or Network. Carry Business Cards. Flaunt Your Professional Credentials Proudly.

Talking to strangers comes naturally to health professionals. Every new patien–client is first a stranger. Everyone should practice their introduction and ask themselves what they want people to remember about them. They should shake hands and make eye contact. It helps to repeat a person's name when ending a conversation (this does two things: it endears one to him or her because people like hearing their name, and it

helps one remember the other person's name). Activists should exchange business cards—which should include credentials! Strangers cease to be strangers when their business cards become part of a phone list or database to be used for political action or fund-raising. Following up with an e-mail or "nice to meet you" card endears the sender to his/her new network member. It really becomes a small world when strangers talk to strangers and become friends.

In garnering support/opposition for issues or candidates, no one is a stranger to health professionals. These professionals should print "RN" or other credentials on their checks so that candidates who receive them will know they have received hard-earned money.

6. Money Is the Mother's Milk of Politics. Give It Early, and If You Don't Have It, Raise It . . . Even If You Do Have It, Raise It!

The invention of television, allowing candidates to speak directly but not personally to voters, heralded the elimination of the importance of political parties as the mechanism for establishing party philosophy and disseminating political messages to the electorate (DeLaney, 1995). Television has not changed who has the right to run for office (any citizen can run and only the president must be a native-born citizen of the United States), but it has changed who wins. Candidates who cannot afford television time invest in the next best (and still costly) method of communicating with voters, targeted direct mail, to bring their message directly to voters' mailboxes in well-planned, nonsubstantive glossy brochures. Targeted direct mail lists are purchased from campaign consultants, who purchase them from the registrar of voters and sort them by any number/combination of fields depending on the target audience. For example, the list may be sorted by citizens who voted in the last three elections (called likely or perennial voters), political party, sex, age, those who vote by mail, those who own homes/rent homes, neighborhood, etc. The strategy in direct mail campaigning focuses on projecting how many votes are needed from the target audiences and then tailors the message to that audience.

Campaigns require money and more money, hence the saying, "Money is the mother's milk of politics." The amount of money candidates raise early in campaigns determines a candidate's viability early in a race. The American Nurses Association (ANA) Political Action Committee (PAC) is an example of a political organization that supports candidates who support nursing's positions on issues. It has raised (from members, in contributions averaging $40) and contributed more than $1 million dollars in each congressional election since 1994. In evaluating candidates before primaries (when there are often several candidates in the field) for possible early endorsement, the ANA political staff compiles information on how much money each candidate has raised and how much is projected to be spent. How much money has been raised is a measure of the candidate's viability. (If someone said he or she had to lose 25 pounds before a class reunion, and the reunion was only two weeks away, most people would not take him or her seriously—so, too, with raising money.) The PAC does not support candidates who cannot raise the money to win their election. If some candidates have not raised much money, and others have, the field of possible endorsements is narrowed to those who are serious about winning. EMILY's list is an example of a national fundraising effort for pro-choice

Democratic women candidates. EMILY stands for "early money is like yeast" because contributing to women candidates early helps them establish their viability as credible candidates, and therefore, to raise other funds. People and organizations that provided early financial support are always remembered once politicians get elected because they know they would not have been elected without them. Relationships made early in campaigns have exponential returns because elected officials usually run for higher office and those early relationships are forever.

Nurses and other health professionals often bemoan the fact that they are not affluent and cannot afford to make large contributions; this is where networking—the fifth commandment—comes into play. Professional credibility allows them to call friends, relatives, and colleagues to collect $10–$50 from each contact. Collecting eight $25 contributions raises $200. Volunteering to help make fund-raising calls is a key campaign activity.

Most individuals can afford a contribution of $45 per year (less than $5 per month) to health PACs and to their state associations to ensure that their voice is heard. Raising funds for and contributing money to friends of particular professional organizations are important both for the candidate and for the organization. Candidates, even those in safe seats (where the voter registration favors their party) who are likely to be elected or reelected, need to assist other allies in other parts of the state/country in getting elected. This will ensure that they have friends elected into the body into which they are being elected (more to follow in commandment 8), and will not only help them gather support for the legislation they introduce, but will also help them pave the road to a leadership position within their party in the legislature, council, and Congress. This is especially true in situations in which the number of terms an elected official may serve is limited by statutory term limits; this requires the official to climb to a leadership position much faster.

7. *Negotiate Visibility. Take Credit; Take Control.*

Throughout history it seems that the profession of nursing, while held in high regard by the public, has not been given (or has not taken) credit for the essential role of nurses within healthcare systems. Nurses have little control over the systematic decisions being made by health corporations and the physicians who often control them. Taking control requires taking credit, whether in the healthcare system or in politics. When Nurses for _____ for Congress raises $1,000 and produces 10 volunteers every Saturday, it must negotiate visibility for nursing or for a few key health professionals in the campaign. Credit may take the form of listing nurses (or other professionals) on every piece of campaign literature, getting 10 seats at a large fund-raising dinner instead of only five, or being included in the candidate's policy kitchen cabinet. Visibility is never offered, it must be asked for and negotiated. First-time candidates and candidates in competitive races never forget individuals and constituencies who were visible in difficult races.

8. *Politics Has a Chit Economy, So Keep Track. Seniority Counts.*

Commandment 3 requires an ability to communicate, and in some instances, to ask for help, and then to count votes. Most people like to help. However, help has a price. The exchange of votes, help lining up votes, raising money,

or mobilizing volunteers to walk precincts all accrue chits. For elected officials, chits are exchanged for appointments to key committees and for leadership positions. At the federal level, the longer the tenure of the legislator the higher his or her rank regardless of his or her status as a member of the majority or minority party. Seniority is given consideration in committee assignments so it is to a district's or state's advantage to reelect incumbent legislators who have good voting records. For individuals, chits mean access when requesting appointments to boards and commissions or for assistance with legislative issues.

9. *Reputations Are Permanent.*

In politics as in life, there is nothing more important to success than a positive reputation. No one assigns reputations; they are earned and remembered. A key ingredient in developing a positive reputation is dependability. Dependable people deliver promptly what has been promised whether it is an article, names and addresses of possible supporters, campaign funds, or volunteers. They answer questions honestly and directly, and offer to research unknown information. They return calls and respond to requests for assistance. Those who identify themselves as a member of an organization leave a reflection of the profession and/or the organization they say they represent.

For example, in a congressional election for an open seat (no incumbent running), an RN activist promised to provide the American Nurses' Association position statements on issues to assist with the candidate's platform development after the candidate had been endorsed by the ANA PAC. Within 2 days, the RN activist was drafting the candidate's statements on health care and later became a staff member to that member of Congress. If the RN activist had failed to follow through on the promise of assistance, her credibility and nursing reputation would have been tarnished.

10. *Don't Let 'Em Get to Ya.*

"Sticks and stones may break your bones but names will never hurt you." Activists facing criticism should use the mantra: "I'm glad I'm here, I'm glad you're here, I know what I know, and I care about you," or just picture those who mock them or challenge their positions sitting on a bedside commode in a hospital patient gown. (Nobody is attractive in a patient gown!)

Eleanor Roosevelt once said: "No one can make you feel inferior without your permission," yet often, a sense of inadequacy and inferiority has been part of the socialization of women and nurses. To overcome this ingrained subliminal sense, when addressing hostile audiences (or any audiences for that matter) the mantra in the previous paragraph does two things—it causes people to smile because it sounds so corny, and that smile warms the audience and makes them more friendly. This is as true of 2-year-olds as it is of adults.

In political campaigns, a common strategy today is: "Go negative on your opponent before he goes negative on you" (DeLaney, 1995). We unfortunately live in a world that thrives on crises and negativity. Negative comments are going to be made and reported. Rebuttals are not always possible and are often wasted on hysterical, angry responses. The best defense is a good offense. It is important to know that comments will be misinterpreted and reported and measure one's response just as one did on the playground in grade school. Activists should correct the misinterpretation, refute the allegation, and repeat over and over to themselves: "Sticks and stones may break my bones, but names will never hurt me."

Conclusion

Health professionals have a unique and broad perspective of the healthcare delivery needs of individuals and populations. Health professionals have excellent communication skills and organizational skills. Health professionals are well suited to be activists, lobbyists, leaders, and legislators. Failure to apply these skills and unique expertise in politics is to fail their professional organization and the patients who rely on them. Nursing has a legacy of advocates and activists. Margaret Sanger, a graduate public health nurse who studied with Lillian Wald at the Henry Street Settlement House in the early 1900s and who founded Planned Parenthood, once said: "If one is to truly live, one must put one's convictions into action." So everyone must get involved!

Discussion Questions

1. Discuss each of the 10 political strategies and cite local examples and experiences of each.
2. Choose a current healthcare policy issue or concern and prepare talking points regarding its impact on advanced practice nursing to present to policy makers, healthcare providers, and consumers.

References

DeLaney, A. (1995). *Politics, for dummies*. Foster City, CA: IDG Books Worldwide.

Webster's ninth new collegiate dictionary. (1984). Springfield, MA: Merriam-Webster.

Part III

Quality and Information for Advanced Practice Nursing

With specialized knowledge and practical application of that knowledge to influence patient outcomes, nurses in advanced practice have the fiduciary responsibility not only to provide and/or manage quality care, but also to take the leadership within the practice setting to promote a culture of quality. As we saw in Part II, quality is one of the major triads of health care along with cost and access. In this part, we will consider quality issues and the intersection of quality and information technology.

There are many definitions of quality and many perspectives on what healthcare quality means. Consumers, providers, payers, and regulators may all have differing viewpoints about what healthcare quality is and how it should be measured and reported. However, with the national, healthcare industry, and societal interest in the costs of health care and the outcomes of that care, the Institute of Medicine's definition (2001) of quality is a well accepted one and the one used for this book. Healthcare quality is "The degree to which health services for individuals and populations increase the likelihood of desired health outcomes and are consistent with current professional knowledge."

Further, in their report, *Crossing the Quality Chasm*, the IOM (2001) has described six quality aims stating that health care should be:

1. Safe
2. Effective
3. Patient centered
4. Timely
5. Efficient
6. Equitable

These characteristics of quality should be foremost in mind as readers study Part III.

Patient safety is one of the top, if not the top, current quality issues politically and professionally; however, one should think broadly about healthcare quality beyond just safety and keep foremost in one's thinking all of the aforementioned characteristics of quality.

With the recent emphasis on patient safety as a result of the 2000 Institute of Medicine (IOM) report, *To Err Is Human*, a concerted, ongoing effort focused on assessing and improving patient safety has been a major driver in health care. In this report, the IOM documented the serious and pervasive nature of the nation's overall patient safety problem, concluding that over 98,000 deaths per year occurred due to medical error, and the healthcare system has a severe problem. In Chapter 15, Sullivan introduces the work of the IOM regarding patient safety, and Chapter 16 is a more detailed analysis of this important national issue. In addition, many regulatory bodies are supporting the efforts to improve healthcare quality. These bodies and their responses to the patient safety reports are discussed in Chapter 16.

Prior to these initiatives, healthcare organizations have adopted programs of total quality improvement. Although always important, they have taken on new meaning and importance since quality and patient safety have become national issues. In Chapter 15, Sullivan traces the history of quality initiatives in health care from quality to assessment to today's performance improvement. This chapter is both informative about quality programs and health care and practical with strategies for measuring quality and forming quality teams.

In the final chapter in Part III, Godin first describes the basic components of information technology and security issues that arise from computerized medical records. Although these information systems have multiple uses from financial reporting and analysis to documenta-tion of care, perhaps most important to the advanced nurse practitioner is using clinical systems to analyze patient outcomes and improve quality.

References

Institute of Medicine. (2000). *To err is human: Building a safety health system.* Washington, DC: Author.

Institute of Medicine. (2001). *Crossing the quality chasm: The IOM health care quality initiative.* Washington, DC: Author.

Part

III

Quality and Information for Advanced Nursing Practice

CHAPTER 15   Health Care Quality

CHAPTER 16   Contributions of the
              Professional, Public, and
              Private Sectors in Promoting
              Patient Safety

CHAPTER 17   Information Technology for
              Advanced Nursing Practice

Health Care Quality

Dori Taylor
Sullivan

CHAPTER OBJECTIVES

1. Trace the history of quality and performance improvement approaches in healthcare organizations.
2. List the major principles of quality and performance improvement.
3. Discuss the role that the management of information and information technology play in achieving the best results from improvement efforts.
4. Relate the concept of evidence-based practice to quality improvement in general and the role of the advanced nurse practitioner.
5. List the significant accrediting and regulatory bodies influencing quality measurement in health care and discuss their focus.

Introduction

In this chapter, quality improvement is presented along with ways to build a culture of quality. The advanced nurse practitioner plays a major role in identifying priorities for improvement, establishing and maintaining quality standards, participating in data collection activities for regulatory and accreditation purposes, and assuring that improvements are evaluated for safety, efficacy, and effectiveness. As a role model, the advanced nurse practitioner can play a key role in creating a quality of culture or a commitment to continuous improvement in the organization.

This chapter provides an overview of the evolution of performance improvement in health care followed by the major principles of quality and performance improvement common to all the major approaches. Regardless of the specific quality improvement program that an organization has selected or developed, most of the principles will be applicable. For example, the commitment to data-driven decisions for improvement is universal. While the initial focus of performance improvement was on administrative processes, the practice rapidly spread to clinical systems and outcomes; so we discuss this as a special case of performance improvement.

The chapter suggests how evidence-based practice is related to performance improvement and particularly the impact of the quality of available data to inform identification of best practices. Finally, the chapter presents a summary of what the major regulatory and accreditation agencies are requiring related to quality improvement, patient safety, and outcomes of care.

Introduction of Continuous Quality Improvement to Health Care

Sometime around 1980, the concept of quality assurance (QA) began to be popular in clinical settings in acute care hospitals. Early QA efforts were mostly a counting activity and, while carried out with the best intentions, tended to focus on aspects of care that were relatively easy to count rather than processes or outcomes of most interest to practitioners. These early QA activities received a lukewarm reception from most disciplines and were met with relative disdain from physicians. As is often noted by measurement experts, it seems that the easy things to measure are relatively unimportant, while those things that would really make a difference are difficult to measure and interpret. The fact that the focus of QA tended to be determined and imposed by a central authority was another strike against these early efforts. The result was general compliance with the mandates but little enthusiasm and limited use of the findings.

The Quality Movement and Its Translation into Health Care

During the 1980s, the work of Deming (1986) was noticed by healthcare leaders. Deming is considered the ultimate guru of total quality management (TQM), based on his work rebuilding the manufacturing businesses of war-torn Japan beginning around 1950. Deming promoted what he termed *constancy of purpose* and *systematic analysis*, with measurement of process steps in relation to capacity or outcomes. The TQM approach incorporated the view, as the name implies, that the entire organization must be committed to quality and improvement to achieve the best results—and to promote joy in work.

The staggering success of these improved Japanese businesses was first recognized by some industries in the United States, including manufacturing; slowly other sectors took note. Health care was a natural extension given the concerns about quality and cost of care that were beginning to accelerate. Soon after gaining popularity in health care, the quality improvement movement was translated into public and higher education. While some were quick to label quality improvement as a fad, it has flourished in health care and education and has become a business standard for success.

Besides Deming, other experts quickly gained national prominence. New and existing consulting firms created or added quality and performance improvement consulting and education services to assist the many healthcare organizations eager to introduce these powerful methods. Juran (1988) and Joiner (1994) are two other widely recognized experts in quality improvement, both of whom lead international consulting firms devoted to quality management principles, culture, and techniques. Today the field is comprised of hundreds of trademarked approaches to quality, making it impossible to cover them all. We can, however, identify and discuss the most important principles of quality and performance improvement.

Language of Quality Improvement

First, a word about the jargon of quality improvement (QI). Over time, different terms became popular and then faded away as newer terms were embraced. The relatively early *TQM* was somewhat displaced by *continuous quality improvement (CQI)* and then by *performance improvement (PI)*. Although there are distinctions made by the originators of these and other terms, for our purposes we will use *quality* and *performance improvement* to describe a comprehensive and formal system of principles, methods, and techniques to systematically measure and improve processes and outcomes. Also, how quality is defined differs somewhat among various approaches; however, virtually all definitions of quality include meeting or exceeding customer needs, decreasing variation, and minimizing or eliminating defects or errors from products or services.

Quality improvement may focus on enhancing existing processes or designing quality processes. When existing processes are believed to be incapable of yielding the desired results, redesign or reengineering of a process is undertaken. Hammer and Champy (1993) explained reengineering as the "fundamental rethinking and radical redesign of processes to achieve dramatic improvements in critical, contemporary measures of performance, such as cost, quality, service, and speed" (p. 22). While there are clearly differences in improving versus redesigning a work process,

we will use the term *quality improvement (QI)* to describe all such efforts.

Principles of Quality and Performance Improvement

Scholtes (1988) aptly notes that many elements of quality leadership have "appeared separately in fads that swept through business schools and organizations (pp. 1–10)," such that many are unfamiliar with a comprehensive approach to performance improvement that has been termed "a new way of doing business." The principles shown in Table 15–1 and described in the following pages, as presented by Scholtes about the Joiner model, may be worded differently in various approaches, but their meaning is the same.

Customer Focus

The customer is the center of quality efforts as an organization strives to meet or exceed customer goals and provide value. Quality approaches recognize external customers (the users of products or services) and internal customers (those within the organization that receive goods or services from other departments).

The translation of QI principles into health care requires that we think about the term *customer* a bit differently. In a strict business sense, customers are the ones who pay for the service or product they receive. The case in health care is more complex, since much of the cost of health care is borne by third parties, including employers, insurance companies, and the government as opposed to clients themselves. And, frequently the goals and desires of clients are in conflict with those of the payers. Some have referred to the client as the ultimate customer, so as not to confuse where our primary obligation lies. That said, most healthcare organizations and their

---

Table 15–1 PRINCIPLES OF QUALITY LEADERSHIP

1. Customer focus
2. Obsession with quality
3. Recognizing the structure in work
4. Freedom through control
5. Unity of purpose
6. Looking for faults in systems
7. Teamwork
8. Continued education and training

Source: Scholtes, 1988, pp. 1–11.

clinical managers typically try to identify and balance the needs of these major customers, which sometimes are conflicting.

A related principle in this customer focus is to measure, not assume or guess about, what customers need and want. This focus on data and information recurs in many of the quality principles.

OBSESSION WITH QUALITY

Everyone in an organization must be obsessed with quality! This principle may be best defined by the phrase *building a culture of quality* where the norm becomes the relentless pursuit of quality products and services through efficient and effective methods of execution. Building a culture of quality requires attention to staff education, clear communication of goals and expectations, provision of necessary resources, organizational systems that are efficient and effective, and alignment of performance and rewards systems.

RECOGNIZING THE STRUCTURE IN WORK

All work is comprised of processes that are structured, not random. The structure and

processes must be studied, measured, analyzed, and improved systematically to achieve the best results. Quality improvement includes specific tools and techniques to quantify and understand work, providing the data needed to create improvements.

To best understand the structure of work, management and staff must work together since each brings valuable information to the activity. We must appreciate that the people directly involved in the work have the best information about how that work is performed—and how it could be done better. In addition, the focus on work rather than individual performance engages staff in a positive way. This approach fundamentally changes the relationship between staff and management and fosters trust, respect, and empathy. One should recognize these as elements of transformation leadership.

FREEDOM THROUGH CONTROL

Quality improvement embraces the idea of quality control and reducing variation to produce regular desired results. Standardizing processes and ensuring that everyone uses those standards should make work processes more efficient and effective. The increase in productivity should allow for more freedom to develop new ideas for the business, enhance service to the customer, and improve skills in key areas. For example, in a clinical service area, if the scheduling procedure for clients is a refined and effective process, the scheduler or receptionist should not have to spend as much time on the telephone or negotiating with patients or providers, freeing up time for other important activities.

UNITY OF PURPOSE

Unity of purpose speaks to a clear and widely understood vision for the organization that unites or aligns all who work there. It is the vision that guides quality improvement efforts and provides criteria for decision making and problem solving when issues or opportunities arise. In a truly patient-centered healthcare organization, we would expect to see tangible efforts to promote comfort, safety, and timeliness. During a recent visit to an ambulatory surgery facility, the following actions were noted. A sign in the reception area asked patients to come up to the desk if they had been waiting longer than 15 minutes to be called for registration. Upon changing into a hospital gown, patients were provided with two warmed bath blankets. While awaiting surgery, patients were asked if they wanted fresh warmed blankets, and blankets were also wrapped around a family member who was chilled. No one in that organization raised questions about the cost of providing this service, as patient satisfaction data clearly supported how much this amenity was valued, both for its physical comfort and communication of caring at a stressful time.

LOOKING FOR FAULTS IN SYSTEMS

The QI philosophy and culture specifies aggressive continuous improvements of all work systems. The most important factor underlying this principle is accepting that systems rather than individual people are responsible for 80–85% of the results achieved (claims made by Deming and Juran, and supported by the Pareto principle, or 80/20 rule). Loosely translated, the Pareto principle says that 80% of the poor results or troubles come from 20% of the problems. Or, as some managers like to say, 20% of their staff causes 80% of the problems!

Realistically, we cannot work on all systems at the same time, so a way to identify priorities for improvement is essential. This is usually done through the collection of performance data on critical indicators across the organization (sometimes called a dashboard report or report card). In addition, departments create function-specific performance indicators that reflect improvement foci for specific areas. There needs to be some alignment or relationship between organization-wide goals and focus and those of the departments, since it is at the point of service within the departments that quality happens or doesn't happen. An example of this alignment might be an organizational commitment to improving turnaround time. For radiology, this might mean the reading of reports. In the lab, the measure would be time until test results are available. In the rehabilitation department, it might relate to readying special rooms or equipment between clients so there would be decreased waiting time and more appointments possible during a day.

TEAMWORK

There are few if any important work tasks that people do completely by themselves. Thus, we rely on others who play a part in supplying us with the products and services (including information) that we need to do our jobs well—or who need to work collaboratively with us to achieve the desired results. Teamwork differs from individuals or groups in that teams are defined by having members who are committed to working toward a common goal or vision. The best team results are achieved when there is a diversity of ideas and relevant skills on the team that represent the important aspects of the work to be improved.

CONTINUED EDUCATION AND TRAINING

An ongoing commitment to education and training across the organization is critical to keeping the culture of quality alive and thriving. There are always new techniques and ideas to be shared and enhanced skills for obtaining, managing, measuring, analyzing, and using information for improvement. Furthermore, education tends to make staff feel valued and important while enhancing their skills in a concrete way.

Tools and Techniques for Improving Quality and Performance

Improving quality and performance in any organization requires attention to three major areas: leadership, skills for gathering and using information related to work analysis, and the people factor. The Joiner triangle (Scholtes, Joiner, & Streibel, 2003, p. xxi) in Figure 15–1 shows the relationship of these elements where quality leadership and the scientific approach represent the skills and tools for work analysis and improvement and all one team represents the people factor. Teamwork is at the heart of most QI efforts because teamwork reflects how work is typically accomplished and because more brainpower with different perspectives usually develops better solutions. We next present an overview of each of these areas so that you can consider the implications for your role as an advanced nurse practitioner.

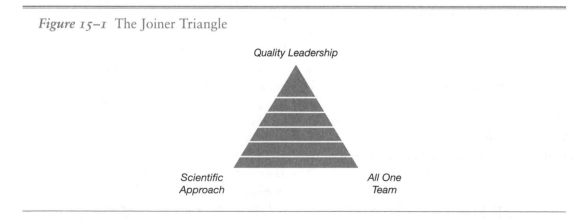

Figure 15–1 The Joiner Triangle

Quality Leadership

Scientific Approach

All One Team

Source: In Scholtes, P., Joiner, B., Streibel, B. (2003). *The TEAM Handbook* (3rd ed.). Madison, WI, Oriel Inc., p. xxi.

Leadership for Quality

The role of leaders in an organization endeavoring to create a culture of quality and continuous improvement cannot be underestimated. Any serious initiative to create a quality organization must be sincerely embraced at the senior levels of the organization as well as by nurse managers and advanced nurse practitioners and be constantly reinforced through actions and reward structures, or what has been called walking the talk. Staff are experts at identifying inconsistencies in leader behavior, and they use any incongruence to decide whether to believe and invest in what is being proffered.

Scholtes (1988) identified six steps needed for quality leadership and a continuous improvement culture. Senior leadership must first commit to a rigorous education program for their team. The program must address all three elements of the triangle. Second, they should define the organizational culture characteristics and values that they wish to develop that are consistent with continuous improvement. Third, senior leaders should develop a multiyear improvement strategy (2 years is recommended) so that a pathway is clearly defined. The next step is a plan for educating the entire workforce, usually done in phases for logistical and cost reasons. This is a significant undertaking that when well done yields powerful results by introducing a new way of thinking about work improvement and relationships. Fifth, a formal network of support and guidance (often defined as access to quality facilitators with advanced knowledge of QI techniques) should be established and communicated. Finally, the specific improvement projects should be identified and initiated.

As an advanced nurse practitioner, you will be called on to be a formal and/or informal leader for quality improvement initiatives. Knowing the process of quality improvement can assist you to be more effective in this role.

Using the Scientific Method

In simple terms the scientific method can be used to test our assertions. More precisely, the scientific method is a set of orderly, systematic, controlled procedures for acquiring dependable, empirical—typically quantitative—information about a topic or question (Polit & Beck, 2004). This method involves four steps after identifying a question or, in our case, a work process, to focus on: assessment and data collection, problem identification, interventions, and evaluation (Table 15–2).

SCIENTIFIC METHOD TOOLS FOR QI

Some commonly used tools for data collection, analysis, and problem identification have evolved from the quality movement: traditional statistical control processes (mostly from manufacturing)

Table 15–2 STEPS IN THE SCIENTIFIC METHOD

1. Assessment and data collection
2. Problem identification
3. Selection of interventions or solutions
4. Evaluation of results

and the discipline of management engineering. For our purposes, we describe only the most frequently used tools so that readers can get a feel for this skill set. Our purpose is to introduce readers to the tools. Readers can build their knowledge base by searching the Internet and/or working with a quality improvement department. Readers' charge is to determine the specific quality approach, methods, and tools used in their own organization so that their knowledge and skill development target those specific areas.

Flowcharts. A flowchart is a diagram that uses standardized symbols to create a paper picture of steps and decisions that make up a work process. There are several variations of flowcharting but each serves the purpose of defining the detail and order of a process. Flowcharts may be developed as a team activity, or individuals may be assigned to create a flowchart based on their understanding of the work process. There are often conflicting opinions about process flowcharts, so one of the major purposes they serve is to develop a common view of an existing or proposed process, a first step in reducing variation.

Pie Charts and Pareto Charts. Most people are familiar with pie charts, which display the percentage of categories or responses using the wedges of a circle that look like slices of pie. The size of the wedge reflects the frequency or size of that category. Similarly, Pareto charts use the same information as a pie chart but depict the categories or responses in a bar graph that orders the named categories from highest to lowest in terms of frequency or impact. The purpose of the Pareto chart is to determine whether in each case the rule holds true, that is, 20% of the categories will explain 80% of the problems.

Cause and Effect (Fishbone) Diagrams. Fishbone diagrams are used to categorize and analyze possible problem causes related to a desired or problematic effect or outcome. The shape of the diagram resembles a fish with bones, thus the name. The fishbone diagram is a picture of lists with increasing amounts of detail as more "bones" are added to the descriptions of possible causative factors. As with flowcharts, cause and effect diagrams may be developed by the team or by individual/small group efforts and then compared.

Operational Definitions. Operational definitions specify a concept or element and how it will be measured. For example, a definition of good turnaround time for a pathology report could be more precisely stated as a typed, signed, final report delivered to the ordering physician within 72 hours of receipt of the specimen. Without precise definitions of effects or outcomes, it becomes difficult to measure the impact of various work process steps or issues.

Run Charts (Time Plots) and Control Charts. A run chart or time plot depicts a series of observations or measures of a work process over time. The purpose of seeing variations over time is to look for patterns that could lead to understanding causes of variation or diminished performance so that effective improvement strategies can be created. Recall that one of the first steps in QI is decreasing variation; the run chart shows the amount of variation over time. For example, the clinical manager of an emergency clinic wishes to see the number of patient visits by day of week so that he can develop a better staffing plan. A 2-week run chart shows that visits are much higher on Thursdays, Fridays, and Saturdays. The next step might be to analyze time of day of visits for those days on a second run chart. A control chart is a run chart with boundaries for expected variation drawn into the display. The values for these boundaries are calculated from statistical control formulas that a quality expert could assist in determining. Variation within the boundaries is referred to as common cause or normal variation. Points of variation outside the boundaries are termed special cause and require further investigation.

Checksheets. Checksheets are forms developed to facilitate collection of observed data about a work process step or element. Checksheets should be as simple as possible with the goal of showing patterns or amounts easily. As an example, consider the case of a courier service that provides service to a freestanding nutrition center. The center might develop a checksheet to document whether the courier is on time and how many items he is delivering. This data could be used to decrease the service and reduce costs or to investigate an improved method of accomplishing this activity.

Gap Analysis. A gap analysis is used to assess the nature and amount of difference between the current state and the desired state of designated characteristics or outcomes. The best gap analyses incorporate measurement data to support the description of the current state and definition of the desired future. For instance, if a goal is to have active participation in shared governance of a department, one could count the number of staff participating on councils.

Root Cause Analysis. Root cause analysis is a formalized investigation and problem-solving approach focused on understanding the underlying causes of an event as opposed to focusing on symptoms of a problem. Root cause analysis seeks to determine what happened, how it hap-

pened, and why it happened, with the overall goal of making recommendations for prevention of future events. The four steps in root cause analysis are data collection, causal factor charting, identification of root causes, and generation of recommendations and implementation of changes (Rooney & Vanden Heuvel, 2004). A root cause summary table may be used to summarize the findings and recommendations of the analysis.

The People Factor and Teams

Each of us has probably experienced an unproductive or uncomfortable group meeting, where differing opinions and dialogue did not result in a consensus or decision. Consensus may be defined as an idea or proposal that all team members can positively support, even though it may not be their personal first choice or preference. Achieving consensus is generally preferred to majority rules voting or an authoritarian decision because it promotes better solutions and improved team relationships as well as buy-in from members.

TEAM COMMUNICATION AND DECISIONS

Using structured communication and decision-making tools improves team functioning and outcomes. The tools and techniques described below are designed to promote efficient presentation of ideas and opinions after which agreements can be developed for how to proceed.

Brainstorming. Brainstorming is a technique that enables a group to generate and list many ideas within a short time period. It also promotes relatively equal participation, assuring that talkative members do not monopolize the discussion.

Participants contribute one item in order with no comments about the ideas allowed. People may pass if they have nothing to add during that round, and the session is stopped by time or lack of additional ideas. The group then clarifies their understanding of each idea and may combine similar items. The next steps are for the group to agree on criteria for evaluating these ideas or how to reduce the list to the best ideas to make it manageable.

Multivoting. Multivoting allots a certain number of votes to each participant that each uses for their most preferred items from a brainstorming or other list. Multivoting reduces the list of ideas by retaining only those items with the higher number of votes. It is often used following a brainstorming session to focus the team on one or more items. After combining similar items, the remaining items are numbered. Each member is given a specified number of votes. Items with the lowest vote totals are eliminated and another multivoting session may be conducted; this process can be repeated as many times as needed.

Nominal Group Technique. This technique is a more formalized approach to determine priorities from a list generated by participants. It combines elements of brainstorming as participants write down their ideas independently in response to a question or topic. A master list of the ideas is compiled on a flip chart. Each participant is then asked to assign a rating or number of points to a specified number of the ideas presented. This technique is helpful for relatively new teams or controversial topics.

Affinity Diagrams. Creating an affinity diagram is an action strategy to develop categories or see how numerous elements might be related based on perceptions of a group. Each member is instructed to write down three to five responses to a question, writing each response on a separate sticky note. The individual notes are then posted on a large wall by all participants. Participants are instructed to group the sticky notes together as best makes sense to them without speaking to others. Each individual can move the sticky notes into whatever configuration he or she prefers, but the next person can come along and undo it. After a period of time the group tends to arrive at a good enough solution. The clusters of notes depict a number of broad categories or themes that emerge. This activity can promote enhanced understanding of underlying causes of issues.

Lessons Learned for Promoting QI Team Effectiveness

In addition to the structured QI tools just discussed, consideration must be given to how to structure team activities for the best outcomes, acknowledging that individuals have needs and motivations that may detract from team effectiveness. As a culture of quality develops in a unit or organization, the norm is to question and improve everything and defensiveness decreases. However, to promote optimal team functioning and outcomes, attention must be given to establishing a clear charge, selecting the team members, and assigning roles. These recommendations apply whether the team is from one unit or comprised of several departments across the organization, so it is important to make the appropriate adjustments depending upon the type of team.

Team Charge

Most organizations create a formal mechanism for deciding upon improvement priorities relying on appropriate performance data and quality indicators. Once the decision is made that a cross-functional team (comprised of staff from multiple departments or areas) should be convened to address an improvement opportunity, a formal charge to the team is prepared. This charge should include the specific nature of the improvement opportunity and the desired outcomes, timelines, resources available, team members, and any other parameters or assumptions the team needs to accomplish its charge. A team charge is similar to a team charter, differing only in how much detail is fleshed out by the person or group creating the team.

Selection of Members

The selection of team members is crucial to team success. Individuals who have process owner status, meaning that they have primary responsibility for this work, must be included both for their knowledge and to promote buy-in for recommended improvements. If one wants to establish a team on one's unit to improve the response time of the night shift and there is a night charge person, it is essential to have the charge person on the team. Staff who actually perform the work and are closest to the provision of services should also be team members. Those who supply information, products, or services (suppliers) as well as internal and possibly external customers should also be represented, either as team members or through invitations to join certain meetings. The size of a QI team varies among organizations and projects, but most experts seem to agree that between seven and nine is the best number for team effectiveness.

Team Roles

There are six basic roles in a QI team: team leader or chair, team member, recorder, timekeeper, facilitator or quality adviser, and executive cham-

pion. Depending on the size of the team, some of these roles may be combined or even rotated; whatever the plan, the team needs to ensure that all the functions are assigned and carried out.

TEAM LEADER

The team leader is formally in charge of the team's efforts including meeting schedules and agendas, between-meeting assignments, maintenance of the formal team records, and communication with others regarding the team's work (unless this is specifically assigned to a team member for specific requests). The team leader role may be performed by cochairs if desired. The team leader works closely with the facilitator for guidance and feedback on team performance and next steps. Whenever possible, the next meeting's agenda and between-meeting assignments should be reviewed and documented near the end of the meeting.

TEAM MEMBER

Team members accept responsibility for sharing their ideas and information, preparing for meetings, completing between-meeting assignments, committing to continued learning, and contributing to overall team effectiveness.

RECORDER

It is highly recommended that the team's work be captured on flip charts or smart boards so that all members can see and assist with what is being recorded. In addition, this method of recording eliminates the need to spend time writing minutes after the meeting, as meeting documentation can be typed from the recording sheets. Any reports or charts prepared may also be attached and distributed to foster the team's work progress. The recorder function may be assigned to a specific team member or, more often, it is rotated among members.

TIMEKEEPER

As the name suggests, this team role is responsible for helping the team manage its time. Agendas should include suggested time allocations for each agenda item and/or the team should discuss how to best use the available time at each meeting. The timekeeper notifies the team when the allocated time has elapsed, at which point the team can decide to stop the discussion or agree to continue for an amount of time.

FACILITATOR

The facilitator or quality adviser may be from the quality or education department or it could be a colleague who has received in-depth quality training. The facilitator has three main responsibilities. First and foremost, the facilitator works with the team leader to plan out the team's work and consider which QI tools or methods might be most helpful at different stages of the project. Second, the facilitator attends team meetings to observe and make recommendations to the team about its level of effectiveness and its enhancement. Many facilitators take 5 minutes at the end of each meeting to elicit members' perceptions of what went well and facilitated work versus what could be done better for the next time. Third, the facilitator is an expert in QI and provides formal or just-in-time training as needed to foster team progress.

CHAMPION

Each QI team should have a senior leader appointed as the executive champion of the team's project. For unit teams, the advanced nurse practitioner would be identified as the champion. Frequently, the team leader and the facilitator encounter issues or barriers that require assistance or advice from senior administration. And while the champion does not attend all team meetings, that person does establish regular communication, and this provides information to show that the team is on track to meet the improvement goals. Table 15–3 provides a summary of QI tools and techniques, and Table 15–4 lists the team decision methods.

Ground Rules

Ground rules (or rules of engagement) evolve from team discussions about how members wish to behave with one another to promote member satisfaction and team success. Ground rules often include expectations related to prompt attendance, participation, interruptions (pagers

---

Table 15–3 SUMMARY OF QI TOOLS AND TECHNIQUES

QI Tools	QI Techniques
Flowchart	Brainstorming
Pie chart/Pareto chart	Multivoting
Cause and effect (Fishbone) diagram	Nominal group technique
Operational definitions	Affinity diagrams
Run and control charts	Structured discussion
Checksheets	
Root cause analysis	

Table 15-4 SUMMARY OF QI TEAM CONCEPTS
Team charge (opportunity, outcomes, timelines, resources, assumptions)
Selection of members
Size of team
Team roles (leader, member, recorder, timekeeper, facilitator, executive champion)
Ground rules

and phones), decision making, conversational courtesies (such as no interrupting when others are speaking), and confidentiality agreements when appropriate. Once ground rules are established through consensus, it is easier to hold members accountable for compliance.

What Makes Quality Improvement Successful?

The traditionalist QI approaches developed by Deming, Juran, and Joiner, among others, remain the method of choice in numerous healthcare organizations. Others have opted to follow two newer models: General Electric's (GE) Six Sigma and Work Out (GE, n.d.) and Studer Group's Pillars of Excellence (Studer Group, n.d.). The Six Sigma and Pillars of Excellence approaches have been adopted by growing numbers of healthcare organizations. These approaches, while evolutionary in terms of QI, retain the core principles presented earlier in this chapter.

Many QI approaches have led to spectacular organizational successes. The major factors in this success may be summarized into three themes. First is the commitment of leadership to the fundamental principles of quality, improvement, measurement, empowerment, and involvement. Leaders must visibly, powerfully, and continuously talk and walk the talk!

Second, a clear and consistent model for QI should be selected and refined for use in an organization; this would also be used at the unit level. The QI field is cluttered with jargon and people become easily frustrated if the language changes all the time. Staff want to master QI skills, and that is more difficult to do without a clear model, terms, and processes. Third, there must be an investment in building a quality infrastructure to provide the human and material resources required for QI success. An advanced nurse practitioner needs to assure that staff teams have sufficient resources and direction for success. Members of a staff may also be asked to develop additional QI skills to support efforts throughout the organization.

Benchmarking is a term denoting the use of information from other organizations to use as a comparison or benchmark in evaluating an organization's performance. Benchmarking may be a relatively informal, collegial process or, more often, an extensive and detailed project. The utility of benchmarking data is enhanced when there are common operational definitions for key data elements and metrics for reporting. It also works better when the organizations, or at least the specific area or work process being benchmarked, share important characteristics.

Recently the emphasis in benchmarking has been on best or better practices. For example, if a hospital is trying to reduce length of stay for patients having total knee replacements, it should access information from a hospital having the lowest lengths of stay and excellent quality outcomes. This comparison yields two helpful things. It provides a reality-based sense of the possible in the current environment, and it allows for learning about how the length of stay reduction is achieved.

Many healthcare organizations belong to proprietary benchmarking service companies or groups and can regularly access performance data in areas of interest such as patient satisfaction. These comparisons may also facilitate the identification of organizational or departmental improvement priorities if there is a major difference in efficiency and/or effectiveness of the care or services under study.

Benchmarking is discussed in more detail in the section on accrediting and regulatory agencies' quality initiatives. We now turn our attention to the special case of clinical improvement and the related concept of evidence-based practice.

Clinical Process Improvement and Evidence-Based Practice

The successes in administrative and support processes using QI skills led to transferring this approach to clinical processes and outcomes. While QI was largely driven by administrators at the beginning, physician leaders and other clinicians recognized the opportunities that a structured approach to improvement provided. Further, given the long tradition of a research-based approach to care, a renewed interest in using research evidence to guide care decisions and protocols developed. The term *evidence-based medicine* or *practice* was coined and reflects this

renewed emphasis by medicine, nursing, and other health disciplines. We also note how advances in information technology have accelerated and supported clinical improvement and evidence-based practice.

Clinical-Process Improvement

Clinical-process redesign or improvement means "the effective design of the continuum of care to satisfy customers, improve patient outcomes, maximize efficiencies, and improve the organizational climate" (Strongwater & Pelote, 1996, p. ix). The specific outcomes of general interest specified by these authors include clinical outcomes, functional outcomes (physical, social, and quality of life), patient satisfaction, and organizational climate (staff satisfaction and readiness to change), along with cost and utilization indicators.

As individual healthcare organizations identified clinical-process improvement as a major strategic goal, entities that support hospitals and other agencies developed clinical-improvement programs and resources to assist their constituencies. For example VHA, Inc., a national membership organization for community hospital systems, and the University Healthsystems Consortium (UHC), a member organization for academic medical center hospitals and systems, each created divisions for clinical improvement. VHA, Inc. and UHC added physicians, nurses, and other quality experts to their staffs to provide consultation and other resources to support their members' efforts. The development of comparative databases for benchmarking and creating peer relationships for learning and improvement blossomed during the 1990s, and entire conferences were regularly held to advance this area.

At about the same time, the Agency for Healthcare Research and Quality (AHRQ) came into being and began assimilating research to issue practice guidelines with the expectation of improving patient outcomes. The stated mission of AHRQ is to improve the quality, safety, efficiency, and effectiveness of health care for all Americans (AHRQ, n.d.). The AHRQ develops consensus around evidence-based best practices for priority healthcare concerns like pain, incontinence, and others. This brings us to evidence-based practice.

Evidence-Based Practice

Evidence-based practice (EBP) is the integration of best research evidence with clinical expertise and patient values to deliver optimal care (Sackett, Straus, Richardson, Rosenberg, & Haynes, 2000). Best research means clinically relevant, patient-centered research studies. Clinical expertise refers to the role of clinical skills and experience as well as unique patient presentations. The inclusion of patient values reflects the need to individualize care to meet individual preferences, needs, and concerns to best serve that patient. These authors further assert that to carry out EBP there must be sufficient research published on the specific topic

of interest, the health practitioner must have skills in accessing and critically analyzing research, and last, that the practice must allow for implementing changes based on the evidence. Table 15–5 summarizes a five-step process for EBP.

The evaluation of evidence is often done using a system for grading or leveling the quality of the evidence according to accepted research standards. There are several systems for grading evidence with one example being the following three-grade system:

- Level I or A—a multisite randomized clinical trial or several single-site randomized studies
- Level II or B—a quasi-experimental study
- Level III or C—a correlational or descriptive study

While EBP in health care is not totally new, the emphasis and widespread commitment to its use, facilitated by exploding and more readily available evidence, continues to grow and has become the standard of care. Another factor contributing to EBP is the time pressure experienced by most

Table 15–5 SUMMARY OF EBP AND THE FIVE-STEP PROCESS

Evidence-based practice (EBP) is the integration of best research evidence with clinical expertise and patient values to optimize clinical outcomes and quality of life (Sackett, Straus, Richardson, Rosenberg, & Haynes, 2000, p. 1).

1. Formulate a question arising from patient clinical problems based on current knowledge and practice.
2. Search for and access relevant evidence or research.
3. Evaluate the evidence using established criteria for scientific merit.
4. Choose interventions or changes in practice, justifying the selection with the most valid evidence for the patient population to which it will be applied.
5. Implement the change(s) and evaluate the results.

healthcare providers. Instead of having to go to a library, clinicians can use their PDAs or a computer with Internet access to quickly locate current research data and critical reviews on a particular topic. There are also evidence-based clinical guidelines available for purchase to guide practice in the field.

Recognizing that patient outcomes result from the efforts of numerous disciplines, the most effective EBP models combine the interventions of the involved disciplines for various patient conditions, although each discipline retains responsibility for assessing its own professional practice. For further information about and examples of current evidence-based improvement initiatives, refer to the Web sites for the Institute for Healthcare Improvement (www.ihi.org) and ZYNX (www.zynx.com).

Despite its popularity, some barriers to EBP have been identified, most commonly accessibility of research findings, anticipated benefits of using research, organizational support to use research, and support from others (Retsas, 2000). Healthcare organizations need to find ways to foster the culture of quality and support systems to make EBP a way of life to provide the best and most cost-effective care. Advanced nurse practitioners will be expected to use research knowledge and skills to promote safe, high-quality care. Those who have not already done so, should consider taking a formal or continuing education course to enhance their competence in this area.

Managing Information and Information Technology

The evolution of computerization and information technology (IT) in health care is a complex and interesting topic. For our purposes, we comment on the critical role of IT and some of the issues and decisions that will critically affect our ability to improve quality and enhance efficiency using IT advances. We expect that all readers have some experience with IT systems in their organizations whether it be for managing staffing or supplies, scheduling visits or procedures, tracking records, entering medical orders, or using electronic medical records.

One of the major issues in health care is the jigsaw puzzle approach to computerization in most healthcare organizations. For a variety of reasons, different departments or functions were automated at different times, after which more comprehensive software systems became available. Decisions related to interfacing abilities (getting the systems to talk to one another and share information) versus extinction of the original system in favor of wider benefits are quite common. Comprehensive software systems can now be purchased for many healthcare setting needs related to client medical records, tracking, services, payments, and outcomes; financial matters; staff and patient scheduling; and many others.

Automation tends to improve information access, communication, and documentation; decrease redundancy of data entry; facilitate the use of data for research and QI; and promote easier compliance with regulatory requirements. Initial and ongoing costs of these systems along with information security can be significant challenges. Another challenge is called data integrity or verifying that the data in the system is accurately coded, entered, and available. While many healthcare organizations are making progress in implementing a fully automated medical record, most are still working at this process.

Leapfrog Group is a conglomerate of nonhealthcare Fortune 500 company leaders committed to modernizing the current health-care system (Milstein, 2000). This increasingly influential group has identified three evidence-based initiatives it believes will dramatically improve outcomes: (1) computerized physician order entry (CPOE), (2) evidence-based hospital referrals (EHR), and (3) intensive care unit physician staffing (IPS) (Hudon, 2003, p. 233). We discuss the first two, since they directly relate to subsequent content.

Implementation of a CPOE system addresses several components of medical errors related to medications, namely the legibility of orders, completeness of information, and the ability to use a clinical decision support system (CDSS) to cross-check for dangerous drug interactions or contraindications. Although evidence clearly supports improved quality and financial outcomes related to CPOE, the initial expenses are substantial. These statements could apply to many software systems available to healthcare agencies. Another factor is that most would agree that computerization often does not save professional time but does improve the quality and availability of data.

The EHR recommendation supports that consumers should have access to quality and outcome data for specific conditions and procedures so that they can make informed choices regarding where to seek care. We address this in more detail in the section on regulatory and accrediting quality initiatives.

Advanced nurse practitioners will need to be involved in the implementation of systems that include their areas or serve their areas specifically. And it is generally recommended that representative advanced nurse practitioners and the staff on the front line participate in the selection of software systems to provide the end-user perspective. Thus, enhancing knowledge of infor-mation technology systems and capabilities will lead to better use of information for evidence-based practice and quality, financial, and other purposes.

Accreditation and Regulatory Focus on Quality

The major accreditation and regulatory entities in health care have taken significant steps to promote quality and safety in the delivery of health care. Although many of the efforts focused on hospitals, they noted that other settings would likely have similar issues. Recommendations for assessing other settings (like nursing homes, ambulatory care, and home care) to identify differences and effective solutions were frequently encouraged. In this chapter, we review some of the major changes and recent requirements that focus on improving the quality of care and patient safety with attention to cost effectiveness and service utilization, changes that have significant impact on advanced nurse practitioners in most settings.

Joint Commission Performance Improvement and Safety Standards

The Joint Commission on the Accreditation of Health Care Organizations (JCAHO), provides voluntary accreditation services to hospitals, home-care agencies, ambulatory care, long-term care, behavioral health, laboratories, and office-based surgery, among others. The JCAHO should be credited for an early effort to require contemporary QI activities of their accredited facilities. As early as 1987, JCAHO's Agenda for Change called for demonstration of systematic QI efforts including closing the loop by evaluating the impact of improvement strategies. At the same time, JCAHO began development of performance measures that evolved into the ORYX initiative, a requirement for benchmarking clinical outcomes of selected conditions.

Since 1999, the Joint Commission has met with stakeholder groups to develop a set of hospital core measures. Three initial major diagnoses were selected for testing after extensive pilot testing, feedback from pilot hospitals, and information derived from the Centers for Medicare and Medicaid Services (CMS) of the United States Department of Health and Human Services (HHS). The three diagnoses are: acute myocardial infarction (AMI, 9 measures), heart failure (HF, 4 measures), and community-acquired pneumonia (CAP, 5 measures). A fourth area, pregnancy and related conditions (PR), was added later as was the measure for surgical infection prevention (SIP). Additional measures are under development with the stated intent to stay consistent with CMS goals and initiatives.

Two other Joint Commission requirements deserve mention in the context of quality and safety. The Joint Commission calls for a patient safety plan that reflects a comprehensive approach for reporting, analyzing, and preventing medical errors through a variety of actions. Specific attention is given to sentinel events, defined as "an unexpected occurrence involving death or serious physical or psychological injury, or the risk thereof" (www.jcipatientsafety.org). In an assessment of 2,966 hospital sentinel events reported between 1995 and 2004, JCAHO listed the top five root causes of sentinel events from all categories as communica-

tion, orientation and training, patient assessment, staffing, and availability of information.

For our purposes and because of the role hospitals play in the current system, we have used the Joint Commission accreditation of hospitals as an exemplar to illustrate how quality and safety requirements have evolved. Advanced nurse practitioners should become knowledgeable of the Joint Commission or other accreditation agency standards for their areas, many of which have headed in similar directions. The next section summarizes reports from the Institute of Medicine (IOM) and highlights the information that drove some of these changes.

IOM Reports

Three reports among the many issued by the IOM of the National Academies fueled the focus on measuring and reporting quality and safety in health care. Each of these reports is briefly presented with the major recommendations.

The first of the three reports, *To Err Is Human* (IOM, 2000), drew major headlines with its finding that as many as 98,000 deaths each year in the United States were due to medical errors. This number surpasses the number of deaths from motor vehicle accidents, breast cancer, and AIDS. It was also reported that the cost of one category of these errors, preventable adverse drug reactions, was about $2 billion. The goal of the report was to break what was called the "cycle of inaction" and improve the quality and safety of the delivery of health care in the United States. A four-tiered set of recommendations was made, including:

1. A national focus to create leadership, resources, tools, and protocols to increase the knowledge base on health-care safety.

2. Identification and learning from errors with mandatory reporting of events.
3. Raising standards and expectations for improving safety among oversight organizations, purchasers of care, and professional groups.
4. Creation of safer systems in healthcare organizations leading to safe practice at the level where care is delivered—the ultimate goal of all the recommendations.

The next pivotal IOM report, *Crossing the Quality Chasm* (IOM, 2001), called for fundamental changes to the healthcare system to increase the benefits of care while decreasing harm. It acknowledged that the current system does not make the best use of resources due to the impact of errors and overuse. The report also stated that the system is plagued by outmoded systems of work and called for public and private purchasers of care, healthcare organizations, clinicians, and patients to work together to redesign healthcare processes. Six aims for redesign of the healthcare system were established, indicating the new system should be safe, effective, patient-centered, timely, efficient, and equitable. The IOM also suggested that HHS take a role in identifying priority conditions and foster research and improvements in care delivery based on this knowledge. Finally, the report listed 10 principles to guide the redesign of the healthcare system:

1. Care should be based on continuous healing relationships.
2. Care should be customized based on patient needs and values.
3. Patients should have control with shared decision making.
4. There should be shared knowledge and a free flow of information.

5. Evidence-based decision making should be evident.
6. Safety should be designed in as a system priority.
7. There should be transparency to promote informed decision making.
8. The system should anticipate patient needs, not just respond.
9. There should be a continued decrease in waste within the system.
10. There needs to be cooperation among clinicians.

In its 2004 report, *Keeping Patients Safe: Transforming the Work Environment of Nurses*, the IOM was asked by AHRQ to conduct a study with two aims: (1) identify key aspects of the work environment for nurses that were likely to have an impact on patient safety, and (2) recommend potential improvements in nurses' work conditions that would likely increase patient safety. This report emphasized the critical role that nurses play in patient safety and confirmed that the evidence supported that aspects of nurses' work environments were threats to patient safety. The IOM specifically noted the impact of reengineering or redesign in health care as detrimental by decreasing nurses' trust in administration and diminishing the voice of nurses in patient care at multiple levels. *Keeping Patients Safe* contains a wealth of detailed research evidence about many aspects of work environments and is worth reading in its entirety. Although the report targets nurses, many of the principles and recommendations can be applied to other healthcare providers. The report identified transformational leadership and evidence-based practice for management as two important concepts for improving work environments.

Specific recommendations were made in the areas of:

- Nurse staffing ratios and practices
- National data reporting of staffing
- Increased resources for knowledge and skill development from orientation through length of tenure
- Support for interdisciplinary activities that promote collaboration
- Limits on hours worked
- Design of work environments and care processes with a recommendation to first focus on medication administration and hand washing
- Creating an overall culture of safety within healthcare organizations

The later IOM reports built upon the work of the prior reports and had substantial impact on the healthcare system and professional communities. The imprint of the IOM report recommendations can be seen in later health initiatives.

CMS Initiatives

In November 2001, HHS and CMS announced the quality initiative designed to measure and report on healthcare quality for consumer use with the support of Medicare's quality improvement organizations. The CMS launched the Hospital Quality Initiative in 2003, which aimed to define and standardize hospital data for collection, data transmission requirements, and performance measures. A 10-measure starter set focused on acute myocardial infarction (AMI), heart failure (HF), and pneumonia (PNE). Another 12 measures are under discussion under the auspices of the Hospital Quality Alliance (CMS, 2004).

Building on the Hospital Quality Initiative and work related to nursing home quality, pilot testing of improved measures for nursing home quality occurred in 2002 and 2003. It was reported that about 3 million elderly and disabled Americans received care in approximately 17,000 Medicare and Medicaid certified nursing homes in 2001. As of January 2004, the CMS Nursing Home Quality Initiative listed 14 quality measures on its Nursing Home Compare Web site for comparison in the areas of delirium, pain (acute and chronic), pressure sores, decline in activities of daily living, bedfast, worsening anxiety or depression, incontinence, indwelling catheters, mobility decline, physical restraints, urinary tract infections, and weight loss. New initiatives in the creation of staffing quality measures and background checks for employees are under development.

The CMS Home Health Quality Initiative was launched in 2003 to assess and report on quality measures for the significant number of individuals receiving home care services. About 3.5 million elderly and disabled Americans received care from nearly 7,000 Medicare certified home health agencies in 2001 (CMS, 2003). The home care quality indicators rely heavily on data provided from the Outcomes and Assessment Information Set (OASIS) introduced in the late 1990s to fulfill provisions of the Balanced Budget Act (BBA) of 1997 related to prospective payment for Medicare patients. The OASIS assessment purports to include core items of a comprehensive assessment for an adult home care patient and provide data for purposes of outcome-based quality improvement. The National Quality Foundation (NQF) is working with CMS on additional measures that are likely to include improvements related to ambulation, bathing, transferring, managing oral medications, pain interfering with activity, dyspnea, urinary incontinence, acute care hospitalization, discharge to community, and emergent care.

In the ambulatory care domain, CMS is again working with the NQF to endorse a set of standards, building on work initiated by the CMS and the American Medical Association's Physician Consortium for Performance Improvement, of the National Committee for Quality Assurance. The standards are expected to address asthma and respiratory illness, depression and behavioral health, bone conditions such as osteoporosis, arthritis, diabetes, heart disease, hypertension, prenatal care, and prevention/immunization/screening activities (CMS, n.d.).

Additional quality measures for other healthcare settings are in the Joint Commission and CMS standards as well as in other accrediting and regulatory bodies' published information. Advanced nurse practitioners should access these other quality standards relevant to their areas. We have presented an array of current activities to underscore the wide and intensive efforts under way to measure and report quality, since it is a major responsibility of healthcare leaders.

Medicare Pay for Performance Initiatives

CMS is developing and implementing a set of pay for performance initiatives to support QI in the care of Medicare beneficiaries. CMS is focusing first on hospitals, physicians, and physician groups to be followed by home health and dialysis. As part of a demonstration project, incentive payments will be made to hospitals that demonstrate high quality based on data from 34 quality measures relating to five clinical conditions. A similar demonstration project began in

selected physician practices across the country in spring 2005. More information about other pay for performance proposals can be accessed on the CMS Web site.

In summary, there is increasing evidence that the healthcare system is fragmented, unacceptably unsafe, and costly. The mounting evidence and public attention have led to unprecedented cooperation among major accrediting, regulatory, and professional groups to address this evolving crisis in health care. As you consider the information just presented, please reflect on the congruencies among the priority areas identified by major agencies like the Joint Commission, AHRQ, and CMS. Today, evidence-based management and decision making are identifying clearer priorities for healthcare improvement. In addition, there is a comprehensive effort to include all settings where health care is delivered, which is especially important considering the shift of services outside of hospitals in recent years.

Conclusion

With advanced knowledge and skills, advanced nurse practitioners must be at the cutting edge in assimilating and acting on quality and performance standards driven by external forces (primarily accrediting and regulatory agencies) and internal mandates (health system corporate entities and organization-wide goals). Success in this area calls for balancing scientific or data-driven changes for improvement with the human side of the equation, recognizing that it takes time for people to embrace change. The creation of a culture of quality can enhance the staff's ability to positively improve care, control costs, and accelerate the pace of change that is needed.

An advanced nurse practitioner will need to hone his or her skills and commitment to mastering the skills of QI so that he or she can serve as a resource and role model to nursing staff. He or she will also be called upon to have an up-to-date knowledge of the current and expected quality measures that relate to clinical expertise and the area in which he or she is employed. The detailed planning for compliance with quality reporting depends heavily upon information management and technology, both system-wide applications and unit-based software systems.

While all these changes in QI and public reporting can feel a bit overwhelming, they are introducing a new era of excitement by refocusing health providers on our mission through outcomes-based QI and enhancing the care delivered to clients. The systematic use of evidence to support or redefine how to best provide care is energizing and supports interdisciplinary collaboration. This focus on quality care and outcomes is assisting healthcare organizations to reinvent themselves and cut through the status quo system (or existing system) that no longer serves us or our patients well.

Discussion Questions

1. What is the culture of your organization as it relates to QI?
2. Describe and name the overall approach to QI that is used in your organization. What is the nature of your participation in QI?
3. What are the most significant external quality standards or measures for your area(s), and from which accrediting or regulatory bodies are they derived?
4. Identify a current quality concern or improvement opportunity within your scope of responsibility and then consider if there is evidence to support considering a change.

References

AHRQ (Agency for Healthcare Research and Quality). (n.d.). *Mission statement*. Retrieved May 10, 2005, from http://www.ahrq.gov/about/profile.htm

CMS (Centers for Medicare and Medicaid Services). (2003, March 21). *Home health quality initiative overview*. Retrieved from http://www.cms.hhs.gov/quality/

CMS (Centers for Medicare and Medicaid Services). (2004, January). *Nursing home quality initiative*. Retrieved from http://www.cms.hhs.gov/quality/

CMS (Centers for Medicare and Medicaid Services). (2004, November 22). *Building on the foundation:*

Hospital measures for public reporting, CMS fact sheet. Retrieved from http://www.cms.hhs.gov/quality/

Deming, W. E. (1986). *Out of the crisis*. Cambridge, MA: MIT Center for Advanced Engineering Study.

GE (General Electric). (n.d.). *Six sigma*. Retrieved May 5, 2005, from http://www.ge.com/sixsigma/keyelements.html

Hammer, M., & Champy, J. (1993). *Reengineering the corporation: A manifesto for business revolution*. New York: HarperCollins.

Hudon, S. (2003). Leapfrog standards: Implications for nursing practice. *Nursing Economics, 21*(5), 233–236.

IOM (Institute of Medicine). (2000). *To err is human: Building a safer health system*. Washington, DC: National Academy Press.

IOM (Institute of Medicine). (2001). *Crossing the quality chasm: A new health system for the 21st century*. Washington, DC: National Academy Press.

IOM (Institute of Medicine). (2004). *Keeping patients safe: Transforming the work environment of nurses*. Washington, DC: National Academy Press.

Joiner, B. L. (1994). *Fourth-generation management: The new business consciousness*. New York: McGraw-Hill.

Juran, J. M. (1988). *Juran on planning for quality*. New York: The Free Press.

Milstein, A. (2000). *Statement on behalf of the business roundtable*. Retrieved May 16, 2005, from http://www.brtable.org/document.cfm/372

Polit, D., & Beck, C. T. (2004). *Nursing research: Principles and methods* (7th ed.). Philadelphia: Williams & Wilkins.

Retsas, A. (2000). Barriers to using research evidence in nursing practice. *Journal of Advanced Nursing, 31*(3), 599–606.

Rooney, J. J., & Vanden Heuvel, L. N. (2004, July). Root cause analysis for beginners. *Quality Progress*, 45–53.

Sackett, D. L., Straus, S. E., Richardson, W. S., Rosenberg, W., & Haynes, R. B. (2000). *Evidence-based medicine: How to practice and teach EBM* (2nd ed.). Edinburgh: Churchill Livingstone.

Scholtes, P., Joiner, B., & Streibel, B. (2003). *The TEAM Handbook* (3rd ed.). Madison, WI: Oriel Inc.

Strongwater, S. L., & Pelote, V. (1996). *Clinical process redesign: A facilitator's guide*. Gaithersburg, MD: Aspen.

Studer Group. (n.d.). *Health care flywheel*. Retrieved May 15, 2005, from http://www.studergroup.com/$spindb.query.2flywheel.studview

Contributions of the Professional, Public, and Private Sectors in Promoting Patient Safety

Evelyn D. Quigley

CHAPTER OBJECTIVES

1. Identify the major organizations that have identified patient safety as a top priority for health care and explain how they are responding to improve patient safety.
2. Explore options to improve systems to promote patient safety.
3. Discuss the role of the advanced nurse practitioner in identifying safety issues and improving quality of care.

Introduction

Patient safety has become a national priority. The purpose of this article is to discuss the contributions of the professional, public, and private sectors regarding patient safety and to explore options in creating improved systems for this pressing issue. With the increased complexity of the healthcare system, workforce shortages, decreased reimbursement, and more demand for services, the imperative to find solutions for safer care is even more urgent. The pace of work has increased considerably,

along with greater interdependence among healthcare professionals and in the various healthcare settings. This interdependent relationship calls for more frequent transfer of care from one professional to another, presenting frequent occasions for system failure and communication breakdown.

Additionally, due to the lack of integrated technology and appropriate decision support applications, steps to identify and reduce medical errors in healthcare have been impeded. Since the traditional reporting practice of healthcare settings has been to report one incident at a

Source: Promoting patient safety. (2003, September 30). *Online Journal of Issues in Nursing, 8*(3), manuscript 1. Available at www.nursingworld.org/MainMenuCategories/ANAMarketplace/ANAPeriodicals/OJIN/TableofContents/Volume82003/Num3Sep30_2003/ContributionsinPromoting.aspx. Reprinted with permission.

time, errors have been treated as singular incidents without regard to the frequency or intensity of impact. Due to malpractice and confidentiality concerns, the healthcare industry acknowledges that errors are generally underreported. Based on the unique response of individuals to medical treatment, medical errors can be difficult to recognize.

Strategies to create a safe care environment are being advanced from the professional, public, and private sectors. New safety standards will push healthcare institutions to be proactive rather than reactive in identifying and preventing potential sources of patient risk. How do healthcare organizations assist patients, families, and clinicians to deal with errors, failures, and accidents that result in harm? How do healthcare leaders cope with advocating open disclosure about errors and accidents in an industry that experiences negative publicity and high exposure to legal liability? An exploration of the contributions of various diverse constituencies will be conducted in pursuit of the potential for greater interaction with one another.

Responses by Professional Associations

American Nurses Association Response

While nursing has had patient safety as a primary focus, a coordinated and comprehensive system for patient safety has not existed. Various organizations have drawn attention to the need for the development and support of an integrated and comprehensive system that identifies and manages medical errors and rewards healthcare systems for positive outcomes. It was the American Nurses Association (ANA) Board of Directors that instituted the Nursing's Safety & Quality Initiative in 1994 (ANA, 1999). Given the fact that considerable restructuring was occurring in the healthcare industry, this multiphase initiative gave direction to the study of the impact of these changes on safety and quality of patient care as well as nursing. Numerous projects were launched from the investigation. Key focus was placed on educating registered nurses about "quality measurement, informing the public and purchasing/regulating constituencies about safe, quality healthcare, and investigating research methods and data sources to empirically evaluate the safety and quality of patient care" (ANA, 1999, p. 1).

Of primary importance was the creation of a National Database of Nursing-Sensitive Quality Indicators (NDNQI). ANA defined nursing-sensitive quality indicators as "those indicators that capture care or its outcomes most affected by nursing care" (ANA, 1999, p. 4). In 1998, ANA funded the development of the national database for the nursing-sensitive quality indicators. The database was located at the Midwest Research Institute (MRI) in Kansas City, Missouri. The MRI and the University of Kansas School of Nursing jointly managed the database. The purpose of the NDNQI was to "promote and facilitate the standardization of information submitted by hospitals across the United States on nursing quality and patient outcomes" (ANA, 1999, p. 8). Hospitals have used the results from the database to make internal comparisons of their nursing quality and patient outcomes while also making comparisons of their performance with like organizations. Because healthcare organizations accredited by the Joint Accreditation of Healthcare Organization (JCAHO) are required to meet JCAHO 2002 staffing effectiveness standards, this database serves as an invaluable tool for nurse executives to effectively compare staffing patterns and methods with clinical outcomes (Runy, 2003). Presently, the NDNQI is housed at the University of Kansas School of Nursing with fiscal/legal support from the MRI and a participation of over 347 hospitals in 48 states and the District of Columbia.

Current studies validate the link between nurse staffing and outcomes of patient care. Aiken, Sean, Sloane, Sochalski, and Silber (2002) found links between high patient-to-nurse ratios, increased mortality rates among surgical patients, and the increased likelihood of nurse burnout and dissatisfaction. The study reported that mortality rates among surgical patients increased 7% for every additional patient added to the average nurses' workload. The additional patient assignment contributed to a 23% increase in the odds of nurse burnout. Needleman, Buerhaus, Mattke, Stewart, and Zelevinsky (2002) concluded that a higher proportion of care provided by registered nurses and a greater number of hours of care by nurses per day are associated with positive patient care results. Some of the outcomes found were shorter lengths of stay, fewer urinary tract infections, and fewer cases of upper gastrointestinal bleeding for hospitalized patients.

American Medical Association Response

Another organization to study patient safety was the American Medical Association (AMA). By establishing the National Patient Safety Foundation in 1997, the AMA commissioned the Foundation to conduct a national survey to address patient safety issues in the healthcare

environment (Harris & associates, 1997). The findings from the national telephone survey of 1,513 respondents indicated that "the healthcare environment was perceived by the general public as 'moderately' safe" (Harris & associates, p. 3). The respondents stated that "carelessness or negligence on the part of healthcare professionals was the main cause of errors"; while, "the second most cited reason for medical errors was related to healthcare professionals being overworked, hurried and stressed" (Harris & associates, p. 5). It was noted that 95% of the respondents would report a medical mistake if they encountered one (Harris & associates). Recommendations were proposed for preventing medical mistakes. The major suggestions were to improve oversight of caregivers; ensure appropriate qualification and training of healthcare professionals; provide physician information to consumers; create an independent organization to examine the causes of medical mistakes; and increase the public's awareness of the issues surrounding errors (Harris & associates). Organizations may consider replicating this survey in order to have a greater understanding of their customer needs.

First Institute of Medicine Report and Responses

The most significant study that not only galvanized the healthcare industry but elevated the awareness of the public on patient safety was the Institute of Medicine (IOM) report on medical errors, entitled *To Err Is Human: Building a Safer Health System* released in 1999 (Kohn, Corrigan, & Donaldson, 2000). The findings of the report produced a substantial media, public, congressional, and departmental response regarding concern for patients' health and safety.

According to the IOM report, in-hospital errors account for as many as 44,000 to 98,000 deaths each year in the United States. The IOM provided the following definition: "An error is defined as the failure of a planned action to be completed as intended (i.e., error of execution) or the use of a wrong plan to achieve an aim (i.e., error of planning)" (Kohn et al., 2000, p. 28). The study addressed errors in acute care hospitals but did not include data about care delivered in clinics, homes, rehabilitation centers, psychiatric facilities, or long-term care settings. It reported that in 1 year, more people die from medical errors than from breast cancer, AIDS, or motor vehicle accidents. Errors also caused injuries to patients; adverse events occurred in 3–4% of hospitalized patients, while 1 in 10 resulted in death. Errors occurred in virtually every hospital in the country. According to the study, medical errors were also costly. Total national costs were projected between $17 and $29 billion each year. Medication errors, which were among the most common errors, tacked on an additional $4,700 to the average hospital bill each time they occurred. Most importantly, over half of all errors investigated were preventable. A major finding of the IOM report was that these errors occurred because of system failures rather than people problems; and preventing errors required designing safer systems of care (Kohn et al., 2000).

To help improve systems of care, the IOM report recommended a four-part plan for government and healthcare settings. The plan set forth the following recommendations:

- Establish a national center for patient safety
- Develop reporting systems to identify and learn from errors
- Raise standards for safety through regulatory and market forces
- Create safety systems in healthcare organizations at the care delivery level (Kohn et al., 2000)

This first IOM report prompted considerable debate regarding the accuracy of the actual number of errors. Since the focus of the report was placed on errors occurring in hospitals, little is known regarding the number of errors or frequency of occurrence in home care, ambulatory care, nursing homes, or hospice settings. In addition, the report left the accountability for error management unclear by recommending both internal and external oversight. Porter-O'Grady and Malloch (2003) proposed that managing errors closest to the point of occurrence resulted in performance improvement, especially when a standardized national repository exists. In contrast, the authors indicated that external control reinforced a culture of blame.

On the other hand, the IOM report generated action from both the public and private sector. Within the public sector, President Clinton immediately ordered a government feasibility study. Based on the findings of the study in 2000, the President mandated that the IOM recommendations be implemented. Specifically, a 50% reduction in medical errors was to be achieved within the next 5 years. To further advance these directives, the President mandated that all 6,000 hospitals participating in the Medicare program implement patient-safety initiatives, including medications and safety-oriented approaches (Kimmel & Sensmeier, 2002).

Agency for Healthcare Research and Quality Response

As described in the IOM report, a recommendation was made for the Agency for Healthcare Research and Quality (AHRQ) to create a Center for Patient Safety having accountability to the President and Congress (Kohn et al., 2000). To promote the patient safety agenda, the AHRQ received a $50 million grant to fund error-reduction research. It is interesting to note that the amount allocated by Congress for safety research in 2002 was less than half of 1% of the National Institute of Health budget for important medical research (Leape, Berwick, & Bates, 2002). The first effort of the AHRQ to investigate patient safety from an evidence-based medicine approach was published in a report titled *Making Healthcare Safer: A Critical Analysis of Patient Safety Practices* (Shojania, Duncan, McDonald, & Wachter, 2001). The report was a result of a commissioned group of 40 researchers, including experts in patient safety, evidence-based medicine, and various areas of clinical medicine, nursing, and pharmacy (Shojania, Duncan, McDonald, & Wachter, 2002). The research was conducted from a systemic approach addressing diseases and procedures. Results were reported by opportunities for safety improvement and for research. Evidence-based medical approaches were found to be as vital for advancing the patient safety agenda as were the advances proposed in the nonmedical field, such as bar-coding, simulation, and computerized physician order entry. The report called for greater emphasis on engaging the clinicians in the workplace to decrease risks attributed to care practices (Shojania et al., 2002).

The report received considerable attention. Some opposition surfaced regarding applying the principles of evidence-based medicine to patient safety practices. The method for the prioritizing of action items to improve patient safety were challenged and recommended for future research (Leape et al., 2002). However, there was agreement that the practice of anesthesia was an outstanding example of how a high level of safety could be achieved in healthcare. The success of this achievement was based on a broad range of changes in process, technological advances, training, and teamwork.

The Leapfrog Response

In addition to government agencies, the private sector also responded to the first IOM report. The Business Roundtable (BRT) formed a new program called "The Leapfrog Group," a coalition of Fortune 500 companies and other large private and public healthcare purchasers. Under Leapfrog, employers have agreed to base their purchase of healthcare on principles encouraging more stringent patient safety measures. These measures included computerized physician order entry, evidence-based hospital referral, and intensive care unit staffing by physicians trained in critical care medicine (Birkmeyer, Birkmeyer, Wennberg, & Young, 2000). There has been a positive response from the marketplace. Recently, the Leapfrog Group has been joined by JCAHO, increasing the original membership of 60 purchasers to more than 90 and now representing 25 million beneficiaries (Kimmel & Sensmeier, 2002).

Quality Interagency Coordination Task Force Response

The Quality Interagency Coordination Task Force (QuIC), which received direction from the President, reported more progress on the IOM recommendations. In order to consider all the important implications of medical errors, the QuIC proposed an expansion of the IOM's definition of medical errors. The QuIC defined an error as "the failure of a planned action to be completed as intended or the use of a wrong plan to achieve an aim. Errors can include problems in practice, products, procedures, and systems" (U.S. Department of Health and Human Services [U.S. DHHS], 2003b, p. 3435). The Center for the Medicare and Medicaid Services (CMS), an agency of the Department of Health and Human Services (U.S. DHHS), adopted the revised definition and published the results in the Federal Register (U.S. DHHS, 2003b). This expanded definition allowed for the identification of possible factors leading to errors, such as seclusion, restraints, equipment failures, and blood transfusions.

In the AHRQ evidence report, the term "error" was not included in the definition in order to minimize a negative connotation and because of the difficulties in specifying what constitutes a medical error. Rather, the authors defined a patient safety practice as a "type of process or structure whose application reduces the probability of adverse events resulting from exposure to the healthcare system across a range of diseases and procedures" (Shojania et al., 2002, p. 508).

For years, patient errors have primarily been addressed through malpractice litigation. Prior to the publication of the 1999 IOM report, the emphasis on having patients actively involved in error prevention was minimal. Organizations lack the processes to make the transition from a risk management environment of identification and discipline of individuals to a cooperative, system-based pursuit of improvement (Kohn et al., 2000). Because risk management is typically framed as a professional approach, organized medicine on one side, and the trial bar on the other, with patients the object of discussion and seldom involved in the process, the method for consistent patient involvement has not been designed (Sage, 2002). Forging stronger links with customer satisfaction and the clinical safety focus of the health system could be a start. In the review of several studies, Sage proposed that reducing lawsuits requires preventing errors and not just placating patients. Approaching legal aspects from a customer-focused perspective would not only control legal costs, but would also aid in conducting more reliable statistical analysis of medical practices in order to seek opportunities for improvement. With greater emphasis on advanced technology, "acting on the signals offered by patient complaints, therefore, can reduce both physician and interpersonal harm to patients" (Sage, 2002, p. 3004).

As was previously found in the AMA study, consumers offered several recommendations for preventing medical errors. Healthcare organizations are challenged to create innovative systems for engaging patients and their families in efforts to take action on steps following errors or on reporting near misses. Most recently, hospitals have endorsed polices and procedures to disclose such situations when they occur. However, a considerable amount of focus needs to be placed on moving from an adversarial, legal approach to a more inclusive, collaborative approach with the patient and family. Tools are available to assist healthcare organizations to assess their performance in this area. One such instrument, The

Patient Safety Organizational Assessment Tool, developed by Wilson, provides a systematic method to evaluate current processes and systems and measure ongoing progress in establishing a safer environment (Sarudi, 2001).

Second IOM Report and Responses

In March 2001, the Committee on the Quality of Care in America produced the second IOM report, *Crossing the Quality Chasm: A New Health System for the 21st Century*. The focus of this IOM publication was a call for action to improve the nation's healthcare delivery system. With the aging of America, greater demand for services, and advanced technology and drugs, healthcare costs were increasing as resources were being overutilized. This report, like the first IOM report, repeatedly addressed patient safety problems with a major emphasis on redesign of the system. Six specification areas were recommended as significant when revamping the healthcare delivery model. These specification areas are: "patient safety, patient-centered care, efficiency, effectiveness, timeliness, and equity" (Committee on Quality of Healthcare in America, 2001, p. 6).

Medicare Response

Again, the public sector responded when the CMS promulgated a new rule instructing hospitals to develop and implement quality assessment and improvement programs (QAIP) to identify patient safety issues and to decrease medical errors. The rule, Medicare Conditions of Participation (CoP), for hospitals went into effect on January of 2003 (U.S. DHHS, 2003a). U.S. DHHS Secretary Tommy G. Thompson said:

This rule will encourage a greater emphasis on patient safety in hospitals. This serves as another step toward bringing improved patient safety, accountability and quality to the forefront of medical practice. Ultimately, we hope to create an environment where hospitals and other providers compete based on the quality of care that they provide to their patients. (U.S. DHHS, 2003a, p. 1)

Specifically, the QAIP of hospitals must reflect the complexity of the organization and services, be organizational-wide, focus on maximizing quality of care outcomes, and include preventative measures to promote patient safety. The expectation of the mandate is to ensure uniformity in quality standards for all Medicare-participating hospitals.

National Nursing Home Response

In November of 2002, CMS released nationwide data on quality measures of each nursing home in the United States. This national Nursing Home Quality Initiative (NHQI) was introduced to assure higher quality of care provided to Medicare and Medicaid beneficiaries. In addition to the previous reporting requirements, CMS contracted with the National Quality Forum (NQF) to develop 10 quality measures for consumers to compare the quality of nursing homes (NDHCRI, 2002). It is interesting to note that many of these indicators are descriptive of the nursing-sensitive indicators developed by the ANA. A comparable initiative requiring home health agencies to measure patient safety outcomes is expected to be announced by CMS in 2003 (U.S. DHHS, 2003a).

Joint Efforts

The demand for improvement in patient safety has been validated by the public, private, and regulatory sectors. Responding to the challenge offered by IOM, groups such as JCAHO, Leapfrog Group, AHRQ, and the Institute for Safe Medication Practice (ISMP) have all taken action to elevate the importance of patient safety and in some instances have points of intersection from their various recommendations. One such agreement was the need for greater education and training as it related to look alike/sound alike drugs. All addressed the big challenge of transforming the internal environment into a culture that embraced safety and delivered high reliability services. Additionally, transforming the external environment into a collective model of accountability was proposed to be equally challenging. With the recent alliance between JCAHO and the Leapfrog Group, healthcare leaders are faced with having to meet the new patient safety standards set by regulatory agencies and the marketplace.

JCAHO Response

Over the past years, JCAHO has answered the call by the IOM for greater accountability. One of the actions taken was to redesign the accreditation process. The direction of the revised process has been to concentrate on systemic recommendations and promote a nonprescriptive approach with the exception of sentinel review and reporting. JCAHO defined sentinel events as "unexpected occurrences involving death or serious physical or psychological injury, or risk thereof, which signal the need for immediate investigation or response" (Levy, 2001, p. 10). In 2001, JCAHO put into effect new standards requiring organizations to create a culture of safety; to implement a safety program with a specific visible administrative leader assigned the accountability for patient safety; and to disclose to patients the outcome of their care. Disclosure followed an earlier standard, when hospitals were required to report any incident of patient harm or death related to medical error, and to conduct an intensive review of the case. The methodology for analyzing these sentinel events was called a "root cause analysis" (RCA) and was grounded in industrial safety methodology (Kirkpatrick, 2003). The purpose of an RCA review was for hospitals to develop an action plan to ensure that the factors leading up to the sentinel event were resolved. Additionally, the JCAHO published the *Sentinel Event Alert*, which described actual cases and was intended to educate hospitals regarding errors that were occurring. The publication was also intended to stimulate a proactive stance so that organizations would examine their work processes and make the necessary changes. Levy (2001) indicated that perhaps the most controversial aspect of the redesigned approach by JCAHO is the requirement for healthcare givers to inform patients and their families when results of a procedure or action is not what was expected.

Based on a rigorous review of the reported sentinel events, the JCAHO in 2002 approved its first set of six National Patient Safety Goals (JCAHO, 2003b). These six goals with measurable objectives were intended to standardize the risk-reduction tactics used by healthcare organizations. Kirkpatrick (2003) indicated that by having organizations approach patient safety in a uniform way, JCAHO would be able to measure the effectiveness of setting key strategies. All hospitals will be required to comply with the six patient safety goals in future JCAHO surveys starting in 2003. "Failure to implement one or more of the recommendations (or acceptable alternatives) will result in a single special Type I recommendation" (JCAHO, 2003b, p. 2). The six key issues determined for compliance include accurate patient identification, effective communication, safe use of high-alert medication, elimination of wrong-site surgery, safe use of infusion pumps, and safe use of clinical alarms (Kirkpatrick, 2003). Each of the six standards and their implications for nursing practice will be described below.

Nursing's Role

Nursing practice will influence all of the new standards on patient safety and outcomes of care. Nurses, by the very nature of their professional knowledge and skill, are critical resources to the organization. Nurses need to be given a strong and rightful place in decision making about issues relating to clinical practice. Nurses will affect patient safety in all healthcare settings. While the focus of the IOM study has been on acute care settings, nurses serve as the patient and family advocate no matter what setting of healthcare is required. With the advent of more procedures taking place in ambulatory settings, the potential for more injury to patients exists. Today, 65% of all surgical procedures do not involve a hospital stay (Lapetina & Armstrong, 2002). The intent of developing the nursing-sensitive indicators was to provide nurse executives with more definitive data to demonstrate the clear linkages between nursing interventions, staffing levels, and positive patient outcomes (ANA, 1999). The importance of advancing the nursing-sensitive quality measures for use in publicly available report cards cannot be over emphasized. As previously noted, the Nursing Home Quality Initiative mandated by the CMS

is an example of the power of ANA's Nursing Safety & Quality Initiative of 1994.

Nurses will provide considerable leadership to the implementation of the JCAHO patient safety goals. The first standard, accuracy of patient identification, has two components. First, organizations are required to establish two patient identifiers, other than the patient room, such as patient's name, date of birth, or hospital identification number. The other component of this goal is to have a rigorous verification process followed on any surgical or invasive procedure to ensure correct patient, procedure, and site. Involving key stakeholders, such as nurses, in formalizing the two patient identifiers provides the opportunity for the organization to clearly establish indicators and measurement criteria at the same time. Standardizing the current (manual) process would increase understanding and support so hospitals could prepare for future bar coding technology.

Kirkpatrick (2003) stressed the fact that nurses needed to be more assertive when carrying out the second component of the identification requirement. Nurses need a routine method to ensure that the appropriate patient, the appropriate procedure, and the appropriate procedure site are verified in a consistent manner prior to the start of any surgical or other invasive procedure.

Nursing's role is critical in meeting the intent of the effective communication standard on orders and symbols, the second safety standard. This standard requires the accurate transcription of verbal and telephone orders, and the appropriate interpretation of difficult or unclear written orders. The relationship between the nurse and the provider giving the order contributes considerably to the success of this standard, since nurses are required to read back any verbal or telephone orders given. Kirkpatrick (2003) reported that hospitals would be required to formalize an approved abbreviation, acronym, and symbol listing, as well as to formalize a list of abbreviations that are not permitted, with clearly defined consequences for those not complying. The most controversial aspect of this standard is to define the consequences of noncompliance when physicians, nurses, and pharmacists are deviating from the organization policies and procedures.

Well-defined protocols developed by physicians, pharmacists, and nurses ensure safer use of high-alert medications. High-alert medications are those drugs which when misused have a "high risk of injury or death" (Cohen & Mandrack, 2002, p. 371). Because of their greater risk, special considerations are required when administering these drugs. Cohen and Mandrack (2002) reported that these high-alert medications are packaged differently with visible warnings, stored differently so that they are separated from other medications, prescribed differently with standardized orders, and administered by requiring independent double-checking. Standardized protocols promote consistency of dosing calculation and methods of administration. Additionally, limiting the number of drug concentrations places additional control over medication errors. By standardizing the concentration of a medication, the dosing calculations are the same from one case to the other. Initiating protocols would not only provide direction for nurses in the administration of drugs, but also contribute to the development of educational tools and methods to verify consistency for patient and family education.

Previous reference was made to ensuring the correct identifier for the right patient. The major focus of the fourth safety standard is to eliminate wrong-site, wrong-patient, and wrong-procedure surgery. While the patient is very much involved with the process of site marking, another aspect of the standard is the verification process in the operating room. There are many similarities between the airline industry and surgical safety procedures. Airline safety processes include standardized procedures, checklists, explicit cross-checking, redundant checks, and a culture of equal accountability. Based on hundreds of little changes in work procedures, training, and system processes, aviation safety has established a strong safety culture (Leape et al., 2002).

Improving the safe use of infusion pumps is the fifth standard. The goal, specifically, requires infusion pumps to have a built-in protection from free-flowing fluids. Organizations can achieve this safety goal by involving nurses in the selection of products, setting minimum specifications for product evaluation, and defining the competencies required for nursing proficiency. Nursing education can schedule frequent educational skill development events to increase awareness of the safety features and ensure nursing proficiency through demonstration efforts. In addition, meeting this standard calls for a rigorous organizational maintenance program to serve as a check-and-balance system.

The sixth safety standard was designed to improve the effectiveness of clinical alarm systems. With the advanced technology, numerous alarms are available in patient care settings such as ventilator alarms, bed alarms, and pagers, to name a few. A major deterrent in meeting this standard is the potential to mute an alarm to create a quiet environment for the patient. To meet the intent of the sixth safety standard, organizations would need to validate that an active preventive maintenance program exists, and that the alarms are activated appropriately. Reviewers would call for evidence of compliance such as logs, records, usage, and training of healthcare workers. As was detailed in the fifth standard, organizations have the prerogative to define minimum specifications and educational requirements for their users. Nursing has an opportunity to work closely with other departments within the healthcare setting as purchasing decisions are made and maintenance programs are established.

Close attention to meeting the patient safety goals will be ongoing. JCAHO has announced its 2004 national patient goals. The new release reported that all of the 2003 goals will be continued with the addition of a new goal that will concentrate on reducing the risk of acquired infections in healthcare settings (JCAHO, 2003a).

Conclusion

There has been a convergence of thought among professional, private, and governmental healthcare decision makers that agree with the basic premise: patient safety will be a top priority agenda item for healthcare providers now and in the future. Various constituencies have contributed to the definition and detailed examination of the issues surrounding patient safety. In exploring the unique contributions of the major professional, public, and private groups, there are similarities and differences in the recommendations about the pathways to patient safety. All groups have validated the demand for improvement in patient safety. One agreement stated was the need for greater education and training as it related to look alike/sound alike drugs. Many of the constituencies addressed the big challenge of transforming the internal environment into a culture that embraced safety and delivered highly reliable services. Additionally, transforming the external environment into a collective model of accountability was proposed to be equally challenging.

The potential for these groups to interact with one another in order to create an even stronger infrastructure for patient safety is enormous. In fact, organizations that exemplify best practices in patient safety will be rewarded by the purchasers of health care and by accreditation agencies. Forging stronger links with the consumer is an untapped opportunity. Furthermore, linking consumer needs with the clinical safety focus of the healthcare system has the potential to decrease the risk of malpractice and enhance relationships. Nursing has a major role in providing leadership in the creation of solutions to advance patient safety standards.

Discussion Questions

1. Go the Web sites of the major organizations discussed in this chapter and update the status of each. What is new? What is the evidence, if any, to demonstrate that any of the initiatives are working?
2. How has your current workplace responded to the patient safety issues discussed in this chapter?
3. What role can you play currently and in the future to improve patient safety as an individual practitioner and with the multidisciplinary team?

References

Aiken, L. H., Clarke, S. P., Sloane, D. M., Sochalski, J., & Silber, J. H. (2002). Hospital nurse staffing and patient mortality, nurse burnout, and job dissatisfaction. *The Journal of the American Medical Association, 288*(16), 1987–1993.

American Nurses Association [ANA]. (1999). Nursing facts: Nursing-sensitive quality indicators for acute care settings and ANA's safety & quality initiative. Retrieved June 2, 2003, from www.nursingworld.org/readroom/fssafe99.htm

Birkmeyer, J. D., Birkmeyer, C. M., Wennberg, D. E., & Young, M. P. (2000). *Leapfrog safety standards: Potential benefits of universal adoption* [Monograph]. Washington, DC: The Leapfrog Group.

Cohen, H., & Mandrack, M. M. (2002). Application of the 80/20 rule in safeguarding the high-alert medications. *Critical Care Nursing Clinics of North America, 14*, 369–374.

Committee on Quality of Healthcare in America, Institute of Medicine. (2001). *Crossing the quality chasm: A new health system for the 21st century.* Washington, DC: National Academy Press.

Harris, L., & associates. (1997). *Public opinion of patient safety issues: Research findings.* Commissioned for the National Patient Safety Foundation at the American Medical Association, September, 1997. Retrieved June 23, 2003, from www.npsf.org/download/1997survey.pdf

Joint Commission on Accreditation of Healthcare Organizations. (2003a). *Joint Commission announces 2004 national patient safety goals.* Retrieved July 25, 2003, from www.jcaho.org/news+room/news+release+archieves/nsg04.htm

Joint Commission on Accreditation of Healthcare Organizations. (2003b). *Facts about patient safety.* Retrieved on June 6, 2003, from http://www.jcaho.org/accredited+organizations/patient+safety/facts+about+patient+safety.htm

Kimmel, K. D., & Sensmeier, J. (2002). A technological approach to enhancing patient safety [Monograph]. *Healthcare Information and Management Systems Society, 1*–7.

Kirkpatrick, C. (2003). Safety first: The JCAHO introduces new patient safety goals. *NurseWeek, 4*(2), 19–20.

Kohn, L. T., Corrigan, J. M., & Donaldson, M. (Eds.). (2000). *To err is human: Building a safer health system.* Washington, DC: National Academy Press.

Lapetina, E. M., & Armstrong, E. M. (2002). Preventing errors in the outpatient setting: A tale of three states. *Health Affairs, 21*(4), 26–39.

Leape, L. L., Berwick, D. M., & Bates, D. W. (2002). What practices will most improve safety? Evidence-based medicine meets patient safety. *Journal of the American Medical Association, 288*(4), 501–507.

Levy, D. (2001). New standards enable nurses to shape patient policy. *NurseWeek, 2*(9), 10–11.

Needleman, J., Buerhaus, P., Mattke, S., Stewart, M., & Zelevinsky, K. (2002). Nurse-staffing levels and the quality of care in hospitals. *The New England Journal of Medicine, 346*(22), 1715–1722.

Porter-O'Grady, T., & Malloch, K. (2003). *Quantum Leadership: A textbook of new leadership.* Sudbury, MA: Jones and Bartlett.

North Dakota Healthcare Review, Inc. (2002). Quality counts: Nursing Home Quality Initiative. (2002). *Quality initiative to be conducted in nursing homes* (ND-6SOW-O2-QP-32) [Brochure]. Author.

Runy, L. A. (2003). Staffing effectiveness: A toolkit for JCAHO new standards. *Hospitals & Health Networks, 77*(3), 57–63.

Sage, W. M. (2002). Putting the patient in patient safety: Linking patient complaints and malpractice risk. *Journal of American Medical Association, 287*(22), 3003–3005.

Sarudi, R. (2001). Keeping patients safe. *Hospitals & Health Networks, 75*(4), 42–46.

Shojania, K. G., Duncan, B. W., McDonald, K. M., & Wachter, R. M. (Eds.). (2001). *Making health care safer: A critical analysis of patient safety practices.* Evidence Report/Technology Assessment, No. 43. Prepared by the University of California at San Francisco-Stanford, Evidence-based practice center under contract No. 290-97-0013 for Agency for Healthcare Research and Quality. Retrieved June 9, 2003, from www.ahcpr.gov/clinic/ptsafety/

Shojania, K. G., Duncan., B. W., McDonald, K. M., & Wachter, R. M. (Eds.). (2002). Safe but sound: Patient safety meets evidence-based medicine.

Journal of the American Medical Association, 288(4), 501–512.

U.S. Department of Health and Human Services. (2003a). *CMS issues final quality assessment and performance improvement conditions of participation for hospitals.* Washington, DC: Center for Medicare and Medicaid Services.

U.S. Department of Health and Human Services. (2003b). *Medicare and Medicaid conditions of participation: Quality assessment and performance improvement.* (U.S. DHHS Publication No. 42 CFR Part 482). Washington, DC: U.S. Government Printing Office.

Chapter 17

Information Technology for Advanced Nursing Practice

Michelle Godin

CHAPTER OBJECTIVES

1. Understand basic computer concepts and components.
2. Appreciate security issues that have evolved as a result of the introduction of technology in health care.
3. Discuss the implications of the Health Insurance Portability and Accountability Act for advanced practice nursing.
4. Discuss the use of information systems for the storage and retrieval of data for individual clients and for populations.
5. Discuss the use of technology for initiating a line of inquiry into a comprehensive database in order to improve patient outcomes.

Introduction

The use of information technology in today's health care is inescapable. More and more healthcare organizations and provider practices are computerizing patient data for easy retrieval and data analysis. It is essential for advanced nurse practitioners to be knowledgeable about information technology and how it can best be utilized in their daily practice not only for the care of the individual patient but also to evaluate quality, safety, and costs of care.

This chapter will start with the basic computer concepts of the hardware and software components. The chapter will then discuss the concept of information privacy and confidentiality. With the advent of technology, controls over the access to patient data became an all-important national concern. The enactment of the Health Insurance Portability and Accountability Act (HIPAA) created rules to govern the access and release of health information. The chapter will end with information on specific categories of computer applications with which nurses in advanced practice should be the most familiar.

Basic Computer Concepts

There are two major components with any computer system: the hardware and the software. The hardware component is defined as the physical component of the system. The software component is defined as the elements responsible for the operation of the system and the performance of specific tasks.

Hardware

The hardware of the computer systems is made up of four separate elements. The first element is the central processing unit (CPU). The CPU decides where and when to send information. It functions with the internal clock, which sets the speed. The clock speed of a computer will be identified by its megahertz. Many of the computers today have speeds in gigahertz (1 gigahertz is equal to 1,000 megahertz). The speed to process information is identified by bytes, but you will probably see information listed as KB, or kilobytes, which is 1,000 bytes.

The CPU is where the "brains" and the computer memory reside. There are three types of memory: random access memory, read-only memory, and cache. Random access memory (RAM) is the primary working memory of the computer. Think of it as a scratch pad to do the current work. The data is temporarily stored in this area and is deleted from the system when the computer is shut off. The read-only memory (ROM) is the section where there is permanent storage of information. This section is where the actual programs and instructions for the computer are stored. Cache is a special memory that allows for rapid access to information based on what information is used repeatedly.

Input devices are the second element of the hardware components. The computer system needs a means to receive the data. There are a variety of devices currently available: keyboards, light pens, mice, touch screens, bar code readers, microphones, scanners, cameras, and biometrics scans (retinal or fingerprint). The variety of devices allows for the input of information to be performed under different circumstances. A light pen, touch screen, and bar code reader have an advantage over a keyboard at a patient's bedside, while a mouse or keyboard work better at the nursing station when one is putting in physician orders. When deciding on the type of input device, it is important to assess not only the type of data being entered but the environment in which the entry is occurring.

The third element of the hardware component is the output. The reason for entering data into a computer system is the ability to store, analyze, and retrieve it. The main output device is the screen display. The screens have advanced greatly over time. Depending upon the data to be displayed, the screen size can be from a few inches for handheld devices such as personal digital assistants (PDAs), to 20 inches for desktop monitors that display patient tracking information. The decision on the type of display is usually dependent upon the type of data being displayed. For instance, clinical documentation with large volumes of data are difficult to display on small handheld screens but can be viewed with greater ease on larger desktop monitors. Some applications will make recommendations on screen size to maximize the functionality of the application.

Printers, which display the collected data in a printed form, are also considered output devices. Most organizations today use either laser or inkjet printers and many of them print in both black and white or color. The advent of the multifunctional device has also brought a new output device into the healthcare setting. These devices allow for not only the printing of information but the copying, scanning, or faxing of the information as well. The decision on which type of printer to select is usually based on the primary output requirements. The use of color printing can be based on financial constraints since the current cost of color toner for the printer is significantly higher than the black toner.

The last element of the hardware is the storage devices. Disks, tapes, flash or jump drives, CDs, and DVDs are all different types of storage devices. These devices can serve as both input and output devices. The purpose is to retain information in a storage space separate from the main computer memory. This allows for portability and backup capability of the data.

Software

There are two categories of software utilized by computer systems. The first category is the operating system. This category of software is responsible for the tasks that make the computer work, such as what keys were struck and in what order, sending messages to printers, and identifying errors and problems. DOS, GUI, UNIX, and LINUX are some of the terms referring to this category. The larger category of software is the applications. These are the individual programs developed to perform specific functions. Most computers will have as basic features a word processing product (for typing documents and memos) and a spreadsheet product (for calculating numbers and analyzing data). Depending

upon the job requirements of the user, a computer may also have a presentation product (used to create slides and posters) and a database management product (for categorizing and analyzing large amounts of data).

Security Considerations

When using any type of computer in a healthcare setting, there are two levels of security to protect patient information. The first type is the physical security of the device(s) which possess a dilemma. Workstations should be positioned in such a way to protect them from unauthorized access while at the same time be visible. However this must be balanced with safety concerns to avoid interruptions of staff when using the computer and should not be in direct view of unauthorized users. A computer in a staff lounge or locker room might be great for staff to access their hospital e-mail, but it should not have software that would allow access to patient information. Mobile devices should be stored in locked areas when not in use to prevent theft as well as unauthorized access.

The second type of security is password security. In order to protect access to data and information, multiple layers of passwords are essential. The more sensitive the data is, the more layers that should be required to access the data. Application passwords grant a user access to a specific application. An example would be that advanced nurse practitioners need access to a program to document patient care but the housekeeping staff would have no reason for access to that application. The next layer of the password security is location. In this layer, the user's access to the application is limited by the department or location of the device. As with the previous example, while all nurses have access to document, only those nurses who work on the psychiatric unit will be able to access and document those particular patient records. The last layer of security is based on the job requirement. Access to an application is given but only to the specific sections of the application that are necessary for the user to perform his or her job. An example of this is a nurse's aide, whose job requires him or her to document vital signs. He or she is given access to document that particular element of the patients' care, but will not be able to access any other part of the patient record.

The use of all the layers of security allows an organization to maintain the integrity of the patient information and protect the privacy and confidentiality of the data. The main focus of the security is to give access to individuals based on what their job requirements are and only what they need to perform that job efficiently and effectively.

Information Privacy and Confidentiality Issues

The Health Insurance Portability and Accountability Act (HIPAA) was enacted by the U.S. Congress in 1996. It is comprised of two titles or sections. Title I addresses the issue of healthcare access, portability, and renewability.

The focus of this section is on the rules governing an individual's ability to obtain healthcare coverage. Table 17–1 outlines the details.

Title II addresses preventing healthcare fraud and abuse. The second title is of particular importance to healthcare organizations and their employees, including the advanced nurse practitioner. It is broken down into five sections: privacy rule, transactions and code set rule, security rule, unique identifiers rule, and the enforcement rule. The privacy rule became effective on April 14, 2003 and established the regulations for the use and disclosure of protected health information (PHI). PHI is any information about health status, provision of health care, or payment for health care that can be linked to an individual. It requires reasonable effort to disclose only the minimum amount of information and the use of reasonable steps to ensure the confidentiality of communication with others. This rule also requires organizations to appoint a privacy officer and a person responsible for receiving complaints and to train all members of the workforce in the proper care of PHI.

The transactions and code set rule became effective on October 6, 2004, and required that all medical providers who file claims electronically would have to file the claims using HIPAA standard codes in order to be paid. These codes

---

Table 17–1 HIPAA TITLE I HIGHLIGHTS

- Regulates the availability and breadth of group and individual health insurance plans.
- Prohibits any group health plan from creating eligibility rules or assess premiums for individuals in the plan based on health status, medical history, genetic information, or disability.
- Limits restrictions that a group health plan can place on benefits for preexisting conditions.
- Forbids individual health plans from denying coverage or imposing preexisting condition exclusions on individuals who have at least 18 months of creditable group coverage under any group, state, or federal health plans at the time they seek individual insurance.

Table 17-2 HIPAA SECURITY RULE CONTROL SAFEGUARDS

Administrative Safeguards	Physical Safeguards	Technical Safeguards
• Designation of a privacy officer. • Indication of classes of employees who have access to PHI (must be restricted on a need to know basis). • Demonstrate ongoing training and education. • Document the process involved in auditing records. Audits should be both on a routine basis and when an event occurs.	• Oversight of addition and removal of hardware and software from the network. • Equipment with PHI should be monitored. • Hardware and software must be limited to properly authorized individuals. • Workstations should be removed from high traffic areas and monitor screens should not be in direct view of the public.	• Utilization of encryption software must be used to protect information. • Ensuring that data is not altered in an unauthorized manner.

were developed to force a standardization of the data stream from each organization to the insurance companies.

The security rule was implemented on April 21, 2005 and complements the privacy rule by outlining three types of security safeguards necessary for compliance. The administrative safeguards are policies and procedures designed to show how an organization will comply with the act. Physical safeguards work to control physical access to protect against the inappropriate access to protected data. Technical safeguards allow for the control of access to computer systems and protect communications containing PHI transmitted electronically. See Table 17–2 for some of the specific controls that an organization must have in place to comply with this specific rule.

The enforcement rule went into effect on March 16, 2006, and set a monetary penalty for violating the HIPAA rules. The last rule is the estab-

lishment of unique identifiers. This rule went into effect on May 23, 2007, and established a unique national provider identifier (NPI) for every healthcare provider who files healthcare forms. Every healthcare organization and provider must possess an NPI number when submitting claims.

The enactment of HIPAA has forced each and every healthcare entity to review and reassess their controls over who has access to information. The auditing of patient records is not limited to who accessed a specific patient record. It goes to the level of whether or not an individual had reason to access the individual record and the specific information.

Hospital Information Systems

Computers have been around since the 1930s, but it was not until the 1950s that hospitals began to utilize the technology. Not surprising, financial and statistical calculations were the first applications to be utilized within the hospital setting. Patient charges, payroll, inventory control, and patient statistics (birth and death rates) were more easily and rapidly calculated utilizing the computer than by manual methods. The first hospital computer was developed in the late 1960s to address clinical applications and was very unsuccessful. Hardware and software were expensive and inflexible, and the input devices were expensive and unreliable.

A hospital information system (HIS) refers to computer systems that support patient care. There are two categories of systems within a hospital setting: clinical systems that allow the organization to provide, monitor, and evaluate patient care; and administrative systems that allow the organization to monitor the quality of care as well as the revenue and expenditures related to the delivery of care.

Clinical Systems

Nursing Information Systems

A nursing information system (NIS) is one of the major types of clinical systems. This type of system allows for the assessment of the patient and the documentation of the care and teaching delivered. There are two approaches to documentation. The first is menu-driven screens that present content in prearranged categories that allow the practitioner to select the most applicable items. The categories are designed around the nursing process from admission through to discharge based on the nursing diagnosis. Most are modeled after the paper forms currently in use. The second approach is to utilize care protocols. In this type of documentation, a specific protocol is selected based on the admission diagnosis. The protocol lists the elements of care to be initiated and monitored during each patient day. The documentation is related to the ability of the patient to achieve the established daily protocol goals. There are many advantages to an NIS, but there are also some disadvantages, as can be seen in Table 17–3.

Clinical Information Processing Systems

Another major type of clinical system is the clinical information processing system. These systems are responsible for recording and storing patient data from a variety of clinical settings. Many departments have specific systems that facilitate their own unique activities (medical records, operating room, emergency department, home care, etc.). Other systems cross departments to assist in the delivery of patient care. The specific systems of order entry, patient monitoring, radiology, laboratory, and pharmacy systems will be reviewed in more detail.

The beginning point of these systems is the order entry process. Orders are entered into a computer system, which processes the orders and sends information to specific departments requesting services. The receiving departments, through requisitions, process the order and perform a test or deliver a service.

ORDER ENTRY

There are two methods of order entry. One is simple data entry by selecting items from menus. The other method is to utilize sets of orders based on clinical guidelines or best practices. This type of order entry can be quicker

Table 17–3 ADVANTAGES AND DISADVANTAGES IN UTILIZING AN NIS

Advantages

- Increased observation due to forced recall.
- Increased accuracy and reliability of observations. If done in real time, no need to write on paper and then transcribe. No time to forget.
- Legibility with less time required to read and interpret accurately.
- Decrease time in writing notes.
- Available for statistical analysis. Elements already coded and can be selected.
- Teaching tool to guide observations. Can develop specific elements to help the staff with what they need to look for.
- Errors and omissions are decreased or eliminated with protocol followed.

Disadvantages

- Charting may be longer due to need for review of content prior to selection.
- Wording may not be common to user's language. Standard dictionaries are not readily available.
- Preestablished content and need to make sure protocols are individualized for patients with comorbidities.

depending upon the amount of flexibility in completing individual orders. Many orders sets will have multiple orders covering items such as antibiotics or pain medication to allow the practitioner to individualize the type and dose of drug most appropriate for a specific patient. The order sets can also include directions for other departments such as holding meals when a specific radiology exam is ordered and having pharmacy send the preparations for tests.

An advantage of an order entry system is the rapid initiation of orders. Orders are entered and transmitted, and the receiving department will be notified of the request for services in real time. Additionally, as the orders are entered, the system can prompt for prerequisite pieces of information that must be entered before an order can be initiated. An example would be the requirement for the medical reason for an exam

on a radiology order before the order is sent to radiology to be performed, therefore documenting the medical necessity. This assures that important pieces of data regarding the patient are recorded and communicated.

As a response to the patient safety issues discussed in the two previous chapters, the trend in today's healthcare environment is for physician order entry. This type of order processing requires the physician to input the orders directly into the computer system, thereby eliminating any transcription errors. With this method there is an additional advantage in the ability of an order entry system to provide the physician with alerts regarding such things as allergies and medication interactions. These alerts warn a physician of a potential problem and offer options for the physician to change the orders before they are initiated.

PATIENT MONITORING

Patient monitoring systems include all types of devices that automatically collect data regarding the patient condition. Cardiac monitors, IV pumps, pulse oximeters, and blood pressure cuffs are some examples of these devices. The advantage of this type of system is the ability to quickly detect a deviation in a patient's condition and alert the appropriate personnel, freeing up clinicians from watching the monitors and focusing on the patient.

RADIOLOGY

A radiology imaging system allows for the processing of an exam from the scheduling of exams to the storage of images. Most systems today provide for the images using digital technology rather than film. Providers can be sitting at any desktop anywhere and view the images on the monitor. This allows for rapid turnaround in the treatment of injuries especially during the evening and night hours. On-call physicians can view images from their homes to immediately begin initiating treatment plans.

LABORATORY

A laboratory information system allows for the processing of lab specimens. These systems receive the request from the order entry system and provide the results to the clinicians. Many of these systems report the results directly into an HIS system. Within the HIS system, a patient's data can be readily viewed and trended over time and can be viewed from any computer. Inherent in the system is avoidance of duplication of tests within predetermined time frames and alerts for results outside established parameters (both high and low). These alerts can be tied directly to many communication

tools such as PDAs to immediately alert clinicians of potential problems and allow for rapid treatment.

PHARMACY

The ability to track the ordering, dispensing and administration of drugs is at the heart of a pharmacy information system. Beginning with the ordering of the pharmaceuticals, the pharmacy systems have been extremely beneficial to assist in the delivery of quality care. The primary advantage of these systems is the prevention of medication errors. Once orders are entered into the system, the orders are reviewed and verified by pharmacists. The orders are checked against the patient's allergy profile, a drug interaction profile, and available laboratory results to assure that any foreseeable problems from the drugs will be avoided. Medication dispensing devices both within the pharmacy and on the nursing units creates a system where the proper drug is selected. In the pharmacy, the robotic system selects the drug based on the order and delivers it to the nursing unit. On the nursing unit, the nurse selects the drug from the dispensing device by selecting the correct patient and drug. The device then only opens a drawer where the drug is contained. This allows for accurate record keeping of administration of medications and can keep the pharmacy aware of drug levels in the devices.

Administrative Systems

Administrative systems assist the organization in supporting the patient care process and can be used to monitor patient outcomes to improve quality and safety. Table 17–4 lists a variety of systems that are considered administrative systems.

A specific type of administrative system used in most healthcare organizations is a staffing and scheduling system. This system allows for the efficient and effective scheduling of both patients and staff. Patient scheduling systems allow the organization to schedule appointments for services that maximize the equipment and the staff in the best possible manner. Staff scheduling systems perform a similar function. Staff scheduling systems have two components, a scheduling component and a staffing component. The scheduling component develops a plan for when the staff will be working. Most schedules are developed 4–6 weeks in advance, balancing employee days on and off with requests for vacation and holiday. The staffing component uses a patient volume indicator (visits, patient days, acuity, or hours per patient

day) to determine what the required staff needs for a department.

Decision support systems are specialized administrative systems that bring together all the data that has been collected in the clinical systems as well as the administrative systems. The data can then be used by administrators or clinicians to help in the decision-making process by identifying trends, developing models for future endeavors, and demonstrating the financial position of projects.

The ability to utilize a decision support lies in the ability to query the database effectively. The first step in the query is to get the question right. What is or are the specific data elements that are necessary? The ability to identify the exact elements that are needed is crucial. Time can be wasted running and rerunning database

Table 17–4 CATEGORIES OF ADMINISTRATIVE INFORMATION SYSTEMS AND THEIR USES

System	Uses
Human resources	Track applicants and employee information regarding work status, credentials, and performance evaluation
Payroll	Time and attendance with salary data for proper accounting of pay
Risk management	Occurrence and incident tracking for a variety of issues involving patients and employees
Quality management	Review of patient outcome data to help identify trends and make performance improvements
Financial systems	Includes accounting and contract management for reimbursement
Material management	Manages the charging and inventory of supplies for the organization

queries if the elements are not correct. Another question to be asked is in which database are the elements located? If the elements are not in the same database, additional querying skills might be required to achieve the right elements.

Educational Applications

There is an additional computer application that can be useful for any professional—applications developed specifically for educational functions. The use of computers and the Internet have changed the face of education and training forever. Many individuals use the Internet daily, seeking information that now can come from anywhere in the world. The use of educational applications, either on a computer or through the Internet, allows individuals to gain knowledge at their own pace and at a time that is convenient for the individuals.

Educational applications have three main uses: to provide education, to evaluate education, and to determine the competency.

Provide Education

Education applications provide education in a variety of methods, including the following:

- Drills and practice sessions—The computer serves as a supplement for the teacher. The main concepts and new material are presented by the teacher while the computer allows the student to practice.
- Tutorial—This method provides certain original portions of the content. It relies on coaching the student through a situation in sequences in which the student can discover the correct answers.
- Simulation and gaming—This is used when a student has received the basic

information about a topic and then uses the information with the computer to gain a deeper understanding. This method enables the student to explore situations that might be too expensive, dangerous, or time consuming in real life, in which the ramifications of wrong answers can endanger or hurt patients.

Evaluate Education

Using the computer to evaluate education allows the instructor or student to determine whether the content of educational lessons has been learned. The programs are geared to the specific tasks, abilities, and progress of the student. The systems have the ability to provide feedback and reinforcement to the student regarding their performance. For the instructors, reports from the system can be used to assess the progress of the student and where there are potential areas that need improvement.

Determine Competency

The last step in the educational process is to determine competency in the subject matter. The Nursing Competency Licensing Exam (NCLEX) is a perfect example of that process in action. Graduate nurses take a computerized exam in which the computer determines if they have reached a level of knowledge to allow a professional license to be issued.

One of the advantages of an educational computer system is that the applications can be used for both staff and patients. They can be used to orient new staff and train staff and patients on the functionality of new equipment. Since the applications are programmable they can be adapted for any skill level and in any language that is required. This is of great benefit for patients who may have limited medical background and would like to review information privately and at a time of their own convenience.

There is another advantage, which is the effect the applications have on teaching itself. Educational applications have helped shift the emphasis from the teacher and teaching to the learner and learning. Students can be independent and supplement their learning with additional methods that are more suited to their learning style.

Instructors also benefit since they are able to allow the educational applications to provide content better suited to the computer simulation and focus on the students. Some educational applications have also assisted in teaching content where there is no faculty staff that possesses expertise in the content. These same applications can also assist in presenting specific disease situations in which there is a lack of clinical exposure.

Conclusion

This chapter presented a look into the growing and ever-changing world of information technology. Every day one hears about a new device or application that has been developed. Each practitioner must evaluate that information and determine what is usable in their practice to maintain good quality patient outcomes.

Discussion Questions

1. Describe the current hardware components that you currently use in practice. Based on the text in this chapter, what are the strengths and weaknesses of the current system?
2. Describe the current software components that you currently use in practice. Based on the text in this chapter, what are the strengths and weaknesses of the current system?
3. What security issues have you faced in your practice and/or what opportunities for improvement exist in your current system?
4. How will HIPAA affect your role as an advanced practice nurse? How does this differ for each of the various advanced nursing practice roles?
5. Consider a current clinical issue or concern in your practice. What information do you need to better understand the scope of the issue? Is there data stored in the system that would help you understand the issue? If so, how can you retrieve it? If not, what new data would you need to enter the system?

Theoretical Foundation and Research for Advanced Nursing Practice

The chapters included in Part IV are not intended to be a summary of major nursing theories, but rather provide a foundation for understanding, critiquing, evaluating, and using theory for advanced practice. A fundamental question posed by Cody in Chapter 19 is "Why do nurses need theory to guide their practice?" The answer, although seemingly simple, is that theory can provide a framework about what nurses know, do, and think and can guide the advanced practice nurse to know what to ask, what to observe, what to focus on, and what to think about (Chinn & Kramer, 1995).

The terminology and definitions surrounding theory can be confusing for the novice advanced practice nurse to fully understand. Further, scholars of nursing theory do not consistently agree on the definitions, thus there is a lack of clarity in this field of study. As way of introduction to Part IV, the generally agreed-upon definitions of terms to provide the foundation for the chapters in this part are presented here.

What is theory? As with many concepts, there are a variety of definitions of theory, but they have a set of common characteristics. For our purposes, theories are organized systems that describe, explain, predict or prescribe phenomenon. They are composed of concepts (constructs or variables) and propositions (hypotheses) that specify relationship among the concepts. Further theories are substantiated by and derived from established evidence and can be repeatedly confirmed by observation and testing.

There are four types of theory that are derived from the aforementioned definition:

1. Descriptive theories describe concepts of a discipline.
2. Explanatory theories explain how the concepts relate to each other.
3. Predictive theories predict the relationships between the concepts of a phe-

nomenon and predict under what conditions it will occur.

4. Prescriptive theories prescribe interventions and the consequences of interventions.

Additionally there are four levels of theory that can be placed on a continuum from very abstract and broad metatheory, to very specific and narrow, referred to as practice theories.

1. Metatheory is the most abstract and cannot be easily tested. There are no theories labeled as such in nursing. The most commonly cited examples of metatheory are the big bang and evolution.

2. Grand theories define broad perspectives for nursing practice and are less abstract than metatheory. As such they can be tested. Some of the more well-known nursing theories classified as grand theory are those proposed by Nightingale, Parse, Lenninger, Benner, and Henderson. But there are many more, and a search of the Internet can lead to a long list of nursing grand theories.

3. Middle range theories are moderately abstract and have a limited number of concepts. They can be tested directly. Mid-range theories can predict and prescribe nursing interventions and patient outcomes. Many new mid-range nursing theories have been proposed over the last two decades. They are often used for both nursing research and practice. Some examples are uncertainty, comfort, pain, social support, and quality of life. A search of the Internet can reveal many nursing middle range theories useful to the advanced practice nurse.

4. Practice theory traces the outline for practice. Objectives are set and actions are set to meet the objectives.

Another important fundamental understanding of nursing theory is needed before reading the chapters in Part IV. In 1984, Fawcett presented a seminal paper on the metaparadigms of nursing. It is now widely accepted, but not universally, that the metaparadigms for nursing theory are:

- Nursing
- Health
- Person
- Environment

As you read Part IV, these terms will be referred to frequently.

Theory, practice, and research are intertwined. Theory informs practice as practice informs theory. Research is used to test the theory while at the same time can be used to develop and refine theory. As nursing goes forward as a discipline and as consumers and policy makers demand effective, cost-conscious, evidence-based practice, we must understand and use theory and research to guide practice while at the same time analyzing and critiquing our practice to generate new theories that can be tested by research.

The first chapter in this section, Chapter 18, by Kenney, provides a foundation to appreciate the value and relevance of theory from both nursing and other disciplines and applying them to practice. In Chapter 19, Cody presents a brief history of nursing theory development and then provides a provocative distinction between value-based and evidence-based care.

Chapter 20 is a classic and often cited article from Carper. Her distinction of four ways of knowing, empirics, esthetics, ethics, and personal knowing, have and will continue to inform nursing theory, thought, practice, and research for decades. In Chapter 21, White reviews, critiques, and updates Carper's work. Since Carper's work in 1978, nursing has embraced qualitative methodologies including phenomenology as one way to discover new knowledge and extend knowing. In Chapter 22, Tingen compares and contrasts empirics and interpretative paradigms in nursing science. This will provide a basic understanding of the two major research paradigms students will further discuss and use in research courses.

Nursing theory and research are intertwined, therefore this part concludes with an overview of health sciences research in general (Chapter 23) and nursing research specifically (Chapter 24). The AACN recommends separate course work in research and an informal survey of Master of Science in Nursing curricula demonstrates that most often research is done in separate courses in advanced nurse practice programs. Thus it is not the intention of this book to lay forth the research process and methods, but rather to put the need for health research and nursing research into a broader context so the reader can appreciate how research improves practice and informs decision making.

References

Chinn, P. L., & Kramer, M. K. (1995). *Theory and nursing: A systematic approach* (4th ed.). St. Louis, MO: C. V. Mosby.

Fawcett, J. (1984). The metaparadigms of nursing: Present status and future refinements. *Image, 16(3),* 84–87.

Part IV

Theoretical Foundation and Research for Advanced Nursing Practice

CHAPTER 18   Theory-Based Advanced
Nursing Practice

CHAPTER 19   Values-Based Practice
and Evidence-Based Care:
Pursuing Fundamental
Questions in Nursing
Philosophy and Theory

CHAPTER 20   Fundamental Patterns of
Knowing in Nursing

CHAPTER 21   Patterns of Knowing:
Review, Critique, and
Update

CHAPTER 22   Multiple Paradigms of
Nursing Science

CHAPTER 23   Research: How Health
Care Advances

CHAPTER 24   Knowledge Development
in Nursing: Our
Historical Roots and
Future Opportunities

Chapter 18

Theory-Based Advanced Nursing Practice

Janet W. Kenney

CHAPTER OBJECTIVES

1. Describe the value and relevance of theory-based nursing for advanced practice nurses.
2. Discuss issues for applying theories in nursing practice.
3. Discuss the structure of nursing knowledge and the transformative process for theory-based practice.
4. Explain the relationship of theory and critical thinking.
5. Discuss the process for selecting and applying appropriate nursing, family, and other disciplines' models and theories to advanced nursing practice.

Introduction

All professional disciplines are based on their unique knowledge, which is expressed in models and theories that are applied in practice. The focus of nursing knowledge is on humans' health experiences within the context of their environment and the nurse–client relationship. Theory-based nursing practice is the application of various models, theories, and principles from nursing science and the biological, behavioral, medical, and sociocultural disciplines to clinical nursing practice. Conceptual models and theories provide a broad knowledge base to assist

nurses in understanding and interpreting the client's complex health situation and in planning nursing actions to achieve desired client outcomes. "Explicit use of conceptual models of nursing and nursing theories to guide nursing practice is the hallmark of professional nursing"; it distinguishes nursing as an autonomous health profession (Fawcett, 1997, p. 212).

This chapter describes the value and relevance of theory-based nursing for advanced practice nurses and discusses some underlying concerns about applying theories in nursing practice. The structure of nursing knowledge and the transformative process for theory-based practice are explained, along with the importance of critical thinking. An overview of various models and theories of nursing, family, and other disciplines is provided. Finally, the process for selecting and applying appropriate models and theories in nursing practice is thoroughly described.

Relevance of Theory-Based Practice in Nursing

The value of theory-based nursing practice is well documented in numerous books and journal articles. Although many articles illustrate the application of a nursing model or theory to clients with a specific health problem, Alligood (1997b) reviewed the nursing literature and found that about 68% of the articles reflect a medical approach to nursing. She also noted that most nurses described their practice in terms of a specialty area, types of care or health problems, and nursing interventions.

All nurses use knowledge they acquired during their formal education and clinical experience to guide their practice. Some nurse practitioners consistently use models and theories to guide their practice, but most nurses are unaware of existing theories and models or do not know how to apply them. Many nurses are not aware of what knowledge they use or where they learned it; thus, their implicit knowledge tends to be fragmented, diffused, incomplete, and greatly influenced by the medical model (Fawcett, 1997). Although graduate nurse practitioner students learn about nursing models and theories, their education often emphasizes application of medical knowledge as the base for their nursing practice. Thus, the use of medical knowledge and policies of healthcare delivery

systems has replaced nursing knowledge and influenced some nurses to become "junior doctors," instead of "senior nurses" (Meleis, 1993).

Theories and models from nursing and behavioral disciplines are used by advanced practice nurses to provide effective, high quality nursing care. Many nurses believe that use of nursing theories would improve the quality of nursing care but that they do not have sufficient information about them or the opportunity to use them (McKenna, 1997b). According to Meleis (1997), theories improve quality of care by clearly defining the boundaries and goals of nursing assessment, diagnosis, and interventions and by providing continuity and congruency of care. Theory also contributes to more efficient and effective nursing practice and enhances nurses' professional autonomy and accountability. Aggleton and Chalmers (1986) claim that providing nursing care without a theory base is like "practicing in the dark." Kenney (1996) reported that professional nurses can effectively use theories and models from nursing and behavioral disciplines to:

- collect, organize, and classify client data
- understand, analyze, and interpret clients' health situations
- guide formulation of nursing diagnoses
- plan, implement, and evaluate nursing care
- explain nursing actions and interactions with clients
- describe, explain, and sometimes predict clients' responses
- demonstrate responsibility and accountability for nursing actions
- achieve desired outcomes for clients

The healthcare revolution requires that nurses demonstrate efficient, cost-effective, high-quality care within organized delivery systems. "Nursing theory-based practice offers an alternative to the dehumanizing, fragmented, and paternalistic approaches that plague current delivery systems" (Smith, 1994, p. 7). With changes in the current third-party reimbursement systems, nurses will be paid for effective theory-based practice that enhances clients' health and their quality of life. To accomplish this, nurse practitioners must use critical thinking skills combined with theory-based knowledge and clinical expertise to achieve desired client outcomes.

Issues Related to Theory-Based Nursing Practice

In recent years, the enthusiasm for using nursing models and theories in practice has waned due to criticisms about the theory–practice gap and the lack of relevance to clinical practice. Also, there are philosophical concerns about whether only nursing models should guide practice and whether models and theories of nursing and other disciplines may be integrated in practice. This section discusses some of these issues.

The theory–practice gap refers to the lack of use or inability of nurses to use nursing and other theories in clinical practice. McKenna (1997b) claims that theories are not being used in a systematic way to guide nursing practice, although using theories may improve the quality of care. He believes nurses do not use nursing theories because they do not know about them, understand them, believe in them, know how to apply them, or are not allowed to use them. Professional nursing practice more often reflects the medical or organizational model of

care than application of relevant nursing models or theories.

According to Rogers (1989, p. 114), "Nursing knowledge . . . is often seen as being unscientific, intuitive, and highly subjective." Some nurses believe that conceptual models and theories are too abstract to apply in nursing practice; they do not provide sufficient information to guide nursing judgments, are subject to different interpretations, are incomplete, and lack adequate testing and refinement (Field, 1987; Firlet, 1985). Others argue that some nursing theories were never meant to be directly applied in nursing practice but were intentionally abstract to stimulate thinking, provide new insights, and develop creative ways of viewing nursing (McKenna, 1997b).

As a practice discipline, nursing models and theories should be useful in practice, or their value is questionable. When models and theories are logical and consistent with other validated theories, they may provide the rationale and consequences of nursing actions and lead to predictable client outcomes. There are numerous articles and chapters describing application of various models to clinical nursing practice. However, rigorous research studies on how nursing models and theories contribute to desirable nursing actions and client outcomes are lacking.

Another issue is whether only nursing models and theories are appropriate for the discipline, as nursing is an applied science. Most professional nurses are familiar with theories from other disciplines, such as systems theory, family theories, developmental theories, and others; in clinical practice, nurses often combine their nursing and medical knowledge with theories from other disciplines. Some nurse scholars argue that nursing practice must be based on nursing models and theories, as they are consistent with nursing's view of human science and provide the structure for explaining nursing's unique contribution to health care (Cody, 1996; Mitchell, 1992). Because nursing models or theories represent the theorist's unique beliefs about persons, health, and nursing and guide how nurses interact with clients, McKenna (1997b) believes that an eclectic approach, combining theories from nursing and other disciplines, may compromise nursing theories if the concepts are removed from their original context and interwoven with other theories.

In contrast, Meleis (1997) argues that because nurses study other disciplines, nursing theory tends to reflect a broad range of perspectives and premises. Many nursing theorists have incorporated or borrowed theories from other disciplines and then transmuted them to fit within the context of nursing so that their nursing theories comprise shared knowledge used in a distinctive way (Timpson, 1996).

A related issue is whether professional nurses should consistently use only one nursing model or use various models and theories from nursing and other disciplines in their practice. Most professions, like nursing, have multiple theories that represent divergent and unique perspectives about the phenomena of concern to their practice. Within nursing, conceptual models and theories range from broad conceptual models, or grand theories, to specific practice theories. There are advantages and disadvantages to using one or more theories in clinical practice. Depending on the nurse's knowledge and clinical practice area, some nursing models and theories may be more appropriate than others. However, some would argue that use of only one nursing theory limits the nurse's assessment to only those things addressed by the theory, and the nurse may be forced to fit the client situation to the theory.

Others believe that nurses should consider a variety of nursing theories and select the model or theory that best fits the client's health problems. The majority of early nursing theories were based on traditional scientific methods and reflect a reductionistic perspective of humans as passive beings, consisting of elementary parts that respond to external stimuli in a linear, causal, and predictive way (Benner & Wrubel, 1989). Nursing models based on this perspective ultimately dehumanize individuals into disparate parts and systems and lead to fragmented, nonholistic nursing care (Aggleton & Chalmers, 1986). More contemporary nursing models view humans as continuously changing during reciprocal interactions with their environment, thus individual reactions to nursing care are not predictable, nor can they be controlled. However, these newer nursing models are more abstract than earlier models and are less likely to offer specific guidelines for nursing actions. Professional nurses are expected to develop unique, creative nursing actions suitable for each client's health problem and lifestyle, and theories from other disciplines may be integrated to complement and strengthen some limitations in both early and contemporary nursing models.

Cody (1996) contends that eclecticism, or selecting the best theory from other sources, is not necessarily wrong, but constantly borrowing theories from other disciplines does not contribute to the science of nursing or differentiate nursing from other professions. He believes that nursing practice ought to reflect a coherent, nursing theoretical base to guide practice in specific ways and contribute to the quality of care.

Since professional nurses provide health care for a variety of clients, each of whom is unique yet may have similar health concerns, nurses must use a broad knowledge base from nursing and other disciplines to select and apply relevant models and/or theories that are congruent with the client's situation. Health care, based on appropriate nursing models and theories, that integrates appropriate family, behavioral, and developmental theories, is most likely to achieve desired client health outcomes.

Structure of Nursing Knowledge and Perspective Transformation

Advanced practice nurses must first understand the structure of nursing knowledge and the process of transforming nursing models and theories into useful perspectives prior to implementing theory-based practice. Fawcett (1995) described the structural hierarchy of nursing knowledge or nursing science. Nursing's metaparadigm, which includes the major concepts of person, health, environment, and nursing, provides the foundation from which nursing philosophies, conceptual models, and theories are derived. Each nurse theorist developed unique definitions of her major concepts, based on her education, practice, and personal philosophy (values, beliefs, and assumptions) about humans, health, nursing, and environment. The theorist's philosophy also influenced her conceptual model, which describes how the concepts are linked; the model explains the relationships among client–health–nursing situations (Sorrentino, 1991). Conceptual nursing models are usually called "grand theories" because they are broad and abstract and may not provide specific directions for nursing actions. Some nurse theorists have developed midrange

or practice theories from their models, which describe specific relationships among the concepts and suggest hypotheses to be tested.

According to Rogers (1989), an individual's personal meaning perspective or conceptual model provides a frame of reference or lens that influences how one perceives, thinks, and behaves in the world, yet most people are not aware of how their perspective influences and affects their view of themselves, others, and their world because underlying beliefs are held in the unconscious mind. In practice, nurses' perceptions, thoughts, feelings, and actions are guided by their personal framework or perspective of nursing, which provides a cognitive structure based on their assumptions, beliefs, and values about nursing (Fawcett, 1995). Many nurses unconsciously use a medical or institutional model as their perspective for organizing care. The prevalent values of such models or perspectives are efficiency, standardized care, rules, and regulations, such as "critical care pathways" (Rogers, 1989). As nurses become aware of the differences between the present and potential possibilities of nursing practice, they experience a cognitive dissonance or discomfort from an awareness of what is versus what could be (Rogers, 1989). Thus, only when nurses experience cognitive dissonance in practice will they change their frame of reference and use nursing models and theories.

For professional nurses to apply conceptual nursing models and theories, a dramatic change, or perspective transformation, must occur (Fawcett, 1995; Rogers, 1989). Perspective transformation is the process of moving from one frame of reference or perspective to another when unresolved dilemmas arise and create dissonance in one's current perspective (Mezirow, 1979). It is a process of critical reflection and analysis of other explanations or perspectives that might resolve the dilemma and explain or guide one's understanding and actions. The process involves gradually acquiring a new perspective that leads to fundamental changes in the way nurses experience, interpret, and understand their world and their relationships with others (Fawcett, 1995).

Fawcett (1995) describes nine phases leading to perspective transformation. Initially, the prevailing stability of the current nursing practice is disrupted when use of a nursing conceptual model or theory-based practice is introduced. Dissonance occurs as nurses consider their own perspective for practice and the challenge of changing to a new conceptual model or theory. Some nurses identify discrepancies between their current practice and how the new model or theory could affect their practice. Confusion may follow as nurses struggle to learn about the model or theory and how to apply it in practice. Nurses often feel anxious, angry, and unable to think during these phases and may grieve the loss of familiar perspectives of nursing. Their former perspective no longer seems useful, yet they have not internalized the new model or theory well enough to use it effectively. While dwelling with uncertainty, nurses acknowledge that their confusion is not due to personal inadequacy, and as their anxiety diminishes, they begin to critically examine former practice methods and explore the possibilities of implementing a new model or theory (Fawcett, 1995; Rogers, 1989).

With the discovery that a new model or theory is coherent and meaningful, synthesis occurs. As ways to apply the new model become clearer, new insights assist nurses to understand the usefulness of the conceptual model or theory in nursing practice (Fawcett, 1995). Resolution occurs as nurses become comfortable using the new model; they may feel a sense of empowerment and view their practice differently. Gradually, nurses consciously change their practice during reconceptualization; they shift from their former patterns to new ways of thinking and acting within the new model or theory. The final phase, return to stability, occurs when nursing practice is clearly based on the new nursing model or theory. Acceptance of a new perspective or paradigm, along with the corresponding assumptions, values, and beliefs, concludes the transformation process.

Models and theories from nursing and other disciplines provide the cognitive structures that guide professional nursing practice. This body of knowledge helps nurses explain what they know and the rationale for their nursing actions that facilitate the client's health (Fawcett, 1997). Theory-based nursing practice depends on the depth of nurses' knowledge of models and theories and their understanding about how to apply them in practice (Alligood, 1997a). Nursing models and theories represent ideal, logical, unique perspectives or maps of the person and health. They provide a structure and systematic approach to examine clients' situations, identify relevant information, interpret data for nursing diagnoses, and plan effective nursing care through critical thinking, reasoning, and decision making (Alligood, 1997a; Mayberry, 1991; Timpson, 1996).

Nurses must use critical thinking skills to apply models and theories to their clients' health concerns. Paul and Nosich's (1991) definition of critical thinking, which follows, is a commonly accepted one.

> Critical thinking is the intellectually disciplined process of actively and skillfully conceptualizing, applying, analyzing,

synthesizing, or evaluating information gathered from, or generated by, observation, experience, reflection, reasoning, or communication, as a guide to belief and action. (p. 4)

According to Cradock (1996), it is not what they know that makes nurses advanced practitioners, but how they use what they know. They must make expert clinical decisions based on reflection, complex reasoning, and critical thinking to apply theoretically based knowledge to diverse client situations (Spiracino, 1991). Critical thinking incorporates ideas from both models or theories with clinical experience and provides the structure for unique, creative nursing practice with each client (Alligood, 1997a; Field, 1987; Mayberry, 1991; Sorrentino, 1991). Several nurse authors believe that nursing theories will become the stimuli for reflection and critical thinking, leading to realms for creative expressions in nursing practice (Chinn, 1997; Marks-Moran & Rose, 1997). Theory-based nursing and critical thinking are the foundations of advanced nursing practice (Mitchell, 1992). Specific critical thinking skills for each component of the nursing process are identified in Table 18–1.

Models and Theories Applicable in Advanced Nursing Practice

Theory-based nursing practice is the creative application of various models, theories, and principles from nursing, medical, behavioral, and humanistic sciences. Models and theories from relevant disciplines provide the knowledge base to understand various aspects of the client's health concerns and guide appropriate nursing management. In advanced nursing practice, the client may be an individual, families, or an aggregate, such as a community or special population. Knowledge of relevant models and theories from nursing and other disciplines enables the nurse to select those that best fit each client. This section provides a brief overview of some nursing, family, community, and other models and theories that may be relevant and useful to nurse practitioners.

Nursing Models and Theories

Numerous nursing models and theories have been reported in the literature since the 1950s. Some well-known nurse theorists' works are cited; readers are encouraged to seek other sources for more information about their models and theories. The early nurse theorists' conceptual models focused on individual clients and described nursing goals and activities. Peplau's interpersonal model described a goal–directed, nurse–client interpersonal process to promote the client's personality and living. Orlando's model explained a deliberative nursing approach to understand nurse–patient relationships and the communication process. Hall's core-care-cure model expanded and clarified nursing actions to promote clients' health. Levine's model identified four principles of human conservation to guide nursing activities.

More contemporary nursing theories have been published since 1970, when Rogers introduced her science of unitary man. She described mutually evolving relationships between humans and their environment that are expressed as changing energy fields, patterns, and organization. Orem's self-care model identified requisites for an individual's self-care and specific nursing systems to deliver care according to the client's

Table 18–1 APPLICATION OF CRITICAL THINKING SKILLS TO THE NURSING PROCESS

Components and Definitions	Critical Thinking Skills and Activities
Assessment An ongoing process of data collection to determine the client's strengths and health concerns	Collect relevant client data by observation, examination, interview and history, and reviewing the records Distinguish relevant data from irrelevant Distinguish important data from unimportant Validate data with others
Diagnosis The analysis/synthesis of data to identify patterns and compare with norms and models A clear, concise statement of the client's health status and concerns appropriate for nursing intervention	Organize and categorize data into patterns Identify data gaps Recognize patterns and relationships in data Compare patterns with norms and theories Examine own assumptions regarding client's situation Make inferences and judgments of client's health concerns Define the health concern and validate with the client and health team members Describe actual and potential concerns and the etiology of each diagnosis Propose alternative explanations of concerns
Planning Determination of how to assist the client in resolving concerns related to restoration, maintenance, or promotion of health	Identify priority of client's concerns Determine client's desired health outcomes Select appropriate nursing interventions by generalizing principles and theories Transfer knowledge from other sciences Design plan of care with scientific rationale
Implementation Carrying out the plan of care by the client and nurse	Apply knowledge to perform interventions Compare baseline data with changing status Test hypotheses of nursing interventions Update and revise the care plan Collaborate with health team members
Evaluation A systematic, continuous process of comparing the client's response with the desired health outcomes	Compare client's responses with desired health outcomes Use criterion-based tools to evaluate Determine the client's level of progress Revise the plan of care

self-care needs. King designed a systems model that included the individual, family, and society, then developed her theory of goal attainment, which described nurse–patient transactions to achieve the client's goals. Roy's adaptation model identified three types of stimuli that affect a patient's four modes of functioning. She described how the nurse identifies maladaptive behaviors and alters stimuli to enhance the client's adaptation. Paterson and Zderad developed a model of humanistic nursing. Leininger's transcultural nursing model explained differences between universal and cultural-specific views of health and healing, and how nurses can provide culturally congruent health care. According to Watson, nursing is the art and science of human care; nurses engage in transpersonal caring transactions to assist persons to achieve mind–body–soul harmony. Johnson's behavioral systems model focused on nurturing, protecting, and stimulating the individual's seven subsystems to maintain balance and stability. Neuman designed a complex health care systems model that identified different types of stressors and levels of defense; nursing actions were based on three levels of prevention. Parse developed a man–living–health theory in which nurses assist individuals to explore their past, present, and future life experiences and illuminate possible lifestyle choices to enhance their health and lives. Newman's theory of health as expanding consciousness considers disease as part of health, and explores time and rhythm pattern recognition with changes in life and health.

Family Models

Although most nursing models were originally designed to focus on individual clients, a few are applicable to families. King views the family as a social system or group of interacting individuals and family health as dynamic life experiences. Roy views the family as part of the client's immediate social environment, whereas Neuman's concept of family is harmonious relationships among family members. These nurse theorists focused on the individual client with the family seen as context. If the family is viewed as the client, the nurse must decide what the model should focus on—family development, interactions and stress, family systems, structure and function, or a combination of these models, such as the Calgary family model.

Family development models are based on the premise that the life cycle of families follows a common sequence of events from marriage through child rearing, retirement, and bereavement. Most are based on the typical nuclear two-parent family and emphasize the stages and adult's responsibilities to accomplish desired goals. Duvall's (1977) model is well known, and Stevenson (1977), a nurse theorist, also designed a family model.

Family interactional models view family members as a unit of interacting personalities within a dynamic life process. These models focus on how members' perceptions and interpretations of themselves and other family members determine their behaviors and actions. Also, these models consider how members' roles affect their interaction with others. Satir's family interaction model is an example. Family stress and coping models, based on the work of Lazarus and Folkman, were developed by Moos and Billings (1982) to identify how the family appraised the situation, dealt with their problems, and handled the resulting emotions. McCubbin and McCubbin (1993) designed the double ABCX model, which examines family life stressors and resources, along with changes that affect their adaptation to health problems and their ability to manage family crises. Curran's (1985) healthy family model identified characteristics of healthy families and common stressors affecting families.

Family systems models view the whole family as greater than and different from the sum of its parts or members. These models focus on the family with a hierarchy of subsystems (mother–father, parent–child) and supersystems in the community (social, occupational, recreational, and religious networks) that interact with the family system. Olson, Russell, and Sprenkle's (1983) model identifies 16 types of family systems based on the premise that a balance must be maintained in family cohesion, so that members do not become too enmeshed or too distant, and on adaptability, wherein too much change creates chaos and too little change leads to rigidity. Communication between family members is the third dimension. The Beavers system model (Beavers & Voeller, 1983) examines the structure, flexibility, and competence of a family and its members. Centripetal families enjoy close family relationships, while centrifugal families seek satisfaction outside the family.

Family structural–functional models view the family as a social system composed of nuclear and extended family members, and their social–communicative interactions to achieve family functions. According to Friedman (1992), the structural components include family composition, values, communication patterns, members' roles, and the power structure. Functional components of this model include physical necessities and care, economic, affective, and reproductive behaviors, socialization and placement of family members, and family coping abilities. The structural and functional components are interrelated, and each part is affected by changes in other parts.

A model that combines many of the aforementioned models is the Calgary family model, developed by Wright and Leahey (1994). The major components include the internal and external family structure, similar to Friedman's (1992) model, along with family context, such as race, ethnicity, social class, religion, and environment. Family functions are viewed as instrumental or daily living activities, and expressive activities, including communication (emotional, verbal, and behavioral), problem solving, roles, influences, beliefs, and alliances or coalitions. Family developmental stages and tasks, similar to Duvall's (1977), are also part of this comprehensive model.

Any family model may be combined with and complement a nursing model because nursing practice may involve individual clients or families. Nurses with knowledge of various family models are more likely to select the most appropriate and relevant one to meet the family's health concerns.

Community Models

There are many community models that are useful to nurses, but they differ according to whether community is considered a target population or aggregate or a geographic area. McKay and Segall (1983) described an aggregate model, in which the focus is on a group of individuals who share common characteristics, but may not interact with each other. Shamansky and Pesznecker (1981) identified three interdependent factors that constitute a geographical community: (1) persons who reside in an area; (2) space and time, which includes the community's history and environmental features; and (3) purpose factors that explain functional processes such as government policies, educational services, and forms of communication.

The community-as-client model, designed by Anderson, McFarlane, and Helton (1986), combines both the aggregate and geographical community. It addresses the following eight subsystems of the aggregate in the community: physical environment, education, safety and transportation, politics and government, health and social services, communication, economics, and recreation. A community nursing process model was developed by Goeppinger, Lassiter, and Wilcox (1982). It examines the following eight processes in a community: commitment of members, awareness of others' views, articulation of community needs, effective communication within and among members, conflict containment and accommodation, participation in organizations, management of relations with the larger society, and mechanisms to facilitate participant interactions and decision making. Knowledge of several community models facilitates selection of the most appropriate one.

Other Useful Models and Theories

Nurses and theorists in other disciplines have developed many relevant models and theories that are useful in advanced nursing practice. Some of these models include Maslow's hierarchy of needs, Erikson's stages of development, Piaget's cognitive development of children, Pender's (1987) health promotion/disease prevention model, and Loveland-Cherry's (1989) family health promotion model. In addition, there are numerous theories of stress, crises, coping, grief, bereavement, death, and dying developed in psychology and behavioral disciplines. Nurses have transformed some of these theories to encompass a health–illness context. Nurses who are cognizant of a variety of nursing, family, community, and behavioral models and theories are more likely to select the best fitting model for their clients.

Selection of Relevant Models and Theories

This section provides an overview of several nurse scholars' criteria and guidelines for selecting models and theories. Meleis (1997) identified six criteria to guide selection of suitable models and theories for practice. McKenna (1997a) described seven selection criteria based on a review of the literature. Kim (1994) constructed a framework for practice theories with four dimensions to consider in selecting nursing models and theories. Fawcett and associates (1992) suggested that nurses consider three questions to determine the best fit between the client's health concerns and various models and theories. Relevant criteria from these scholars' work were integrated with the author's prior work to delineate five guidelines for selecting appropriate models and theories (Christensen & Kenney, 1996).

Meleis (1997) wrote that selecting models and theories for nursing practice is both a subjective and objective process. She identified the following six criteria for nurses to consider in the selection process:

1. Personal—the nurse's comfort with the theory and congruency with the nurse's own philosophical views of life
2. Mentor—the model or theory learned from a nurse mentor or educator
3. Theorist—their reputation in the discipline and degree of recognition
4. Literature—support the amount of literature available about the theory and the theory's significance for one's specialty

5. Sociopolitical congruency—the model or theory's acceptability within the nurse's workplace and whether major structural or practice changes are required
6. Utility—the ease in which nurses can understand and apply the model or theory in practice settings

McKenna (1997a) reviewed the literature and identified the following seven criteria for selecting models and theories.

1. The type of client—The client's needs should direct the choice because the theory provides guidelines to achieve the client's goals.
2. Healthcare setting—The type of clinical setting and nursing practice are contextual factors that affect selection of theories.
3. Parsimony/simplicity—Simple and realistic theories are more likely to be understood and applied in practice.
4. Understandability—Nurses must understand a theory if they expect to use it.
5. Origins of the theory—The credibility, prior use, and testing of the theory should also be considered.
6. Paradigms as a basis for choice—Nurses must decide between the totality or simultaneity paradigm, as each provides a different view of clients and nursing actions.
7. Personal values and beliefs—The theory must be congruent with the nurse's own views about humans, health, and nursing.

In her article on practice theories, Kim (1994) defined two dimensions of theories, which include four sets of practice theories relevant to selecting models and theories. One dimension is the target, which addresses both the philosophy of care for the person and the philosophy of therapy for the client's problems. The other dimension is the nurse-agent, which includes two phases—deliberation and enactment. The four sets of practice theories serve to guide nurses in choosing theories that will (1) explain the patient's problems and ideas about therapy for the problems; (2) provide ideas about how the nurse should approach the patient, such as through communication, caring, or empowerment; (3) explain how to make decisions about appropriate nursing actions for the patient; and (4) explain what happens during enactment of nursing actions. Kim proposed that a science of nursing practice could be developed from this framework.

Fawcett and associates (1992) identified questions to guide nurses' selection of appropriate theories and models. The nurse must understand the differences among various models and theories in nursing and other disciplines to answer these questions. The following three questions will help the nurse identify the most appropriate model:

1. Does the theory or model address the client's problems and health concerns?
2. Are the nursing interventions suggested by the model consistent with the client's expectations for nursing care?
3. Are the goals of nursing actions, based on the model or theory, congruent with the client's desired health outcomes?

These questions help nurses decide which models and theories will assist them to organize the data into patterns, identify other health concerns, and determine congruency of the client's and nurse's view of nursing and health.

The first step toward theory-based nursing practice is the conscious decision to use theories in practice (Fawcett, 1997). The second step is recognizing that use of conceptual nursing models and theories requires a major change in how the nurse thinks about and interacts with clients to alleviate their health concerns. This change, referred to earlier as a perspective transformation, occurs gradually as the nurse discards one framework of practice and learns another perspective. Adopting and applying new models and theories in practice depends on nurses having knowledge of various models and theories and understanding how these models and theories relate to each other (Alligood, 1997a).

Guidelines for Selecting Models and Theories for Nursing Practice

After deciding to implement theory-based nursing practice, the author believes that each nurse must engage in the five steps described here:

1. Consider personal values and beliefs about nursing, clients, health, and environment. Each nurse has a personal frame of reference or perspective of nursing practice, based on his/her conscious or unconscious assumptions, beliefs, and values about nursing. One's perspective of nursing provides a cognitive structure that guides one's perceptions, thoughts, feelings, and nursing actions (Fawcett, 1995). Clarifying one's own values and beliefs about clients, health, and nursing practice is necessary before a perspective transformation can occur.

2. Examine the underlying assumptions, values, and beliefs of various nursing models, and how the major concepts are defined. After clarifying one's own values and beliefs, the nurse examines the definitions of major concepts in various models and theories to determine whether they are congruent with one's own beliefs (Alligood, 1997a). Nursing models and theories are based on different values and beliefs about the nature of the client's behaviors and abilities, what is health and environment, and what nursing actions facilitate clients' health. Each nursing model and theory provides a unique view for specific nursing practice. Some nursing models reflect a totality paradigm and view humans as having separate biological, social, psychological, and spiritual parts that respond to environmental stimuli or change, and the nurse's role is to facilitate adaptation or equilibrium to maintain health. Other nursing models reflect a simultaneity paradigm and propose that humans are intelligent beings, capable of making informed decisions about their lives, and that they continuously engage in a dynamic, mutual interaction with their environment. In this paradigm, the nurse's role is to guide clients in choosing lifestyles and/or therapies that are acceptable to them and facilitate their growth and life–health process.

3. Identify several models that are congruent with one's own values and beliefs about nursing, clients, and health. Each nurse must consider whether the theorist's underlying values are congruent with one's own personal values and beliefs about clients, health, and nursing

because the theorist's values guide the nurse's critical thinking and reasoning processes (Alligood, 1997a). Models and theories reflect the theorist's views about people and nursing. They directly affect how nurses approach their clients, what information they gather, how that information is processed, what nursing activities are appropriate, and what client outcomes are expected based on the model. For example, some traditional nursing models define the person as a bio-psycho-social being who responds to environmental stimuli, and health results from nursing actions that lead to predictable changes. These models would be incongruent for contemporary nurses who believe that people are free agents, dynamically interacting with their environment as a whole and capable of making rational decisions, and that the nurse's role is to assist clients to explore various options and choose ones that are acceptable with their values and lifestyle.

4. Identify the similarities and differences in client focus, nursing actions, and client outcomes of these models. Nursing models and theories consist of concepts with specific definitions and statements that describe how the concepts are interrelated. Some propose specific nursing actions and expected client outcomes. The major concepts guide what data is collected during the assessment and how the data is organized to identify and interpret bio-behavioral patterns and determine nursing diagnoses. Nursing models also guide development of the nursing care plans and designate desired outcomes to evaluate. By comparing various models, nurses recognize which ones are congruent with their values and beliefs about nursing and offer the best fit with the client's health concerns.

5. Practice applying the models and theories to clients with different health concerns to determine which ones best fit specific situations and guide nursing actions that will achieve desired client outcomes. The nurse explores specific models in depth and may analyze their usefulness before implementing them. By comparing several models and examining the attributes of the client, the focus of nursing actions, and the proposed outcomes, the nurse will acquire a more in-depth understanding of different models. Each nursing model describes different areas for assessment, unique nursing diagnoses, and specific nursing interventions to assist the client toward health. The nurse must decide which models and theories are most appropriate for each client. Which one offers the best fit for the client's health concerns? Selecting appropriate models and theories for each unique client health situation requires nurses to use their broad knowledge base from various disciplines, critical thinking skills, clinical expertise, and intuition to identify the best fit between the client's health concerns and nursing models (Fawcett et al., 1992).

Application of Theory-Based Nursing Practice

The choice of theories and models suitable to the client's health concerns occurs during the initial data assessment process. The initial data focus on the client's primary expressed concerns and how they are related to or affect the client's lifestyle and patterns of living. These data assist the nurse to identify and understand the client's common and unique patterns. The client's view of health, along with past and present lived experiences and future lifestyle and health concerns, are also considered. Using this information, the nurse considers various models and theories from nursing and other disciplines that are relevant to the client's unique health concerns and congruent with the nurse's own beliefs. Then, the nurse selects those models and other theories that best fit the client's situation and health concerns and will systematically direct nursing practice.

The major concepts of the chosen models and theories guide each component of the nursing process, as shown in Table 18–2. The concepts serve as categories to guide additional data collection. They suggest, either directly or indirectly, what information is relevant and should be collected. The models and theories assist the nurse to organize, categorize, and interpret pertinent data that illustrate the client's bio-behavioral patterns and identify appropriate nursing diagnoses that are linked to relevant etiological factors.

Nursing and other models and theories guide development of a care plan by suggesting appropriate types of nursing interventions and specific nursing actions. Desired client outcomes are derived from the models and theories and define what changes in the client should be evaluated. For example, if Roy's model is chosen, data about the client's physiological needs, self-concept, role mastery, and interdependence, along with related stimuli, would be collected and used to identify adaptive and maladaptive

behavioral patterns. The nurse who uses Orem's self-care model would assess and judge clients' ability to meet their universal and developmental self-care requisites and whether they had any health deviations. From analysis of this data, the nurse would diagnose self-care deficits and determine appropriate nursing plans for partial, compensatory, or health education nursing care. Nursing care plans are based on the model and describe the client's desired outcomes, along with nursing actions to achieve the client's outcomes. Nurses who use Johnson's behavioral systems model would consider ways to nurture, protect, or stimulate the client to facilitate health, whereas the Neuman's healthcare systems model assists the nurse to explore ways to reduce stressors within the three levels of disease prevention.

Some nurses believe that family models complement nursing models and provide a more holistic and comprehensive perspective of clients and their health concerns. Selection of a family model occurs after the nurse gathers preliminary data about the family and identifies its unique and common patterns. Then the nurse decides whether the family as context or family as client would be more appropriate and best fit the client's situation. Also, the nurse's perception and definition of family and health guide the selection of a family model. For example, a pediatric nurse who works in an outpatient clinic may choose Orem's self-care model to guide care of a 9-year-old child with an ear infection and the mother's treatment of the child. Friedman's family system model may complement Orem's model and enhance understanding of the family's structure and functions. The nurse may also use Erikson's developmental framework to help the mother recognize and encourage her child's normal developmental

Table 18–2 THEORY-BASED NURSING PRACTICE

Component	Nursing Process Use	Nursing Model Use
Assessment	Describes how to collect data	Guides what data to collect
Diagnosis	Describes how to process data	Guides organizing, categorizing, and interpreting data
	Provides format for nursing diagnosis	Provides concepts for nursing diagnosis
	Describes *how* to plan	Guides *what* to plan
	Facilitates development of care plan unique to client	Designates appropriate types of nursing interventions
		Directs model-specific nursing actions
Implementation	Describes phases of implementation	
		Guides *what* to evaluate
Evaluation	Identifies *how* to evaluate	
		Enhances accountability of theory-based practice
General	Requires accountability through use of systematic approach to nursing practice	
	Process enhances continuity of care	Provides a comprehensive, coherent approach to care of client

behaviors. Pain management theories may also be applied to reduce the child's earache.

This example illustrates how nurses examine and judge the value of various models and theories and select those that are most congruent and useful and best fit the client's health concerns and the nurse's perspective of practice. Gradually, nurse practitioners develop an expertise in selecting theories and models that are appropriate and relevant to their client's

health concerns and congruent with their own views of advanced practice.

Conclusion

This chapter described the importance and value of applying models and theories from nursing and other disciplines in advanced nursing practice. Issues related to the nursing theory–practice gap were discussed, along with concerns about using only one nursing model in practice and about integrating models and theories from other disciplines with nursing models and theories. The structure of nursing knowledge was explained, as was the need for a perspective transformation to occur prior to implementing theory-based nursing practice. Critical thinking, logical reasoning, and creatively applying nursing models and theories were emphasized. Different types of nursing, family, community, and other models and theories were discussed. Finally, the process of selecting and applying models and theories was thoroughly described.

In the last few decades, the emergence of nursing models and theories has illuminated several nursing paradigms and explicated their underlying assumptions, beliefs, and values that guide nursing practice. The science of nursing and empirical patterns of knowing is represented by these nursing models and their theories. Application of models and theories from nursing and other disciplines depends on nurses having a broad knowledge base and understanding how models and theories are interrelated. Empowerment of nurses through perspective transformation and the use of nursing models and theories is essential. They provide the framework for critical thinking within the context of nursing and guide the reasoning that professional nurses need to survive in an era of cost containment and evidence-based practice. Use of models and theories from nursing and related health disciplines enables nurses to demonstrate accountability for their decisions and actions through scientific explanation and provides a coherent approach to theory-based nursing practice.

Discussion Questions

1. List the reasons to apply nursing, family, and other theories to advanced practice. What are some underlying concerns about applying theories in nursing practice?
2. Based on the review in this chapter of nursing, family, and other disciplines' theories, choose at least one theory to investigate further. Use the five guidelines for selecting models and theories for nursing practice and evaluate the theory's applicability for your current practice. Was the theory applicable or do you need to search for a different one?
3. How does the structure of nursing knowledge relate to nursing's metaparadigms?
4. How can applying theory to practice enhance one's critical thinking skills?
5. What is the process and what are the pitfalls of the process for selecting and applying appropriate nursing, family, and other disciplines' models and theories to advanced nursing practice?

References

Aggleton, P. J., & Chalmers, H. (1986). *Nursing models and the nursing process.* Basingstoke, UK: Macmillan.

Alligood, M. R. (1997a). Models and theories: Critical thinking structures. In M. R. Alligood & A. Marriner-Tomey (Eds.), *Nursing theory: Utilization & application* (pp. 31–45). St. Louis, MO: C. V. Mosby.

Alligood, M. R. (1997b). Models and theories in nursing practice. In M. R. Alligood & A. Marriner-Tomey (Eds.), *Nursing theory: Utilization & application* (pp. 15–30). St. Louis, MO: C. V. Mosby.

Anderson, E. T., McFarlane, J. M., & Helton, A. (1986). Community as client: A model for practice. *Nursing Outlook, 3*(5), 220.

Beavers, W. R., & Voeller, M. N. (1983). Family models: Comparing and contrasting the Olson circumplex model with the Beavers systems model. *Family Process, 22*, 85–98.

Benner, P., & Wrubel, J. (1989). *The primacy of caring.* Menlo Park, CA: Addison-Wesley.

Chinn, P. L. (1997). Why middle-range theory? *ANS, 19*(3), viii.

Christensen, P. J., & Kenney, J. W. (1996). *Nursing process: Application of conceptual models* (4th ed.). St. Louis, MO: C. V. Mosby.

Cody, W. K. (1996). Drowning in eclecticism. *Nursing Science Quarterly, 9*(3), 86–88.

Cradock, S. (1996). The expert nurse: Clinical specialist or advanced practitioner? In Gary Rolfe (Ed.), *Closing the theory-practice gap: A new paradigm for nursing.* Oxford, UK: Butterworth-Heinemann Ltd.

Curran, D. (1985). *Stress and the healthy family.* Minneapolis, MN: Winston Press.

Duvall, E. M. (1977). *Marriage and family development* (5th ed.). Philadelphia: Lippincott.

Fawcett, J. (1995). Implementing conceptual models in nursing practice. In J. Fawcett (Ed.), *Analysis and evaluation of conceptual models of nursing* (3rd ed.). Philadelphia: F. A. Davis.

Fawcett, J. (1997). Conceptual models of nursing, nursing theories, and nursing practice: Focus on the future. In M. R. Alligood & A. Marriner-Tomey (Eds.), *Nursing theory: Utilization & application* (pp. 211–221). St. Louis, MO: C. V. Mosby.

Fawcett, J., Archer, C. L., Becker, D., Brown, K. K., Gann, S., Wong, M. J., et al. (1992). Guidelines for selecting a conceptual model of nursing: Focus on the individual patient. *Dimensions of Critical Care Nursing, 11*(5), 268–277.

Field, P. A. (1987). The impact of nursing theory on the clinical decision making process. *Journal of Advanced Nursing, 12*, 563–571.

Firlet, S. I. (1985). Nursing theory and nursing practice: Separate or linked? In J. McCloskey & H. K. Grace (Eds.), *Current issues in nursing* (pp. 6–19). Boston: Blackwell Scientific Publications.

Friedman, M. M. (1992). *Family nursing: Theory and practice* (3rd ed.). New York: Appleton & Lange.

Goeppinger, J., Lassiter, P. G., & Wilcox, B. (1982). Community health is community competence. *Nursing Outlook, 30*(8), 464.

Kenney, J. W. (1996). Relevance of theory-based nursing practice. In P. J. Christensen & J. W. Kenney (Eds.), *Nursing process: Application of conceptual models* (4th ed., pp. 1–23). St. Louis, MO: C. V. Mosby.

Kim, H. S. (1994). Practice theories in nursing and a science of nursing practice. *Scholarly Inquiry for Nursing Practice: An International Journal, 8*(2), 145–158.

Loveland-Cherry, C. J. (1989). Family health promotion and health protection. In P. Bomar (Ed.), *Nurses and family health promotion: Concepts, assessment, and interventions.* Baltimore, MD: Williams & Wilkins.

Marks-Moran, D., & Rose, P. (Eds.). (1997). *Reconstructing nursing: Beyond art and science.* Philadelphia: Bailliere Tindall.

Mayberry, A. (1991). Merging nursing theories, models, and nursing practice: More than an administrative challenge. *ANS, 15*, 44.

McCubbin, M. A., & McCubbin, H. I. (1993). Families coping with illness: The resiliency model of family stress, adjustment and adaptation. In C. B. Danielson, B. Hamel-Bissell, & P. Winstead-Fry (Eds.), *Families, health and illness: Perspectives on coping and intervention* (pp. 21–65). St. Louis, MO: C. V. Mosby.

McKay, R., & Segall, M. (1983). Methods and models for the aggregate. *Nursing Outlook, 31*(6), 328.

McKenna, H. (1997a). Choosing a theory for practice. In H. McKenna (Ed.), *Nursing theories and models* (pp. 127–157). New York: Rutledge.

McKenna, H. (1997b). Applying theories in practice. In H. McKenna (Ed.), *Nursing theories and models* (pp. 158–189). New York: Rutledge.

Meleis, A. I. (1993). *Nursing research and the Neuman model: Directions for the future.* Panel discussion conducted at the Fourth Biennial International Neuman Systems Model Symposium, Rochester, NY.

Meleis, A. I. (1997). *Theoretical nursing: Development and progress* (3rd ed.). Philadelphia: Lippincott.

Mezirow, J. (1979). Perspective transformation. *Adult Education, 28*(3), 100–110.

Mitchell, G. (1992). Specifying the knowledge base of theory in practice. *Nursing Science Quarterly, 5*(1), 6–7.

Moos, R. H., & Billings, A. G. (1982). Conceptualizing and measuring coping resources and processes. In L. Goldberger & S. Breznitz (Eds.), *Handbook of stress.* New York: Free Press.

Olson, D. H., Russell, C. S., & Sprenkle, D. H. (1983). Circumplex models of marital and family systems: VI. Theoretical update. *Family Processes, 22*, 69–83.

Paul, R. W., & Nosich, G. M. (1991). *Proposal for the national assessment of higher-order thinking* (revised version). Washington, DC: The United States Department of Education Office of Educational Research and Improvement, National Center for Education Statistics.

Pender, N. J. (1987). *Health promotion in nursing practice.* New York: Doubleday.

Rogers, M. E. (1989). Creating a climate for the implementation of a nursing conceptual framework. *Journal of Continuing Education in Nursing, 20*(3), 112–116.

Shamansky, S. L., & Pesznecker, B. (1981). A community is . . . *Nursing Outlook, 29*(3), 182–185.

Smith, M. C. (1994). Beyond the threshold: Nursing practice in the next millennium. *Nursing Science Quarterly, 7*(1), 6–7.

Sorrentino, E. A. (1991). Making theories work for you. *Nursing Administration Quarterly, 15*(3), 54–59.

Spiracino, P. (1991). The reciprocal relationship between practice and theory. *Clinical Nurse Specialist, 5*(3), 138.

Stevenson, J. (1977). *Issues and crises during middlescence.* New York: Appleton-Century-Crofts.

Timpson, J. (1996). Nursing theory: Everything the artist spits is art? *Journal of Advanced Nursing, 23*, 1030–1036.

Wright, L. M., & Leahey, M. (1994). *Nurses and families: A guide to family assessment and intervention* (2nd ed.). Philadelphia: F. A. Davis.

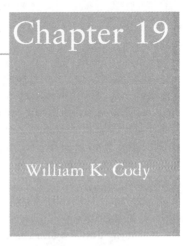

Chapter 19

Values-Based Practice and Evidence-Based Care: Pursuing Fundamental Questions in Nursing Philosophy and Theory

William K. Cody

CHAPTER OBJECTIVES

1. Trace a brief history of nursing theory development.
2. Distinguish between values-based and evidence-based care.
3. Identify values and beliefs that inform personal practice for advanced nursing practice.

Introduction

Florence Nightingale is hailed throughout the English-speaking world as the founder of modern nursing. As she was a woman of action and a great advocate for improvements in health care in the 19th-century British Empire, it is often forgotten that Florence Nightingale was primarily a writer. Her great and lasting influence in health care came about through the power of her ideas laid out in prose and circulated in official reports, essays, and books.

Nightingale is sometimes thought of as the first nurse theorist (Tomey & Alligood, 2002), although it is doubtful that she would have understood what the term meant, had she heard

it in the 1850s. Focusing largely on hygiene, nutrition, and rest, Nightingale (1859/1969) created a system for delivering effective care to patients in the context of her time. She created schools for the training of women called to do this work, and she recorded her ideas in writing for preservation and dissemination. Formal schools modeled more or less on the Nightingale model grew up rapidly in the late 19th century. The trend spread to America, where it proliferated. Although its progenitor was unquestionably an intellectual giant of her time, nursing was not viewed by many, over the ensuing decades, as a highly intellectual pursuit. The Anglo-American tradition of nursing, from Nightingale's time until very recently, was construed largely as vocational rather than professional, as applied rather than basic science, and as a subordinate category of labor, rather than a distinct and learned discipline.

Nursing history reflects a number of important events in the first century after Nightingale opened her schools, such as the emergence of formalized public health nursing and university education for nurses. The creation of new models of nursing and the dissemination of eloquent discourse about concepts and principles of nursing were hardly expected during that era, however, and developments in nursing philosophy and theory were few and far between. It was not until the publication of Hildegarde Peplau's *Interpersonal Relations in Nursing* in 1952 that a work of scholarship named as a theory of nursing by its author was published. Slowly, additions to the literature on philosophy and theory in nursing began to appear.

Considerable nursing theoretical literature in the 1950s and 1960s focused on simply naming what many nurses believed to be present in the content and context of the best nursing (e.g., Henderson, 1966). A feature of the evolving literature was the borrowing and application of theories and concepts from other disciplines, which can be detected to some extent in most of the various frameworks put forth (see Tomey & Alligood, 2002). The whole interesting project of the creation of theory to guide nursing practice became a popular topic in the scholarly nursing literature. Such endeavors came to be viewed as extremely important to nursing's future among nurse scholars who laid the groundwork for the nursing theory-based practice movement that continues in force today.

Perhaps the most salient feature of the nursing theoretical literature that arose in the 1960s

was the notion that the whole person and health in all its dimensions, taken together, comprise the proper focus of nursing care. When this idea first arose, it was taken for granted that the proper approaches for study or care planning would be to merely alternate or combine extant biological, psychological, sociological, and spiritual concepts and methods. In 1970, Martha Rogers put forward a radically different vision of nursing science as a new emergent in human history with a new and unique single focus: the unitary human being, more than and different from the sum of parts, and knowable only as unitary, not through particulate approaches. Thus, a new paradigm of nursing was born.

The 1970s and 1980s were an exciting time in the evolution of nursing philosophy and theory. During those decades, at least 20 significant nursing frameworks intended to guide practice were published; the notion that a nurse, a nursing unit, and a nursing school should have an explicit theoretical framework for practice was popularized; research to test and expand the extant frameworks became more common and proliferated in doctoral programs in nursing; and thus, discourse about philosophy and theory in nursing became a permanent and indispensable constituent of nursing scholarship. Through the early 1990s, the literature was rife with spirited dialogue and debate around issues of nursing philosophy and theory.

In the last decade, much of the scholarly dialogue and debate in nursing centered around issues of practice and research in which the preceding discourses about philosophy and theory seemingly played little part. Master's programs in nursing increasingly turned into practitioner programs largely teaching medical knowledge, and schools with doctoral programs in nursing increasingly focused on research that would bring in government funding, which was rarely framed in a context of nursing's disciplinary knowledge. Nevertheless, there is today a sense that a critical mass has been achieved, a corner has been turned, and a milestone has been passed. Now, rooted precisely in the philosophy and theory of nursing, there are very real reasons that a talented person might choose to become a nurse rather than a physician, a psychologist, or a social worker. Further, there are intriguing ideas in nursing philosophy and theory that can be explored more thoroughly through nursing scholarship than through any other means. There are also challenges to human betterment that nursing may well be the discipline best suited philosophically to meet. Whether or not nurse scholars make extensive use of nursing's extant theories or fervently embrace nursing's stated paradigms, most nurse scholars today would agree with these assertions. The distinctiveness of nursing's disciplinary knowledge base is a reality that cannot be ignored.

Possibly the single most important philosophical question to be posed within a practice discipline is "what guides practice?" In nursing, historically, a long list of traditions and rules from a variety of sources served to guide practice before (and since) the advent of nursing theories. In science, traditionally, the short answer to the question "what guides practice?" usually has been rendered as theory, and nursing has developed a strong body of theories; however, many powerful and subtle forces influence choices in practice. By reflecting on the manifold influences on one's choices in practice, the practitioner can construct a personal answer to the fundamental question "what guides my practice?"

A clear understanding of what guides practice helps the practitioner to pursue useful knowledge more efficiently, to represent one's disciplinary perspective more articulately, and to communicate more effectively with clients and the multidisciplinary team. This section of the book is concerned with philosophical and theoretical perspectives to guide nursing practice. It is important to note that nursing could not take its place in the academic sun and be recognized as the distinct discipline that it is today until it could point to a domain of human knowledge specific to the discipline, knowable only through the formal study of nursing (Coyne, 1981). This domain was mapped through the creative, deliberative construction of nursing theories over the past 50 years.

Value-Laden Theory and the Fallacy of Value-Free Science

A theory's power is proportionate to the breadth of situations and events it can encompass. There are a number of frameworks in nursing that are capable of guiding nursing practice across a range of situations and events, which reflects the maturity of nursing's knowledge base. Some nurse scholars have expressed doubt that these frameworks can guide practice broadly because they are abstract or because they are humanistic in orientation or because they include nonobjective dimensions or because many have not been extensively tested under controlled conditions. Grounding of a theoretical framework in an underlying philosophy, however, strengthens the theory as a guide to practice by making explicit the assumptions and values that form its underpinnings. Many nursing frameworks have explicitly incorporated values such as caring, profound respect for all persons, and attentive presence into their conceptualizations and propositions. Learning these frameworks has profoundly changed the lives of many advanced practice nurses.

In the mid-20th century, a movement for value-free science rooted in the philosophies of science known as positivism, logical positivism, and logical empiricism wielded pervasive influence. This movement in its various guises sought essentially to purge science of all thought not arising from either empirical observation or strict rules of logic. Its influence on the sciences has lingered despite subsequent developments in philosophy of science that weakened or refuted most of its claims (Proctor, 1991). The fact that scientists are human means that science cannot be value free. Values are fundamental constituents of the human lifeworld. Indeed, there is warrant to say even that science itself is a value. That nursing's body of theory is heavily and explicitly value laden can today be seen as a strength, not a weakness, of our body of knowledge.

The hopes and expectations that grew strong in the 1980s, that nurses, nursing units, and nursing schools would adopt, use, support, and grow nursing's own theories have today been somewhat diminished by the influences of other forces converging upon the practice of nursing. These forces are multifarious and include the advent of prospective payment systems, shortened hospital lengths of stay, digitization of healthcare documentation, higher education of influential nurses in nonnursing disciplines, and the persistent need for 2-year nursing programs to meet workforce demands. Along with all of these factors, the attenuated growth of the nursing theory movement can also be attributed to the failure of many members of our own disci-

pline to recognize the uniqueness and value of our own body of knowledge and to face down criticisms from other quarters courageously.

The Clarion Call for Evidence-Based Practice

In contemporary nursing, there is a persistent clarion call to adopt evidence-based practice, implement it, teach it, study it, and standardize it (Melnyk & Fineout-Overholt, 2004). Many nurse leaders holding advanced degrees would answer the question, "what guides nursing practice?" today by saying without hesitation, "Evidence." Evidence-based practice refers, in the main, to the use of rigorously derived empirical findings preferentially as the basis for intervention and nonintervention. It is not unique to nursing. The nomenclature for this movement varies, and one sees literature referring to evidence-based practice and literature referring to evidence-based care. In this chapter, a basis for differentiating the two will be proposed.

The evidence-based practice movement, although centered on the findings of empirical research and the findings of integrative reviews of empirical research, includes proponents of various kinds of evidence, including ethical considerations and other dimensions of life (Goodman, 2003). The movement is not without its internal controversies and divergent views (e.g., Franks, 2004; Timmermans & Berg, 2003; Welsh & Lyons, 2001). Still, for the most part, the movement and the vast majority of the related literature focus on the use of rigorous and replicable research findings to inform or even determine questions of intervention and nonintervention in health care.

Standards of care can be said to approximate the state of the art in evidence-based practice. Note here the difference in terminology (standards of care), which is significant. A set of standards of care is typically based on multiple research studies accumulated over time. It is constructed by large panels of experts to provide practitioners with a well thought-out synthesis of the available evidence for intervention and nonintervention. These standards of care adhere predominantly to the medical model in their approach, but they are commonly used by nurses, health educators, and others. Some sets of standards achieve such familiarity among practitioners across disciplines that they are known chiefly by brief acronyms such as *JNC-7*, which is the *Seventh Report of the Joint National Committee on Prevention, Detection, Evaluation and Treatment of High Blood Pressure* (U.S. Department of Health and Human Services, 2004). Equivalent sets of guidelines exist for many diseases and conditions. It would be difficult to argue against such standards of care within the parameters for which they are designed because they represent feats of combined intellectual achievement that no one person could conceivably match. They help to ensure the availability of the consensus of best reasoned options for care to millions of people.

The evidence base for many of the conventions of tradition-laden and routinized health care, however, the truth be told, can be rather weak. Also, for any number of possible unique acts of intervention or care giving, there may be no research evidence at all. Does this mean, then, that we have no guide for practice in human situations in which there is insufficient research to support recommendations? Or does it mean that knowledge resources other than strongly conclusive research must be brought to bear on situations as guides to practice? Goodman (2003) proposes dealing with uncertainty (as to treatment) in medicine through "management, acknowledgement, and reduction [of the uncertainty]" (p. 131). Interestingly, Goodman does not turn to values for guidance in the absence of convincing evidence one way or another. One aim of the evidence-based practice movement is to minimize bias, and attention to the values of the practitioner can be read as an open invitation to allow bias to rule. Such an interpretation of the dynamics of personal and professional values in practice ignores the fact that many or most healthcare practitioners in fact have a value (i.e., a bias) for objective evidence of efficacy and for the use of good evidence in planning care. With or without evidence, it is the practitioner's values that drive her or his performance in providing care.

In reality, no formal guide to practice or any body of knowledge in any discipline can be both broad and specific enough to guide all actions in every situation. Practitioners are human, and life is complex, ever-changing, and unpredictable. Historically, this philosophical problem has been discussed in the discourse concerned with praxis.

Understanding Praxis

The discourse on evidence-based practice in nursing could benefit from an exploration of the literature on praxis, a concept that has been well examined from ancient times to the present. In demurring from engagement with the literature on praxis, the proponents of evidence-based practice limit discussion of considerations other than evidence that have a strong bearing on practice.

Praxis has been defined and described in several different ways. Aristotle related praxis to human situations requiring practical reasoning to inform action. Habermas (1973), Freire (1993), and Bernstein (1999), in the 20th century, have contributed to our contemporary understandings of praxis, which always unfolds embedded in human situations replete with the complications of multidimensional human interactions, the uncertain, and the unknowable. Persons pursue reasoning related to their peculiar situations based on an understanding of what is good and what contributes to human well-being. Praxis and practical reasoning always unfold in a context that is profoundly interpersonal and relatively unpredictable. The end is not predetermined, and as possible ends evolve situationally, possible means evolve as well. Thus, praxis is creative and dialogical. In political and pedagogical discourse, praxis has even been explicated as the practice of freedom.

Practice as Praxis

If practice is examined in the light of this voluminous literature of over 2,000 years, it must be viewed as driven by far more than scientific evidence alone. Even the most diehard logical positivist would concede, at a minimum, the need for a code of ethics to provide parameters of conduct for science-based practice. Many considerations other than scientific evidence can be identified as reasons for action and as knowledge to guide practice.

The practice of nursing is intentional and deliberate action, guided by nursing science and other sources of knowledge, performed by nurses, and intended for the benefit of persons and society. In this regard, it is comparable to other professional practices. The moment-to-moment acts of nursing practice are chosen from a wide variety of options by each individual nurse in the ever-unfolding and unpredictable context of interrelationships with persons, families and communities, their meanings to the persons involved, and the values that are interwoven among the meanings. The animus underlying nursing practice is the intention to benefit people. However, the actions, behaviors, and words that provide the benefits change from moment to moment with the situation.

Each nurse is responsible for her or his own practice in a fundamental and inescapable way. The actions entailed in professional nursing practice are also the responsibility of, and occur under the stewardship of, the nursing profession itself, by way of its regulatory bodies and professional associations. These bodies determine the expectations of all the nurses within their spheres of influence, and these expectations are laid out in accord with conventions such as the nursing process and standards of ethics. In short, practice is predominantly driven by the personal and professional values of the nurse. It is owned and controlled by the individual nurse to a great extent although governed by certain bodies representing the profession and the state.

Care

Human care is a recognizable and structured interaction in human societies through which persons give and receive assistance with basic human needs, in wellness and in illness, across the lifespan, before birth, throughout life, and beyond death. Specialized care of various kinds is delivered by professionals and is largely deemed to be deliverable only by such professionals. In contemporary society, human care, hereinafter care, should be and is largely consumer driven. Care delivery is governed, at the individual level, largely by the recipient of care or the guardian or designee of the recipient, who has the right to accept or refuse whatever care is offered.

It is axiomatic across healthcare disciplines that clients have a right to be offered care based on the best evidence available. It is not for the practitioner to decide ultimately what intervention, if any, the client will receive; rather, this decision rests with the client, who has the right to be well informed about the evidence and to make a choice. What evidence is most valued by the practitioner varies from one practitioner to the other, but all are expected to adduce evidence to justify their recommendations and offerings to clients. It is important to note that from the practitioner perspective care is offered and, within the bounds of ethics, not ordered, required, or forced, because care, in a fundamental sense, belongs to the consumer. It is the consumer's to request, accept, or reject in accord with personal values. It is the professional's responsibility to offer that for which there is best evidence. As demonstrated above, this expectation is exemplified in the standards of care that delineate the best knowledge that the health sciences have to offer at a given time.

Differentiating Practice and Care

The discourse on evidence-based practice does not differentiate clearly between practice and care. This conflation of what should be two distinct concepts is especially troubling in nursing, wherein scholars have emphasized nursing's special commitment to care and caring for generations. Upon reflection, however, one can discern a fundamental difference between the nature and structure of professional practice on the one hand and the care that is delivered by professionals on the other. In Table 19–1, four ways of differentiating practice and care are specified.

Practice belongs to the practitioner and is driven by values. Only the actor has the agency to initiate and cease deliberate actions. The practitioner is assumed to have control over her or his own actions and to be responsible for them. Nothing can remove the onus of individual responsibility from any professional practitioner, neither haste in service to one's charges, nor pressure from one's hierarchical superiors, nor lack of key information. This responsibility and relative autonomy is further emphasized at the societal level by assigning

Table 19–1 DIFFERENTIATING PRACTICE AND CARE

Practice	Care
Belongs to the practitioner	Belongs to the consumer
Controlled by the practitioner, by the profession, and by society	Controlled by the consumer, by rules/laws, and by society
More discipline specific, since it is more practitioner driven	More interdisciplinary, since it is more consumer driven
Values based	Evidence based

control and governance of the profession largely to the members of the profession itself. Professional practice is governed by the individual practitioner, her or his discipline, the governments of states and countries, laws, and societal norms. Professional practice is relatively discipline specific in that education and licensure to perform complex and sophisticated tasks to benefit others, for pay, is typically regulated in a context of disciplinary knowledge, expertise, socialization, and customary expectations.

Practice is necessarily and profoundly practitioner driven. The knowledge base and decision-making capacity of the practitioner are among the very defining factors of professional practice. Practice, as stated before, is highly contextual and situational. Many factors impinge on moment-to-moment decision making in practice. No external resource for decision making can be absorbed by the practitioner thoroughly and rapidly enough to inform all action or inaction in situation to an extent equal to individual knowledge and experience. This immediacy of intention and action is in the nature of all multidimensional, deliberative interactions among human beings.

That which most fundamentally drives one's practice is one's values. Values are by definition the cherished beliefs that prompt and inspire choices and actions over time. Making similar choices repeatedly and performing similar actions repeatedly over time confirms the value as an abiding cherished belief within one's world of meaning (Parse, 1998). The way a nurse practices and the way she or he provides care to persons reflects her or his personal and professional values (Woodbridge & Fulford, 2003). Spending time with clients may reflect a value for offering attentive presence. Frequently urging clients to make changes in health maintenance routines may reflect the values of norms or problem solving. One's values are constituents of who one is and thus are reflected in all that one does.

Care is the prerogative of the consumer and is structured by evidence. Only the consumer/client (or her/his legitimate designee) has the right to accept or reject care, even though typically care is designed and prescribed or recommended by others (i.e., professionals). This assertion is an outgrowth of the ongoing paradigm shift toward person-centered care, attending to the whole person, and respect for individual and cultural differences. The professional caregiver's responsibility is to see that the consumer's choice of care is informed and that the delivery of care is carried out competently. Legal protections and social sanctions exist to ensure that the consumer's rights to be well informed and to receive competent care are protected.

As described earlier, standards of care represent something close to the consensus state of the art of evidence-based care. All clients of healthcare professionals have the right to expect that care that is structured to the extent possible in accord with broadly recognized standards of care will be offered.

Values-Based Practice and Evidence-Based Care

We live our values. The strongest confirmation of a value is to act on it repeatedly, which also describes rather precisely how we construe professional practice. The practitioner chooses how to practice based on personal values. The client chooses what care to receive based on personal values. The practitioner offers care to address the client's needs and desires, care that is structured based on the best evidence available.

As the philosopher Raz (2003) has pointed out in his book, *The Practice of Value*, "Concepts of false values cannot have instances" (p. 24). This is another way of saying essentially that we live our values. To frame this proposition more colloquially, if you don't live it, it's not your value. In contrast, there can be false evidence. Indeed, the history of science is replete with instances of evidence misinterpreted and misunderstood. Evidence is a phenomenon that emerges only as evidence of something. The answer is already halfway there when the question is posed.

Standards of care are rewritten periodically based on newly emergent evidence, and it is not unusual for standards to seesaw back and forth between yea and nay to certain procedures between one edition of guidelines and the next. Surely something more substantial, lasting, and meaningful to both nurse and client must underpin nursing practice. To this author's way of thinking, that underpinning is found in the interface of personal meanings and values with the meanings and values structured in a theoretical framework for nursing practice. Readers are invited to use this text to assist them in identifying the values and meanings that inform and inspire their practice.

Discussion Questions

1. Do you agree with the historical development of theory in which several theories are used for practice versus the adoption of a single theory? Why?
2. How can both values and evidence guide your practice? Think about a time when these were in conflict and describe the situation and how it was or was not resolved.
3. What values underpin your practice?

References

Bernstein, R. J. (1999). *Praxis and action: Contemporary philosophies of human activity.* Philadelphia: University of Pennsylvania Press.

Coyne, A. B. (1981). Prologue. In R. R. Parse (Ed.), *Man–living–health: A theory of nursing* (pp. vii–xii). New York: John Wiley.

Franks, V. (2004). Evidence-based uncertainty in mental health nursing. *Journal of Psychiatric and Mental Health Nursing, 11,* 99–105.

Freire, P. (1993). *Pedagogy of the oppressed* (M. B. Ramos, Trans.). New York: Continuum.

Goodman, K. W. (2003). *Ethics and evidence-based medicine: Fallibility and responsibility in clinical science.* Cambridge, UK: Cambridge University Press.

Habermas, J. (1973). *Theory and practice* (J. Viertel, Trans.). Boston: Beacon.

Henderson, V. (1966). *The nature of nursing: A definition and its implications for practice, research, and education.* New York: Macmillan.

Melnyk, B. M., & Fineout-Overholt, E. (2004). *Evidence-based practice in nursing and healthcare: A guide to best practice.* Philadelphia: Lippincott Williams & Wilkins.

Nightingale, F. (1969). *Notes on nursing: What it is and what it is not.* New York: Dover. (Original published in 1859).

Parse, R. R. (1998). *The human becoming school of thought: A perspective for nurses and other health professionals.* Thousand Oaks, CA: Sage.

Peplau, H. E. (1952). *Interpersonal relations in nursing.* New York: G. P. Putnam's Sons.

Proctor, R. (1991). *Value-free science? Purity and power in modern knowledge.* Cambridge, MA: Harvard University Press.

Raz, J. (2003). *The practice of value.* Oxford, UK: Oxford University Press.

Rogers, M. E. (1970). *An introduction to the theoretical basis of nursing.* Philadelphia: F. A. Davis.

Timmermans, S., & Berg, M. (2003). *The gold standard: The challenge of evidence-based medicine and standardization in health care.* Philadelphia: Temple University Press.

Tomey, A. M., & Alligood, M. R. (Eds.). (2002). *Nursing theorists and their work* (5th ed.). St. Louis, MO: C. V. Mosby.

U.S. Department of Health and Human Services. (2004). *Seventh report of the Joint National Committee on Prevention, Detection, Evaluation and Treatment of High Blood Pressure.* Rockville, MD: Author.

Welsh, I., & Lyons, C. M. (2001). Evidence-based care and the case for intuition and tacit knowledge in clinical assessment and decision making in mental health nursing practice: An empirical contribution to the debate. *Journal of Psychiatric and Mental Health Nursing, 8,* 299–305.

Woodbridge, K., & Fulford, B. (2003). Good practice? Values-based practice in mental health. *Mental Health Practice, 7*(2), 30–34.

Chapter 20

Fundamental Patterns of Knowing in Nursing

Barbara A. Carper

CHAPTER OBJECTIVES

1. Examine four patterns of knowing that provide different perspectives and significance to the practice of nursing.
2. Apply each of the four patterns of knowing to nursing practice.

Introduction

It is the general conception of any field of inquiry that ultimately determines the kind of knowledge the field aims to develop as well as the manner in which that knowledge is to be organized, tested, and applied. The body of knowledge that serves as the rationale for nursing practice has patterns, forms, and structure that serve as horizons of expectations and exemplify characteristic ways of thinking about phenomena. Understanding these patterns is essential for the teaching and learning of nursing. Such an understanding does not extend the range of knowledge, but rather involves critical attention to the question of what it means to know and what kinds of knowledge are held to be of most value in the discipline of nursing.

Identifying Patterns of Knowing

Four fundamental patterns of knowing have been identified from an analysis of the conceptual and syntactical structure of nursing knowledge (Carper, 1975). The four patterns are distinguished according to logical type of meaning and designated as (1) empirics, the science of nursing; (2) esthetics, the art of nursing; (3) the component of a personal knowledge in nursing;

---

and (4) ethics, the component of moral knowledge in nursing.

Empirics: The Science of Nursing

The term *nursing science* was rarely used in the literature until the late 1950s. However, since that time, there has been an increasing emphasis, one might even say a sense of urgency, regarding the development of a body of empirical knowledge specific to nursing. There seems to be general agreement that there is a critical need for knowledge about the empirical world, knowledge that is systematically organized into general laws and theories for the purpose of describing, explaining, and predicting phenomena of special concern to the discipline of nursing. Most theory development and research efforts are primarily engaged in seeking and generating explanations that are systematic and controllable by factual evidence and that can be used in the organization and classification of knowledge.

The pattern of knowing that is generally designated as "nursing science" does not presently exhibit the same degree of highly integrated abstract and systematic explanations characteristic of the more mature sciences, although nursing literature reflects this as an ideal form. Clearly, there are a number of coexisting, and in a few instances competing, conceptual structures—none of which has achieved the status of what Kuhn calls a scientific paradigm. That is, no single conceptual structure is as yet generally accepted as an example of actual scientific practice "which include[s] law, theory, application, and instrumentation together . . . [and] . . . provide[s] models from which spring particular coherent traditions of scientific research" (Kuhn, 1962, p. 10). It could be argued that some of these conceptual structures

seem to have greater potential than others for providing explanations that systematically account for observed phenomena and may ultimately permit more accurate prediction and control of them. However, this is a matter to be determined by research designed to test the validity of such explanatory concepts in the context of relevant empirical reality.

New Perspectives

What seems to be of paramount importance, at least at this stage in the development of nursing science, is that these preparadigm conceptual structures and theoretical models present new perspectives for considering the familiar phenomena of health and illness in relation to the human life process; as such, they can and should be legitimately counted as discoveries in the discipline. The representation of health as more than the absence of disease is a crucial change; it permits health to be thought of as a dynamic state or process that changes over a given period of time and varies according to circumstances rather than a static either/or entity. The conceptual change in turn makes it possible to raise questions that previously would have been literally unintelligible.

The discovery that one can usefully conceptualize health as something that normally ranges along a continuum has led to attempts to observe, describe, and classify variations in health, or levels of wellness, as expressions of a human being's relationship to the internal and external environments. Related research has sought to identify behavioral responses, both physiological and psychological, that may serve as cues by which one can infer the range of normal variations of health. It has also attempted to identify and categorize significant etiological factors that serve to promote or inhibit changes in health status.

Current Stages

The science of nursing at present exhibits aspects of both the "natural history stage of inquiry" and the "stage of deductively formulated theory." The task of the natural history stage is primarily the description and classification of phenomena that are, generally speaking, ascertainable by direct observation and inspection (Northrop, 1959), but current nursing literature clearly reflects a shift from this descriptive and classification form to increasingly theoretical analysis, which is directed toward seeking, or inventing, explanations to account for observed and classified empirical facts. This shift is reflected in the change from a largely observational vocabulary to a new, more theoretical vocabulary whose terms have a distinct meaning and definition only in the context of the corresponding explanatory theory.

Explanations in the several open-system conceptual models tend to take the form commonly labeled functional or teleological (Nagel, 1961). For example, the system models explain a person's level of wellness at any particular point in time as a function of current and accumulated effects of interactions with his or her internal and external environments. The concept of adaptation is central to this type of explanation. Adaptation is seen as crucial in the process of responding to environmental demands (usually classified as stressors) and enables an individual to maintain or reestablish the steady state, which is designated as the goal of the system. The developmental models often exhibit a more genetic type of explanation in that certain events, the developmental tasks, are believed to be causally relevant or necessary conditions for the normal development of an individual.

Thus, the first fundamental pattern of knowing in nursing is empirical, factual, descriptive, and ultimately aimed at developing abstract and theoretical explanations. It is exemplary, discursively formulated, and publicly verifiable.

Esthetics: The Art of Nursing

Few, if indeed any, familiar with the professional literature would deny that primary emphasis is placed on the development of the science of nursing. One is almost led to believe that the only valid and reliable knowledge is that which is empirical, factual, objectively descriptive, and generalizable. There seems to be a self-conscious reluctance to extend the term *knowledge* to include those aspects of knowing in nursing that are not the result of empirical investigation. There is, nonetheless, what might be described as a tacit admission that nursing is, at least in part, an art. Not much effort is made to elaborate or to make explicit this esthetic pattern of knowing in nursing—other than to associate vaguely the "art" with the general category of manual and/or technical skills involved in nursing practice.

Perhaps this reluctance to acknowledge the esthetic component as a fundamental pattern of knowing in nursing originates in the vigorous efforts made in the not-so-distant past to exorcise the image of the apprentice-type educational system. Within the apprentice system, the art of nursing was closely associated with an imitative learning style and the acquisition of knowledge by accumulation of unrationalized experiences. Another likely source of reluctance is that the definition of the term *art* has been excessively and inappropriately restricted.

Weitz (1960) suggests that art is too complex and variable to be reduced to a single definition.

To conceive the task of esthetic theory as definition, he says, is logically doomed to failure in that what is called art has no common properties—only recognizable similarities. This fluid and open approach to the understanding and application of the concept of art and esthetic meaning makes possible a wider consideration of conditions, situations, and experiences in nursing that may properly be called esthetic, including the creative process of discovery in the empirical pattern of knowing.

Esthetics Versus Scientific Meaning

Despite this open texture of the concept of art, esthetic meanings can be distinguished from those in science in several important aspects. The recognition "that art is expressive rather than merely formal or descriptive," according to Rader (1960), "is about as well established as any fact in the whole field of esthetics" (p. xvi). An esthetic experience involves the creation and/or appreciation of a singular, particular, subjective expression of imagined possibilities or equivalent realities that "resists projection into the discursive form of language" (Langer, 1957). Knowledge gained by empirical description is discursively formulated and publicly verifiable. The knowledge gained by subjective acquaintance, the direct feeling of experience, defines discursive formulation. Although an esthetic expression required abstraction, it remains specific and unique rather than exemplary and leads us to acknowledge that "knowledge—genuine knowledge, understanding—is considerably wider than our discourse" (Langer, 1957, p. 23).

For Wiedenbach, the art of nursing is made visible through the action taken to provide whatever the patient requires to restore or extend his [sic] ability to cope with the demands of his [sic] situation (Wiedenbach, 1964), but the action taken, to have an esthetic quality, requires the active transformation of the immediate object—the patient's behavior—into a direct, nonmediated perception of what is significant in it—that is, what need is actually being expressed by the behavior. This perception of the need expressed is not only responsible for the action taken by the nurse but reflected in it.

The esthetic process described by Wiedenbach resembles what Dewey (1958) refers to as the difference between recognition and perception. According to Dewey, recognition serves the purpose of identification and is satisfied when a name tag or label is attached according to some stereotype or previously formed scheme of classification. Perception, however, goes beyond recognition in that it includes an active gathering together of details and scattered particulars into an experienced whole for the purpose of seeing what is there. It is perception rather than mere recognition that results in a unity of ends and means that gives the action taken an esthetic quality.

Orem (1971) speaks of the art of nursing as being "expressed by the individual nurse through her creativity and style in designing and providing nursing that is effective and satisfying" (p. 155). The art of nursing is creative in that it requires development of the ability to "envision valid modes of helping in relation to 'results' which are appropriate" (p. 69). This again invokes Dewey's (1958) sense of a perceived unity between an action taken and its result—a perception of the means of the end as an organic whole. The experience of helping must be perceived and designed as an integral component of its desired result rather than conceived separately as an independent action imposed on an independent subject. Perhaps this is what is meant by the concept of nursing the whole patient or total patient care. If so, what are the qualities that enable the creation of a design for nursing care that eliminate or would minimize the fragmentation of means and ends?

Esthetic Pattern of Knowing

Empathy—that is, the capacity for participating in or vicariously experiencing another's feelings— is an important mode in the esthetic pattern of knowing. One gains knowledge of another person's singular, particular, felt experience through empathic acquaintance (Lee, 1960; Lippo, 1960). Empathy is controlled or moderated by psychic distance or detachment in order to apprehend and abstract what we are attending to and in this sense is objective. The more skilled the nurse becomes in perceiving and empathizing with the lives of others, the more knowledge or understanding will be gained of alternate modes of perceiving reality. The nurse will thereby have available a larger repertoire of choices in designing and providing nursing care that is effective and satisfying. At the same time, increased awareness of the variety of subjective experiences will heighten the complexity and difficulty of the decision making involved.

The design of nursing care must be accompanied by what Langer (1957) refers to as sense of form, the sense of "structure, articulation, a whole resulting from the relation of mutually dependent factors, or more precisely, the way the whole is put together" (p. 16). The design, if it is to be esthetic, must be controlled by the perception of the balance, rhythm, proportion, and unity of what is done in relation to the dynamic integration and articulation of the whole. "The

doing may be energetic, and the undergoing may be acute and intense," Dewey (1958) says, but "unless they are related to each other to form a whole," what is done becomes merely a matter of mechanical routine or of caprice.

The esthetic pattern of knowing in nursing involves the perception of abstracted particulars as distinguished from the recognition of abstracted universals. It is the knowing of a unique particular rather than an exemplary class.

The Component of Personal Knowledge

Personal knowledge as a fundamental pattern of knowing in nursing is the most problematic, the most difficult to master and to teach. At the same time, it is perhaps the pattern most essential to understanding the meaning of health in terms of individual well-being. Nursing considered as an interpersonal process involves interactions, relationships, and transactions between the nurse and the patient–client. Mitchell points out that "there is growing evidence that the quality of interpersonal contacts has an influence on a person's becoming ill, coping with illness and becoming well" (Mitchell, 1973, p. 4950). Certainly the phrase "therapeutic use of self," which has become increasingly prominent in the literature, implies that the way in which nurses view their own selves and the client is of primary concern in any therapeutic relationship.

Personal knowledge is concerned with the knowing, encountering, and actualizing of the concrete, individual self. One does not know about the self; one strives simply to know the self. This knowing is a standing in relation to another human being and confronting that human being as a person. This "I–Thou" encounter is unmediated by conceptual categories or particulars abstracted from complex organic wholes (Buber, 1970). The relation is one of reciprocity, a state of being that cannot be described or even experienced—it can only be actualized. Such personal knowing extends not only to other selves but also to relations with one's own self.

It requires what Buber refers to as the sacrifice of form, that is, categories or classifications, for a knowing of infinite possibilities, as well as the risk of total commitment.

> Even as a melody is not composed of tones, nor a verse of words, nor a statue of lines— one must pull and tear to turn a unity into a multiplicity—so it is with the human being to whom I say You. . . . I have to do this again and again; but immediately he is no longer You (Buber, 1970, p. 59).

Maslow refers to this sacrifice of form as embodying a more efficient perception of reality in that reality is not generalized nor predetermined by a complex of concepts, expectations, beliefs, and stereotypes (Maslow, 1956). This results in a greater willingness to accept ambiguity, vagueness, and discrepancy of oneself and others. The risk of commitment involved in personal knowledge is what Polanyi (1964) calls the "passionate participation in the act of knowing" (p. 17).

The nurse in the therapeutic use of self rejects approaching the patient–client as an object and strives instead to actualize an authentic personal relationship between two persons. The individual is considered as an integrated, open system incorporating movement toward growth and fulfillment of human potential. An authentic personal relation requires the acceptance of others in their freedom to create themselves and the recognition that each person is not a fixed entity, but constantly engaged in the process of becoming. How then should the nurse reconcile this with the social and/or professional responsibility to control and manipulate the environmental variables and even the behavior of the person who is a patient in order to maintain or restore a steady state? If a human being is assumed to be free to choose and chooses behavior outside of accepted norms, how will this affect the action taken in the therapeutic use of self by the nurse? What choices must the nurse make in order to know another self in an authentic relation apart from the category of patient, even when categorizing for the purpose of treatment is essential to the process of nursing?

Assumptions regarding human nature, McKay (1969) observes, "Range from the existentialist to the cybernetic, from the idea of an information processing machine to one of a many splendored being" (p. 399). Many of these assumptions incorporate in one form or another the notion that there is, for all individuals, a characteristic state which they, by virtue of membership in the species, must strive to assume or achieve. Empirical descriptions and classifications reflect the assumption that being human allows for prediction of basic biological, psychological, and social behaviors that will be encountered in any given individual.

Certainly empirical knowledge is essential to the purposes of nursing, but nursing also requires that we be alert to the fact that models of human nature and their abstract and generalized categories refer to and describe behaviors and traits that groups have in common. However, none of these categories can ever encompass or express the uniqueness of the individual encountered as a person, as a "self." These and many other similar considerations are involved in the realm of personal knowledge, which can be broadly characterized as subjective, concrete, and existential. It is concerned with the kind of knowing that promotes wholeness and integrity in the personal encounter, the achievement of engagement rather than detachment, and it denies the manipulative, impersonal orientation.

Ethics: The Moral Component

Teachers and individual practitioners are becoming increasingly sensitive to the difficult personal choices that must be made within the complex context of modern health care. These choices raise fundamental questions about morally right and wrong action in connection with the care and treatment of illness and the promotion of health. Moral dilemmas arise in situations of ambiguity and uncertainty, when the consequences of one's actions are difficult to predict and traditional principles and ethical codes offer no help or seem to result in contradiction. The moral code that guides the ethical conduct of nurses is based on the primary principle of obligation embodied in the concepts of service to people and respect for human life. The discipline of nursing is held to be a valuable and essential social service responsible for conserving life, alleviating suffering, and promoting health, but appeal to the ethical "rule book" fails to provide answers in terms of difficult individual moral choices, which must be made in the teaching and practice of nursing.

The fundamental pattern of knowing identified here as the ethical component of nursing is focused on matters of obligation or what ought to be done. Knowledge of morality goes beyond simply knowing the norms or ethical codes of the discipline. It includes all voluntary actions that are deliberate and subject to the judgment of right and wrong—including judgments of moral value in relation to motives, intentions, and traits of character. Nursing is deliberate action, or a series of actions, planned and implemented to accomplish defined goals. Both goals and actions involve choices made, in part, on the basis of normative judgments, both particular and general. On occasion, the principles and norms by which such choices are made may be in conflict.

According to Berthold (1968), "Goals are, of course, value judgments not amenable to scientific inquiry and validation" (p. 196). Dickoff, James, and Wiedenbach (1968) also call attention to the need to be aware that the specification of goals serves as "a norm or standard by which to evaluate activity . . . [and] . . . entails taking them as values—that is, signifies conceiving these goal contents as situations worthy to be brought about" (p. 422).

For example, a common goal of nursing care in relation to the maintenance or restoration of health is to assist patients to achieve a state in which they are independent. Much of the current practice reflects an attitude of value attached to the goal of independence and indicates nursing actions to assist patients in assuming full responsibility for themselves at the earliest possible moment or to enable them to retain responsibility to the last possible moment. However, valuing independence and attempting to maintain it may be at the expense of the patient's learning how to live with physical or social dependence when necessary—for example, in instances when prognosis indicates that independence cannot be regained.

Differences in normative judgments may have more to do with disagreements as to what constitutes a "healthy" state of being than lack of empirical evidence or ambiguity in the application of the term. Slote (1966) suggests that the persistence of disputes, or lack of uniformity in the application of cluster terms, such as health, is due to "the difficulty of decisively resolving certain sorts of value questions about what is and is not important." This leads him to conclude, "That value judgment is far more involved in the making of what are commonly thought to be factual statements than has been imagined" (p. 220).

The ethical pattern of knowing in nursing requires an understanding of different philosophical positions regarding what is good, what ought to be desired, what is right; of different ethical frameworks devised for dealing with the complexities of moral judgments; and of various orientations to the notion of obligation. Moral choices to be made must then be considered in terms of specific actions to be taken in specific, concrete situations. The examination of the standards, codes, and values by which we decide what is morally right should result in a greater awareness of what is involved in making moral choices and being responsible for the choices made. The knowledge of ethical codes will not provide answers to the moral questions involved in nursing, nor will it eliminate the necessity for having to make moral choices, but it can be hoped that

> The more sensitive teachers and practitioners are to the demands of the process of justification, the more explicit they are about the norms that govern their actions, the more personally engaged they are in assess-

ing surrounding circumstances and potential consequences, the more "ethical" they will be; and we cannot ask much more (Greene, 1973, p. 221).

Using Patterns of Knowing

A philosophical discussion of patterns of knowing may appear to some as a somewhat idle, if not arbitrary and artificial, undertaking having little or no connection with the practical concerns and difficulties encountered in the day-to-day doing and teaching of nursing, but it represents a personal conviction that there is a need to examine the kinds of knowing that provide the discipline with its particular perspectives and significance. Understanding four fundamental patterns of knowing makes possible an increased awareness of the complexity and diversity of nursing knowledge.

Each pattern may be conceived as necessary for achieving mastery in the discipline, but none of them alone should be considered sufficient. Neither are they mutually exclusive. The teaching and learning of one pattern do not require the rejection or neglect of any of the others. Caring for another requires the achievements of nursing science, that is, the knowledge of empirical facts systematically organized into theoretical explanations regarding the phenomena of health and illness, but creative imagination also plays its part in the syntax of discovery in science, as well as in developing the ability to imagine the consequences of alternative moral choices.

Personal knowledge is essential for ethical choices in that moral action presupposes personal maturity and freedom. If the goals of nursing are to be more than conformance to un-examined norms, if the "ought" is not to be determined simply on the basis of what is possible, then the obligation to care for another human being involves becoming a certain kind of person—and not merely doing certain kinds of things. If the design of nursing care is to be more than habitual or mechanical, the capacity to perceive and interpret the subjective experiences of others and to imaginatively project the effects of nursing actions on their lives becomes a necessary skill.

Nursing thus depends on the scientific knowledge of human behavior in health and in illness, the esthetic perception of significant human experiences, a personal understanding of the unique individuality of the self, and the capacity to make choices within concrete situations involving particular moral judgments. Each of these separate but interrelated and interdependent fundamental patterns of knowing should be taught and understood according to its distinctive logic, the restricted circumstances in which it is valid, the kinds of data it subsumes, and the methods by which each particular kind of truth is distinguished and warranted.

The major significances to the discipline of nursing in distinguishing patterns of knowing are summarized as (1) the conclusions of the discipline conceived as subject matter cannot be taught or learned without reference to the structure of the discipline—the representative concepts and methods of inquiry that determine the kind of knowledge gained and limit its meaning, scope, and validity; (2) each of the fundamental patterns of knowing represents a necessary but not complete approach to the problems and questions in the discipline; and (3) all knowledge is subject to change and revision. Every solution of an existing problem raises new and unsolved questions. These new and as yet unsolved problems require, at times, new methods of inquiry and different conceptual structures; they change the shape and patterns of knowing. With each change in the shape of knowledge, teaching and learning require looking for different points of contact and connection among ideas and things. This clarifies the effect of each new thing known on other things known and the discovery of new patterns by which each connection modifies the whole.

Discussion Questions

1. What does it mean "to know?"
2. What kinds of knowledge are held to be of most value in the discipline of nursing?
3. Reflect on a specific nursing situation with a client and discuss this case from the four perspectives of knowing: (1) empirics, (2) esthetics, (3) personal knowledge, and (4) ethics. How did analyzing the situation from all four ways of knowing inform your practice? What were the similarities and differences? If you had looked at the situation only from the empirical perspective, what information would you be missing? Ask this same question for each of the four perspectives.

References

Berthold, J. S. (1968, May–June). Symposium on theory development in nursing: prologue. *Nurse Researcher, 17*, 3.

Buber, M. (1970). *I and thou*. (W. Kaufman, Trans.). New York: Charles Scribner and Sons.

Carper, B. A. (1975). *Fundamental patterns of knowing in nursing*. PhD dissertation, Teachers College, Columbia University, New York.

Dewey, J. (1958). *Art as experience*. New York: Capricorn Books.

Dickoff, J., James, P., & Wiedenbach, E. (1968, September–October). Theory in a practice discipline: Part I. *Nurse Researcher, 17*, 422.

Greene, M. (1973). *Teacher as stranger*. Belmont, CA: Wadsworth Publishing Co., Inc.

Kuhn, T. (1962). *The structure of scientific revolutions*. Chicago: University of Chicago Press.

Langer, S. K. (1957). *Problems of art*. New York: Charles Scribner and Sons.

Lee, V. (1960). Empathy. In M. Rader (Ed.), *A modern book of esthetics* (3rd ed.). New York: Holt, Rinehart and Winston.

Lippo, T. (1960). Empathy, inner imitation and sense-feeling. In M. Rader (Ed.), *A modern book of esthetics* (3rd ed.). New York: Holt, Rinehart and Winston.

Maslow, A. H. (1956). Self-actualizing people: A study of psychological health. In C. E. Moustakas (Ed.), *The self*. New York: Harper and Row.

McKay, R. (1969, September–October). Theories, models and systems for nursing. *Nurse Researcher, 18*, 5.

Mitchell, P. H. (1973). *Concepts basic to nursing*. New York: McGraw-Hill Book Co.

Nagel, E. (1961). *The structure of science*. New York: Harcourt, Brace and World, Inc.

Northrop, F. S. C. (1959). *The logic of the sciences and the humanities*. New York: The World Publishing Co.

Orem, D. E. (1971). *Nursing: Concepts of practice*. New York: McGraw-Hill Book Co.

Polanyi, M. (1964). *Personal knowledge*. New York: Harper and Row.

Rader, M. (1960). Introduction: The meaning of art. In M. Rader (Ed.), *A modern book of esthetics* (3rd ed.). New York: Holt, Rinehart and Winston, 1960.

Slote, M. A. (1966, April 14). The theory of important criteria. *Journal of Philosophy, 63*.

Weitz, M. (1960). The role of theory in aesthetics. In M. Rader (Ed.), *A modern book of esthetics* (3rd ed.). New York: Holt, Rinehart and Winston.

Wiedenbach, E. (1964). *Clinical nursing: A helping art*. New York: Springer Publishing Co., Inc.

Chapter 21

Patterns of Knowing: Review, Critique, and Update

Jill White

CHAPTER OBJECTIVES

1. Discuss each of the patterns of knowing as first defined by Carper.
2. Explore the extension of the patterns of knowing as developed by the Jacobs-Kramer and Chinn model.
3. Assess how the current view on knowing influences advanced nursing practice.

Introduction

In 1978 Barbara Carper published "Fundamental Patterns of Knowing in Nursing" in the first edition of *Advances in Nursing Science*. Based on her doctoral work, the article described her typology of patterns of knowing in nursing. These patterns she named empirics, esthetics, ethics, and personal knowing.

Carper's patterns of knowing have been much cited and commented on, albeit somewhat uncritically, in the writing of nurses over the ensuing years. As with much of nursing's written heritage, there is little connection between the number of citations and the extent of critical development that has taken place. An important

exception to this, however, is the work of Jacobs-Kramer and Chinn (1988) a decade after Carper's article first appeared. Jacobs-Kramer and Chinn extended Carper's framework by producing a model that elucidated their understanding of the creation and development, the expression and transmission, and the assessment of each of Carper's patterns of knowing. Their intention was for such an elucidation to facilitate the integration of these patterns of knowing in nursing into clinical practice.

The lack of recent dialogue about the patterns themselves or about the model may reflect the decreased interest in the use of models generally in nursing, part of a move from reductionist thinking. The continued citation of

Source: White, J. (1995). Patterns of knowing: Review, critique, and update. *Advances in Nursing Science, 17*(4): 73–86. Reprinted with permission from Lippincott, Williams & Wilkins.

both Carper and Jacobs-Kramer and Chinn, however, suggests their work is still being used in teaching.

The "patterns" of Carper (1978) and "model" of Jacobs-Kramer and Chinn (1988) do provide convenient conceptual organizers for introducing students to different ways of knowing in nursing. The patterns and model can be used to facilitate exploration of nursing practice and to enhance understanding of the rich history of modern nursing writing. They enable the contributions of nurses from the past to be analyzed in terms of the dominant social, political, and philosophical contexts of their time and enable nurses to trace with understanding the cumulative and disparate knowledge development that contributes to the discipline of nursing.

Given that the patterns and the model are still being used in education, it is appropriate that they be reviewed and critiqued within the context of nursing knowledge development in the mid-1990s. This article offers such a review, critique, and update.

In her seminal article, "Fundamental Patterns of Knowing in Nursing," Carper (1978) identified the following patterns:

- empirics, or the science of nursing
- ethics, or the moral component
- the component of personal knowledge
- esthetics, or the art of nursing

In this article the author explores each of these patterns in turn, looking first at what Carper had to say, then at the extension of this pattern within the Jacobs-Kramer and Chinn model, and finally at questions that arise with references to the current literature and each particular pattern. Table 21–1 summarizes the essential elements of Jacobs-Kramer and Chinn's model of nursing knowledge.

Empirics: The Science of Nursing

Carper described empirics as

> knowledge that is systematically organized into general laws and theories for the purpose of describing, explaining, and predicting phenomena of special concern to the discipline of nursing. . . . The first fundamental pattern of knowing in nursing is empirical, factual, descriptive, and ultimately aimed at developing abstract theoretical explanations. It is exemplary, discursively formulated, and publicly verifiable (Carper, 1978, pp. 14–15).

The key element here is that the "ultimate aim" of this knowing is "theory" development. Inherent in theory development is the ontological position that nature has a single or dominant reality commonly experienced and about which one can draw generalizable abstract explanations. This clearly encompasses the traditional view of scientific knowledge with its stance of objectivity and context-free replicability. This view was the dominant one in the nursing research and writing at the time of Carper's doctoral work. However, it is debatable at this time whether this pattern encompasses all research-based knowing, which Jacobs-Kramer and Chinn (1988) expressed as "facts, theories, models and descriptions that impart understanding" (p. 132).

The realist ontological position, whose assumptions allow generalization, may also be seen as including grounded theory and ethnographic research, which generate generalizable abstractions. However, the relativist position of the interpretive paradigm as represented by

---

Table 21–1 SUMMARY OF ESSENTIAL ELEMENTS: MODEL OF NURSING KNOWLEDGE

Dimension	Empirics	Ethics	Personal	Esthetics
Creative	Describing	Valuing	Encountering	Engaging
	Explaining	Clarifying	Focusing	Interpreting
	Predicting	Advocating	Realizing	Envisioning
Expressive	Facts	Codes	Self: Authentic	Art-act
	Theories	Standards	and disclosed	
	Models	Normative-ethical theories		
	Descriptions to impart understanding	Descriptions of ethical decision making		
Assessment: Critical question	What does this represent?	Is this right?	Do I know what I do?	What does this question mean?
	How is this representative?	Is this just?	Do I do what I know?	
Process-context	Replication	Dialogue	Response and reflection	Criticism
Credibility index	Validity	Justness	Congruity	Consensual meaning

phenomenology, for example, also seeks to provide "descriptions that impart understanding" but would not be consistent with Carper's (1978) definition of having an ultimate aim of developing abstract theoretical explanations that could be "systematically organized into general laws and theories" (p. 14).

It is therefore suggested that the definition of the empirical pattern of knowing needs to be modified to accommodate the relativist ontological positions of knowledge development using methodologies such as phenomenology. If

not modified, nursing needs to acknowledge the limitations of this definitions in encompassing empirical knowing that seeks not to generalize, but rather through interpretation or description to put before the reader context-embedded stories whose purpose is to enrich understanding.

The inclusion of the word "understanding" by Jacobs-Kramer and Chinn (1988) within the aim of the empirical pattern of knowing may be confusing; "understanding" is more commonly associated with the aim of research within the interpretive paradigm. The ontological position of the interpretive paradigm embraces the notion of multiple realities that cannot be generalized and puts this paradigm outside Carper's definition of this pattern of knowing. As discussed later, interpretive and critical research is encompassed more appropriately elsewhere.

Jacobs-Kramer and Chinn's (1988) model suggests that the pattern of empirics is expressed through "facts, theories, models and descriptions" (p. 132). This expressive dimension may be extended to include the common mode of expression and transmission via books for academic theoretical instruction and professional journals for stimulation of professional debate.

Jacobs-Kramer and Chinn's (1988) assessment dimension asks the critical questions, "What does this represent?" and "How is it representative?" The process of assessment is by replication, and the index of credibility they suggest is validity—that the knowledge can be demonstrated to be what it is thought to be. The assessment dimension is dealt with in their article in a brief paragraph that makes it somewhat difficult to fully grasp the intent of the critical questions; a critical question, one would assume, inquires about the relationships between the variables under study and the generalizability of the relationships.

In the case of grounded theory, a critical question would be the relationship to the core concepts of the other concepts and the nature of these relationships. The process of judging the trustworthiness of the results would require both sufficient detail to enable replication and application and the seeking out and offering up to professional debate of the findings. As Kuhn (1970) said, "There is no standard higher than assent of the relevant community" (p. 94). The remaining process for ascertaining credibility is the "fit" of the new knowledge with the extant knowledge in the area at the time.

It is within this assessment dimension that the case for empirics, not including work using the interpretive or critical paradigm, gains credence. Here, clearly, the standards of credibility are not related to validity, replication, or relationships between variables or categories. If the empirical pattern were to be expanded to accommodate knowledge created through interpretive or critical work, an entirely new assessment would be required with different critical questions, processes, and credibility indices (Sandelowski, 1993). Possible modifications to the pattern of empirics within the model of nursing knowledge are proposed in Table 21–2.

Ethics: The Moral Component

"The fundamental pattern of knowing identified here as the ethical component of nursing is focused on matters of obligation or what ought to be done" (Carper, 1978, p. 20). In exploring this pattern Carper acknowledged the important place of knowledge of norms and ethical codes: "The examination of the standards, codes, and values by which we decide what is morally right should result in a greater awareness of what is involved in making moral choices and being responsible for the choices made" (p. 21).

However, Carper (1978) goes on to caution that the complexity of the ethical issues in modern health care practice means that "moral choices to be made must be considered in terms of specific actions to be taken in specific concrete situations" (p. 21). In extending this caution, Carper represents one of the earliest nursing writers to speak of the situational and

Table 21–2 EMPIRICS: ESSENTIAL ELEMENTS

Dimension	Original Model[a]	Modifications
Creative	Describing	Describing
	Explaining	Explaining
	Predicting	Predicting
Expressive	Facts	Facts
	Theories	Theories and models described in books and
	Models	professional journals
	Descriptions to impart understanding	Descriptions that indicate relationships
Assessment:	What does this represent?	What relationships were found?
Critical question	How is it representative?	Under what conditions do these relationships hold?
Process-context	Replication	Replication and application
		Professional debate
		Fit with extant knowledge
Credibility index	Validity	Validity
	Reliability	Reliability

[a]Jacobs-Kramer & Chinn, 1988.

relational importance of moral decision making, which has become fundamental to the ethic of care now so prevalent in the nursing literature.

There has been a plethora of publications in the area of moral knowing. Principal among these are the works of Benner (1984; 1991), Benner and Wrubel (1989), Bishop and Scudder (1985; 1990), Cooper (1990; 1991), and Watson (1985; 1990). Not directly within nursing but highly relevant are the works of Gilligan (1979; 1982), Noddings (1984), Pellegrino (1982; 1985), and Zaner (1985; 1988).

Much of this work has its origins in Gilligan's (1979) critique of Kohlberg's (1981) hierarchy of moral decision making. Gilligan challenged Kohlberg's contention that believing in "the primacy and universality of individual rights" was the highest form of moral development and that this represented a morally superior position to Kohlberg's penultimate stage, which embodies a "very strong sense of being responsible to the world" (Gilligan, 1979, p. 444). Gilligan suggested that the focus on individual justice is a predominantly male orientation, whereas women more commonly adopt the contextual, relational, care orientation that focuses on social and moral good.

Moss (1992) provided an excellent exploration of the impact of Gilligan's work over the past 15 years, particularly in relation to nursing.

Together with Moss, Bishop and Scudder (1990), Benner (1991), and Watson (1985; 1990) suggested that the moral ideal of doing what is good (that is, adopting a caring orientation), rather than that which is just, will most fruitfully be revealed through the exploration of practice rather than simply through reference to "rule-books." This, they suggested, will happen through processes of reflection, discussion, and storytelling of life and nursing practice (Benner, 1991; Bishop & Scudder, 1990). Bishop and Scudder made a particularly salient point for nurses within this discussion by questioning the notion that moral decision making is about "solving" dilemmas at all: "One way in which the moral sense differs from traditional nursing ethics is that it directs us to moral dilemmas which cannot be solved but must be lived with and, when possible, ameliorated" (1990, p. 124).

Zaner (1985), with reference to physicians but equally applicable to nursing, suggested "Moral life is essentially communal at its root, and it is mutuality (in all its complex forms), not autonomy, that is foundational. Nowhere is this more plainly evident than in the contexts of clinical situations dealing with ill persons" (p. 292). Zaner went on to say that "autonomy and rights" inhibit moral decision making within health care, which requires, foundationally, cooperation and collaboration.

Cooperation is also emphasized in the work of Gadow (1980) on existential advocacy. She reinforced the importance of collaboratively making "the effort to help persons become clear about what they want to do, by helping them discern their values in the situation and on the basis of that self examination, to reach decisions which express their reaffirmed, perhaps recreated, complex of values" (p. 44). Gadow put this effort forward as a moral ideal, not duty, norm,

or prescription. It is a moral enterprise through situated engagement.

Jacobs-Kramer and Chinn (1988) focused on justice in their assessment dimension of this pattern. An expansion of the assessment dimension is required to accommodate an ethic of care as well as an ethic of justice. Thus, potential modifications to the ethical pattern of knowing are listed in Table 21–3.

The discussion about ethics shows how intimately linked the patterns of moral and personal knowing are. Moral knowing requires fundamentally an authentic interpersonal involvement for its development.

Personal Knowing

The pattern of personal knowing is concerned with "the knowing, encountering and actualizing of the concrete individual self. One does not know about self; one strives simply to know the self. This knowing is a standing in relation to another human being and confronting that human being as a person" (Carper, 1978, p. 18). The pattern of personal knowing develops when the nurse approaches the patient not as an object or category of illness, but strives instead "to actualize an authentic personal relationship between two persons" (Carper, 1978, p. 19). This pattern requires the nurse to allow the person who is the patient–client to "matter." It involves engagement as opposed to detachment.

Mayeroff, whom Carper (1978) cited as a source for her notion of personal knowing, saw a special feature of caring for a person as being "able to understand [the person] and his world as if I were inside it" (Mayeroff, 1971, p. 42). For Mayeroff, relationship is about reciprocity, about helping the other "grow" and through

Table 21-3 ETHICS: ESSENTIAL ELEMENTS

Dimension	Original Model[a]	Modifications
Creative	Valuing	Valuing the moral idea of caring
	Clarifying	Critically appraising values
	Advocating	Existential advocacy[b]
		Sensitizing to other value positions
		Fostering articulation of everyday notions of good[c]
Expressive	Codes, standards	Codes, standards
	Normative theories	Normative theories
	Descriptions of decision making	Observation
		Storytelling to explore embedded notions of good
Assessment: Critical question	Is it right?	Is it good?
	Is it just?	Is it just?
		Is it right?
		Does it embody caring?
Process-context	Dialogue	Dialogue
		Critical reflection
		Collaborative values elaboration
Credibility index	Justness	Justness
		Goodness
		Caring
		Congruence with personal values of patients

[a]Jacobs-Kramer & Chinn, 1988.
[b]Gadow, 1980.
[c]Benner, 1991.

this, growing oneself. However, Mayeroff's words harbor subtle paternalism: "I want it to grow in its own right . . . and I feel the other's growth as bound up with my own sense of well-being" (1971, p. 8). Such a position mitigates against genuine reciprocity.

Mayeroff's reciprocity was elaborated on and refined in the works of Watson (1985) in describing her concept of "transcendental moment," by Taylor (1992) in her exposition of the "ordinariness" of nursing, in Morse's (1991) work on nurse–patient relationships, and in Moch (1990) in her exploration of "personal knowing," and probably most well known within nursing is Benner's (1984) seminal work *From Novice to Expert*. Benner's notion of involvement and engagement was further developed collaboratively with Tanner (Benner & Tanner, 1987) on intuition and with Wrubel (Benner & Wrubel, 1989) on the primacy of caring.

The idea of "being-with," of presence, of letting the person matter and being open to help that person make meaning out of his or her experience, is an essential feature of nursing practice. Without this knowing of self that allows an openness to the knowing of another person, nursing is only technical assistance, not involved care. In Carper's words, "It is concerned with the kind of knowing that promotes wholeness and integrity in the personal encounter, the achievement of engagement rather than detachment, and it denies the manipulative, impersonal orientation" (1978, p. 20).

In the model of nursing knowledge described by Jacobs-Kramer and Chinn (1988), the pattern of personal knowing is seen as being created by "experiencing the self-encountering and focusing on self while realizing the realities and potentialities" (p. 135). It also involves "experiencing, encountering and focusing" (p. 135). These are not easy concepts to grasp. Carper herself said of this pattern that it "is the most problematic, the most difficult to master and to teach. At the same time, it is perhaps the pattern most essential to understanding the meaning of health in terms of individual well-being" (Carper, 1978, p. 18).

The creation of personal knowing may be enhanced through the use of art, poetry, literature, and storytelling in an endeavor to more truly "understand [the person] and his world as if I were inside it" (Mayeroff, 1971, p. 42). An example of this is poetry about childbirth that helps the midwife "see" inside the patient's world; poems such as Sharon Doubiago's "South American Mi Hija" (in Chester, 1989) show the intensity that can allow the soul to grow, whereas stories such as Anais Nin's "Birth" (in Chester, 1989) illuminate the potential for the soul to shrivel if a woman is not supported by the right kind of caring. Poems such as "Sunshine Across Living Centre" in Krysl and Watson (1988) help nurses "see" the humanity of nurse and patient in interaction. The expressive dimension is the self as authentic (privately known) and disclosed (revealed to others): "Personal knowledge is expressed as ourselves, through the self" (Jacobs-Kramer & Chinn, p. 135).

The assessment of this pattern comes through the "focus on the self as privately known and expressed to others. Assessment of self is a process carried out by the self through a rich inner life" (Jacobs-Kramer & Chinn, p. 135). The critical questions involve exploration for congruence between knowing what we do and doing what we know, between the authentic and disclosed self. The process through which this assessment is made is the reflection and response of others to us, which we reflect on in turn. Agan (1987) put it succinctly by suggesting that "credibility of this type of knowing is determined through individual reflection that is informed by the responses of others" (p. 70). The credibility index is therefore congruence with the authentic and disclosed self.

Although the volume of literature in this area has provided much clarification and extension of the notion of personal knowing, the "essential elements" identified by Jacobs-Kramer and Chinn (1988) are still pertinent. An elaboration could include, within the creative dimension, some examples of the means by which "encountering, focusing and realizing" might be facilitated (e.g., poetry, art, literature, and storytelling) and within the process-context dimension, reflection informed by the response of others (see Table 21–4).

Table 21–4 EMPIRICS: PERSONAL KNOWING

Dimension	Original Model[a]	Modifications
Creative	Encountering Focusing Realizing	Encountering, focusing, and realizing through practice and through art, literature, poetry, and storytelling
Expressive	Self: Authentic and disclosed	Self: Authentic and disclosed
Assessment: Critical question	Do I know what I do? Do I do what I know?	Do I know what I do? Do I do what I know?
Process-context	Response and reflection	Reflection informed by the response of others and our reflection on our response to the life-world of others
Credibility index	Congruity	Congruity

[a]Jacobs-Kramer & Chinn, 1988.

Esthetics: The Art of Nursing

Carper (1978) suggested that the delay in explicating the esthetic pattern of knowing is associated with nursing's attempt to see itself as scientific and to "exorcise the image of the apprentice-type education system" (p. 16). This delay has certainly been overcome, and there has been intense interest in this pattern recently. The pattern had its beginnings in the works of many early nursing writers. Wiedenbach (1985) suggested that esthetic practice is making "visible through action" the nurse's perception of what the patient needs. Orem (1971) spoke of the "creativity and style in design" of the provision of care. Orem also mentioned as necessary in artful practice the ability to "envision" models of helping with regard to the appropriate

outcomes. Benner (1984) was foremost in the development of the notion of perceiving the whole of a situation, without reference to rational processes, in her work on expert nursing practice. The concept of "intuitive" knowing developed by Benner and Tanner (1987), Rew (1988), and Agan (1987) (and mentioned earlier as part of personal knowing) is an important component of perceiving and envisioning.

The design of the art-act combines all patterns of knowing in its esthetic form—it is all of and more than the other patterns: "The design, if it is to be esthetic, must be controlled by the perception of balance, rhythm, proportion and unity of what is done in relation to the dynamic integration and articulation of the whole" (Carper, 1978, p. 18).

Carper named "empathy" as an important mode in the esthetic pattern of knowing; however, there is currently debate in the nursing literature over the appropriateness of this concept for nursing. Morse, Bottorff, Anderson, O'Brien, and Solberg (1992) suggested that "empathy was uncritically adopted from psychology and is actually a poor fit for the clinical reality of nursing practice" (p. 273). They recommended exploration of other communication strategies that have been devalued, such as sympathy, pity, consolation, compassion, and commiseration. To these Taylor (1992) might add affiliation, fun, and friendship.

Whatever the definitional outcome, the basic requirement of effective and authentic interpersonal engagement remains. This is highlighted in the recent Australian work of Taylor (1992) and in the innovative work of Lumby (1993) in her development of a critical feminist methodology for exploring nursing.

According to Jacobs-Kramer and Chinn,

> Esthetic knowledge finds expression in the art-act of nursing. Like personal knowledge, the expression of esthetic knowledge is not in language. We can unfold our art and retrospectively recollect and write about its features, and we can record it using electronic media, but the knowledge form itself is not what we write or record. The knowledge form is the art-act (1988, p. 137).

They then proceeded to raise an important issue, albeit indirectly, that experience is an important component of esthetic knowing:

> As practice contexts are encountered, processes within the creative dimension of esthetics are initiated. Through the process of engagement, interpreting, and envisioning, "past" knowledge is enfolded into esthetics, and clients are uniquely cared for.

As caring processes continue, new knowledge merges (Jacobs-Kramer & Chinn, 1988, pp. 137–138).

In putting forward experience as a necessary condition to esthetic practice, it may be necessary to include this context-specific experience as part of the creative and generative dimension, suggested by Jacobs-Kramer and Chinn as including "engaging, interpreting, and envisioning." The addition of experience, particularly context-specific experience, suggests that these acts are cumulative, aligning with Benner's (1984) position that expertise is context specific and not a transferable skill.

In exploring the assessment dimension within Carper's model of knowledge, Jacobs-Kramer and Chinn followed her inclusion of notions of esthetic appreciation from other art forms. They suggested that the critical question is, "What does this mean?"

Criticism requires empathy and an intent to fully appreciate what the actors meant to convey. As the art-act is criticized, credibility is discerned by reaching for consensus—a full and rich understanding of the art-act that brings together the perspectives of a community of co-askers who construct and confer meanings (Jacobs-Kramer & Chinn, 1988).

Table 21–5 presents the essential elements for the esthetic pattern.

The major point of Jacobs-Kramer and Chinn's model development appears to be the unfolding of a story that suggests that each pattern may be seen by "examination of the art-act that integrates all knowledge patterns as expressed in practice . . . [as it] provides a comprehensive, context-sensitive means for enfolding multiple knowledge patterns" (p. 138). This, they suggested, leads nursing away from

Table 21–5 ESTHETICS: ESSENTIAL ELEMENTS

Dimension	Original Model[a]	Modifications
Creative	Engaging	Cumulative experience by engaging, interpreting,
	Interpreting	and envisioning and including the "artful
	Envisioning	enfoldment" of all other patterns
Expressive	Art-act	Art-act
Assessment:		
Critical question	What does this mean?	What does this mean?
Process-context	Criticism	Exhibition and criticism
		Recognition as authentic to other nurses
Credibility index	Consensual meaning	Consensual meaning

[a]Jacobs-Kramer & Chinn, 1988.

"a quest for structural truth and towards a search for dynamic meaning" (p. 138).

The model and its exposition of essential elements provide critical questions that may structure our process of inquiry, processes by which the inquiry might take place, and credibility indices to which claims of rigor may be addressed. If it is to be useful in the process of our practice-based inquiry, the model must adequately account for all patterns of knowing and their appropriate processes of inquiry.

Sociopolitical Knowing: Context of Nursing

The patterns and inquiry processes in Jacobs-Kramer and Chinn's (1988) model appear adequate to the description of the nurse–patient relationship and the persons of the nurse and the patient. What appears to be missing is the context—the sociopolitical environment of the persons and their interaction. This represents a fifth pattern of knowing essential to an understanding of all the others.

The other patterns address the "who," the "how," and the "what" of nursing practice. The pattern of sociopolitical knowing addresses the "wherein." It lifts the gaze of the nurse from the introspective nurse–patient relationship and situates it within the broader context in which nursing and health care take place. It causes the nurse to question the taken-for-granted assumptions about practice, the profession, and health policies.

Sociopolitical knowing may be conceptualized as including understandings on two levels: (1) the sociopolitical context of the persons (nurse and patient), and (2) the sociopolitical context of nursing as a practice profession, including both society's understanding of nursing and nursing's understanding of society and its politics.

The sociopolitical context of the persons of the nurse–patient relationship fundamentally concerns cultural identity, for it is in culture that "self" is intrinsically located. This cultural location influences each person's understanding of health and disease causation, language, identity, and connection to the land. Such understanding goes well beyond Carper's (1978) or Mayeroff's (1971) notion of personal knowing. It is related to deeply embedded historical issues of connection to and dislocation from land and heritage.

Chopoorian (1986) suggested that "nursing ideas lack an archaeology of the social, political, and economic worlds that influence both client states and nursing roles" (p. 41). She claimed that unequal class structure, power relationships, and political and economic power produce sexism, racism, ageism, and classism, which in turn affect health and result in illness. Chopoorian continued, "Nursing practitioners continually confront the human responses to the underlying social dynamics of poverty, unemployment, undernutrition, isolation and alienation precipitated through the structures of society" (pp. 40–41).

Violence, drug dependence, and diabetes are examples of responses to what are inherently political rather than simply personal problems, and nurses' efforts to deal with them require nurses to articulate what they see resulting from societies' structures. Stevens (1989) suggested that nurses must provide a "critique of domination within fundamental social, political and economic structures and the analysis of how domination affects the health of persons and communities" (p. 58). This effect includes the position and visibility of nursing in policy planning and decision making about health issues.

To have a voice in these decisions, nurses must both be articulate about what they know and do and be recognized by others as having something to contribute to debate. Nurses must have an understanding of the gatekeeping mechanisms within the political arena and their function. It is a paradox that when people are involved with nurses and nursing as patients or as concerned friends, the contribution of nurses is prized. Why then is it so quickly forgotten when these same people are influencing healthcare decisions? Diers and Fagin (1981) suggested that the reason is visible in the metaphors the public associates with nursing, which include nurturance, dependence, and intimacy. These images are often reminders of personal pain and vulnerability, the natural reaction to which is suppression. To resurface an understanding of nursing is to resurface the context and all that is associated with it. Nurses must find a way of helping people remember, when they are well and politically able, what they knew of nursing when in crisis. Nurses must find the intersections between the health-related interests of the public and nursing and must become involved and active participants in these interests.

A sociopolitical understanding in which to frame all other patterns of knowing is an essential part of nursing's future in an increasingly economically driven world. Nurses must explore and expose alternative constructions of health and health care, find means of enabling all concerned to have a voice in this care provision, and develop processes of shared governance for the future. Table 21–6 illustrates how the sociopolitical dimension might be added to the model of knowing.

As Chinn (1991) said of nursing in the next century, "it is time to construct critical analyses of our present that are informed by the ethical and political ideals that we seek. It is time to

Table 21–6 SOCIOPOLITICAL KNOWING: ESSENTIAL ELEMENTS	
Dimension	Characteristics
Creative	Exposing and exploring alternate constructions of reality
Expressive	Transformation
	Critique
Assessment: Critical question	Whose voice is heard?
	Whose voice is silenced?
Process-context	Critique and hearing all voices
Credibility index	Shared governance, enlightenment
	Movement toward equality

begin to envision what our future nursing might be like and to create knowledge and skills that we need to begin to make it happen" (p. 56). Understanding the context of nursing practice is fundamental to this endeavor. Appreciation and exploration of all the patterns of knowing in nursing and their interactions can contribute to the future articulation and development of nursing practice and nurses' place in determining the future of nursing practice and of health care.

Discussion Questions

1. Assess how each of the patterns of knowing has developed over time.
2. What is the current understanding of these patterns as developed by the Jacobs-Kramer and Chinn model?
3. Relook at the practice situation you discussed in Chapter 20 and assess how your understanding of this situation has changed using the new thinking.

References

Agan, R. D. (1987). Intuitive knowing as a dimension of nursing. *Advances in Nursing Science, 10*(1), 64–70.

Benner, P. (1984). *From novice to expert: Excellence and power in clinical nursing practice.* Menlo Park, CA: Addison-Wesley.

Benner, P. (1991). The role of experience, narrative, and community in skilled ethical comportment. *Advances in Nursing Science, 14*(2), 1–21.

Benner, P., & Tanner, C. (1987). Clinical judgment: How expert nurses use intuition. *The American Journal of Nursing, 87,* 23–31.

Benner, P., & Wrubel, J. (1989). *The primacy of caring: Stress and coping in health and illness.* Menlo Park, CA: Addison-Wesley.

Bishop, A., & Scudder, J. (Eds.). (1985). *Caring, curing, coping.* University, AL: University of Alabama Press.

Bishop, A., & Scudder, J. (1990). *The practical, moral and personal sense of nursing.* Albany: State University of New York Press.

Carper, B. (1978). Fundamental patterns of knowing in nursing. *Advances in Nursing Science, 1*(1), 13–23.

Chester, L. (Ed.). (1989). *Cradle and all.* Boston: Faber & Faber.

Chinn, P. (1991). Looking into the crystal ball: Positioning ourselves for the year 2000. *Nursing Outlook, 39*(6), 251–256.

Chopoorian, T. (1986). Reconceptualizing the environment. In P. Moccia (Ed.), *New approaches in theory development.* New York: National League for Nursing.

Cooper, M. (1990). Reconceptualizing nursing ethics. *Scholarly Inquiry for Nursing Practice, 4*(3), 209–218.

Cooper, M. (1991). Principle-oriented ethics and the ethic of care: Creative tension. *Advances in Nursing Science, 14*(2), 22–31.

Diers, D., & Fagin, C. (1981). Nursing as a metaphor. *New England Journal of Medicine, 309*(2), 116–117.

Gadow, S. (1980). Existential advocacy: Philosophical foundation of nursing. In S. Spicker & S. Gadow (Eds.), *Nursing: Images and ideals—Opening dialogue with the humanities.* New York: Springer.

Gilligan, C. (1979). In a different voice: Women's conception of self and morality. *Harvard Educational Review, 47*, 481–517.

Gilligan, C. (1982). *In a different voice.* Cambridge, MA: Harvard University Press.

Jacobs-Kramer, M., & Chinn, P. (1988). Perspectives on knowing: A model of nursing knowledge. *Scholarly Inquiry for Nursing Practice, 2*(2), 129–139.

Kohlberg, L. (1981). *The philosophy of moral development.* San Francisco: Harper & Row.

Krysl, M., & Watson, J. (1988). Existential moments of caring: Facets of nursing and social support. *Advances in Nursing Science, 10*(2), 12–17.

Kuhn, T. (1970). *The structure of scientific revolutions.* Chicago: University of Chicago Press.

Lumby, J. (1993). *A woman's experience of illness: The emergence of a feminist method for nursing.* Geelong, Victoria, Australia: Deakin University.

Mayeroff, M. (1971). *On caring.* New York: Harper & Row.

Moch, S. (1990). Personal knowing: Evolving research and practice. *Scholarly Inquiry for Nursing Practice, 4*(2), 155–165.

Morse, J. (1991). Negotiating commitment and involvement in the nurse–patient relationship. *Journal of Advanced Nursing, 16,* 455–468.

Morse, J., Bottorff, J., Anderson, G., O'Brien, B., & Solberg S. (1992). Beyond empathy: expanding expressions of caring. *Advanced Nursing, 17,* 809–821.

Moss, C. (1992). Has Gilligan's "Different Voice" made a difference? In *Nursing research: Scholarship for practice.* Geelong, Victoria, Australia: Deakin Institute of Nursing Research, Deakin University.

Noddings, N. (1984). *Caring—A feminine approach to ethics and moral education.* Berkeley: University of California Press.

Orem, D. (1971). *Nursing: Concepts of practice.* New York: McGraw-Hill.

Pellegrino, E. (1982). Being ill and being healed. In V. Kestenbaum (Ed.), *The humanity of the ill.* Knoxville: University of Tennessee Press.

Pellegrino, E. (1985). The caring ethic. In A. Bishop & J. Scudder (Eds.), *Caring, curing, coping.* University, AL: University of Alabama Press.

Rew, L. (1988). Intuition and decision-making. *Image—The Journal of Nursing Scholarship, 20*(3), 150–154.

Sandelowski, M. (1993). Rigor or rigor mortis: The problem of rigor in qualitative research revisited. *Advances in Nursing Science, 16*(2), 1–8.

Stevens, P. (1989). A critical social reconstruction of environment in nursing: implications for methodology. *Advances in Nursing Science, 11*(4), 56–68.

Taylor, B. (1992). Enhancement of the nursing encounter through a shared humanity. In *Nursing research: Scholarship for practice.* Geelong, Victoria, Australia: Deakin Institute of Nursing Research, Deakin University.

Watson, J. (1985). *Nursing: Human science and human care.* Norwalk, CT: Appleton-Century-Crofts.

Watson, J. (1990). The moral failure of the patriarchy. *Nursing Outlook, 28*(2), 62–66.

Wiedenbach, E. (1985). *Clinical nursing: A helping out.* New York: Springer-Verlag.

Zaner, R. (1985). How the hell did I get here? In A. Bishop & J. Scudder (Eds.), *Caring, curing, coping.* University, AL: University of Alabama Press.

Zaner, R. (1988). *Ethics and the clinical encounter.* Englewood Cliffs, NJ: Prentice Hall.

Chapter 22

Multiple Paradigms of Nursing Science

Elizabeth J. Monti
and
Martha S. Tingen

CHAPTER OBJECTIVES

1. Compare and contrast empiricism and interpretative paradigm.
2. Debate the pros and cons of adapting a single paradigm versus multiple paradigms of nursing science.

Introduction

A discipline is a community of interest that is organized around the accumulated knowledge of an academic or professional group (Donaldson & Crowley, 1997). The discipline of nursing represents the body of knowledge related to the study of caring in human health that encompasses both the science and art of nursing (Donaldson & Crowley, 1997; Newman, Sime, & Corcoran-Perry, 1991). Within the discipline, nursing science is devoted to answering questions of interest to the profession and adding to the body of knowledge. Nursing practice represents the art of the discipline.

The unique perspective of the discipline is exemplified by the metaparadigm, which describes, from a global perspective, the concepts and themes chosen as the focus of the discipline and those that differentiate it from others (Fawcett, 1989). The metaparadigm concepts of nursing generally are agreed to be person, environment, nursing, and health; however, these are not exclusive (Chinn & Kramer, 1995; Fawcett, 1984; Fawcett, 1989; Newman et al., 1991). The metaparadigm also reflects the shared values and beliefs of the discipline. For example, nurses subscribe to common values and beliefs, including respect for persons, caring, autonomy of persons, health promotion, illness prevention, professional competence, and ethical conduct (Donaldson & Crowley, 1997; Gortner, 1990).

While nursing scientists are in general agreement about the metaparadigm, they often are in

Source: Monti, E. J., & Tingen, M. S. (1999). Multiple paradigms of nursing science. *Advances in Nursing Science, 21*(4): 64–80. Reprinted with permission from and copyright © 1999 Aspen Publishers, Inc.

disagreement about the paradigms of the discipline. This disagreement stems in part from failure to agree on a single definition of the term; as a result, writers often are describing different concepts. However, the debate also stems from the idea that the discipline must have a predominant paradigm in order to demonstrate progress as a legitimate science. Because primary paradigms in nursing are considered to represent fundamentally different patterns of knowing and perspectives of reality (Fawcett, 1989), these disagreements also focus on the ability of paradigms to answer questions and to explore reality in different ways, the relevance of different types of knowledge for the discipline, and the congruence between paradigm and metaparadigm concepts.

Of the many controversies that have accompanied the growth of nursing as a discipline, few have been debated as long or as vigorously as the question of which paradigm should guide nursing science. Despite more than 20 years of discussion, the question remains unresolved. This article discusses the concept of paradigm, explores the paradigms that influence nursing science, and compares and contrasts the advantages and disadvantages of theoretical unification and multiparadigmism. In addition, the implications and consequences of multiparadigmism for the present and future development of nursing as a science within a practice discipline are presented.

The Nature of Paradigms

Many definitions of the word "paradigm" exist. Webster defines it first as "a pattern, example, or model" and secondarily as "an overall concept accepted by most people in an intellectual community, as a science, because of its effectiveness in explaining a complex process, idea, or set of data" (Webster's, 1988, p. 979). A paradigm also has been described as an abstract view or perspective of a discipline, a set of systematic beliefs, a worldview, and a theory (Kuhn, 1970). Kuhn (1970), who popularized the term, provided multiple descriptions of a paradigm in the first edition of his book, yet failed to precisely define it. In an effort to resolve the confusion that arose from his varying uses of the term, Kuhn later provided two definitions for a paradigm. In the primary sense of the word, a paradigm is a "disciplinary matrix," the ordered elements of which are held by the practitioners of a discipline. According to this definition, a paradigm includes symbolic generalizations (laws and definitions), shared beliefs, and shared values. In an alternate use, Kuhn defines paradigms in a more circumscribed manner as exemplars or shared examples. Exemplars are a part of the disciplinary matrix by which students learn to solve problems through the application of concrete solutions.

Nursing authors also have contributed to a lack of coherence about paradigms. Fawcett (1984) stated that ". . . paradigms are represented by diverse conceptual models of nursing that provide distinctive contexts for the metaparadigm concepts and themes" (p. 2). Newman (1992) states that paradigms are pervasive in nature and that a paradigm's values are deeply embedded in its followers. Kim (1997) defines paradigms as ". . . general scientific perspectives and traditions," because nursing science is developing from various research traditions and the discipline's problems require different perspectives. Lincoln and Guba (1985) define a paradigm as ". . . a systematic set of beliefs, together with their accompanying methods" (p. 15). Hardy (1997), citing Kuhn, defines the paradigm as a gestalt or worldview, a metaparadigm that is broader than theory and precedes it. The definition of paradigm as a worldview or philosophy that reflects the values and beliefs embraced by a segment of the discipline does not seem useful for the development of nursing science because values and beliefs seldom are amenable to change and the nature of science is about change. The authors of this article prefer Kim's definition because it infers methods that scientists apply to solve problems regardless of their philosophy and perspective or lens through which phenomena can be viewed. Kim's definition of paradigm is used throughout this article.

Paradigms are important to scientific communities because they not only answer the discipline's most important questions—or puzzles, as Kuhn (1970) called them—but also shape the way scientists "do" research. The ontological and epistemological assumptions of a paradigm drive its methodologies. Scientists who share a paradigm ". . . are committed to the same rules and standards for scientific practice" (Kuhn, 1970, p. 11). A paradigm is useful in that it provides scientists with a general orientation to phenomena, a way of organizing perceptions, criteria for selecting problems, guidelines for investigations and methods, and limitations on possible solutions. Thus, a paradigm provides a guiding framework for resolving problems, conducting research, and deriving theories and laws. For nursing scientists, paradigms direct the perspective from which research questions are asked, problems are investigated, research is designed as well as what methods are used and how data are collected, analyzed, and interpreted (Newman et al., 1991).

Paradigms in Nursing

Nursing science is characterized by two predominant paradigms that are broadly classified as the empiricist and the interpretative. These two paradigms represent fundamentally opposing views of knowledge development and reality. Several conceptual frameworks of nursing depict the metaparadigm concepts from the perspective of the different paradigms. The contribution of the primary paradigms to nursing science will be discussed, and examples of conceptual frameworks that are derived from them will be presented. The cardinal features of the two paradigms are presented in Table 22–1.

Empiricism is based on the assumption that what is known can be verified through the senses (Chinn & Kramer, 1995). The ontological assumption of empiricism is that there is one reality, which is out there somewhere and can be validated through the senses. In the empiricist paradigm, knowledge is developed through sense observation of the natural world in order to verify and justify theories that describe, predict, and prescribe. Research studies in this tradition focus on the context of justification. Theories depicting reality are reduced into components that can be either validated or disproved empirically in order to justify the relationships set forth. Empiricism also has been described as reductionistic because parts rather than the whole of phenomena are examined and because of the positivistic emphasis on theory reduction.

Empiricism has its roots in the logical positivist school of philosophy. Logical positivism, also called logical empiricism and the received view, was espoused by a group of philosophers known as the Vienna school (Lincoln & Guba, 1985; Jacox & Webster, 1997; Suppe & Jacox,

Table 22–1 A COMPARISON OF THE EMPIRICIST AND INTERPRETATIVE PARADIGMS

	Empiricism	Interpretative
Alternative names	Mechanistic Positivism	Organismic
Nursing	Particulate–deterministic	Unitary–transformative
Paradigms	Totality	Simultaneity
Ontology	One reality Reality is independent of context Truth can be determined Certainty is possible	Multiple realities Composite reality Meaning is grounded in experience Truth can never be determined
Epistemology	Reality can be verified by the senses Value-free observations Cognition and perception are separate entities	Knowledge is derived from experience, art, ethics Value-laden observations Cognition, perception and experience affect what is seen or conceptualized Shared meaning
Purpose	Verification and justification Theory testing Identify cause and effect	Discovery and meaning Theory generating Increase understanding and knowledge of lived reality
Human beings are:	Machines The sum of their parts Closed systems	Living organisms Holistic beings Greater than the sum of their parts Open systems
Researcher is	Observer Objective Uninvolved	The instrument Co-creating Involved in the process
Phenomena	Can be reduced to parts	Holistic view Irreducible Context dependent
Behavior	Predictable, linear	Probabilistic Unpredictable
Movement	Organism is passive or at rest Exterior forces cause movement	Active From within organism

Table 22–1 A COMPARISON OF THE EMPIRICIST AND INTERPRETATIVE PARADIGMS (CONTINUED)

	Empiricism	Interpretative
Methodologies	Quantitative Observation Control	Qualitative Attention to context and interpretation Interview, observation
Research question	What is the relationship of A and B? What is the effect of A on B? Hypothesis testing	What is the meaning of . . . ? What is the structure of the lived experience?
Designs	Experimental Quasi-experimental	Emergent Phenomenology Grounded theory
Sample	Random selection Random assignment Convenience	Purposive Theoretical Volunteer
Data collection techniques	Instrumentation Observation	Interviews Observation Analysis of art, literature, documents
Data analysis	Deductive Statistical analysis	Inductive Interpretation Constant comparative method

1985). Positivists disavowed religious and metaphysical explanations of reality and analyzed theories for logical patterns of reasoning that could be verified in reality (Suppe & Jacox, 1985). Logical positivism, however, was an extremist variant of empiricism because it espoused the idea that the only reality was that which could be observed in the world (Jacox & Webster, 1997; Poole & Jones, 1996). Thus, the mind was not an object of study unless the mind could be associated with a physical reality, a position reminiscent of Descartes' theory of mind–body dualism. Positivism also was associated with an antiquated view of the universe that equated it with a machine operated by laws

understood only by God (Jacox & Webster, 1997). The purpose of science was to discover these laws, or products, in order to be able to explain and predict events in the world. Theories describing reality in formal language either could be verified or disproved by observation of objects in the world. Thus, science resulted in a product, a theory, that could be used to describe, predict, and prescribe.

Positivism fell into disfavor in the 1960s when it was criticized for using defective methods of analysis and having little to do with actual science (Suppe & Jacox, 1985). Although discredited and recognized as a dead movement since the 1960s (Gortner, 1990; Silva &

Rothbart, 1997), many nursing scientists continue to react to contemporary empiricism as though positivism were flourishing. Gortner (1990) feels that empiricism has been given short shrift in nursing, because of ". . . continued fallacious identification with logical positivism" (p. 482). Modern empiricism, also called postpositivism, incorporates a historical approach to science along with empirical methods (Gortner, 1990).

Historicism is concerned with the values and beliefs of scientists as well as the sociological and historical context in which decisions regarding scientific research are made (Silva & Rothbart, 1997). Historical approaches incorporate the ideas of philosophers such as Laudan, who thought that science should be judged by the number of problems it solved rather than whether or not theories were verified (Silva & Rothbart, 1997). Thus, postpositivist empirical research retains the empiricist elements of precision, deductive reasoning, objectivity, theory testing, and substantiation of theoretical claims with valid data (Weiss, 1995), while recognizing the impossibility of verification and the value-laden qualities of theory and observation (Gortner, 1990; Poole & Jones, 1996). However, postpositivists also recognize that the purpose of scientific investigation in nursing is patient care; that the meaning of relationships can be clarified; that generalizable patterns can be ascertained without full prediction and control; that the conditions or context in which the phenomenon occurs is important; and that the researcher must prevent personal biases from influencing the outcomes of research (Weiss, 1995).

The method associated with empiricism is the scientific method. This method focuses on the experiment, control, objectivity, precise measurement, quantification of data, and description of results in statistical terms. Because empiricists believe that the senses can be used to verify reality, observation is the preferred method of data collection. The scientist uses tools and instruments to measure the phenomenon of concern while remaining a detached observer in order to prevent personal biases from influencing the study results (Burns & Grove, 1997). Numerical values are assigned to data in order to test relationships using statistical methods. The empiricist paradigm is necessary if nursing science is to substantiate claims regarding nursing care and the responses of persons in health and illness situations, provide explanatory models, and test and generate theory (Gortner, 1990; Weiss, 1995). The value of the empirical approach to knowledge development lies in its ability to test hypotheses, compare interventions, produce generalizations, and generate confidence intervals that uncover influences (Poole & Jones, 1996). The ability to test hypotheses allows the relationships in theories to be tested and validated (Burns & Grove, 1997). Although no one study ever can verify a relationship, the data collected can offer strong support for the presence of a relationship. Establishment of valid relationships enables theories to be used to explain, predict, and prescribe notions that are essential and relevant for clinical practice (Schumacher & Gortner, 1992). Control limits the problem being researched and attempts to limit extraneous factors so that relationships can be examined more precisely. Random assignment of subjects or treatments also allows factors that may affect the variable of interest to be equally distributed (Poole & Jones, 1996). Generalizability is an important goal of empirical research, as it allows relationships to be extrapolated to a larger population or different situation, a factor that is advantageous in nursing practice (Burns & Grove, 1997). Statistical methods allow for both exploratory and confirmatory analyses of data to describe the data and search for potential relationships (Burns & Grove, 1997). However, discovery of statistical significance does not indicate necessarily clinical significance (Poole & Jones, 1996).

Criticisms of Empiricism

Objectivity and control are aspects of empiricism that have been criticized severely by many nursing researchers. In empirical investigations, researchers control extraneous or confounding variables in order to increase the validity of study results. However, when studying humans, it is impossible to control many factors that might affect the outcome of a study. In addition, excessive control of variables in human studies can remove important contexts that influence a situation and contribute to its meaning. Excessive control produces an artificial situation that bears no resemblance to reality and thus decreases generalizability. Objectivity is also seen as preventing ". . . full recognition of the other as a person" (Holmes, 1990) while experimental conditions can decontextualize the human experience. Thus, the traditional experimental method, in which persons respond to the environment like a machine rather than interacting with the environment, is seen as having a dehumanizing effect (Holmes, 1990).

Some nursing scientists criticize positivism because it does not recognize other forms of knowing besides that that can be verified. Nurses always have recognized the knowledge embedded in practice. Carper (1997) identified four fundamental patterns of knowing in nursing: empirics, ethics, esthetics, and personal knowledge. Empirics, or the science of nursing, is concerned with describing, explaining, and predicting phenomena of concern. Esthetics, or the art of nursing, is the expressive and perceptive aspect of nursing that can defy expression. Ethics focuses on moral questions of right and wrong and what ought to be done. Personal knowledge ". . . is concerned with the knowing, encountering, and actualizing of the concrete, individual self" (Carper, 1997, p. 251). The four are not isolated entities but interrelate to form a whole that is greater than the sum of the parts. Thus, knowledge acquisition does not occur as a result of one isolated way of viewing the world but through the simultaneous interaction of the four patterns. Logical positivism ignored aspects of nursing knowledge that were acquired through means other than empirical methods and thus negated a rich source of nursing knowledge.

Prior to the 1950s, nursing research activities were limited (Burns & Grove, 1997). In the 1950s and 1960s, empiricism was the predominant approach to developing nursing knowledge. Strongly influenced by the medical model and education in other disciplines, early nursing scientists favored the empiricist paradigm because they were eager to establish the scientific basis of the profession and demonstrate that nursing was a unique, professional discipline (Munhall, 1993). However, many nursing scientists became frustrated with the positivistic approach and began questioning its use because it often did not reflect the values and beliefs of nursing nor the discipline's focus on holism, person-centered care, and understanding of human experiences in health and disease. Desiring a more humanistic approach that could address the concerns of nurses and their patients, many researchers turned to the methods proposed by phenomenological and existential schools of philosophy that are concerned with the meaning of human experience and understanding the day-to-day experience of individuals (Holmes, 1990).

The Interpretative Paradigm

The interpretative paradigm in nursing science evolved for several reasons. First, many early nurse scientists were educated in disciplines such as philosophy, sociology, and anthropology that exposed them to alternate ways of viewing the world and the methodologies associated with those paradigms. Second, to some nurse scientists, empiricism did not recognize the esthetic, ethical, and personal knowledge inherent in nursing. Interpretative traditions acknowledge that reality has multiple meanings and that knowledge can be derived from sources other than the senses. Thus, other patterns of knowing important to nursing are given credence by interpretative approaches. Third, the interpretative approach was seen as more congruent with the language and beliefs of nursing. Where nursing spoke of holism, individualism, autonomy, and self-determination, the dominating scientific/medical model spoke of reductionism, objectivity, manipulation, prediction, and control (Munhall, 1993). A fourth reason for embracing the interpretative paradigm is that nursing wished to establish a theoretical base for the discipline. The interpretative paradigm provided methods for generating theory that are representative of nursing views rather than borrowed from other professions (Munhall, 1993). Finally, a qualitative approach offers new perspectives and methodologies for answering

the questions of the discipline (Bramlett, Gueldner, & Boettcher, 1993).

The interpretative paradigm is characterized by the ontological assumptions that reality is complex, holistic, and context dependent (Boyd, 1993; Lincoln & Guba, 1985). The focus of investigation is on human experience: thus, subjectivity rather than objectivity is emphasized (Hardy, 1997). Because reality and human experience are variable, multiple ways of knowing are valued to uncover the knowledge that is embedded in human experience. Tacit or intuitive knowledge is recognized in addition to that which is expressed in language or can be observed (Lincoln & Guba, 1985). Therefore, the method includes techniques that result in extended contact of the researcher with the participant and in mutual interaction. A natural setting is selected because ". . . wholes cannot be understood in isolation from their contexts . . ." (Lincoln & Guba, 1985, p. 39), nor can they be separated into parts for study. Inductive reasoning is used to identify patterns of meaning in the data (Lincoln & Guba, 1985).

Broadly grouped under the term *qualitative research*, interpretative methods include phenomenology, hermeneutics, grounded theory, ethnography, and others. The general goal of interpretative methods is to understand and derive meaning from the human experience; however, instrumentation and conceptualization are other identified purposes (Boyd, 1993). Common features of these research traditions are a holistic approach to questioning, a focus on human experience, purposive sampling, sustained contact with participants, the involvement of the researcher in the process, emergent design, negotiated outcomes, and special criteria for trustworthiness (Lincoln & Guba, 1985). In-depth interviews with open-ended questions and participant observations are used for data collection. Data analysis proceeds through analysis of written narratives to extract the meaning of the experience (Boyd, 1993).

A strength of the interpretative paradigm is the usefulness of this approach for generating theories. When little is known about a subject, qualitative methods are useful in identifying patterns of experiences and the relationships between them. Relational statements reflecting these relationships can be written and used to develop new theories (Burns & Grove, 1997). For example, grounded theory methods can identify basic social structures or processes (BSP) through the method of constant comparative analysis. These BSPs are then linked into a theory (Boyd, 1993).

Criticisms of the Interpretative Paradigm

Although antipositivist perspectives have been embraced by many nursing researchers, they are not without their limitations for developing knowledge in nursing. While the interpretative paradigm emphasizes humanistic approaches, it ignores the reality of physiological problems that are an integral part of a discipline that deals with health and disease (Downs, 1989; Gortner, 1990). Nursing is not a social science and must acknowledge that physiological and psychosocial phenomena are at the core of the discipline. Nursing science must address the complex clinical problems that practicing nurses deal with daily. Research traditions that rely solely on interpretation and gaining understanding are not amenable to testing theory (Gortner, 1990). Practitioners need theories that help guide their practice and answer questions posed by clinical situations. Although qualitative methodologies such as grounded theory can present theories describing the knowledge embedded in practice, testing of these nascent theories by empirical methods is required.

Interpretative methodologies have been criticized for a lack of rigor, primarily on the basis of criteria used to judge quantitative studies (Burns & Grove, 1997). However, quantitative criteria are inappropriate for evaluating the rigor of qualitative studies (Burns & Grove, 1997; Lincoln & Guba, 1985). Issues that have been cited as reflecting a lack of rigor include failure to adhere to the philosophy of the method being used, inadequate time spent collecting data, failure to identify values and beliefs that may impinge on the study, and poorly developed methods (Burns & Grove, 1997). Credibility, transferability, dependability, and confirmability are the appropriate criteria for judging qualitative methodologies (Lincoln & Guba, 1985).

The results of qualitative studies have been characterized as ". . . a set of interesting stories" that result in isolated findings that do not advance the discipline because they do not form the basis for further work (Downs, 1989). Although nursing is concerned with the uniqueness of individuals, in daily practice, nurses must identify patterns, look for commonalities, and establish priorities. While the results of qualitative research may serve to uncover some of the esthetic, ethical, and personal knowledge of nurses, practice demands that this knowledge also be put to use. Knowledge that does not help nurses meet society's needs, understand and explain the concepts and relationships of the metaparadigm and conceptual models, and predict events and effects does not contribute to the discipline.

Various writers have suggested other names for the empiricist and interpretative worldviews in nursing. Parse characterized the worldviews of the empiricist and interpretative paradigms as the totality and simultaneity paradigms (Fawcett, 1989; 1993). The simultaneity worldview regards the person as more and different than the sum of its parts, an open being, free to choose, in rhythmic interaction with the environment (Fawcett, 1989; 1993). In the totality paradigm, the person is the sum of bio–psycho–social–spiritual parts and interacts with the environment in a linear manner (Fawcett, 1993). Newman (1992) proposed the particulate–deterministic, interactive–integrative, and unitary–transformative perspectives. In the first worldview, phenomena can be viewed as isolated, reducible entities with measurable properties that have an orderly relationship. The second paradigm is related to the first except that the context of phenomena is considered and reality is understood to be multidimensional. In the third paradigm, human beings are considered to be evolving as unitary self-organizing fields (Newman, 1992). Fawcett (1993), attempting to integrate these different models, coined the reaction, reciprocal interaction, and simultaneous action worldviews. Despite the differences in names, the totality, particulate–deterministic, interactive–integrative, and reaction worldviews are representations of the empiricist or mechanistic paradigm, whereas the others are derived from the interpretative or organismic tradition.

Is Nursing Science a Mature Science?

Does the fact that nursing science lacks a predominant paradigm mean that nursing is not a mature science? Nurses too often attempt to measure the success of the discipline with criteria proposed by others that only serve to highlight the limitations of nursing science and fail to acknowledge its successes (Meleis, 1997). Zbilut (1997) states that "perhaps nursing has become a full-fledged professional discipline inasmuch as it succumbs to academic fashion" (p. 188). Many nursing scientists subscribe to Kuhn's (1970) depiction of a mature science. Kuhn (1970) characterized science as having three distinct phases: pre-paradigmatic, normal science or postparadigmatic, and transformative periods that he calls "revolutions." The preparadigmatic stage is characterized by ". . . debates over legitimate methods, problems and standards of solution . . ." (Kuhn, 1970, p. 48) and the lack of primacy of a particular worldview. Change from preparadigm to postparadigm science is characterized by multiple schools of thought giving way to one and science finding a more satisfactory method of "solving puzzles." A period of "normal science" exists when one paradigm emerges as the predominant way of solving problems, members of a scientific community accept the paradigm as foundational, and use the worldview espoused by the predominant paradigm to solve problems. Debates about methods, questions for study, and ways of answering questions disappear during periods of normal science. Revolutions occur following a crisis, when scientists begin to see the world differently and debates emerge about the paradigm. Gradually, one paradigm supplants that previously in favor and a new period of normal science begins.

Mature science develops through revolutions that provide a transition from one paradigm to another (Kuhn, 1970). According to Kuhn (1970), a mature science is characterized by

1. the scientific community's acceptance of a paradigm.

2. approaches to solving the discipline's problems that are driven by the paradigm.
3. the presentation of knowledge as research articles in scientific journals rather than books.
4. the development of a language that is unintelligible to the uninitiated.

A predominant paradigm is the most important criterion.

Using these criteria, nursing science is at a preparadigmatic stage because several paradigms are extant. There is a vigorous, ongoing debate within the nursing scientific community about the appropriateness of philosophies and methodologies for directing and conducting research as well as about the questions of relevance to the discipline. However, nursing does meet Kuhn's requirements for shared values, a unique language, scientific journals, and reporting of research findings in articles. A review of the numerous scientific nursing journals indicates that nursing has developed a language of its own and that a significant body of scholarly activity has been accumulated. However, Kuhn (1970), a physicist by training, has been criticized as providing an inaccurate account of the history of science and evaluating science from a positivist perspective due to his emphasis on facts, empiricism, experimentation, and natural science. This positivist perspective is inappropriate and too narrow for a human science such as nursing that confronts a variety of problems (Fry, 1995; Meleis, 1997). Other ways of evaluating scientific progress may be more useful to nursing science.

Meleis (1997) proposed a theory of integration for evaluation of progress in nursing science that is more congruent with the tortuous path

by which the discipline has developed. Diversity, theory development, competition, creativity, innovation, openness, flexibility, and change are characteristics of a mature discipline according to Meleis. She states that nursing has achieved disciplinary status when evaluated by these criteria.

Fawcett (1984) identified three areas of success in nursing research and suggested yardsticks for measuring future progress in nursing science. She recognized "hallmarks of success" that nursing has achieved as identification of the boundaries of research, the types of research required by the discipline, and the types of research activities appropriate for nurses with different educational preparation. Goals for the 21st century are elimination of obstacles to nursing research, acceptance of multiple methods of inquiry, and utilization of research findings in practice. Whether or not nursing science achieves these goals or nursing scientists are in agreement about these criteria, they are important because they provide a nursing perspective of what is important to the discipline rather than applying qualifications developed by those unfamiliar with the history and advances of nursing science.

Single or Multiple Paradigms?

Kuhn's (1970) conceptualization of an overarching paradigm that directs the scientific endeavors of a discipline is the basis for the idea of theoretical unification in nursing. This idea is reminiscent of the positivist philosophy of theoretical reduction and reflects his philosophical underpinnings. Paradigmatic supremacy represents the outmoded positivist viewpoint that considers theory reduction an important goal of science (Silva & Rothbart, 1997). This philosophy assumes that there is one inclusive theory that can reveal the characteristics of reality (Silva & Rothbart, 1997). However, the concept of unification suggests the mingling of paradigms rather than the dominance of one over the other. Given that the empiricist and interpretative paradigms represent opposing ontological and epistemological views, it is impossible to reconcile the differences underlying the two paradigms to form a unified paradigm.

Several authors suggest that theoretical unification is beneficial to the profession. The advantage of one paradigm lies in its simplicity and parsimony, as there are fewer concepts and relationships to be examined (Silva & Rothbart, 1997). Hardy (1997) suggests that one possible reason for adopting a predominant paradigm is to define the boundaries of the profession or "turf." Others believe that a unified focus ". . . has the potential for claiming the shared vision of nursing" (Newman, 1991, p. 5). Reed (1995) believes that accepting multiple paradigms is contrary to the idea of holism and ". . . nursing may be sacrificing coherence for diversity" (p. 78). Reed (1995) advocates a "meta-narrative" or overarching ideal of nursing to direct knowledge development in the profession. While a metanarrative offers potential for discourse and reflection, it does not offer resolution for the differences between the interpretative and empiricist paradigms.

A disadvantage of theoretical unification or the ascendancy of one worldview is the narrowness of vision afforded by such a perspective. Kuhn (1970) describes the paradigm as an "inflexible box" (p. 24) which directs periods of normal science. In this respect, the purpose of normal science is not to examine new phenomena; rather, the aim of normal science is to articulate ". . . the phenomena and theories that the paradigm already supplies" (p. 24). Because a paradigm directs the work of a community of scientists, selection of one perspective narrows the focus of vision to examining in detail only those phenomena it recognizes. However, when the paradigm becomes too restrictive, scientists "behave differently" and change the nature of their research problems. Thus, theoretical unification can be likened to the idea of the young child who enthusiastically scribbles in a coloring book, only to be told to stay within the lines. Initial enthusiasm for the task quickly becomes discouragement. The challenges confronting practitioners of nursing art and science are too numerous and pressing to permit disenchantment for change or challenge to occur by the unqualified acceptance of a single paradigm.

The existence of multiple paradigms in nursing science indicates a strong and flourishing science. Multiple paradigms are indicative of a "healthy" scientific community because they encourage creativity, stimulate debate and the exchange of ideas, provide diversity of views (Kim, 1997; Ramos, 1997), promote productivity (Donaldson & Crowley, 1997), and keep open avenues of inquiry (Ramos, 1997).

Creativity is a vital and necessary source of ideas in science. Multiple paradigms stimulate creativity by providing different points of view from which to examine a problem or question (Jacox & Webster, 1997). Because nursing deals with human behavior, one viewpoint is not sufficient to explain the variety of phenomena and relationships nurses encounter (Meleis, 1997). Theoretical unification focuses vision in one plane, like a microscope, but multiple paradigms expand vision, like a wide-angle lens. Because the goal of nursing science is not simply to add to the discipline's knowledge base, but to develop theories that explain, predict, and prescribe numerous ways of conceptualizing ideas and examining phenomena are beneficial. Multiple paradigms encourage "thinking outside the box" rather than in the box like theoretical unification.

Debate is stimulated by the existence of multiple paradigms. According to the theory of integration, it is debate and competition of theories and ideas that make a discipline scholarly (Meleis, 1997). Compendiums of articles such as *Perspectives on Nursing Theory* (Nicoll, 1997) offer a window through which to view debate within the discipline. A review of these articles reveals the intensity with which authors have supported and defended their particular worldview, resulting in clarification, codification, and modification of views. The active exchange of opinions and ideas through discourse stimulates growth and development (Ramos, 1997). Just as a growing organism achieves maturity through rapidly dividing and multiplying, so can a discipline grow through a multiplicity of paradigms. Selection of one worldview can be considered analogous to the loss of variability that accompanies aging and death in complex physiological systems (Lipsitz & Goldberger, 1992).

Diversity of viewpoints has been likened to a cable that is strengthened by multiple strands (Knaft, Pettengill, Bevis, & Kirchhoff, 1988). Nursing is a complex profession with many providers with differing educational preparation and areas of specialization caring for many types of clients in varying situations. How can one paradigm for nursing science possibly reflect this diversity? Just as people have been urged to celebrate their differences, so should nursing science rejoice in the fact that within nursing is a rich and varied assortment of threads that, when woven together, draw a strong, resilient, whole tapestry. The problems of nursing are so diverse that multiple answers and solutions to a question can be appropriate. Multiple perspectives encourage appreciation of the uniqueness of individual nurses and patients by finding multiple answers to common problems. Problems may be erroneously considered solved and questions answered if one perspective for developing knowledge is selected.

Different paradigmatic views may increase productivity. Reliance on one perspective may limit a scientist to repeatedly investigating the same problem from the same approach in different populations. However, applying different viewpoints provides new insights to formulate new ideas to old questions. For example, the continual use of a phenomenological approach will result in many studies about the meaning of an experience. However, for both the discipline and the investigator to advance in knowledge, those studies must be used as a foundation on which to build others that generate and test theory. Other perspectives are needed to channel these initial findings into further studies. In addition to maximizing the strengths and minimizing the weakness of each method, combining or triangulating methods can involve more than one investigator in a research project, resulting in more discussion, more ideas, and more projects (Dzurec & Abraham, 1993).

Premature closure also may result from the selection of one paradigm. Cognitive dissonance may not be noted if only those phenomena that are congruent with a single perspective are examined (Fawcett, 1989). In other words, a single perspective is similar to wearing blinders: phenomena that might attract attention are not seen, as they are outside the field of vision. Thus, opportunities to go somewhere more interesting or follow a different path are thwarted.

Multiple paradigms also have disadvantages for nursing science in that practitioners may become confused and divided over the conflicting claims of different viewpoints (Reed, 1995). Many in the profession find continuing debate over such matters inconclusive, frustrating, and not germane to the business of nursing. Students can become confused if exposed to new, untested ideas, and even experienced practitioners may find the seemingly never-ending debate mystifying (Zbilut, 1997). For example, it is difficult to reconcile the pragmatic aspects of everyday nursing with ideas espoused by interpretative paradigms. If each individual is unique, why are standard care plans devised? What does it mean for a person to be an open system and how can this be evaluated? Why do nurses assess patients systematically if they are holistic beings? How can the accomplishments of empiricism be accepted while its methods are condemned as controlling and dehumanizing? If empiricism is abandoned, what will replace it?

Implications of Multiparadigmism for Nursing Science

A change of perspective is required for nursing science to reconcile the philosophical differences between the two extant paradigms. A perspective that emphasizes inquiry rather than paradigmatic supremacy or unification is more advantageous to nursing as a discipline. Dzurec and Abraham (1993) noted that there were few real differences between quantitative and qualitative methods of research. Although specific techniques may vary between methods, ". . . the

findings generated by both . . . are based on description, probability, and inference" (Dzurec & Abraham, 1993, p. 74). The results of both empirical and interpretative studies are due to interpretation of raw data by the investigator (Dzurec & Abraham, 1993). The authors argue that neither method is more scientific than the other and that the process of inquiry is the same despite the methods used to acquire knowledge. Therefore, nursing scientists can take heart in the thought that careful adherence to the principles and philosophy of the method they chose will result in valid and reliable findings that will add to the body of knowledge of the discipline.

Integration of qualitative and quantitative methods has been suggested as advancing nursing science (Dzurec & Abraham, 1993; Holmes, 1990; Laudan, 1977). Research traditions from the empirical and interpretative paradigms are complementary as each presents a different approach (Poole & Jones, 1996). Qualitative methods can describe phenomenon of interest in nursing and generate theories that propose relationships between identified concepts. Quantitative methods can test the relationships of qualitatively developed theories and suggest whether the theory should be accepted or revised. The different perspectives presented by the empiricist and interpretative paradigms can examine different dimensions of a phenomenon.

Collaboration toward solving problems is more beneficial for the discipline than acrimony and competition over which tradition is most useful (Silva & Rothbart, 1997). Collaboration will result in increased opportunities for all nursing scientists. For example, critical multiplism, a strategy similar to triangulation, has been recommended as an approach for nursing research (Knaft et al., 1988). This strategy is ". . . based on the premise that . . . thoughtful choices are the approach most likely to yield an objective body of knowledge" (Knaft et al., 1988). Multiple multiples are involved: of researchers, institutions, frameworks, research questions, issues, methods, and data collection and analysis modes. The approach increases efficiency by spreading the workload and increases utility by studying more than one question at a time (Knaft et al., 1988). Methods such as this offer greater opportunities for collaboration and discourse than traditional, single-investigator approaches.

When paradigms are associated with values and beliefs, polarization occurs between different views, with little hope of bridging the gulf between the sides. Acceptance of multiple paradigms as perspectives and research traditions rather than as values has the potential to lessen the division between the academic and scientific communities. Practicing nurses often are blind to the relevance of theoretical arguments for the everyday practice of nursing. However, clinicians readily understand that there are many ways to accomplish the same goal and that a nurse uses whatever method he or she is most comfortable with or whatever works best in a particular situation.

Presenting research as a system of inquiry that can be accomplished in several ways may also improve the palatability of research in educational programs. Both baccalaureate and masters students often are overwhelmed by research courses and rate their usefulness to practice as low. However, student interest in research may be spurred by courses that emphasize principles of sound inquiry rather than the vagaries and quirks of different paradigmatic approaches. Just as students learn sound principles of nursing care on which to build their nursing practice, so must they learn basic principles of

inquiry that recognize the equality of all methods. Presenting a system of inquiry rather than a philosophy also will require that instructors provide a more balanced view of different research traditions.

A variety of paradigms allows the development of more theories for nursing. Different perspectives of nursing practice enhance the ability to understand and interpret the meaning in different practice situations, identify relationships, and develop theories. Laudan (1977) recommends a process of integration of different research traditions with the goal of expanding the number of theories in order to solve the problems of the discipline.

The feasibility and importance of a multiparadigmatic approach ultimately will be established through its usefulness in practice. If differing perspectives can generate and test theories that provide faithful representations of practice and are useful in practice settings, they will flourish. As a pragmatic profession, nurses choose the method that works best to provide the critical services clients require. Practice will indicate those aspects of a perspective that are not useful and discard or revamp them into a new variant. Applying different paradigms together in practice situations can help to determine whether the perspective offered by opposing perspectives results in different nursing actions. According to history, often that which is not useful does not survive. If the multiparadigmatic approach is not congruent with practice, it, too, may become obsolete or extinct.

Summary

The discussion about theoretical unification or multiparadigmism is reminiscent of the debate over single or multiple conceptual frameworks for nursing. Interestingly, that debate has been abandoned as the discussion shifts to paradigms. The war of words over single or multiple paradigms cannot be won easily. However, multiparadigmism is an approach to the development of nursing knowledge that offers greater promise for the discipline than theoretical unification. Multiparadigmism recognizes the differences inherent in opposing worldviews while celebrating the possibilities that each offers and the way that each complements the other. Downplaying paradigmatic differences while enhancing the value of scholarly inquiry through multiple approaches is paramount for the advancement of nursing science.

Discussion Questions

1. Choose two research articles, one empirical and one interpretative, and compare and contrast them.
2. Develop a clinical question about your current practice, stating a population, intervention, and outcome. How would you approach answering the question from an empirical perspective? How would you approach the question from an interpretive perspective?
3. What are the pros and cons of each perspective of nursing science discussed in this chapter?
4. Do you agree with the author that multiparadigmism is the best approach to the development of nursing science?

References

Bramlett, M. H., Gueldner, S. H., & Boettcher, J. H. (1993). Reflections on the science of unitary human beings in terms of Kuhn's requirement for explanatory power. *Visions, 1,* 22–35.

Boyd, C. O. (1993). Philosophical foundations of qualitative research. In P. L. Munhall & C. O. Boyd (Eds.), *Nursing research: A qualitative perspective* (2nd ed.). New York: National League for Nursing.

Burns, N., & Grove, S. K. (1997). *The practice of nursing research: Conduct, critique, & utilization* (3rd ed.). Philadelphia: W. B. Saunders.

Carper, B. A. (1997). Fundamental patterns of knowing in nursing. In L. H. Nicoll (Ed.), *Perspectives on nursing theory* (3rd ed.). Philadelphia: Lippincott.

Chinn, P. L., & Kramer, M. K. (1995). *Theory and nursing: A systematic approach* (4th ed.). St. Louis, MO: C. V. Mosby.

Donaldson, S. K., & Crowley, D. M. (1997). The discipline of nursing. In L. H. Nicoll (Ed.), *Perspectives on nursing theory* (3rd ed.). Philadelphia: Lippincott.

Downs, F. S. (1989). New questions and new answers. *Nurse Researcher, 38,* 323.

Dzurec, L. C., & Abraham, I. L. (1993). The nature of inquiry: Linking quantitative and qualitative research. *Advances in Nursing Science, 16,* 73–79.

Fawcett, J. (1984). Hallmarks of success in nursing research. *Advances in Nursing Science, 8,* 1–11.

Fawcett, J. (1989). *Analysis and evaluation of conceptual models of nursing* (2nd ed.). Philadelphia: F. A. Davis Company.

Fawcett, J. (1993). From a plethora of paradigms to parsimony in world views. *Nursing Science Quarterly, 6*(2), 56–58.

Fry, S. T. (1995). Science as problem solving. In A. Omery, C. E. Kasper, & G. G. Page (Eds.), *In search of nursing science*. Thousand Oaks, CA: Sage.

Gortner, S. R. (1990). Nursing's syntax revisited: A critique of philosophies said to influence nursing theories. *International Journal of Nursing Studies, 30*, 477–488.

Hardy, M. E. (1997). Perspectives on nursing theory. In L. H. Nicoll (Ed.), *Perspectives on nursing theory* (3rd ed.). Philadelphia: Lippincott.

Holmes, C. A. (1990). Alternatives to natural science foundations for nursing. *International Journal of Nursing Studies, 27*, 187–198.

Jacox, A. K., & Webster, G. (1997). Competing theories of science. In L. H. Nicoll (Ed.), *Perspectives on nursing theory* (3rd ed.). Philadelphia: Lippincott.

Kim, H. S. (1997). Theoretical thinking in nursing: Problems and prospects. In L. H. Nicoll (Ed.), *Perspectives on nursing theory* (3rd ed.). Philadelphia: Lippincott.

Knaft, K. A., Pettengill, M. M., Bevis, M. E., & Kirchhoff, K. T. (1988). Blending qualitative and quantitative approaches to instrument development and data collection. *Journal of Professional Nursing, 4*, 30–37.

Kuhn, T. S. (1970). *The structure of scientific revolutions* (2nd ed.). Chicago: The University of Chicago Press.

Laudan, L. (1977). *Progress and its problems: Towards a theory of scientific growth*. Berkeley: University of California Press.

Lincoln, Y. S., & Guba, E. G. (1985). *Naturalistic inquiry*. Newbury Park, CA: Sage.

Lipsitz, L. A., & Goldberger, A. L. (1992). Loss of "complexity" and aging: Potential application of fractals and chaos theory to senescence. *Journal of the American Medical Association, 267*, 1806–1809.

Meleis, A. I. (1997). *Theoretical nursing: Development & progress* (3rd ed.). Philadelphia: Lippincott.

Munhall, P. L. (1993). Language and nursing research. In P. L. Munhall & C. O. Boyd (Eds.), *Nursing research: A qualitative perspective* (2nd ed.). New York: National League for Nursing.

Newman, M. A. (1992). Prevailing paradigms in nursing. *Nursing Outlook, 40*, 10–13.

Newman, M. A., Sime, A. M., & Corcoran-Perry, S. A. (1991). The focus of the discipline of nursing. *Advances in Nursing Science, 14*, 1–6.

Nicoll, L. H. (Ed.). (1997). *Perspectives on nursing theory* (3rd ed.). Philadelphia: Lippincott.

Poole, K., & Jones, A. (1996). A re-examination of the experimental design for nursing research. *Journal of Advanced Nursing, 24*, 108–114.

Ramos, M. C. (1997). Adopting an evolutionary lens: An optimistic approach to discovering strength in nursing. In L. H. Nicoll (Ed.), *Perspectives on nursing theory* (3rd ed.). Philadelphia: Lippincott.

Reed, P. G. (1995). A treatise on nursing knowledge development for the 21st century: Beyond postmodernism. *Advances in Nursing Science, 17*, 70–84.

Schumacher, K. L., & Gortner, S. R. (1992). (Mis)conceptions and reconceptions about traditional science. *Advances in Nursing Science, 14*, 1–11.

Silva, M. C., & Rothbart, D. (1997). An analysis of changing trends in philosophies of science on nursing theory development and testing. In L. H. Nicoll (Ed.), *Perspectives on nursing theory* (3rd ed.). Philadelphia: Lippincott.

Suppe, F., & Jacox, A. K. (1985). Philosophy of science and the development of nursing theory. In H. Werley & J. Fitzpatrick (Eds.), *Annual review of nursing research*. New York: Springer.

Webster's New World Dictionary (3rd college ed.). (1988). New York: Webster's New World.

Weiss, S. J. (1995). Contemporary empiricism. In A. Omery, C. E. Kasper, & G. G. Page (Eds.), *In search of nursing science*. Thousand Oaks, CA: Sage.

Zbilut, J. P. (1997). Contradictions of nursing in a postmodern world. *Image, 38*, 188–189.

Chapter 23

Research: How Health Care Advances

Harry A. Sultz and
Kristina M. Young

CHAPTER OBJECTIVES

1. Define and recognize the focus of different types of research and how each type contributes to the advancement of knowledge about health and the healthcare system.
2. Describe the functions and goals of the Agency for Healthcare Research and Quality and how to access information pertinent to advanced nursing practice.
3. Recognize the interface of health research and policy and of research and quality improvement.
4. Discuss future challenges for healthcare research and the impact they will have on advanced practice nursing.

Introduction

The last half of the 20th century saw a remarkable growth of scientifically rigorous research in medicine, dentistry, nursing, and the other health professions. The change from depending on the clinical impressions of individual physicians and other healthcare practitioners to relying on the statistical probability of accurate findings from carefully controlled studies is one of the most important advances in scientific medicine. No longer is the literature of the health professions filled with subjective anecdotal reports of the progress of treatment in one or more individual cases. Now readers of peer-reviewed professional journals can monitor the progress of basic science or clinical or technologic discoveries with confidence, knowing that published findings are, with only rare exceptions, based on research studies that have been rigorously designed and conducted to yield statistically credible results.

In contrast, the ever-growing volume of reports of medical developments that appear in the popular media are often premature and, depending on the source, may be cause for skepticism. The imprudent publication of inadequately proven or unproven therapies, the sensationalizing of minor scientific advances, and the promotion of fraudulent devices and treatments create unrealistic expectations among anxious patients and families that often result in crushing disappointments, mistreatment, and costly deceptions.

From both professional and public perspectives, the continuing research yield of new technologies and clinical advances creates ongoing challenges of evaluation, interpretation, and potential applications.

The Focus of Different Types of Research

Figure 23–1 illustrates the focus of the different types of healthcare research. There are clear distinctions among researchers in terms of focus, methods, and the nature of their subsequent findings. Although the kinds of information derived from each type of research may be different, each knowledge gain is an essential step

in the never-ending quest to create a more efficient and effective healthcare system (Aday, Begley, Lairson, & Slater, 1993).

Research in Health and Disease

Research studies conducted by those in the professional disciplines of health and disease fall into several categories. Basic science research is the work of biochemists, physiologists, biologists, pharmacologists, and others concerned with sciences that are fundamental to understanding the growth, development, structure, and function of the human body and its responses to external stimuli. Much of basic science research is at the cellular level and takes place in highly sophisticated laboratories. Other basic research may involve animal or human studies. Whatever its nature, however, basic science research is the essential antecedent of advances in clinical medicine.

Clinical research focuses primarily on the various steps in the process of medical care—the

Figure 23–1 Variations in Research Focus

Types of Research				
Disciplinary	Biomedical	Clinical	Health Services	Public Health
Theory	Organisms	Patients	System	Community

(Focus — horizontal axis spanning from Disciplinary/Theory to Public Health/Community)

Source: Used with permission from *Evaluating the healthcare system: Effectiveness, efficiency and equity* (3rd ed.). (2004). Aday, Begley, Lairson, & Balkrishnan, Figure 1, page 8. Chicago: Health Administration Press.

early detection, diagnosis, and treatment of disease or injury; the maintenance of optimal physical, mental, and social functioning; the limitation and rehabilitation of disability; and the palliative care of those who are irreversibly ill. Individuals in all of the clinical specialties of medicine, nursing, allied health, and related health professions conduct clinical research, often in collaboration with those in the basic sciences. Much of clinical research is experimental, involving carefully controlled clinical trials of diagnostic or therapeutic procedures, new drugs, or technologic developments.

Clinical trials test a new treatment or drug against a prevailing standard of care. If no standard drug exists or if it is too easily identified, a control group will receive a placebo or mock drug to minimize subject bias. To reduce bias further, random selection is used to decide which volunteer patients will be in the experimental and control groups. In a double-blind study, neither the researchers nor the patients know who is receiving the test drug or treatment until the study is completed and an identifying code is revealed.

Research studies have a number of safeguards to protect the safety and rights of volunteer subjects. Studies funded by governmental agencies or foundations are subject to scrutiny by a peer review committee that judges the scientific merit of the research design and the potential value of the findings. Then a hospital-based or institutional review board checks for ethical considerations and patient protections. Finally, volunteer subjects must receive and sign an informed consent form that spells out in clear detail the potential risks or side effects and the expected benefits of their participation. Volunteers must weigh any potential risks against the likelihood that, by participating in research, they will receive state-of-the-art care and close health monitoring and will contribute to the advancement of science.

Epidemiology

Epidemiology, or population research, is concerned with the distribution and determinants of health, diseases, and injuries in human populations. Much of that research is observational; it is the collection of information about natural phenomena, the characteristics and behaviors of people, aspects of their location or environment, and their exposure to certain circumstances or events.

Observational studies may be descriptive or analytical. Descriptive studies use patient records, interview surveys, various databases, and other information sources to identify those factors and conditions that determine the distribution of health and disease among specific populations. They provide the details or characteristics of diseases or biological phenomena and the prevalence or magnitude of their occurrence. Descriptive studies are relatively fast and inexpensive and often raise questions or suggest hypotheses to be tested. They usually are followed by analytic studies, which try to explain biologic phenomena by seeking statistical associations between factors that may contribute to a subsequent occurrence and the occurrence itself.

Some analytic studies attempt, under naturally occurring circumstances, to observe the differences between two or more populations with different characteristics or behaviors. For instance, data about smokers and nonsmokers may be collected to determine the relative risk of a related outcome such as lung cancer, or a cohort study may follow a population over time, as in the case of a Framingham, Massachusetts, study.

For years, epidemiologists have been studying a cooperating population of Framingham to determine associations between such variables as diet, weight, exercise, and other behaviors and characteristics related to heart disease and other outcomes. These observational studies are valuable in explaining patterns of disease or disease processes and providing information about the association of specific activities or agents with health or disease effects.

Experimental Epidemiology

Observational studies usually are followed by another major type of research: experimental studies. In experimental studies, the investigator actively intervenes by manipulating one variable to see what happens with the other. Although they are the best test of cause and effect, such studies are technically difficult to carry out and often raise ethical issues. Control populations are used to ensure that other non-experimental variables are not affecting the outcome. Like clinical trials, such studies may raise ethical issues when experiments involve the use of a clinical procedure that may expose the subjects to significant or unknown risk. Ethical questions also are raised when experimental studies require the withholding of some potentially beneficial drug or procedure from individuals in the control group to prove decisively the effectiveness of the drug or procedure.

Other Applications of Epidemiologic Methods

Because the population perspective of epidemiology usually requires the study and analysis of data obtained from or about large-scale population samples, the discipline has developed principles and methods that can be applied to the study of a wide range of problems in several fields. Thus, the concepts and quantitative methods of epidemiology have been used not only to add to the understanding of the etiology of health and disease, but also to plan, administer, and evaluate health services; to forecast the health needs of population groups; to assess the adequacy of the supply of health personnel; and, most recently, to determine the outcomes of specific treatment modalities in a variety of clinical settings.

Advances in statistical theory and the epidemiology of medical care make it possible to analyze and interpret performance data obtained from the large Medicare and other insurance databases. Many of the findings of inexplicable geographic variations in the amount and cost of hospital treatments and in the use of a variety of healthcare services resulted from analysis of Medicare claims data and other large health insurance databases.

Health Services Research

Until the last 2 decades, most research addressed the need to broaden understanding of health and disease, to find new and more effective means of diagnosis and treatment, and in effect, to improve the quality and length of life. For the 2 decades after World War II, supply-side subsidy programs dominated federal healthcare policy. Like other subsidy programs, Medicare and Medicaid were politically crafted solutions rather than research-based strategies. Nevertheless, those major healthcare subsidy programs were the driving forces behind the rise of health services research. The continuous collection of cost and utilization data from these programs revealed serious deficiencies in the capability of the health-care system to deliver efficiently and effectively the knowledge and skills already at hand. In addition, evidence was growing that should the large variations in the kinds and amounts of care delivered for the same conditions represented unacceptable volumes of inappropriate or questionable care and too much indecision or confusion among clinicians about the best courses of treatment. Health services research was born of the need to improve the efficiency and effectiveness of the healthcare system and to determine which of the healthcare treatment options for each condition produces the best outcomes.

Agency for Healthcare Research and Quality

Ever since John Wennberg documented large differences in the use of medical and surgical procedures among physicians in small geographic areas in the late 1980s, a number of similar studies brought the value of increasingly more costly health care into serious question. Wennberg noted that the rate of surgeries correlated with the numbers of surgeons and the number of hospital beds, rather than with differences among patients. He found that per capita expenditures for hospitalization in Boston were consistently double those in nearby New Haven (Wennberg, 1986; Wennberg, Freeman, & Culp, 1987; Wennberg, Freeman, Shelton, & Bubolz, 1989). Widely varying physician practice patterns provided little direction as to the most appropriate use of even the most common clinical procedures. In addition, adequate outcome measures for specific intervention modalities generally were lacking.

The problem did not escape the attention of the 101st Congress. The development of new knowledge through research has long been held as an appropriate and essential role of the federal government, as evidenced by the establishment and proactive role of the National Institutes of Health. When it became clear that the indecision about the most appropriate and effective ways to diagnose and treat specific medical, dental, and other conditions was contributing to unacceptably large variations in the cost, quality, and outcomes of health care, federal legislation was passed to support the development of clinical guidelines. The Agency for Healthcare Policy and Research (AHCPR) was established in 1989 as the successor to the National Center for Health Services Research and Health Care Technology. It is one of eight agencies of the Public Health Service within the Department of Health and Human Services.

AHCPR was responsible for updating and promoting the development and review of clinically relevant guidelines to assist healthcare practitioners in the prevention, diagnosis, treatment, and management of clinical conditions. Clinical guidelines are intended to enhance the quality, appropriateness, and effectiveness of health care (Agency for Healthcare Policy and Research, 1990). The authorizing legislation directed that panels of qualified experts be convened by AHCPR or by public and not-for-profit private organizations. These panels were to review the literature that contained the findings of numerous studies of clinical conditions and, after considering the scientific evidence, to recommend clinical guidelines to assist practitioner and patient decisions about appropriate care for specific clinical conditions.

The agency's priority activities included extramural research through the Medical Treatment Effectiveness Program. The Medical Treatment Effectiveness Program funded two types of research projects: patient outcome research teams and literature synthesis projects or meta-analyses. Both the patient outcome research teams and the smaller literature synthesis projects identified and analyzed patient outcomes associated with alternative practice patterns and recommended changes where appropriate. During its decade-long existence, AHCPR supported studies that resulted in a prodigious array of publications focused on patient care and clinical decision making, technology assessment, the quality and costs of care, and treatment outcomes. Although no longer directly involved in producing clinical practice guidelines, the agency assists private-sector groups by supplying them with the scientific evidence that they need to develop their own guidelines.

Within AHCPR there was the Office of the Forum for Quality and Effectiveness in Health Care, which focused on the development and periodic review of practice recommendations. In addition, there were the Centers for Intramural and Extramural Research, the Office of Technology Assessment, and the Office for Data Development, among others (AHCPR, 1990).

Some changes occurred in the mandate of AHCPR since its 1989 inception. The agency narrowly escaped the loss of funding and elimination in 1996 after incurring the wrath of national organizations of surgeons. In keeping with its original mission, AHCPR issued clinical guidelines. One such guideline discouraged surgery as a treatment for back pain on the grounds that it provided no better outcomes than more conservative treatments. Organizations of angry surgeons led a lobbying effort that convinced key members of Congress that the agency was exceeding its authority and establishing standards of clinical practice without considering the expertise and opinions of the medical specialists involved (Stephenson, 1997).

The dispute was resolved when AHCPR agreed to function as a science partner with public and private organizations by simply assisting in developing knowledge that can be used to improve clinical practice. The agency would no longer produce clinical guidelines, but focus instead on funding research on medical interventions and analyzing the data that would underlie the development of clinical guidelines. The guidelines themselves would be generated by medical specialty and other organizations.

Subsequently, the Healthcare Research and Quality Act of 1999 was passed, which retitled the AHCPR to the Agency for Healthcare Research and Quality (AHRQ) and changed the title of the administrator to director. The mission of AHRQ is to (1) improve the outcomes and quality of healthcare services; (2) reduce its costs; (3) address patient safety; and (4) broaden effective services through establishment of a broad base of scientific research that promotes improvements in clinical and health systems practices, including prevention of disease (AHRQ, 2002).

The agency is composed of the following components:

1. Center for Delivery, Organization, and Markets
2. Center for Access, Financing, and Cost Trends
3. Center for Outcomes and Evidence

4. Center for Primary Care, Prevention, and Clinical Partnerships
5. Center for Quality Improvement and Patient Safety
6. Office of Director
7. Office of Communications and Knowledge Transfer
8. Office of Extramural Research, Education, and Priority Populations
9. Office of Performance Accountability, Resources, and Technology (AHRQ, n.d.)

A top priority of AHRQ is getting its sponsored research results and new health information into the hands of consumers. In addition to a number of consumer-oriented publications, the agency provides information to the public over the Internet. Its Web site, www.ahrq.gov, offers a great deal of healthcare information.

Building on concerns about medical errors and the quality of care, Congress and the president have increased support of the AHRQ. If that support continues during the next decade, the agency's greatest contribution to health care may be in the increases in patient care quality and reductions in costs that will result from provider acceptance of its service quality assessments and evidence-based practice recommendations.

Health Services Research and Health Policy

Health services research combines the perspectives and methods of epidemiology, sociology, economics, and clinical medicine; therefore, its curriculum is broader than the research courses taught in most medical schools. Although the basic concepts of epidemiologic research and associated statistics apply, process and outcome measures that reflect the behavioral and eco-nomic variables associated with questions of therapeutic effectiveness and cost benefit are also used. The ability of health services research to address issues of therapeutic effectiveness and cost benefit during this period of fiscal exigency contributed to the field's substantial growth and current value.

The contributions of health services research to health policy within recent years are impressive. Major examples include the Wennberg studies of small area variation in medical utilization, the prospective payment system based on diagnosis-related groups (Fetter, Shin, Freeman, Averill, & Thompson, 1980; Mills, Fetter, Riedel, & Averill, 1976), research on inappropriate medical procedures (Chassin et al., 1987), resource-based relative value scale research (Hsiao & Stason, 1979; Hsaio, Braun, Dunn, Becker, Chen et al., 1988; Hsaio, Braun, Dunn, Becker, DeNicola et al., 1988), and the background research that supported the concepts of health maintenance organizations (HMOs) and managed care.

The RAND Health Insurance Experiment (Newhouse, 1974; Newhouse et al., 1987), one of the largest and longest running health services research projects ever undertaken, began in 1971 and contributed vast amounts of information on the effects of cost sharing on the provision and outcomes of health services. Between 1974 and 1977, the project enrolled families in six sites, representing four major census regions, northern and southern rural areas, and a range of city sizes. Participating families were assigned to one of four different fee-for-service plans or to a prepaid group practice. As might have been expected, individuals in the various plans differed significantly in their rate of use, with little measurable effect on health outcomes. Although the reduced use of hospitals and specialized care by those in HMO plans did not affect their health status, those patients new to HMOs were somewhat less satisfied than the fee-for-service patients. The Health Insurance Experiment was followed by two large research studies: the Health Services Utilization study and the Medical Outcomes study. The findings of both have given impetus to the federal support of outcomes research (Newhouse, 1987).

Determining the outcomes and effectiveness of different healthcare interventions aids clinical decision making, reduces costs, and benefits patients. If the United States is ever able to build political consensus in support of a national health policy, the findings of health services research will underpin the decisions. In the meantime, the findings related to treatment effectiveness guide the cost-containment efforts of managed care organizations.

Quality Improvement

Until the last few years, health care's impressive accomplishments made it difficult for healthcare researchers, policy makers, and organizational leaders to acknowledge publicly that poor quality health care is a major problem within the dynamic and productive biomedical enterprise in the United States. In 1990, after 2 years of study, hearings, and site visits, the Institute of Medicine (IOM) issued a report that cited widespread overuse of expensive invasive technology, underuse of inexpensive caring services, and implementation of error-prone procedures that harmed patients and wasted money (Lohr, 1990; Palmer, 1991).

Although these conclusions from so prestigious a body were devastating in their significance to healthcare reformers, they were hardly news to health service researchers. For decades, practitioners assumed that quality, like beauty, was in the eye of the beholder and, therefore, was unmeasurable except in cases of obvious violation of generally accepted standards. The medical and other healthcare professions had promoted the image of health care as a blend of almost impenetrable, science-based disciplines, leaving the providers of care as the only ones capable of understanding the processes taking place. Thus, only physicians could judge the work of other physicians. Such peer review–based assessment has always been difficult for reviewers and limited in effectiveness. Peer review recognizes that only part of medical care is based on factual knowledge. A substantial component of medical decision making is based on clinical judgment. Clinical judgment means combining consideration of the potential risks and benefits of each physician's internal list of alternatives in making diagnostic and treatment decisions with his or her medical intuition regarding the likelihood of success based on the condition of each patient. Under these complex and often inexplicable circumstances, physicians are repelled by the notion of either judging or being judged by their colleagues.

That is why, until recently, quality assurance, whether in hospitals or by regulatory agencies, was focused on identifying only exceptionally poor care. This practice, popularly known as the bad apple theory, was based on the presumption that the best way to ensure quality was to identify the bad apples and remove or rehabilitate them. Thus, during the 1970s and 1980s, quality assurance interventions only followed detection of undesirable occurrences. For example, flagrant violations of professional standards had to be in evidence before professional review organizations required physicians to begin quality improvement plans. Of course, physicians were guaranteed due process to dispute the evidence.

Focusing on isolated violations required a great deal of review time to uncover a single case that called for remedial action. In addition, it was an unpleasant duty for reviewers to assign blame to a colleague who might soon be on a committee reviewing their records. Most importantly, such an inspection of quality represented a method that implicitly defined quality as the absence of mishap. Clinician dislike of quality assurance activities during the 1970s and 1980s was well founded. The processes were offensive and had little constructive impact.

Specifying and striving for excellent care are very recent quality-assurance phenomena in the healthcare arena. Just as the automobile and other industries were late giving up supervision as a control mechanism and introducing quality circles, or teamwork, so, too, were hospitals and other healthcare organizations that had long focused on peer review committees, incident reports, and other negative quality monitoring activities.

Health services researchers had known for decades that healthcare quality was measurable and that excellent, as well as poor, care could be identified and quantified. In 1966, Avedis Donabedian characterized the concept of health care as divided into the components of structure, process, and outcomes and the research paradigm of their assumed linkages, all of which have guided quality of care investigators to this day.

Donabedian suggested that the number, kinds, and skills of the providers, as well as the adequacy of their physical resources and the manner in which they perform appropriate procedures, should, in the aggregate, influence the quality of the subsequent outcomes. Although today the construct may seem like a simple statement of the obvious, at the time, attention to structural criteria was the major, if not the only, quality assurance activity in favor. It was generally assumed that properly trained professionals, given adequate resources in properly equipped facilities, performed at acceptable standards of quality. For example, for many years, the then Joint Commission on Accreditation of Healthcare Organizations made judgments about the quality of hospitals on the basis of structural standards, such as physical facilities and equipment, ratios of professional staff to patients, and the qualifications of various personnel. Later, it added process components to its structural standards. Aspects of process are the diagnostic, treatment, and patient management decisions and their appropriateness in relationship to current knowledge and practice. These quality assessments were directed to process components and did not attempt to determine what happened to the patients as the result of the medical decisions and interventions. Only recently did the Joint Commission on Accreditation of Healthcare Organizations include outcomes in its accreditation assessments.

Nevertheless, as far back as the 1950s, when Oscar Peterson and his associates at the University of North Carolina reported on a statewide study of general practice physicians, it was known that the quality of health service processes or practices may not reflect the quality of the underlying structural components of training and experience. Looking primarily at process components and using explicit practice quality criteria established in advance by a committee of general practitioners, researchers made onsite observations of each physician's practice behaviors for approximately 1 week. During that time, 44% of the physicians observed showed practice behaviors that were assessed as below average or poor in quality. Actual performance deficiencies may have been even greater because the presence of the observer may have motivated physicians to improve their usual performance temporarily (1956).

Similarly, in the early 1960s, M. A. Morehead conducted a study of the quality of care rendered to members of the Teamsters union in New York City. At that time, the union was spending about $20 million per year for hospital services for its members and their families and wondered whether the quality of the services justified that expense. Unlike the North Carolina study, however, the criteria against which performance was measured were implicit, that is, left to the individual judgments of expert reviewers. Teams of various kinds of specialists reviewed samples of patient records from the large number of hospitals in New York City. Although an examination of outcomes was not part of the study, the researchers did look at the association between structure and process and found strong relationships. Both the level of specialty training of the physicians and the teaching status of the hospitals were associated strongly with high percentages of appropriate admissions and the provision of optimal care (Morehead, 1967).

However, the teams of medical experts making the judgments were themselves board-certified specialists associated with teaching hospitals, so the implicit personal standards they used reflected their own practice styles, values, and beliefs as to what constituted quality care. Clearly, their selection as judges biased

the study in the direction of its subsequent findings—an intrinsic problem when standards are personal and not predefined.

Nevertheless, the findings of the Teamsters' study have been replicated in many others since. In another early study by Peterson, Barsamian, and Eden (1966), the percentage of pelvic surgical procedures with incorrect diagnoses was determined by analyses of the pathologists' examination of the removed tissues. Again, there was a significant difference between major teaching hospitals and other proprietary and not-for-profit institutions. There also was a difference between physicians who were members of the American College of Surgeons and those who were not.

These early landmark quality-of-care studies are noted to illustrate the difference between implicit and explicit normative or judgmental standards. Implicit standards rely on the internalized judgments of the expert individuals involved in the quality assessment. Explicit standards are those developed and agreed on in advance of the assessment. Explicit standards minimize the variation and bias that invariably result when judgments are internalized. More current studies judge the appropriateness of hospital admissions and various procedures and, in general, associate specific structural characteristics of the healthcare system with practice or process variations. The previously noted small area variation studies are typical examples of such research designs.

There is another method for assessing the quality of healthcare practices that is based on empirical standards. Derived from distributions, averages, ranges, and other measures of data variability, information collected from a number of similar health service providers is compared to identify practices that deviate from the norms. A current popular use of empirical standards is in the patient severity-adjusted hospital performance data collected by health departments and community-based employer and insurer groups to measure and compare both process activities and outcomes. These performance report cards are becoming increasingly valuable to the purchasers of care who need an objective method to guide their choices among managed care organizations, healthcare systems, and group practices. The empirical measures of quality include such variables as:

- Timeliness of ambulation
- Compliance with basic nursing care standards
- Average length of stay
- Number of home care referrals
- Number of rehabilitation referrals
- Timeliness of consultation completion
- Timeliness of orders and results
- Patient wait times by department or area
- Infection rates
- Decubitus rates
- Medication errors
- Patient complaints
- Readmissions within 30 days
- Neonatal and maternal mortalities
- Perioperative mortalities

Normative and empirical standards are both used in studying the quality of health care in the United States. For example, empirical analyses are performed to test or modify normative recommendations. Empirical or actual experience data are collected to confirm performance and outcome improvements after the imposition of clinical guidelines derived from studies using normative standards.

Medical Errors

In November 1999, the IOM again issued a report on the quality of medical care. Focused on medical errors, the report described mistakes occurring during the course of hospital care as one of the nation's leading causes of death and disability. Citing two major studies, estimating that medical errors kill some 44,000 to 98,000 people in U.S. hospitals each year, the IOM report was a stunning indictment of the current systems of hospital care. The report contained a series of recommendations for improving patient safety in the admittedly high-risk environments of modern hospitals. Among the recommendations was a proposal for establishing a center for patient safety within the AHRQ. The proposed center would establish national safety goals, track progress in improving safety, and invest in research to learn more about preventing mistakes (Kohn, Corrigan, & Donaldson, 1999). Congress responded by designating part of the increase in the budget for the AHRQ for that purpose.

Evidence-Based Medicine

Evidence-based medicine is defined as "the systematic application of the best available evidence to the evaluation of options and decisions in clinical practice, management and policy-making" (Ware, Snyder, Wright, & Davies, 1983). Although that statement may appear to be a description of the way physicians and other healthcare providers have practiced since the inception of scientific medicine, it reflects a spreading concern that quite the opposite is true. The wide range of variability in clinical practice, the complexity of diagnostic testing and medical decision making, and the difficulty that physicians have in keeping up with the overwhelming volumes of scientific literature suggest that a significant percentage of clinical management decisions are not supported by reliable evidence of effectiveness.

Although it is generally assumed that physicians are reasonably confident that the treatments they give are beneficial, the reality is that medical practice is fraught with uncertainty. In addition, the ethical basis for clinical decision making allows physicians to exercise their preferences for certain medical theories or practices that may or may not have been evaluated to link treatment to benefits (Watanabe, 1997).

Proponents of evidence-based medicine propose that if all health services are intended to improve the health status and quality of life of the recipients, then

> The acid test is whether services, programs and policies improve health beyond what could be achieved with the same resources by different means, or by doing nothing at all. Evidence is the key to accountability; the decisions made by healthcare providers, administrators, policy makers, patients, and the public need to be based on appropriate, balanced, and high-quality evidence (Marwick, 1993).

The evidence-based approach to assessing the acceptability of research findings considers the evidence from randomized clinical trials involving large numbers of participants to be the most valid. Evidence-based medicine advocates dismiss outcomes research that uses large data files created from claim records, hospital discharges, Medicare, or other sources because the subjects are not randomized.

"Outcomes research using claims data is an excellent way of finding out what doctors are doing, but it's a terrible way to find out what doctors should be doing," stated Thomas C. Chalmers, MD, of Harvard School of Public Health, Boston (Watanabe, 1997).

In general, most of the investigations reported in the peer-reviewed medical literature have been preliminary tests of innovations and served science rather than providing guidance to practitioners in clinical practice. Only a small portion of those efforts survive testing well enough to justify routine clinical application (Marwick, 1993).

The situation is changing rapidly, however. Articles on evidence-based medicine are appearing with increasing frequency in the medical literature (Castiel, 2003). Cost-control pressures that encourage efforts to ensure that therapies have documented patient benefit, growing interest in the quality of patient care, and increasing sophistication on the part of patients concerning the care that they receive have stimulated acceptance of the concepts of evidence-based medical practice (Hooker, 1997).

Outcomes Research

Given the huge investment in U.S. health care and the inequitable distribution of its services, do the end effects on the health and well-being of patients and populations justify the costs? Insurance companies, state and federal governments, employers, and consumers are looking to outcomes research for information that will help them to make better decisions about what kinds of health care should be reimbursed, for whom, and when.

Because outcomes research evaluates results of healthcare processes in the real world of physicians' offices, hospitals, clinics, and homes, it contrasts with traditional randomized controlled studies that test the effects of treatments in controlled environments. In addition, the research in usual service settings, or effectiveness research, differs from controlled clinical trials, or efficacy research, in the nature of the outcomes measured. Traditionally, studies measured health status, or outcomes, with physiologic measurements—laboratory tests, complication rates, recovery, or survival. To capture health status more adequately, outcomes research measures a patient's functional status and well-being. Satisfaction with care also must complement traditional measures.

Functional status includes three components that assess patients' abilities to function in their own environment:

1. Physical functioning
2. Role functioning—the extent to which health interferes with usual daily activities, such as work or school
3. Social functioning—whether health affects normal social activities, such as visiting friends or participating in group activities

Personal well-being measures describe patients' senses of physical and mental well-being—their mental health or general mood, their own view of their general health, and their general sense about the quality of their lives. Patient satisfaction measures the patients' views about the services received, including access, convenience, communication, financial coverage, and technical quality.

Outcomes research also uses meta-analyses, a technique to summarize comparable findings from multiple studies. More importantly, however, outcomes research goes beyond determin-ing what works in ideal circumstances to assessing which treatments for specific clinical problems work best in different circumstances. Appropriateness studies are conducted to determine circumstances in which a procedure should and should not be performed. Even though a procedure is proven effective, it is not appropriate for every patient in all circumstances. The frequency of inappropriate clinical interventions is one of the major quality-of-care problems in the system. Research is also under way to develop the tools to identify patient preferences when treatment options are available. Although most discussions about appropriateness stress the cost savings that could be achieved by reducing unnecessary care and overuse of services, it is important to remember that outcomes research may be just as likely to uncover underuse of appropriate services.

It is important to recognize that the ultimate value of outcomes research can be measured only by its ability to incorporate the results of its efforts into the healthcare process. To be effective, the findings of outcomes research must first reach and then change the behaviors of providers, patients, healthcare institutions, and payers. The endpoint of outcomes research, the clinical practice guidelines intended to assist practitioners and patients in choosing appropriate health care for specific conditions, must be disseminated in acceptable and motivational ways. With the healthcare industry in a state of rapid and generally unpredictable change, the need to make appropriate investments in outcomes research has become increasingly apparent. The conclusion is now inescapable that the United States cannot continue to spend over $1.5 trillion a year on health care without learning much more than is now known about what that investment is buying (Reinhardt, Hussey, & Anderson, 2004).

Patient Satisfaction

Patient satisfaction has become an important component of the quality of care. Although the subjective ratings of health care received by patients may be based on markedly different criteria from those considered important by care providers, they capture aspects of care and personal preferences that contribute significantly to perceived quality. It has become increasingly important in the competitive market climate of health care that the providers' characteristics, organization, and system attributes important to the consumers be identified and monitored. In addition to caregivers' technical and interpersonal skills, such patient concerns as waiting times for appointments, emergency responses, helpfulness and communication of staff, and the facility's appearance contribute to patient evaluations of health services delivery programs and subsequent satisfaction with the quality of care received.

A number of instruments have been devised to measure patient satisfaction with health care, and most managed care plans, hospitals, and other health service facilities and agencies have adopted one or more to assess patient satisfaction regularly. Some, like the patient satisfaction questionnaire developed at Southern Illinois University School of Medicine, are short, self-administered survey forms (Marwick, 1993). Others, like the popular patient satisfaction instruments of the Picker Institute of Boston, Massachusetts, may be used as self-administered questionnaires mailed to patients after a healthcare experience or completed by interviewers during telephone surveys (Gerteis, Edgman-Levitan, Daley, & Delbanco, 1993). Whether by mail, direct contact, or telephone interview, questioning patients after a recent healthcare experience is an effective way to both identify outstanding service personnel and uncover fundamental problems in the quality of care as defined by patients. It not only serves the purpose of providing humane and effective care, but is also good marketing to do everything possible to increase patient satisfaction, maintain patient loyalty, and enhance patient referrals.

Research Ethics

In the six decades since World War II, the federal government has invested heavily in biomedical research. The ensuing public–private partnership in health has produced some of the finest medical research in the world. The growth of medical knowledge is unparalleled, and the United States can take well-deserved pride in its research accomplishments.

However, many, if not most, of the sophisticated new technologies address the need to ameliorate the problems of the patients who already have the condition or disease under treatment. Both the priorities and the profits intrinsic to the U.S. healthcare system focus on remedial rather than preventive strategies. Only in the case of frightening epidemics, such as that of polio in the 1940s or AIDS in the 1990s, has there been the requisite moral imperatives to adequately fund abundant research efforts that address public health problems. Clearly, much of the recent funding for medical research has failed to fulfill the generally held belief that the products of taxpayer-supported research should benefit not only the practice of medicine, but also the community at large (Constantine, 1997).

The increasing amount of research funding emanating from pharmaceutical companies is of growing concern. Pharmaceutical companies that pay researchers to design and interpret drug trials have been accused of spinning the results or suppressing unfavorable findings. The conflicts that arise in the testing of new drugs and publishing the results are deepened as more and more of these studies are shifted from academic institutions to commercial research firms (Stevens, 1989).

Commercialism, with its accompanying ethical concerns, has invaded the research laboratory in a big way with the unfolding of the human genome. The scientific importance of being able to read the 3 billion DNA "letters" of the human body is being overshadowed by visions of the technology's commercial potential. The completion of the DNA sequence will revolutionize medicine by giving scientists unprecedented insights into the workings of the human body. Although the benefits of these genetic breakthroughs are years away, debates over whether the technology will stay in the public domain and strategies for profiting from the ability to treat medical conditions through gene manipulation are already under way. Clearly, the admirable advances in understanding and technology resulting from sophisticated medical research are increasingly accompanied by less-than-commendable bending of ethical precepts.

Future Challenges

Much, if not most, of U.S. healthcare research has been directed toward improving the healthcare system's ability to diagnose and treat injury, disease, and disability among those who seek care from the healthcare providers in the vast and complex array of existing health services. For decades, health care has been a complaint and response system, with most patient and provider interactions initiated by ailing patients. Physicians and other health professionals have maintained the mindset that their major, if not sole, duty was to resolve patient problems as expeditiously as possible. Now, largely because of the influences of managed care, research studies are increasingly focused on identifying and improving the health status of populations. Research priorities are shifting from an individual patient perspective to a population orientation and toward continuous scrutiny of the efficiency and effectiveness of the care delivered.

Basic science research will continue to contribute to the diagnostic and therapeutic efficacy of health care by adding to the knowledge about the human body and its functions. In small but critically important increments, basic science research will unlock many of the secrets of aging, cell growth regulation, mental degradation, and other mysteries of immunology, genetics, microbiology, and neuroendocrinology. The propensity of medicine to use newly obtained knowledge to alter certain physiologic processes, as in the several forms of gene manipulation, will produce new ethical, legal, and clinical issues that then will require further research and adjudication.

Massive databases of gene and protein sequences and structure/function information have made possible a new worldwide research effort called bioinformatics. Bioinformatic research probes those large computer databases to learn more about life's processes in health and disease and to find new or better drugs. It is considered the future of biotechnology.

Of particular interest is research in genomics, the study of genetic material in the chromosomes of specific organisms. The sequencing of the human genome will reshape biology and medicine and lead to significant improvements in the diagnosis of disease and individual responses to drugs (George Washington University Medical Center, 2002).

Similarly, certain advances in clinical medicine and the other health disciplines will result in new and particularly disturbing moral dilemmas. Medical achievements, such as those that permit the maintenance of life in otherwise terminal and unresponsive individuals, or the transplantation of organs in short supply that require choosing among recipient candidates when those denied will surely die, generate extremely complex ethical, economic, religious, personal, and professional issues. Thus, much of the basic and clinical research that solves yesterday's problems relating to individual patient care will create new problems to be addressed in the never-ending cycle of discovery, application, and evaluation.

Medical researchers and clinicians are becoming increasingly concerned that health care in the United States is entering a postantibiotic era in which bacterial infections will be unaffected by even the most powerful of available antibiotics. Evidence is accumulating that a growing number of microbes, including strains of staphylococcus and streptococcus bacteria, are becoming resistant to common antimicrobials (Bodenheimer, 2000).

Staphylococcus bacteria are the major cause of hospital infections. According to the Centers for Disease Control and Prevention, these infections are responsible for about 13% of the 2 million infections that occur in U.S. hospitals each year. Overall, those hospital infections result in the deaths of 60,000 to 80,000 patients (Ibrahim, 1985).

Although epidemiologists and clinicians specializing in infectious disease have warned for decades that misuse and overuse of antibiotics would result in a host of deadly drug-resistant pathogens, it appears that neither physicians nor patients took the warnings seriously. Apparently, there was a widespread belief that the constant development of new antimicrobial drugs would keep medicine a step ahead of bacterial resistance. Although the limited development of new antibiotic drugs has failed to keep step with antibiotic resistance, scientists see a promising alternative in bacterial genetics. Introducing synthetic genes into bacteria appears to turn off the bacteria's ability to resist antibiotics (Constantine, 1997).

While researchers address the problems of treatment of these lethal infections, hospitals strive to prevent them. Because bacteria can be transmitted on blankets, clothing, walls, medical equipment, and by hand, hospitals are implementing rigorous infection control and surveillance policies and new education programs for both providers and patients.

Health services research, on the other hand, will continue to focus on the performance of the healthcare system as the basis for proposing or evaluating health policy alternatives. It is interdisciplinary, value-laden research concerned with the effectiveness or benefits of care, the efficiency or resource cost of care, and the equity or fairness of the distribution of care. As the U.S. healthcare system goes through its wrenching adjustment to the competitive, market-driven reforms, health services research becomes more and more central to the development of a logical, well-documented rationale for future healthcare policies and delivery systems. At present, clinical uncertainty is pervasive in the healthcare industry as it defines illness, selects among treatment options, and tries to determine the probabilities of desired and unintended results and to judge the quality of individual outcomes.

Documenting the influence of financial incentives that affect both patient and provider, understanding the important relationships of socioeconomic status to health and health care, determining the effects of the training and experience of the healthcare team and the ability of the members to work together, and understanding how these many influences interact are basic to improving the quality of care. Reducing the monumental quandaries in medicine and health care about what works well in what situations is the challenge of health services research and the key to a more effective, efficient, and equitable healthcare system.

Managed care companies and groups of consumers and businesses are supporting an effort to develop national performance measures for health plans that will help consumers and payers compare plans on measures other than cost. Insurers are increasingly using outcomes research results to refine and improve their reimbursement systems. Hospitals, HMOs, and other organized care systems are incorporating results of outcomes research into their quality review and improvement practices. Results not only provide guidance on what constitutes good care, but also form the basis for discussion among providers and managers about ways of designing more efficient delivery systems.

Public health research is a related research arena that deserves to receive higher priority and significantly increased political support. If health care is ever to develop a true population perspective rather than an individual patient perspective and reap the health and economic benefits of preventive rather than curative medicine, then epidemiology and public health research must be charged with finding ways to understand better and resolve the huge differences in health, health behaviors, health care, and health system effectiveness among communities and the population groups within them. Epidemiology, the core discipline of public health research, relates the health problems and use of healthcare resources to defined populations. It identifies groups that do not present themselves for health care, as well as those that do. Thus, epidemiology can assess the health problems and the provision of health care for the total population rather than just those who are in contact with health services. Surveillance and monitoring of health conditions and assessing the effect of healthcare measures on the entire population are important factors in formulating health policy, organizing health services, and allocating limited resources (Ibrahim, 1985). The strategy for identifying and dealing with real or suspected biological attacks on citizens of the United States will depend heavily on the ability of epidemiologists to identify the common source of such outbreaks, the patterns of transmission, and the outcomes of preventive and remedial efforts.

As health care adds to its traditional focus on theories, disease, and individual patient care, the performance of the healthcare system and the health status of populations, public health, and health services research assume increasing relevance and importance. No matter how well the healthcare system performs for some of the people, it will never be fully satisfactory until it can provide a basic level of care for all.

Discussion Questions

1. Of the various types of research described, which ones are most important to the practice of advanced nursing practice? Which ones will you access to inform your practice and why? Which ones might you actually participate in and how?
2. Go to the Web site of the Agency for Healthcare Research and Quality. Browse the site for updated information. Access one clinical practice guideline of interest to you. What is the evidence that supports the guideline?
3. Find a recent article about a healthcare policy. What research informed the policy? Or what research is needed to support the policy?
4. What future trends will affect your practice in the next 5 years?

References

Aday, L. A., Begley, C. E., Lairson, D. R., & Slater, C. H. (1993). *Evaluating the medical care system: Effectiveness, efficiency, and equity.* Ann Arbor, MI: Health Administration Press.

Agency for Healthcare Policy and Research, U.S. Department of Health and Human Services. (1990). *AHCPR program note.* Rockville, MD: Public Health Service, 1–5.

Agency for Healthcare Research and Quality: Offices and Centers, Agency for Healthcare Research and Quality, Rockville, MD. (n.d.). *Organization and contacts.* Retrieved December 20, 2004, from http://www.ahrq.gov/about/organix.htm

AHRQ Fiscal Year 2003 Budget in Brief, Agency for Healthcare Research and Quality, Rockville, MD. (2002, February). Retrieved August 28, 2002, from http://www.ahrq.gov/about/cj2003/budbrf03.htm

Bodenheimer, T. (2000). Uneasy alliance—clinical investigators and the drug industry. *The New England Journal of Medicine, 342,* 1516–1518, 1539–1544.

Castiel, L. D. (2003, July). The urge for evidence based knowledge. *Journal of Epidemiology and Community Health, 57,* 482.

Chassin, M. R., Kosecoff, J., Park, R. E., Winslow, C. M., Kahn, K. L., Merrick, N. J., et al. (1987). Does inappropriate use explain geographic variations in the use of healthcare services? A study of three procedures. *Journal of the American Medical Association, 258,* 2533–2537.

Constantine, L. M. (1997, October 16). Healthcare providers confront rise in resistant pathogens. *Report of Medical Guidelines and Outcomes Research, 8*(21), 1–5.

Donabedian, A. (1966). Evaluating the quality of medical care. *Milbank Memorial Fund Quarterly, 44,* 166–206.

Fetter, R. B., Shin, Y., Freeman, J. L., Averill, R. F., & Thompson, J. D. (1980). Case-mix definition by diagnosis-related groups. *Medical Care Supplement, 18,* 1–53.

The George Washington University Medical Center. (2002, July). *What is genomics?* Retrieved August 27, 2002, from http://www.gwumc.edu/bioinformatics/about/genomics.htm

Gerteis, M., Edgman-Levitan, S., Daley, J., & Delbanco, T. L. (1993). *Through the patient's eyes: Understanding and promoting patient-centered care.* San Francisco: Jossey-Bass Publishers.

Hooker, R. C. (1997, May 3). The rise and rise of evidence-based medicine. [Letter]. *Lancet, 349*(9061), 1329–1330.

Hsiao, W. C., Braun, P., Dunn, D., Becker, E. R., Chen, S. P., Couch, N. P., et al. (1988). *A national study of resource-based relative value scale for physician services: Final report to the Health Care Financing Administration.* Boston, MA: Harvard School of Public Health.

Hsiao, W. C., Braun, P., Dunn, D., Becker, E. R., DeNicola, M., & Ketcham, T. R. (1988). Results and policy implications of the resource-based relative value study. *New England Journal of Medicine, 319*(13), 881–888.

Hsiao, W. C., & Stason, W. B. (1979). Toward developing a relative value scale for medical and surgical services. *Health Care Financing Review, 1*(2), 23–28.

Ibrahim, M. A. (1985). *Epidemiology and health policy.* Gaithersburg, MD: Aspen Publishers.

Kohn, L. T., Corrigan, J. M., & Donaldson, M. S. (1999). *To err is human: Building a safer health system.* Washington, DC: Institute of Medicine.

Lohr, K. N. (1990). *Medicare: A strategy for quality assurance: Vol. 1.* Washington, DC: National Academy Press.

Marwick, C. (1993, July 14). Federal agency focuses on outcomes research. *Journal of the American Medical Association, 270*(2), 164–165.

Mills, R., Fetter, R. B., Riedel, D. C., & Averill, R. (1976). AUTOGRP: An interactive computer system for the analysis of health care data. *Medical Care, 14,* 603–615.

Morehead, M. A. (1967). The medical audit as an operational tool. *Journal of Public Health, 57,* 1643–1656.

Newhouse, J. P. (1974). A design for a health insurance experiment. *Inquiry, 11*(1), 5–27.

Newhouse, J. P. (1991). Controlled experimentation as research policy. In E. Ginzberg (Ed.), *Health Services Research: Key to Health Policy* (pp. 162–194). Cambridge, MA: Harvard University Press.

Newhouse, J. P., Manning, W. G., Duan, N., Morris, C. N., Keeler, E. B., Leibowitz, A., et al. (1987). The findings of the RAND health insurance experiment—A response to Welch et al. *Medical Care, 25*(2), 157–179.

Palmer, R. H. (1991). Considerations in defining quality of health care, Part I. In R. H. Palmer, A. Donabedian, & G. J. Povar, (Eds.), *Striving for quality in health care: An inquiry into policy and practice* (pp. 1–4). Ann Arbor, MI: Health Administration Press.

Peterson, O. (1956). An analytic study of North Carolina general practice. *Journal of Medical Education, 31*(Suppl., Part 2), 1–165.

Peterson, O., Barsamian, E. M., & Eden, M. (1966). A study of diagnostic performance: A preliminary report. *Journal of Medical Education, 41*(8), 797–803.

Reinhardt, U. E., Hussey, P. S., & Anderson, G. F. (2004, May/June). U.S. health care spending in an international context. *Health Affairs, 23*(3), 10–25.

Stephenson, J. (1997, November 19). Revitalized AHCPR pursues research on quality. *Journal of the American Medical Association, 278*(19), 1557.

Stevens, R. (1989). *In sickness and in wealth.* New York: Basic Books, Inc.

Ware, J. E., Jr., Snyder, M. K., Wright, W. R., & Davies, A. R. (1983). Defining and measuring patient satisfaction with medical care. *Evaluation and Planning, 6,* 247–263.

Watanabe, M. (1997, April 1). A call for action from the national forum on health. *Canadian Medical Association Journal, 156*(7), 999–1000.

Wennberg, J. E. (1986). Which rate is right? *New England Journal of Medicine, 314,* 310–311.

Wennberg, J. E., Freeman, J. L., & Culp, W. J. (1987). Are hospital services rationed in New Haven or over-utilized in Boston? *Lancet, 1,* 1185–1189.

Wennberg, J. E., Freeman, J. L., Shelton, R. M., & Bubolz, T. A. (1989). Hospital use and mortality among Medicare beneficiaries in Boston and New Haven. *New England Journal of Medicine, 321,* 1168–1173.

Chapter 24

Knowledge Development in Nursing: Our Historical Roots and Future Opportunities

Susan R. Gortner

CHAPTER OBJECTIVES

1. Trace the historical development of American nursing research in the past century.
2. Discuss projections for nursing research in the 21st century and how they will influence advanced practice nursing.

Introduction

The purpose of this chapter is to provide an historical overview of nursing research in the past century and to offer projections on where our science will be headed in the 21st century. For the overview, a number of reviews were drawn upon (Abdellah, 1970; DeTornyay, 1976; Gortner & Nahm, 1977; Lindeman, 1975a) with reliance on the last citation, which surveyed published nursing literature from 1900 to 1975. In the last 2 decades, other analyses of published research have been carried out (Brown, Tanner, & Patrick, 1983; Jacobsen & Meininger, 1985; Moody et al., 1988), including an impressive first encyclopedia

of nursing research (Fitzpatrick, 1998). Research agendas and priorities have been developed by the American Nurses Association Commission (American Nurses Association Commission, 1976) and Cabinet on Nursing Research (American Nurses Association Cabinet, 1985), the Academy of Nursing Ad Hoc Group on Knowledge Generation (Oberst, 1986; Stevenson & Woods, 1986b), and by consultant groups to the Division of Nursing's research program (Barnard, 1980; Gortner, 1980a), and to the former National Center for Nursing Research (Bloch, 1988). Research publications of the nursing schools at the University of California–Los Angeles (UCLA; Research, 1998), University of

Source: Reprinted from *Nursing Outlook,* 48(2), Susan R. Gortner, Knowledge Development in Nursing: Our Historical Roots and Future Opportunities, 60–67; copyright 2000, with permission from Elsevier.

California–San Francisco (UCSF; Science, 1999), and the University of Maryland (Advancing the Science) were used to formulate contemporary research questions. As such, they are illustrative rather than representative. Projections for the 21st century have been drawn from the author's reflections on our science (Gortner, 1980a; 1980b; 1984; 1991; Gortner & Schultz, 1988), from Donaldson's seminal paper marking the 25th anniversary of the American Academy of Nursing (1998), and from the latest research agenda of the National Institute of Nursing Research (Grady, 1999). Comments will be made on how our practice has been affected through research and where applications did not occur, when perhaps they should have. Examples will be from projects personally known to the author.

The Early Years

Nursing practice and issues arising from practice have influenced research topics since the time of Nightingale.

While practice issues have varied since then, some early concerns regarding quality of care and qualified caregivers transcended the 19th and 20th centuries into the 21st century. It is no accident that the development of formal programs of nursing education was seen as the means to improve practice. Historical perspectives on nursing and nursing research may be depicted as follows: in the early 1900s, concern was for improvement of the public's health; major communicable diseases of childhood and adulthood were prevalent; maternal/child health had yet to benefit from prenatal care and improved obstetrical practices. Most surgery was done in the home. The literature in our professional journals addressed problems associated with tuberculosis, meningitis, scarlet fever, etc.

In 1913, the committee on public health nursing of the National League for Nursing Education discussed its concern about infant mortality, prevention of blindness, and the problem of unlicensed midwives. The committee believed that the nursing profession should recognize its role in the prevention of unnecessary deaths among infants and in the prevention of unnecessary blindness, and that intelligent care of the sick must involve "some knowledge of the scientific approach to disease . . . causes and prevention. . . ." (Gortner & Nahm, 1977).

During the 1920s, the first case studies appeared; they were used both as a teaching tool for students and as a record of patient progress; nursing care plans for specific patient groups and procedures appeared (e.g., use of turpentine stupes), and continued until recently as a means to standardize and improve practice, medical as well as nursing. The case approach as a major research and teaching model in clinical nursing practice paralleled the use of case studies in medical practice and research. These case studies were used to describe unusual patient situations or symptoms and to report on the effects of nursing and medical therapies with groups of patients. According to personal interviews with the late Lucile Petry Leone,[1] the need for systematic evaluations of nursing procedures had its origins in the post-Depression years. The Depression forced the graduate nurse out of the home and into the hospital and, at the same time, the first postgraduate nursing programs began to develop (Gortner & Nahm, 1977).

The war years prompted the collection of national data on nursing needs and resources (types, numbers, and uses of nurses). In the immediate postwar years, the federal government, assisted by professional nursing organizations and foundations, provided funds and staff to establish resources for nursing, one such being the Division of Nursing Resources of the United States Public Health Service created in 1948. Its staff carried out studies on nurse supply and distribution, job satisfaction and turnover, requirements for public health nursing services, personnel costs, and costs for collegiate nursing education. These studies were widely used throughout the United States, frequently in conjunction with federal staff consultation and training. A 5-year study of nursing functions and activities was begun by the American Nurses Association in 1950, resulting in functions, standards, and qualifications for practice (1959), as well as the publication *Twenty Thousand Nurses Tell Their Story* (Hughes et al., 1958). Also noteworthy during this time was the W. K. Kellogg Foundation Nursing Service Administration Research Project, in which faculty from 12 universities worked with Finer at the University of Chicago to determine needs for administrative science and skills in nursing (Finer, 1952). Thus the period between 1930 and 1960 concentrated on the components of professional nursing practice and how best to secure them.

Focus on the organization and delivery of nursing services was given a boost when the Division of Nursing Resources initiated a small competitive research grant and fellowship program in 1955. Lucile Petry Leone, former director of the cadet nurse corps and then chief nurse officer and assistant surgeon general in the Public Health Service, convinced the surgeon general and the director of the National Institutes of Health to allocate $500,000 for grants and $125,000 for fellowships from the NIH budget. These programs were the precursors to the National Center for Nursing Research and the current National Institute for Nursing Research (Gortner & Nahm, 1977). In 1952, the journal *Nursing Research* came into being; the first few issues contained a section entitled the "Research Reporter," in which areas suitable for research were noted; guest editorials emphasized the need for grassroots support of nursing research by hospitals, agencies, and schools. Lucile Petry Leone's editorial in the Fall 1955 issue summarized the types of studies needed in nursing, based on a staff paper she had prepared earlier. These types included studies of nursing care most essential to patient recovery; the nature of the therapeutic relationship; analysis and optimal use of nursing skills; and efforts to reduce staff turnover rates and student dropout rates. Her thinking provided a visionary public platform for nursing research (Leone, 1955).

Virginia Henderson's 1956 guest editorial noted that studies of the nurse outnumbered studies of practice 10 to 1, that more than half of the doctoral theses were carried out in the field of education, and the "responsibility for designing its methods is often cited as an essential characteristic of a profession. . . ." (Henderson, 1956, p. 99). Six years later, the first Nurse Scientist Graduate Training Grants were awarded to universities offering resources in one or more basic science departments for preparation through the doctorate. The first grant awards were to Boston University School of Nursing for training in biology, psychology, and sociology, and to the University of California School of Nursing for training in sociology. The next fiscal year, three additional grants were awarded, one to the UCLA School of Nursing for study in sociology; one to the University of Washington School of Nursing for graduate study in anthropology, microbiology, physiology, and sociology, and the third to Western

Reserve University School of Nursing for study in biology, physiology, psychology, and sociology.[2] Subsequently, grants were made to schools of nursing at the University of Kansas, Teachers College–Columbia University, University of Pittsburgh, University of Arizona, University of Colorado, University of Illinois, and briefly, New York University (the grant program was terminated in 1975). Required interdepartmental seminars helped to define the boundaries of nursing science for the early grantees. It is not surprising that nurse scientist graduate training settings later developed into PhD programs in nursing (Gortner, 1991).

In the early 1960s, establishment of the American Nurses Foundation grants program helped to address the demand for more practice-related studies. The foundation published the priorities that would guide funding: effects of performance of nursing acts on the patient (i.e., nursing procedures and outcomes); effects on nursing of changing patterns of nursing care and changing health needs; and nursing in different process categories (American Nurses Foundation, 1960).

Ellwynne Vreeland, the first chief of the federal research branch, wrote Chief Nurse Officer Lucile Petry Leone in 1959 that studies were needed to further development of nursing theory by identifying the scientific content of nursing, by seeking and experimenting with new concepts of nursing (e.g., motivation—"finding out why nurses can 'bring back' patients who have given up and who fail to respond to careful medical treatment"), and by careful study of the nursing care given by expert practitioners (the specifics of expert nursing, etc.) (Vreeland, 1959).

Soon the specifics of expert nursing became apparent as several university schools of nursing undertook studies of the nursing process,

patient responses to care, and behavioral phenomena. The Yale study of nursing effects on postoperative vomiting became widely cited because of its experimental design and findings suggesting that nurse counseling had a positive effect (Dumas & Leonard, 1963). UCLA nursing investigators studied recovery stages from myocardial infarction (Coston, 1960) (interviews with cardiologists revealed no clear demarcation of stages appropriate for nursing detection), breastfeeding (Disbrow, 1963), rooming-in (Ringholz & Morris, 1961), and pain relief (Moss & Myer, 1966). These became among the first practice-related studies to be published in the new journal, *Nursing Research*.

At UCSF, sociologists Strauss and Glaser combined talents with nurse investigator Quint to study hospital personnel's views on death and dying (Glaser & Strauss, 1965). Quint's seminal study (1967) of the experiences of women and undergoing radical mastectomies was to launch a scientific career that Donaldson (1998) has termed "pathfinding." Studies at the University of Washington in the early 1960s focused on nursing services for psychiatric, tubercular, alcoholic, and maternity patients; variables included professional attitudes, activities, and accountability for patient care (Gortner & Nahm, 1977). Batey's later expertise in research resource development was an outgrowth of her study with Julian of organizational patterns in psychiatric settings (Batey & Julian, 1964). One of the earliest controlled attempts to document the effects of nursing intervention on the clinical progress of chronically ill adults was carried out by nursing investigators (Little & Carnevali, 1967).

At Presbyterian-University of Pennsylvania Medical Center, a project carried out between 1963 and 1967 in a special facility, the coronary care unit, demonstrated significant reductions in patient morbidity and mortality through continuous monitoring and prompt treatment by expert nurses (Meltzer et al., 1969). This project had been supported by the fledgling research grant program of the Division of Nursing Resources; it was to become the model of coronary care nursing nationwide. It was also among the first reports of nursing research to be published in the *Journal of the American Medical Association*.

Thus the real thrust of nursing research began in the 1960s, a function of the vision of nursing leaders such as Lulu Wolf Hassenplug, Helen Nahm, Mary Tschudin, Hildegard Peplau, Virginia Henderson, Lucile Petry Leone, Ellwynne Vreeland, Faye Abdellah, and Jessie Scott, and the availability of public as well as private funds to support the studies and train nurses in research. I joined the division staff in 1966 to aid in the review of the Nurse Training Act of 1964, and in 1967 was appointed executive secretary to the Research in Patient Care Review Committee, the outside group of scientists charged with determining the scientific merit of research proposals submitted from throughout the United States. During my time as staff scientist and later as branch chief for research grants and fellowships, we attempted to nourish the growing enterprise of nursing research nationwide through staff consultation, conferences, research development grants, nurse scientist graduate training grants, and individual research fellowships. We publicized the grant programs (Gortner, 1973), urged scientific accountability for the profession (Gortner, 1974c) as a practice profession (Gortner, 1974b), and early on attempted to show the contributions of research to patient care with a proposed classification, which named nursing research a "science of practice" (Gortner, Bloch, & Phillips, 1976).

To recapitulate, knowledge development in nursing began in earnest only 40 years ago, primarily in university schools of nursing where nurse scientist graduate training was ongoing in alliance with other disciplines, but also in medical centers such as the City of Hope, where Geraldine Padilla was director of research, at Luther Hospital in Eau Claire, Wisconsin, where Carol Lindeman was in charge, and at the Loeb Center for Nursing at Montefiore under the direction of Gwenrose Alfano. The Loeb Center for Nursing, which demonstrated that cost-effective care could be rendered to elders in a nursing center, was not seen as an innovation until such practice innovations were publicized by the American Academy of Nursing. Why the lag in impact of this research?

Annual research conferences sponsored by the American Nurses Association and later by the regional nursing research societies provided forums for investigators to present their findings and learn the importance of public scrutiny (Gortner & Nahm, 1977). The art of the critique developed gradually; communality and collegiality joined communication and publication as hallmarks of our research efforts, and greater sophistication among nursing's investigators and clinicians resulted in greater intradisciplinary and interdisciplinary collaboration.

The Transition Years

I have termed the period from 1965 to 1985 "transitional" because professional nursing took on major leadership activities to influence federal policy for nursing education and research. The American Nurses Association established a Commission on Research in 1971; the Council of Nurse Researchers was created in 1972. In a paper presented at the first program meeting of the council in 1973, I described the increasing concern that research financed by the federal government be related to major health priorities, stating that ". . . there is no mistaking the trend toward greater legislative specification of science in the health fields" (Gortner, 1974a). The scientist audience was urged to develop research priorities for nursing research.

In response, Lindeman (1975a) undertook a Delphi survey of priorities in clinical nursing research through the Western Interstate Commission on Higher Education, with Division of Nursing support. Respondents identified items on the quality of care, nursing role, nursing process, and the research process. Patient welfare concerns, particularly items related to nursing interventions to mitigate stress and pain, and to provide patient education and support to frail elders also were cited (Lindeman, 1975b).

When the late President Nixon impounded nurse training act, research, and fellowship funds in 1973, all federal support for fellowships and training grants was halted. The president was taken to court by a coalition of nursing organizations and forced to release the funds in 1974. The Division of Nursing held several invitational conferences on nurse scientist graduate training and doctoral personnel needs. Commission members traveled to Washington, D.C. in 1975 to meet with legislators and federal program staff, the first such contacts to be made by what was later to become the nursing research advocacy group. In my capacity as branch chief, I was asked to meet with commissioners to present program needs, vital information for program development and funding that had been embargoed as a result of closure of all public information offices in 1971. Although we could not publish grant and fel-

lowship information, we could respond to requests for information about the programs. To their credit, grantees understood this constraint and found opportunities to request program information. Thus the commission was able to develop priorities for research training and research and set goals for accomplishing them including funding levels (American Nurses Association Commission, 1976).

Health science research training authorization was restored with the passage of the National Research Service Awards Act in 1974; two years later, primarily through Connie Holleran's efforts, the Division of Nursing research training programs were included (Gortner, 1979). Publication of a review of research grants awarded (Abdellah, 1970) was followed by two historical overviews of nursing research (Lindeman, 1975a; DeTornyay, 1976); two new research journals, *Research in Nursing and Health* and *The Western Journal of Nursing Research* appeared in 1978. The 94th Congress specified $5 million for research projects in nursing and $1 million for research fellowships to be spent during 1977 and 1978, the first time funds for nursing research had been earmarked in the appropriation. Until then and since 1964, nursing research funds had been allocated along with nurse training act funds, although that act dealt exclusively with training to address the quality and quantity of professional nurses (Gortner, 1979).

This somewhat awkward allocation process and the difficulty health manpower legislation was experiencing in the 1970s led to open discussions by nurse scientists and educators regarding the need to locate the nursing research programs within the research environment of the National Institutes of Health. The discussions were frank and heated; well-respected deans worried that such a relocation would fracture federal nursing; others worried that nursing research could not mature if not nourished within the institute structure. Legislators were sympathetic and passed legislation (Public Law 99-158) authorizing a new center at the National Institutes of Health; it came into being in 1986 after a successful override of a presidential veto in main attributed to nurse scientist lobbying efforts, including the persuasive efforts of the entire membership of the American Heart Association Council on Cardiovascular Nursing which was meeting in Washington, D.C., at the time. Council Chairperson Marie Cowan adjourned us to go on the Hill. We did, and the entire California delegation was visited (including the senate office of then Senator Pete Wilson who voted to override the veto).

Coincidental with the establishment of the national center was the continuing work both of the American Nurses Association Cabinet on Nursing Research and the scientist group in the American Academy of Nursing. The cabinet published *Directions for Nursing Research: Toward the 21st Century* in 1985, setting goals, priorities, and strategies with dollar amounts to achieve them. The next year the American Academy of Nursing held its annual meeting in Kansas City, with the program theme "Nursing in the Year 2000: Setting the Agenda for Knowledge Generation and Utilization." Stevenson and Woods (1986b) provided a synthesis of the focus group priorities both for the new national center and also for research in the next two decades. These specified fundamental knowledge development about clinical problems, followed by clinical therapeutics to test interventions, and increasing emphasis on health promotion, health status and functioning, on the family, and on vulnerable popula-

tions and age groups. Scientific knowledge synthesis was aided by the beginning of a series of annual reviews of nursing research under the direction of Werley and Fitzpatrick.

Oberst (1986), at the same Academy conference, provided a thoughtful insight for a possible Year 2000 research agenda:

> The heart of the problem may lie in the almost total absence of basic research into the nature of the phenomena we wish to influence. We know very little about patterns of fatigue and sleep or about the nature of immobility, confusion, or anorexia. We cannot expect to intervene to prevent or control a problem such as incontinence, for instance, without basic knowledge of the natural history of that condition in a variety of contexts.

Oberst also spoke to the extreme biophysical derangement associated with organ transplantation, microsurgery, and aggressive chemotherapy protocols, asking whether health providers know the short-term and long-term physical and psychologic effects of these events and their meaning for patients and families. This problem has continued to interest investigators. Mishel and Murdaugh (1987) studied an opportunistic sample of heart transplantation patients and families; this study is one of the finest examples of grounded theory methodology published. Jenkins is among others studying the effects of aggressive protocols on quality of life (Advancing the Science).

The transition years also saw the development of research on primary care and evaluation of nurse practitioner programs. Research was directed toward: (1) understanding the influence of structural variables on nurse practitioner performance (e.g., access to settings), (2) identifying personal and professional characteristics contributing to successful performance as a nurse practitioner, and (3) specifying the nature of clinical judgments used by nurse practitioners and physicians working collaboratively in patient care management to assign patients either to a nurse or to a physician and then reassign responsibilities as changes in health status occur. How do the management plans differ? This last question addresses the elusive nature of the nurse–patient encounter (the initial plan, examination, questioning, priority setting, treatment, and evaluation) (Gortner, 1979). Ford and Silver (1968) evaluated the post-training activities of skilled pediatric nurses and found that these nurses could handle independently three-fourths of clinical visits in a rural station with high patient satisfaction regarding counseling and health monitoring.

Lewis and Resnik (1967) evaluated the use of adult nurse practitioners at the University of Kansas medical clinic with similar findings. To their disappointment, the program was discontinued after grant funding ceased. Veterans Administration (VA) South Hill Clinic in Los Angeles became the site of a second attempt to demonstrate the effectiveness of nurse practitioners in managing adult chronic conditions, this time those of veterans. Charles Lewis had just come to UCLA, Theresa Cheyovich was a visionary nursing chief at the Clinic, and I represented the "Feds" in the first interagency agreement signed by the VA with another federal agency. Two UCLA–trained PRIMEX nurses (UCLA was the original PRIMEX training site), one a former VA clinic nurse, undertook caseloads released by then 33 VA physicians, who had been painstakingly persuaded by Lewis to participate in the project.

One nurse in particular was able to realize major changes in health status and outcomes of her veteran case load. Examining her encounters, we discovered she "contracted" with patients on a weekly basis, and used social persuasion and professional skills to bolster patient confidence in their own health management (Cheyovich, Lewis, & Gortner, 1976). Further, the experiment was so successful that the VA proceeded thereafter to train and place nurse practitioners in many of its settings. Here is still another example of how nursing research has impacted practice.

Nursing Research Becomes Nursing Science

What occurred also during this transition period was a shift in thinking from research to science, a recognition that what we had thought was nursing science was really research, the tool of science. Nursing science was depicted as a human science that had the additional requirement of intervention or clinical therapy. Nursing research was redefined "as the discrete and aggregated investigations that constitute the professions' modes and foci of inquiry . . ." (Gortner, 1980b). The phenomena of interest to nursing were already being documented through research to become tentative propositions about human health and illness, vulnerable population groups (the aged, the chronically ill, women, children, infants), and illness recovery processes and risk factors. The seminal essay by Donaldson and Crowley (1978), "The Discipline of Nursing," clarified our thinking on what might become our knowledge domains and syntax. Meleis' inaugural Helen Nahm lecture (1980) on nursing scholarship heralded both the scientific and theoretical developments that were to occur in the next two decades. Clinical science was seen as focusing on human problems and treatment modalities; fundamental science was characterized as having no immediate utility but devoted to understanding basic processes across a wide variety of disciplines (Gortner, 1980b).

The last period of knowledge development in this century witnessed an explosion of fundamental and clinical science activities in nursing. How these phenomena came about is described next.

Nursing Science Comes of Age

Our science came into maturity during the past decade and a half as a result of several factors. First, emphasis began to shift from discrete studies to aggregates of studies, the precursors of programs of research. This shift initially was encouraged by the Division of Nursing's Nursing Research Emphasis Grant Program, in which areas of concentration, such as vulnerable populations and health across the life span, were suggested as topics to be coupled with graduate education (Holzemer & Gortner, 1988). The program at UCSF concentrated on two of these areas and solicited proposals from faculty that would both extend knowledge and involve and excite graduate students; we were funded and renewed for 5 years. Second, schools of nursing began to recruit doctorally prepared faculty with excellent research preparation and programmatic interests that fit with concentrations of research within the school. University nursing schools featured "centers of excellence," in which faculty effort and talent were aggregated, acknowledging that

selectivity was required to achieve excellence. Third, educational programs in many universities maintained sufficient stability that faculty time and effort could be redirected toward research. That is, curriculum revisions seemed to reach a plateau. Collaboration and colleagueship began to replace competitiveness and solo investigations. Fourth, external competition for research support increased as grant success was forthcoming from both public and private agencies; in the university systems, extramural support is one criterion for advancement up the faculty ranks. At UCSF initially, successful investigators received a bottle of champagne; later beer, and then soda sufficed. Fifth, arguments over appropriate methods, whether experimentation, description, and/or interpretation, waxed heatedly and then seemed to wane, as many of us put our energies into substantive activities, whether empirical investigations or philosophic musings, or both, as was the case with me. Sixth, scientists such as Lindsey, Cowan, Donaldson, Woods, Shaver, Brooten, Norbeck, and Dracup, to name but a few, took the brave step of becoming deans, thus reinforcing the science enterprise in their settings. With this momentum and influx of prepared scientist nurses, some of whom had been exposed to philosophers in their graduate programs, came debate about the nature of nursing science, what should be the prevailing worldview and research approach. We spent a great of time speaking and writing to empiricism, phenomenology (later hermeneutics), critical theory, and feminism, to name but a few. Post-positivists, of which I am one, were maligned for speaking to the components of "good science" such as credibility, reproducibility, and rigor (Gortner, 1991).

The knowledge development group at the American Academy of Nursing program meeting in 1986 attempted to draw a cease-fire between the received and perceived views of science, endorsing pluralism (Stevenson & Woods, 1986a). Meleis (1987) called for a "passion for substance" rather than a passion for method; and I attempted to formulate a philosophy of science for nursing that would embrace values (Gortner, 1990). Notions about nursing research and its substantive activity also have been formulated throughout the years by Ellis (1970), Batey (1971), Barnard (1982), and Shaver (1985). The following represents but one definition of nursing science, drawing on Barnard (1980; Research Spanning, 1998) and Donaldson and Crowley (1998),

> Nursing science as a form of human science, has as its object of analysis the human organism, with particular reference to human response states in health and illness and health across the life span. Its aim is to generate a body of knowledge that can define patterns of behavior associated with normal and critical life events such as catastrophic illness; depict changes in health status and predict how these are brought about; and along with other scientific fields, determine the principles and laws governing life states and processes (Gortner, 1984).

In the decades of knowledge development documented in this review, nursing has identified with tasks and technology and has characterized itself as a compassionate human service; it has taken as its subject matter the ecology of human health and human responses to health illness. While these conceptualizations may appear sequential, based on historical literature, in reality they are concurrent.

The researchable components of human health across the life span comprise indicators of health status, biological and behavioral factors contributing to health and illness, culture, environment, and treatment outcomes. These components were displayed in the National Center for Nursing Research (1988) national nursing research agenda, developed after an invitational conference on research priorities in nursing science at which 50 nurse scientists were present. To establish the agenda, priorities were selected on the basis of the existing knowledge base, opportunities, areas of low emphasis in other institutes, marketability, and available scientific personnel. These priorities were staged as follows: I—"HIV Positive Clients, Partners and Families" and "Prevention and Care of Low Birth Weight Infants"; II—"Long Term Care and Symptom Management and Information Systems"; and III—"Health Promotion" (in which the most critical issues for study are the fundamental psychosocial mechanisms underlying maintenance of health promotion behaviors . . .") and "Technology Dependency Across the Lifespan" (Bloch, 1988).

Ten years later, the National Institute of Nursing Research (NINR) distributed a statement on strategic planning for the 21st century with this definition of research (not science!),

> Nursing research addresses the issues that examine the core of patients' and families' personal encounters with illness, treatment, disease prevention. NINR's primary activity is clinical research and most studies involve patients. The basic science is linked to patient problems.
>
>   . . . Nursing research is essential in defining and confronting the compelling health and illness challenges of the 21st Century (Grady, 1999).

These challenges include risk reduction, promotion of healthy lifestyles, enhanced quality of life for persons with chronic conditions, and care for persons at the end of life. These areas are familiar; they have remained persistent for more than 30 years. The National Institute for Nursing Research stated the following scientific goals for the next 5-year period:

1. Identify research opportunities that will achieve scientific distinction within the scientific and practice communities and within NIH as a result of their significant contributions to health:

    End of life/palliative care research

    Chronic illness experiences

    Quality of life and quality of care issues

    Health promotion and disease
      prevention

    Telehealth interventions

    Implications of generic advances

    Cultural and ethnic considerations
      to decrease health disparities

2. Identify future opportunities for high-quality cost-effective care for patients and contribute to the scientific base of nursing practice through research on:

    Chronic illness (arthritis, diabetes)
      and long-term care, including
      family care

    Health promotion and risk behaviors

    Cardiopulmonary health and critical
      care

    Neurofunction and sensory conditions

    Immune response and oncology

    Reproductive and infant health

3. Communicate research findings

4. Enhance research training opportunities

These initiatives are already displayed in the research programs of many university schools of nursing. I reviewed the research publications from the schools of nursing at the UCLA (Research Spanning, 1998), UCSF (The Science of Caring, 1999), and the University of Maryland (Advancing the Science) in preparation for the original presentation on which this article is based. The scientific topics in these settings include vulnerable populations, cardiovascular and other illnesses, symptom management, chronic pain, health promotion/illness prevention, risk reduction, quality of life, the family in health and illness, women's health, and nursing therapeutics (including intensive cardiac monitoring, coaching for recovery, and "kangaroo care"). As examples:

- Is pain relief universal or are there gender differences? (Miakowski & Levine, UCSF)

- Does an ischemia monitoring protocol result in improved patient outcomes? (Drew et al., UCSF)

- What is the relationship between daytime fatigue and sleep disturbance in women? (Lee, UCSF)

- Does a collaborative intervention (advanced practice nurses and community peer advisors) improve outcomes for cardiac elders? (Rankin, UCSF)

- What is the role of exercise in heart failure patients? (Dracup et al., UCLA)

- Can an intervention with low-income adolescent mothers reduce HIV risk and improve health outcomes? (Koniak-Griffin, UCLA)

- What chromosomal abnormalities result from environmental toxins and affect reproductive health? (Robbins, UCLA)

- What is the quality of life experience of women with differing stages of lung cancer? (Sarna, UCLA)

- Can kangaroo care be as effective in ventilated infants as in premature infants? (Ludington, University of Maryland)
- What are the effects of estrogen on platelet function after cerebral ischemia? (Kearney, University of Maryland)
- How do aggressive treatment modalities affect health status and quality of life? (Jenkins, University of Maryland)

In the study write-ups, investigators often revealed how their interests originated. Many investigators were and are advanced practice nurses. As such, they have credibility both as clinicians as well as scientists. Not surprisingly then, research findings have had an impact on practice by encouraging family sensitive care in several settings;[3] by enhancement of patient self-confidence and self-efficacy through coaching, counseling, and performance;[4] by advocating improved critical care heart monitoring procedures;[5] by early discharge of low-birth-weight infants;[6] and by sensory stimulation of the neonate, including skin-to-skin contact.[7] Whereas nursing investigators have not always received the publicity given medical investigation, this bias is changing slowly as more nurses are appointed and elected to public office and as more become members of scientific and governmental advisory groups. The media recognition awards given annually by the American Academy of Nursing also have been instrumental in raising the veil of public ignorance. Schorr and Kennedy's (1999) splendid pictorial of 100 years of American nursing, just released, is a cause for celebration!

Where the areas of concentration some 20 years ago tended to reflect one dominant knowledge domain, for example, the psychosocial, now the biophysical, particularly biology and genetics, are reflected in the investigations noted above and elsewhere. This phenomenon may have been encouraged by the report of the National Center for Nursing Research biological task force, which stated: "the implications for the interface of nursing science with the biological sciences as a basis for research and its subsequent findings for practice are tremendous" (Hinshaw, Sigmon, & Lindsey, 1991). It also may be a natural development of better understanding that nursing problems cannot be solved within one knowledge domain; most involve multiple and complex factors (Gortner, 1984; Gortner & Schultz, 1988).

Future Opportunities

In preparing for this last section, I queried several colleagues throughout the United States to inquire where the future might lead us. Invariably, the response was: (1) to reexamine the impact of organizational structures on nursing effectiveness, (2) to continue to examine fundamental processes underlying human responses to health and illness, (3) to take the lead with family health, (4) to continue study of end-of-life and palliative care, and (5) to have an impact on health policy. I would add one more to which I would give considerable urgency: (6) to identify the biobehavioral factors (in epidemiologic terms, the host factors) that explain much of illness and associated behavior. These factors will frame why questions (e.g., why is it that personal recovery beliefs are such a powerful predictor of cardiac surgical outcomes along with the usual pathophysiologic markers?) that will bring our science into increasing respect within the greater medical science community at the National Institutes of Health and elsewhere.

Donaldson's "Breakthroughs in Nursing Research" given at the 25th Anniversary of the

American Academy of Nursing in 1998, identified "pathfinders" who created a new realm of nursing research or reconceptualized an existing realm of nursing research (1998). Many were already working in the above areas 30 years ago. Noting that nursing has the "brilliance in family health," she encouraged us to know well the human genotype project, the environment as the social context for health, and to strengthen the bridge between public health and person/family health. To these I would add: strengthen collaboration (between nursing and other disciplines and within nursing) and continue to address fundamental problems at the biobehavioral interface.

Two additional opportunities need mentioning. Nursing has a proud heritage of safe and effective midwifery service that has affected health legislation for Medicaid and rural health but still has not removed barriers to hospital practice (Diers & Burst, 1983). What may be needed here are collaborative teams of obstetrical fellows and midwives in some forward-thinking health science settings who will become "pacesetters" in collaborative practice.

Fagin's (1998) guest editorial in *Nursing Outlook* on the changing burden of care brought on by managed care pleads with us in academia to know what it is like at the bedside. Without documentation of the effects of management on the burden of care, we may not save our workforce. Burden of care has been an issue for us and for housestaff throughout this century. To become clinically refreshed, I undertook a day of practice 20 years ago on a cardiovascular surgery unit. I had forgotten what it was like to leave lunch half eaten in the staff room. What made this experience bearable was the professional support provided by my mentors, two cardiovascular clinical nurse specialists, with whom I collaborated in clinical research on cardiac surgery recovery.[8]

In conclusion, tribute is paid to readers who are pacesetters in clinics, hospitals, private practice, public health, and academia every day of their professional lives. Those of us now white-haired are grateful that you are where you are and are doing what you do. The future is really ours, as it was years ago!

Acknowledgment

I gratefully acknowledge the contribution of Rebecca Wilson-Loots, academic program analyst, Department of Family Health Care Nursing, University of California–San Francisco, for her assistance with the original paper.

Discussion Questions

1. How has the history of nursing research influenced the status of nursing research today?
2. Browse the Web site of the National Center for Nursing Research. What are its current goals and future strategies?
3. Go the Web site of your specialty organization and determine its research agenda for the future. Does the organization publish research studies?

Notes

1. Lucile Petry Leone spent many hours with the author and the late Helen Nahm in the writing of the overview of nursing research. She died on Thanksgiving Day, 1999.

2. The first Doctor of Nursing Science program (in psychiatric nursing) was offered by Boston University; the next was at the University of California–San Francisco. The first PhD program in nursing was begun by New York University, to be followed by the University of Pittsburgh.

3. Suzanne Feetham, Kathleen Dracup, and Catherine Gilliss are among the pioneers in family nursing research, along with Lorraine Wright of Canada, Sally Rankin, Maribelle Leavitt, and Kit Chesla. These and others have studied families in acute and chronic illness.

4. Louise Jenkins and Susan Gortner were among the first to employ self-efficacy as a variable in patient recovery; Sally Rankin, Diane Carroll, Mariead Hickey, Virginia Carrieri, and Marylin Dodd are among others who have studied self-efficacy in clinical populations.

5. Barbara Drew has been the pioneering investigator in this aspect of critical care nursing.

6. Eileen Hasselmeyer, Mary Neal, and Kathryn Barnard were the original pioneers in studies of neonate stimulation, followed by Anderson, Whalberg, and Ludington, among others.

7. Dorothy Brooten is credited for demonstrating the cost effectiveness of low birth weight infants.

8. The author is indebted to Patricia Sparacino, cardiovascular surgery nurse specialist at the Medical Center, University of California–San Francisco, and Julie Shinn, clinical coordinator in cardiovascular surgical nursing at Stanford University Medical Center. Both are internationally known clinicians/scholars and academy members.

References

Abdellah, F. B. (1970). Overview of nursing research 1955–1968. *Nursing Research, 19,* 6–17, 239–252.

Advancing the science of nursing: Vol. 11. (1997–1999). Baltimore: University of Maryland School of Nursing.

American Nurses Association. (1959). *Functions, standards and qualifications for practice.* New York: The Association.

American Nurses Association Cabinet on Nursing Research. (1985). *Directions for nursing research: Toward the twenty-first century.* Kansas City, MO: American Nurses Association.

American Nurses Association Commission on Nursing Research. (1976). *Nursing research: Toward a science of health care. Priorities for research in nursing.* Kansas City, MO: American Nurses Association.

American Nurses Foundation. (1960). Research—pathway to future progress in nursing care. *Nursing Research, 9,* 4–7.

Barnard, K. E. (1980). Knowledge for practice: Directions for the future. *Nursing Research, 29,* 208–212.

Barnard, K. (1982). The research cycle: Nursing, the profession, the discipline. In *Communicating nursing research: Vol. 15. Nursing science in perspective.* Boulder, CO: Western Interstate Commission for Higher Education.

Batey, M. (1971). Conceptualizing the research process. *Nursing Research, 20,* 296–301.

Batey, M., & Julian, J. (1964). Staff perceptions of state psychiatric hospital goals. *Nursing Research, 12,* 89–92.

Bloch, D. (1988). *Report of the national nursing research agenda for the participants in the conference on research priorities in nursing science, January 27–29, 1988* [unpublished]. Bethesda, MD: National Center for Nursing Research.

Brown, J. S., Tanner, C. A., & Patrick, K. P. (1983). Nursing's search for scientific knowledge. *Nursing Research, 32,* 29–32.

Coston, H. M. (1960). Myocardial infarction: Stages of recovery and nursing care. *Nursing Research, 9,* 178–184.

Cheyovich, T. K., Lewis, C. E., & Gortner, S. R. (1976). *The nurse practitioner in an adult outpatient clinic.* Washington, DC: Health Resources Administration. HEW Publication No. (HRA) 76-29.

DeTornyay, R. (1976). *Nursing research in the bicentennial year.* Boulder, CO: Western Interstate Commission for Higher Education.

Diers, D., & Burst, H. V. (1983). Effectiveness of policy related research: Nurse-midwifery as case study. *Image Journal of Nursing Scholarship, 15,* 68–74.

Disbrow, M. A. (1963). Any mother who really wants to nurse her baby can do so. *Nursing Forum, 2,* 39–48.

Donaldson, S. (1998). *Breakthrough in nursing research.* Invited presentation. Proceedings of the 25th Anniversary of the American Academy of Nursing, Acapulco, Mexico.

Donaldson, S., & Crowley, D. (1978). The discipline of nursing. *Nursing Outlook, 26,* 113–120.

Dumas, R. G., & Leonard, R. C. (1963). The effect of nursing on the incidence of postoperative vomiting. *Nursing Research, 12,* 12–15.

Ellis, R. (1970). Values and vicissitudes of the scientist nurse. *Nursing Research, 19,* 440–445.

Fagin, C. (1998). Nursing research and the erosion of care [guest editorial]. *Nursing Outlook, 46,* 259–260.

Finer, H. (1952). *Administration and the nursing services.* New York: Macmillan Company.

Fitzpatrick, J. J. (Ed.). (1998). *Encyclopedia of nursing research.* New York: Springer.

Glaser, B. G., & Strauss, A. L. (1965). *Awareness of dying (Observation series).* Chicago: Aldine Publishing Company.

Gortner, S. R. (1973). Research in nursing. The federal interest and grant program. *American Journal of Nursing, 73,* 1052–1053.

Gortner, S. R. (1974a). The relations of scientists with professional and sponsoring organizations and with society. In M. Batey (Ed.), *Issues in research: Social, professional, and methodological.* Selected papers from the first American Nurses Association Council of Nurse Researchers program meeting. Kansas City, MO: The Association.

Gortner, S. R. (1974b). Research for a practice profession. *Nursing Research, 24,* 193–197.

Gortner, S. R. (1974c). Scientific accountability in nursing. *Nursing Outlook, 22,* 764–768.

Gortner, S. R. (1979). Trends and historical perspective. In F. S. Downs & J. W. Fleming (Eds.), *Issues in Nursing Research.* New York: Appleton-Century-Crofts.

Gortner, S. R. (1980a). Nursing research: Out of the past and into the future. *Nursing Research, 29,* 204–207.

Gortner, S. R. (1980b). Nursing science in transition. *Nursing Research, 29,* 180–183.

Gortner, S. R. (1984). Knowledge development in a practice discipline: Philosophy and pragmatics. In C. Williams (Ed.), *Nursing research and policy formation: The case of prospective payment.* Kansas City, MO: American Academy of Nursing.

Gortner, S. R. (1990). Nursing values and science: Toward a science philosophy. *Image Journal of Nursing Scholarship, 22,* 101–105.

Gortner, S. R. (1991). Historical development of doctoral programs: Shaping our expectations. *Journal of Professional Nursing, 7,* 45–53.

Gortner, S. R., Bloch, D., & Phillips, T. P. (1976). Contributions of nursing research to patient care. *Journal of Nursing Administration, 6,* 22–28.

Gortner, S. R., & Nahm, H. (1977). An overview of nursing research in the United States. *Nursing Research, 26,* 10–32.

Gortner, S. R., & Schultz, P. R. (1988). Approaches to nursing science methods. *Image Journal of Nursing School, 20,* 22–24.

Grady, P. (1999, September 16–18). *Strategic planning for the 21st century.* Proceedings of the National Institute for Nursing Research State of the Science Congress; Washington, DC.

Henderson, V. (1956). Research in nursing practice—When? *Nursing Research, 4,* 99.

Hinshaw, A. S., Sigmon, H. D., & Lindsey, A. M. (1991). Interfacing nursing and biologic science. *Journal of Professional Nursing, 7,* 264.

Holzemer, W. L., & Gortner, S. R. (1988). Evaluation of the nursing research emphasis/grants for doctoral programs in nursing grant program 1979–1984. *Journal of Professional Nursing, 4,* 381–386.

Hughes, E. D. et al. (1958). *Twenty thousand nurses tell their story.* Philadelphia: JB Lippincott Co.

Jacobsen, B. S., & Meininger, J. C. (1985). The designs and methods of published nursing research: 1956–1983. *Nursing Research, 34,* 306–312.

Leone, L. P. (1955). The ingredients of research. *Nursing Research, 4,* 51.

Lewis, C. E., & Resnik, B. A. (1967). Nurse clinics and progressive ambulatory patient care. *New England Medical Journal, 277,* 1236–1241.

Lindeman, C. A. (1975a). Delphi survey of priorities in nursing research. *Nursing Research, 24,* 434–441.

Lindeman, C. A. (1975b). Priorities in clinical nursing research. *Nursing Outlook, 23,* 693–698.

Little, D. E., & Carnevali, D. (1967). Nurse specialist effect on tuberculosis: Report on a field experiment. *Nursing Research, 16,* 321–326.

Meleis, A. I. (1980). *The age of nursing scholarliness: Now is the time. The inaugural Helen Nahm Research Lecture.* San Francisco: University of California, San Francisco School of Nursing.

Meleis, A. I. (1987). Revisions in knowledge development: A passion for substance. *Scholarly Inquiry Nursing Practice Institute Journal,* 1–19.

Meltzer, L. E., Pinneo, R., Ferrigan, M. M., Kitchell, J. R., Ipsen, J., & Bearman, J. (1969). *Intensive coronary care: An analysis of the system and the acute phase of myocardial infarction.* New York: Charles Press.

Mishel, M., & Murdaugh, C. (1987). Family adjustment to heart transplantation. *Nursing Research, 36,* 332–338.

Moody, L. E., Wilson, M. E., Smythe, K., Schwartz, R., Tittle, M., & VanCort, M. L. (1988). Analysis of a decade of nursing practice research: 1977–1986. *Nursing Research, 37,* 374–379.

Moss, F. T., & Myer, B. (1966). The effects of nursing interaction upon pain relief in patients. *Nursing Research, 15,* 303–306.

Oberst, M. T. (1986). Nursing in the year 2000: Setting the agenda for knowledge generation and utilization. In G. Sorenson (Ed.), *Setting the agenda for the year 2000: Knowledge development in nursing.* Kansas City, MO: American Academy of Nursing.

Quint, J. (1967). *The nurse and the dying patient.* New York: Macmillan Company.

Research spanning the life cycle: Vol. 15. (1998, Fall). Los Angeles: University of California, Los Angeles School of Nursing.

Ringholz, S., & Morris, M. (1961). A test of some assumptions about rooming-in. *Nursing Research, 10,* 196–199.

Schorr, T., & Kennedy, M. S. (1999). *100 years of American nursing: Celebrating a century of caring.* Philadelphia: Lippincott Williams & Wilkins.

The science of caring: Vol. 11. (1999, Spring). San Francisco: University of California, San Francisco School of Nursing.

Shaver, J. (1985). A biopsychosocial view of human health. *Nursing Outlook, 33,* 187–191.

Silver, H. K., Ford, L. C., & Day, L. R. (1968). The pediatric nurse practitioner program: Expanding the role of the nurse to provide increased health care for children. *Journal of the American Medical Association, 204,* 298–302.

Stevenson, J. S., & Woods, N. (1986a). Nursing science and contemporary science: Emerging paradigms. In G. Sorenson (Ed.), *Setting the agenda for the year 2000: Knowledge development in nursing.* Kansas City, MO: American Academy of Nursing.

Stevenson, J. S., & Woods, N. (1986b). Strategies for the year 2000: Synthesis and projections. In G. Sorenson (Ed.), *Setting the agenda for the year 2000: Knowledge development in nursing.* Kansas City, MO: American Academy of Nursing.

Vreeland, E. (1959, February). Memorandum to Lucile Petry Leone, chief nurse officer. Some frontiers for nursing research.

Other Core Knowledge for the Advanced Practice of Nursing

The last section of this book will cover two remaining core concepts as recommended by the AACN for advanced practice nursing knowledge—diversity and ethics. Diversity has two complementary issues to consider—diversity of the population cared for by nurses and the diversity of the nursing workforce itself. As we move to a more diverse and pluralistic society in the United States, the nursing profession is challenged to gain greater and greater cultural competence. In Chapter 25, Washington lays a background for understanding the migration patterns which have resulted in a multicultural, multiethnic and multilingual society. The works of two nurse theorists, Leininger and Purnell, have shaped the thinking of the nursing profession related to cultural diversity and cultural competence. Washington reviews their work as a foundation for the reader to apply their theories to practice. Chapter 26 considers diversity from the perspective of African American history and its influence on the nursing profession. Further, Hill integrates the social and nursing history into a discussion of racial and ethnic disparities in health care.

In Chapter 27, Pozgar introduces basic ethics concepts and definitions. Scattered throughout the chapter are examples of ethical situations the reader can use to apply ethical principles to nursing practice. Chapter 28 is a discussion by Twomey of the *ANA Code of Ethics for Nurses*. The readers are encouraged to purchase the entire code with the interpretative statements for their professional libraries.

Part V

Other Core Knowledge for the Advanced Practice of Nursing

CHAPTER 25   Moving Toward a Culturally Competent Profession

CHAPTER 26   Race, Race Relations, and the Emergence of Professional Nursing, 1870–2004

CHAPTER 27   Introduction to Ethics

CHAPTER 28   The Role of Codes of Ethics in Nursing's Disciplinary Knowledge

Moving Toward a Culturally Competent Profession

Deborah Washington

CHAPTER OBJECTIVES

1. Discuss how the current multicultural, multiethnic, and multilingual patient population influences nursing practice.
2. Define cultural competence.
3. Apply Leininger's theory of transcultural nursing to the role of the advanced practice nurse.

Introduction

Historically, nursing has put great effort into establishing itself as a separate and unique discipline. This has meant overcoming challenges to boundaries and functions of practice as well as defining illness and wellness phenomena appropriate to the scope of practice. Over time, the domain of nursing has been clarified through a series of steps, resulting in a recognizable profession with a distinct approach to the delivery of health care.

The 21st century brings a new set of challenges to the ongoing evolution of the nursing profession. In the United States, for example, census data reflect an unprecedented situation in that non-Western cultures are reshaping the national population. The dominant Euro-American culture has shifted to a more pluralistic one. As a consequence, nursing is confronted with a new and provocative undertaking—to explore the professional tenets of nursing as well as to critique whether the United States has a serviceable healthcare system for the current social order. This chapter explores the increasing importance of culture as a direction for growth in clinical practice and discusses how to incorporate theoretical models into patient care. Culture is large in scope and content and has the potential to influence the domain of knowledge unique to nursing as a discipline focused on the phenomenon of care. Although the influence of culture should not change the basic tenets of practice, a determining factor in care is the inclusion of a person-centered approach to the restoration and maintenance of health.

Background

The healthcare setting of the 20th century was the result of conventions that do not reflect the reality of the current millennium. The original healthcare model was designed primarily to serve patients who spoke English, were able to read and write that language, typically had the resources to pay for care, believed in the germ theory of disease, valued biomedical preventive health practices, and acquiesced to the authoritarian model of the patient–healthcare provider relationship. The typical user of health services today no longer matches this image. The current patient population includes a wide array of lifestyles and is multicultural, multiethnic, and multilingual. More specifically, patients may not speak English, much less be able to read or write in their native language. They may be employed, but frequently do not have health insurance. Patients may be refugees, recently arrived immigrants, undocumented workers, or residents not yet acculturated to Western life because of indigenous pride or as a consequence of social isolation.

Human migration continues to be an all-embracing phenomenon. Few countries are unaffected by its trends. In the United States, the foreign-born population increased from 7.90% in 1990 to 11.70% in 2003. Information on immigration in 2003 documents that 305,973 people emigrated from the Americas, 251,296 from Asian nations, and 48,738 from African nations (Global Data Center, 2005). Hispanics surpassed African Americans in the 2000 census and are now the largest minority group in the United States. Non-Hispanic Whites are the slowest-growing group, and some predict they will constitute a smaller percentage of the U.S. population in the future (Day, 2005).

The Diaspora

The diaspora (Greek for "to scatter") of new populations presents challenges to the host culture. Historically, host communities have the unstated expectation that the new arrivals will assimilate into the dominant culture. Adapting to new social norms often requires disengagement from old traditions, customs, and practices and frequently precipitates a loss of heritage-based identity. Culture shock and isolation related to the new environment generate a sense of dislocation, stress, and anxiety. Support services and appropriate resources are necessary to provide for and maintain the mental and physical well-being of groups seeking to establish themselves in new places (Kim, Cho, Klessig, Gerace, & Camilleri, 2002).

Immigrants familiar with health systems and practices in their country of origin face obstacles that can hinder access to care (Leduc & Proulx, 2004). Therefore, informational resources related to health services are of critical importance for new arrivals. The lack of such information influences decision making and compromises timely contact with needed care. Proficiency with English, an understanding of bureaucratic systems, and the ability to acquire health insurance are determining factors with consequences for the clinical encounter. The complexities of providing care to individuals who are unable to cope with these factors can result in culturally insensitive encounters and result in care that is inappropriate and, in some cases, even dangerous.

The inability to communicate and the negative consequences to quality of care have generated both research and awareness among practitioners. Within the paradigm of healthcare disparities, language and communication have been identified as critical additions to a culturally competent healthcare system. In 1999, the U.S. Department of Health and Human Services, Office of Minority Health, proposed national standards for culturally and linguistically appropriate services in order to establish the importance of these criteria as benchmarks for consumers, providers, and health systems. Fourteen recommendations were formulated, five of which explicitly address the need for language support (Table 25–1).

These recommendations are unprecedented. Ramifications for the practice of nursing in all healthcare settings are still to be determined. Safe practice and effective approaches to care are the anticipated outcomes. To include the consumer in full clinical decision making, it is incumbent on the clinician to understand the resource needs of patients from different cultural backgrounds.

Limitations of Multiculturalism

Becoming fluent in cultural mores is not easy and can be compromised by assumptions that all people from one geographic area are the same.

Separating a culture into its component parts as a guide for understanding the whole culture risks reducing complex meanings into formulas. It also is critical to understand people's perceptions of being marginalized as the "other." Canales and Bowers (2001) described the "other" as:

> . . . Someone who is perceived as different from self. Historically, persons labelled as Other, as them, are categorized primarily according to how their differences from the societal norm are perceived. Their Otherness is signified by their relational differences; when compared to the 'ordinary,' 'usual' and 'familiar' attributes of persons, they appear 'different,' as Other. It is persons categorized as Other who often reside at the margins of society. (p. 103)

Additionally, variables such as class, education, gender, and religion significantly influence individuals. Although these factors can be generalized as themes of personhood, care must be exercised to prevent their use as a basis for stereotypes. The importance of identifying this information strongly affects the course of events

---

Table 25–1 CULTURALLY AND LINGUISTICALLY APPROPRIATE STANDARDS (CLAS)

1. Provide all clients with limited English proficiency access to interpreter services.
2. Provide oral and written notices and signage to clients in their primary language, including the right to an interpreter at no cost.
3. Make available patient education and other materials in the language of the predominant group in the relevant service area.
4. Ensure the language proficiency and skills of the interpreter.
5. Ensure that the language preference and self-identified race/ethnicity of the client is included in the organization's information systems.

Source: http://www.omhrc.gov/Assets/pdf/checked/Assuring_Cultural_Competence_in_Health_Care-1999.pdf

that establish quality of care. Access to the best information available as it relates to the patient has significance for length of stay, appropriate discharge planning, and patient satisfaction.

Health Disparities

The constitution of the World Health Organization (WHO) states:

> Health is a state of complete physical, mental and social well-being and not merely the absence of disease or infirmity. The enjoyment of the highest attainable standard of health is one of the fundamental rights of every human being without distinction of race, religion, political belief, economic or social condition. (World Health Organization, 2006)

Decisive evidence of disparities in health care is attracting attention in the literature. The information provided is focused on comparative data that describe a statistical picture of morbidity and mortality, as well as increased awareness of problems of access to care and quality of care. For example, health status and utilization of services by diverse groups have become familiar parts of the discourse on equity in health care. Access and documented health outcomes illustrate a lack of parity between defined populations. However, the lack of national standards in service delivery and the paucity of evaluative research hamper explanations of the causes (Horowitz, Davis, Palermo, & Vladek, 2000). Disparities as an area of concern for healthcare providers is supported by studies that underscore inconsistencies between length of life and quality of life associated with specific cultural groups. The number of excess deaths and the difference between rates of death for minority groups as compared with a reference group reveal a situation in health care that warrants attention (LaVeist, Bowie, & Cooley-Quille, 2000). It is possible to extract issues from current research that indicate the need for close and careful observation of extant conditions. The ability to corroborate the implications of these studies with the daily conventions of clinical practice creates the conditions for strategies to address this dilemma.

Coleman-Miller (2000) emphasized the importance of cultural sensitivity training for healthcare providers to counteract the effects of cultural disregard in the form of poor interpersonal relationships, language with culture-based meanings, and ineffective services. Nontraditional health system designs that serve to improve or advance respectful attention to the needs of a multicultural population must be substantiated with more evaluative research. The significance of this is clear when due consideration is given to the need to delineate the function of factors such as racism and discrimination on health outcomes, despite an inherent discomfort with the concept. A restructuring of the healthcare delivery system driven by budgetary constraints has mobilized entrants into environments where previously they may not have been encountered in great numbers (Williams & Rucker, 2000). This can result in personal and professional challenges for any clinician.

Culture and Western Health Care

Culture can be a facilitator or a barrier to health care (Searight, 2003), and belief systems can sway an individual's use of information (IOM, 2002). Western biomedicine tends to dismiss non-Western approaches to healing because many of them do not base disease causality in germ theory or practice the scientific method. Many non-Western societies find the Western emphasis on pathophysiology and biomedicine to be problematic. The biomedical definition of absence of disease fails to acknowledge the interrelationship of body, mind, and spirit. In *The Spirit Catches You and You Fall Down*, Fadiman (1997) captures this cultural clash. The lack of understanding between doctors and a Hmong family led to tragedy. Lia, a child diagnosed with severe epilepsy, eventually died from complications; her parents did not understand how important the medication was, and the healthcare team did not understand the complex cultural customs of the Hmong.

Cultural interpretations of the value of abandoning natal beliefs in favor of more dominant customs can be life altering. For instance, in Haitian culture, the power of a spirit that rides or possesses a believer is used to explain changes in personality (Holcomb, Parsons, Giger, & Davidhizar, 1996). In Western culture, the ability to medicalize behavior considered outside the norm endows professional experts with civil power (Reddy, 2002).

These differences in belief practices beg several questions:

- What culturally relevant treatments maintain health and well-being?
- Is the definition of health and well-being a moving target—does it mean different things to different cultures?
- Is quality care based on the Western biomedical model? What is the role of the traditional healer?
- What frame of reference does a culturally competent clinician use to answer these questions?

The answers have the potential to place the clinician in an ethical dilemma. The ability to offer a proven best treatment is not simply a function of perspective or worldview. Scientific facts exist and are the basis for evidence-based practice. However, biomedicine does have the capacity to coexist with other belief systems. Therefore, a plan of care that coordinates treatment options, taking into consideration cultural values and customs, can be negotiated.

Nursing Lens of the Multicultural Professional

The impact of culture on nursing must be considered from another perspective if the topic and the profession are to be examined with new vision. The Western model dominates nursing identity and definition (Herdman, 2001). This has evolved into describing the field as science as well as art. In spite of this dual interpretation, however, science and its methods are explicitly positioned as the most desired path to knowledge within the discipline. Observation and experiments are the foundation used to develop tenets of practice, and a knowledge base framed as unique to the profession is the goal of what has become a prolonged endeavor.

Nevertheless, there is also a non-Western perspective on the discipline. From this aspect, nursing can be a formal or an informal concept. This specific differentiation is determined by the infrastructure that validates the role function. When tasks and activities in a particular society are solely the result of an apprenticed experience accepted by the general community, cultural rituals and traditions often dominate. However, when the role is the consequence of an educational regimen controlled by a professional body that confers the status of licensure, there are accustomed methods and procedures resulting from discipline-specific conventions that must be followed. Historically, the scientific approach has carried the designation of modern, and consequently is more highly valued. This has essentially negated the usefulness and importance of learning accessed through the customs, rituals, and traditions of other cultures and societies. These paths to knowledge should be explored for the value they offer to the complementary part of nursing customarily known as its art. The nursing lens of the multicultural professional has much to offer to this part of nursing, which has been deemphasized in the pursuit of its scientific identity.

Ethnic identity influences all of the domains of nursing: person, health, environment, and nursing. In exploring ethnicity as culture, Phinney (1996) suggested that such factors as values and attitudes were assumed to describe the cultural characteristics of a specific group. This perspective was portrayed in a study conducted by Struthers (2001) that explored nursing from a Native American point of view. Here, caring and holism, among other dimensions, were delineated culturally. Caring involved the elements of humor and partnership; holism included balance and the use of nonverbal interaction. Pang and colleagues (2004) compared Chinese, American, and Japanese nurses' understanding of ethical responsibilities. Interestingly, there were different degrees of value placed on statements related to respect. Chinese nurses gave higher marks to language related to respect for nurses, Japanese nurses gave higher marks to respect for patients, and American nurses gave higher value to statements related to respect for individual rights. Pang and colleagues also examined the experience of nursing practice in Chinese culture. The

concept of nursing was rooted in the philosophical principles of the society and the nuances of the associated language. For example, Chinese terms that describe good practice include truthfulness, responsibility, and service, along with understanding and knowledge in conjunction with the actions of protect and interact. Chen (2000) points out that cultural values influenced by relevant philosophical and religious beliefs are by their nature embedded in attitudes related to health in Chinese culture. To merge these cultural ideologies into a universal understanding of the concepts *to nurse* or *to be a nurse* holds great promise for the next steps as the profession continues to develop.

Culturally Competent Care

An overall definition of culture and a description of its basic elements outline the basis for group identity. Leininger and McFarland (2002) offer a broad-based definition that describes culture as a "way of life belonging to an individual or a group that reflects values and customs taught and learned generationally" (p. 9). In her transcultural nursing model, Leininger (2001) includes religious, kinship, social, political and legal, economic, educational, technologic, and cultural values as components of culture.

The individual with a distinct cultural viewpoint has a dynamic and integral relationship with the nurse who provides culturally congruent care. Cultural competence has many definitions in the literature. However, in essence, it is a compilation of the clinical skills and professional behaviors of a healthcare provider focused on the cultural values, beliefs, and perceptions of the consumer while both are engaged in the therapeutic relationship. Cultural competence is an aspect of nursing that will move the profession to its next developmental phase.

Leininger (2001) defines culture care preservation or maintenance as:

> . . . those assistive, supporting, facilitative, or enabling professional actions and decisions that help people of a particular culture to retain and/or preserve relevant care values so that they can maintain their well-being, recover from illness, or face handicaps and/or death. (p. 48)

Nursing has continuously acknowledged the status of the individual. Recognition of the cultural life, values, and beliefs of persons is simply an expansion of that attention. The nursing assessment, problem list, diagnosis, progress note, or discharge plan can only be effective if cultural influences are addressed. This viewpoint is in deference to the concept of cultural autonomy. The dimension of the individual experience is characterized by such concepts as acculturation, the implementation and acceptance of customs different from the primary culture; assimilation, the blending of one culture with another; and cultural autonomy, the ability to retain principal identity in the presence of one or more dominant groups (see Figure 25–1).

Cultural autonomy upholds the importance of the valued presence of customs, conventions, and folkways of all cultures within any given society without the pressure to assimilate. The imperative of one culture should not be the cause for dismissal of another.

In contrast, acculturation denotes an ability to adapt to the rules and conventions of a society different from the country of origin. The newcomer must manage culture shock and develop survival skills that allow for an effective level of function in new and unfamiliar surroundings. Navigating the healthcare system is one of those skills. The culturally competent provider must organize appropriate resources to enable proficient and uncompromising care. Meeting the needs of the unacculturated challenges system design and tests the justification for and the philosophy in support of care delivery. Explanations for professional practice must be grounded in findings more substantive than mere tradition to avoid the entanglements of ethnocentrism. Providing rationale for current methods prompts analysis and objective application of practice principles.

Cultural imposition imposes the way of life of one culture on that of another. It necessitates a belief in the superiority of the prevailing manner of living and conveys compulsory adherence to accepted norms. However, if any culture and its way of life are to endure, the

Figure 25–1 Aspects of Culturally Competent Care

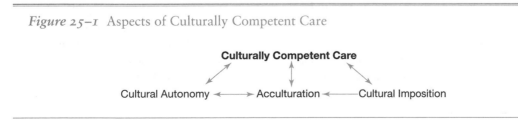

cultural imposition of one group must be off-set by the cultural autonomy of the other. This is the point that underpins the complexities associated with multiculturalism in a pluralistic society. It can be especially problematic in a healthcare situation. In this context, those recently arrived and unaccustomed to the attitudes and values of the culture to which they are not yet accustomed initially present as a problem-solving task in the clinical encounter. Under these circumstances, culturally controlled values and norms can become the focus of intervention as a first step in managing treatment.

The Substance of Nursing: Theory and Culture

Nursing theory is the source of discipline-specific concepts. Theory suggests explanations for what nursing does that differentiate it from other branches of knowledge. Theory explains why nurses act as they do and describes how nurses should use those explanations to assist maintenance or restoration of health and well-being. The influence of culture in this schema deserves exploration.

Transcultural Nursing

Cultural diversity, or multiculturalism, is a social construct of increasing importance to the understanding of healthcare quality. Clarification of the influence of culture on the domains of nursing will be a sign of the next evolutionary stage of the profession. Issues that will move nursing forward include the influence of culture in defin-

ing excellence in patient care and the significance of culture as an applied intervention for the improvement of health.

When the concept of transcultural nursing was introduced in the 1950s, it was not viewed as relevant to nursing practice (Leininger, 1978), perhaps because nursing theory was young or because of the hegemonic views of the Euro-American culture of the time. Because the nursing profession is dynamic, it reflects the social needs and conscience of any given era (Henderson, 1966), thus the profession has come to embrace the pioneering efforts of Madeleine Leininger and her conceptualization of transcultural nursing.

Leininger defined transcultural nursing as "a formal area of study and practice focused on comparative human-care differences and similarities of the beliefs, values and patterned lifeways of cultures to provide culturally congruent, meaningful, and beneficial health care to people" (Leininger & McFarland, 2002, p. 6). Culture is the facilitator through which the nurse can understand and support individual needs. The full range of anthropological constructs (for example, language, group history, religion, and politics) are used as reference for a more fully developed understanding of every person and the circumstances of each individual life.

Transcultural nursing provides a holistic approach to understanding each individual within the context of the various influences on that unique life. The sunrise model includes information on the following factors: education, economic, political and legal, kinship and social, religious and philosophical, and technological. This biographical history captures the important details of a patient's life. These details provide a comprehensive depiction of the individual that serves to enhance care based in knowledge with both depth and abundant detail. Such detail implements a process for increasing familiarity with those who are dissimilar and decreases anxiety related to contact with the unknown for the healthcare provider and patient alike.

Transcultural nursing also possesses an implicit advantage. Many of the concepts that identify a holistic approach to care enable the building of an authentic relationship between patient and provider. In the practice domain, socially sensitive issues related to bias, prejudice, cultural imposition, cultural blindness, and cultural pain become part of the definition of culturally congruent care. Cultural conflict is an expected development when dissimilar groups who have minimal contact find it necessary to interact. Transcultural nursing supplies a knowledge base by which disharmony can effectively be addressed. For example, Leininger (2001) formulated a concept to describe the psychological and emotional distress experienced by patients when healthcare providers demonstrate a lack of concern for the cultural beliefs and customs of others.

As defined by Leininger and McFarland (2002), "cultural pain refers to suffering, discomfort, or being greatly offended by an individual or group who shows a great lack of sensitivity toward another's cultural experience" (p. 52). Understanding an individual within the context of their worldview is the crux of the presence or absence of cultural pain. As an example of emotional distress, cultural pain is associated with hurtful memories, damaging words that evoke those memories, insults, and indignities. It must be acknowledged that what

is considered hurtful from one standpoint may not be understood as such from another. Although inflicting cultural pain is not always intentional or conscious, insensitivity can be enmeshed in a lack of awareness. Concomitant understanding and social blunders often are associated with inadequate knowledge related to cultural triggers that are well known to the insider but less so to the outsider. The resulting distress should not be dismissed by the person hurt simply because the deed was not intended. The prevention of a recurrence is more important and requires an exploration of context and meaning from all relevant perspectives. For example, it is a particular affront to an African American to have his or her smile described as a "big, toothy grin." This can be understood within the context of racist caricatures from the pre–civil rights era. Another example would be the individual who speaks accented English and becomes sensitized to questions about citizenship status.

Understanding the elements of culture in an approach to care that is holistic is a demonstration of cultural competence. As nursing continues to refine the relevance of culturally competent care to its domain of knowledge, an understanding of cultural pain will contribute to an understanding of the impact of diversity on the healthcare system and the clinical encounters that are part of the environment of care.

Elements of culture are a route of communication to generate collaboration between a patient, family, or community and the chosen provider. Separating a culture into its component parts to guide the understanding of a particular people is a more complex process than simple fact finding. Insight that assigns meaning is necessary if the nature and significance of culture are to have value in the care experience.

Purnell's Model for Cultural Competence

The incorporation of cultural skills and knowledge into clinical practice is facilitated by a well-grounded reference, making the gathering of information more manageable. Many culturally based assessment tools for gathering information are very detailed. A busy practitioner would not attempt to collate, at one time, all the information suggested by the instrument. However, the culturally prepared clinician would be mindful of important specifics suggested by these tools that would enhance the quality and usefulness of the information collected.

Larry Purnell developed a conceptual model for the culturally competent provider in 1995 that was originally intended as a nursing assessment tool (Purnell, 2002). His 12 domains of culture (2000) are relevant guideposts for the initial health history (see Table 25–2).

A guide of this nature helps to focus the interview process and draws attention to key elements of each unique cultural perspective. When information is clustered in this way, a useful care plan can be formulated from synthesized information. If this framework is used, some foreknowledge of the cultural group is required to support a focused interview process that remains timely and is not haphazard. Not all questions need to be asked. Clinical judgment should guide the clinician. For example, once the issue of communication has been resolved, for the African American patient with a chief complaint of chest pain the initial assessment would most likely include the domains of healthcare practices and practitioners, high-risk behaviors, biocultural ecology (i.e., physical features), and nutrition to determine the most essential information for this complaint. The culturally prepared practitioner would be aware of the following:

- Prominence of cardiovascular disease among African Americans
- Possibility of traditional practices and self-adjusted dosage of medication
- Ability to metabolize medications
- Soul food
- Social history of African Americans as context for clinical encounter

---

Table 25–2 PURNELL'S MODEL OF CULTURAL DOMAINS

Heritage	Communication
Family roles	Workforce issues
Biocultural ecology	High-risk behaviors
Nutrition	Pregnancy
Death rituals	Spirituality
Healthcare practices	Healthcare practitioners

Conclusion

Cultural diversity, or multiculturalism, is a social construct of increasing importance in understanding healthcare quality. Clarification of the influence of culture on the domains of nursing will be an indication of the next evolutionary stage of the profession. What is the influence of culture in defining excellence in patient care? What is the significance of culture as an applied intervention for the improvement of health? What is the impact of culture on interpersonal and therapeutic relationships?

Culture can be a paradigm for worldviews. In transcultural nursing, these paradigms utilize anthropological concepts to inform a nursing perspective on health and illness beliefs that originate in the cultural life of a given society. Culture is the facilitator through which nurses can understand and support individual needs. The full range of anthropological constructs (e.g., language, group history) is used as a reference for a more fully developed understanding of every person and the context of each individual life and worldview.

Leininger and McFarland (2002) give an orientational definition of worldview as "the way an individual or group looks out on and understands their world about them as a value, stance, picture, or perspective about life or the world" (p. 83). Blacks, Hispanics, Asians, American Indians, and Caucasians have had vastly divergent social experiences in the United States. These experiences are so disparate that perspectives often are polarized. Empathy and increased cultural knowledge of other ethnic heritages are essential to the promotion of positive and more trusting clinical encounters. However, active questions stimulate discourse on Western definitions of what constitutes good care. For example, the Western philosophies of self-care and out-of-bed activity are representative of differing perspectives on wellness behavior.

As a topic of research, the value of culturally competent care to the patient remains unclear and undefined. For example, some practitioners contend that it is possible to generate a sense of well-being for a patient without undue attention to issues of culture. Also, long-established practices reframed as issues of culture (e.g., referrals to spiritual caregivers or dietary consults) can be viewed as standard procedure as opposed to culture-specific care. However, cultural customs that conflict with policy and procedures (e.g., newborn-naming customs of Cambodians call for a wait of one week and the naming is done by grandparents) are clear illustrations that cultural knowledge does indicate the need for new precedents.

Culture is a form of identity. Identity is a complex concept that involves the explication of factors that, among other things, characterize cultural heritage. The ongoing exploration of the meaning of cultural identity is poised to enhance the functioning of our pluralistic society. History has shown cultural heritage can be a highly charged domain of inquiry when it involves race and ethnicity. However, knowledge-based methods of care underpin the type of practice competence that includes awareness of the human dimensions of diversity. The proficient healthcare provider is sensitive to the distinctions of difference and models a nursing process that promotes the reciprocal relationship between culture and quality care.

Discussion Questions

1. Discuss each of the following questions:
   a. What culturally relevant treatments maintain health and well-being?
   b. Is the definition of health and well-being a moving target? Does it mean different things to different cultures?
   c. Is quality care based on the Western biomedical model? What is the role of the traditional healer?
   d. What frame of reference does a culturally competent clinician use to answer these questions?
2. Describe a client situation in which culture misunderstanding and/or differences were evident. What was the influence of culture in achieving or not achieving the patient care outcome? What was the impact of culture on interpersonal and therapeutic relationships?
3. Apply Leininger's theory of transcultural nursing to advanced nursing practice.

References

Canales, M., & Bowers, B. (2001). Expanding conceptualizations of culturally competent care. *Journal of Advanced Nursing, 36*(1), 102–111.

Chen, Y. (2000). Chinese values, health and nursing. *Journal of Advanced Nursing, 36*(2), 270–273.

Coleman-Miller, B. (2000). A physician's perspective on minority health. *Health Care Financing Review, 21*(4), 45–56.

Day, J. C. (2005). National population projections. Retrieved February 2, 2005, from http://www. census. gov/population/www/pop-profile /natproj.html

Fadiman, A. (1997). *The spirit catches you and you fall down.* New York: Farrar, Straus, Giroux.

Global Data Center. (2005). *United States: Inflow of foreign-born population by country of birth, 1986 to 2003.* Available at http://www.migrationinformation.org/ GlobalData/countrydata/data.cfm

Henderson, V. (1966). *The nature of nursing: A definition and its implications for practice, research, and education.* New York: Macmillan.

Herdman, E. (2001). The illusion of progress in nursing. *Nursing Philosophy, 2*(1), 4–13.

Holcomb, L. O., Parsons, L. C., Giger, J. N., & Davidhizar, R. (1996). Haitian Americans: Implications for nursing care. *Journal of Community Health Nursing, 13*(4), 249–460.

Horowitz, C. R., Davis, M. H., Palermo, A. G., & Vladek, B. C. (2000). Approaches to eliminating sociocultural disparities in health. *Health Care Financing Review, 21*(4), 57–74.

Institute of Medicine (IOM). (2002). *Speaking of health: Assessing health communication strategies for diverse populations.* Washington, DC: Institute of Medicine.

Kim, M. J., Cho, H., Klessig, Y., Gerace, L., & Camilleri, D. (2002). Primary health care for Korean immigrants: Sustaining a culturally sensitive model. *Public Health Nursing, 19*(3), 191–200.

LaVeist, T. A., Bowie, J. V., & Cooley-Quille, M. (2000). Minority health status in adulthood: The middle years of life. *Health Care Financing Review, 21*(4), 9–21.

Leduc, N., & Proulx, M. (2004). Patterns of health services utilization by recent immigrants. *Journal of Immigrant Health, 6*(1), 15–27.

Leininger, M. (1978). *Transcultural nursing: Concepts, theories, and practices.* New York: Wiley.

Leininger, M. (2001). The theory. In M. Leininger (Ed.), *Culture care diversity and universality* (pp. 5–68). Sudbury, MA: Jones and Bartlett.

Leininger, M., & McFarland, M. (2002). *Transcultural nursing: Concepts, theories, research, practice.* New York: McGraw-Hill.

Pang, S., Wong, T., Wang, C., Sheng, Z., Zhi Jun, C., Helen, Y., et al. (2004). Towards a Chinese definition of nursing. *Journal of Advanced Nursing, 46*(6), 657–670.

Phinney, J. (1996). When we talk about American ethnic groups, what do we mean? *American Psychologist, 31*(9), 918–927.

Purnell, L. (2000). A description of the Purnell model of cultural competence. *Journal of Transcultural Nursing, 11*(1), 40–46.

Purnell, L. (2002). The Purnell model of cultural competence. *Journal of Transcultural Nursing, 13*(13), 193–196.

Reddy, S. (2002). Temporarily insane: Pathologising cultural difference in American criminal courts. *Sociology of Health and Illness, 24*(5), 667–687.

Searight, H. (2003). Bosnian immigrants' perceptions of the United States healthcare system: A qualitative interview study. *Journal of Immigrant Health, 5*(2), 87–93.

Struthers, R. (2001). A conceptual framework of nursing in Native American culture. *Journal of Nursing Scholarship.* Retrieved August 5, 2004, from the HighBeam Research Database.

Williams, D. R., & Rucker, T. D. (2000). Understanding and addressing racial disparities in health care. *Health Care Financing Review, 21*(4), 75–90.

World Health Organization. (2006). *Constitution of the World Health Organization.* Retrieved November 2, 2007, from http://www.who.int/governance/eb/who_constitution_en.pdf

Chapter 26

Race, Race Relations, and the Emergence of Professional Nursing, 1870–2004

Patricia St. Hill

CHAPTER OBJECTIVES

1. Review social and nursing history of the United States as a backdrop for understanding racial discrimination and healthcare disparity.
2. Suggest future initiatives to increase the numbers of minorities in nursing.
3. Discuss future initiatives for decreasing healthcare disparities.

Introduction

It is widely known that racial and ethnic minorities experience higher rates of illness and disability and die earlier than Whites. The Institute of Medicine, in its 2003 report titled *Unequal Treatment: Confronting Racial and Ethnic Disparities in Healthcare*, stated the obvious—that minorities receive inferior health care. The current national mandate is to end racial and ethnic discrimination in health care by 2010 and to increase the number of minority healthcare providers.

Barriers to ending racial discrimination can best be understood by examining the social history of the United States. Even though health disparities and minority representation in nursing span many races and ethnic cultures, history best documents this for African Americans (Sullivan Commission, 2004). This chapter examines the influence of race and race relations among Blacks and Whites in American society on the developing nursing profession as it emerged from a task-oriented vocation to a profession in its own right. In doing so, the chapter highlights several critical periods and turning points in American history and traces their reverberations and influences on the emerging nursing profession. In closing, the chapter looks to the future and attempts to predict the challenges and rewards faced by professional nursing.

The Civil War Era

A retrospective view of the nursing profession in the United States mirrors the country's existing sociocultural norms, beliefs, and values. Historical documentation of the social climate prior to and during the 1800s explicates the social inequities, unjust laws, and discriminatory practices that Black nurses were subjected to at the dawning of the profession. The works of Carnegie (1986), Staupers (1961), and Hine (1989) make direct linkages between the difficulties and hardships faced by Black nurses in the early years and the prevailing segregationist views of the nursing leadership, nursing organizations, and large segments of American society.

Elmore (1976), speaking to this issue, noted that there are no special records about Blacks from the earliest days of this country and argued that it was difficult to believe that the slave nursemaid did not become the nurse of the time, in her family or her master's family, at least. Similarly, George, Bradford, and Battle (1995) pointed out that a review of nursing history texts showed that Black nurses were rarely mentioned as contributors to the development of the profession.

With the onset of the Civil War, some minor changes occurred, and the historical record, according to Elmore (1976), becomes clearer. During this period, the names of several early Black nurses surface. Among them are Harriet Tubman and Sojourner Truth, both of whom are well known for activities other than nursing, but they also are credited with having cared for wounded soldiers during the Civil War.

Even more widely recognized is Namahyoke Sockum Curtis, who volunteered her services during the Spanish-American War and was assigned as a contract nurse by the War Department. History also shows that she later served as a Red Cross volunteer during the Galveston flood of 1900 and after the San Francisco earthquake in 1906. The ultimate recognition of her work was a government pension and burial at Arlington Cemetery (Elmore, 1976).

Despite the seeming gains and inroads made by this select group of Black nurses, American society remained very much divided along racial lines. In general, the environment for Blacks throughout the 1800s was hostile. In fact, Massey (1934), recounting the sacrifices, struggles, lack of recognition, and adversities faced by Blacks in America, parallels the history of Black nurses in America.

The Segregation Laws and Nursing

Nineteenth-century America was by all measures a hostile, suppressive, and dangerous place for Blacks. The indelible need to dominate and control a perceived inferior group persisted under the guise of the Jim Crow laws, a series of discriminatory laws in the Southern states that called for the separation of the races. Under Jim Crow, segregation of the races was the order of the day. This social custom prevailed and was supported legally in the 1896 Supreme Court ruling of *Plessy vs. Ferguson*. Furthermore, under these laws, the notion of separate but equal was contrived and promulgated to justify the rigid segregation laws that imposed legal punishment on people for consorting with members of another race and that served to divide all of American society, as well as the emerging nursing profession, along racial lines.

The healthcare system post–Civil War to the late 1960s was composed of two separate and unequal systems—one for Whites and a considerably more inferior one for Blacks. As one woman put it:

> Dr. Bailey on Main Street in Greenville was our family physician. There was a separate waiting room for blacks and you had to wait 'til all the white patients were seen before he'd see the blacks. As long as white patients kept coming in, you kept being pushed further and further back. (Smith, 1999, as cited in Sullivan Commission, 2004, p. 32)

Black nursing students, for the most part, were excluded from White hospital-based nursing programs and were relegated to Black-operated schools, whose curricula and programs have been described as deplorable (Pitts-Mosley, 1995). A select few Blacks were provided limited access to White schools in accordance with strictly enforced institutional quotas. It should also be pointed out that educational barriers and challenges existed in both the Northern and the Southern states for Black women interested in pursuing a nursing career. Pitts-Mosley (1995) noted that although Black codes limiting access to practice opportunities and to institutions of learning were legislated and enforced by law in the Southern states, they also were observed and enforced unofficially in the North, a phenomenon frequently referred to as de facto segregation. For example, the New England Hospital for Women and Children in Boston, Massachusetts, although renowned for having graduated America's first Black trained nurse, Mary Mahoney, in 1879, nonetheless employed the quota system, limiting the number of Blacks admitted each year to two. This number was later al-

tered to include one Black and one Jewish student (Carnegie, 1986).

Between 1886 and 1977, 77 schools for Negroes had been established in 20 states and the District of Columbia (Carnegie, 1986). For the women attending Black-operated programs, many of which were, in actuality, led by White superintendents, curricula and programs were less than adequate. Documented evidence points to curricula deficiencies, lack of resources, and inadequately trained teachers. Admittedly, the majority of nursing schools (both Black and White) operating during the late 1800s and early 1900s were plagued by inadequacies, including poorly designed or nonexistent curricula. This prompted the establishment of the American Society of Superintendents of Training Schools of Nurses (the Superintendents' Society) in 1893, which later became the National League for Nursing Education (NLNE), and then the National League for Nursing (NLN).

The purpose of the Superintendents' Society was to improve nursing curricula and develop standards of admissions to schools of nursing (Bullough & Bullough, 1978). These actions contributed to the advancement and professionalization of nursing; however, they were of no benefit to Black nurses. For Black, or Negro, schools, the lack of support and recognition from professional nursing organizations such as the NLNE and the American Nurses Association (ANA) undermined their legitimacy and called into question their professional standing. It was not until 1942 that the NLNE offered individual membership to Black nurses, whose many previous attempts to gain membership had been systematically denied (Champinha-Bacote, 1988). In 1948, six years later, the ANA finally extended its membership to Black nurses.

Nursing Practice Under the Segregation Laws

Upon graduating from nurse training programs, Black nurses faced the challenges of limited practice opportunities and lower wages than their White counterparts. As a general rule, the practice of Black nurses was limited to caring for Black clients either in the home, as private-duty nurses, or in the hospital. The prevailing sentiment was that Black nurses were best suited to care for Black patients (Carnegie, 1986; Staupers, 1961). It was common practice for Black student nurses to care for Black patients in the home, as private duty nurses, without supervision. This practice, although inarguably dangerous and unsafe for both clients and nursing students, was, nonetheless, routine with Black schools that relied on the monies paid to the students (Pitts-Mosley, 1996).

With the establishment of public health nursing at the Henry Street Settlement in 1893, the few Black nurses hired by Lillian Wald, founder and director of the Henry Street Settlement Visiting Nursing Service, were afforded the opportunity to extend their practice into this arena of nursing (Pitts-Mosley, 1996). Still, the pervasive inequities that haunted the profession persisted and were intimately tied to three issues. The first was the educational structure in place for training Black and White nurses separately, which prevented disadvantaged Black nurses from receiving a high-quality education. The second was the administration of separate licensing examinations for Black and White nurses, which served only to further divide the profession along racial lines. The third issue was the exclusion of Black nurses from membership and representation in professional organizations, such as the ANA and the NLNE, hence denying Black nurses and Black nursing practice legitimacy within a system that already had preconceived notions about the competence of Black nursing programs and their graduates.

Racial Quotas and the Wars (1901–1951)

The 20th century was witness to World War I (1914–1918) and World War II (1939–1945), both of which created additional demands for nurses to care for wounded soldiers. Typically, under conditions of a reasonably normal nursing supply, race is one of several characteristics, along with age, education, sex, and marital status, that are taken into account in the hiring and acceptance of nurses. In the face of necessity, such as war, however, the characteristics least relevant to professional performance are dropped, and individuals who can fulfill minimum standards, such as having a license as a professional nurse, get their chance (Goldstein, 1960). In the case of the U.S. military, however, despite its desperate need for nurses to care for wounded soldiers during World War I, the use of Black nurses was not an option. It took the flu epidemic of 1918 to see the first 18 Black nurses accepted and assigned to army camps in Ohio and Illinois, with other assignments to follow (Elmore, 1976).

In 1943, the Cadet Nurse Corps was established to address the acute nursing shortage caused by World War II. Students who signed on would receive reimbursement for tuition, books, uniforms, and a monthly stipend if they agreed to complete one year of military nursing or civilian nursing for the remainder of the war. By 1944, the corps was recruiting both Black and White nursing students, and 2,000 Black nursing students were enrolled. However, even though the National Nursing Council for War Service urged that all qualified nurses—regardless of race—be appointed to military service, most Black nurses were still denied service. The army set a small quota for the number of Black nurses it was willing to accept; by the end of the war in 1945, there were only 479 Black nurses out of 50,000 members of the Army Nurse Corps (Bellafaire, 2000). Notably, all of them were confined to segregated areas of the South or sent overseas to care for Black troops (Kalisch & Kalisch, 2004). Because the War Department set a quota of 10% for Black troops, recruiting more nurses was problematic, as illustrated by this statement in a rejection letter sent to an applicant for the army: "colored nurses are authorized for assignment only to those stations where colored troops predominate" (Kalisch & Kalisch, 2004, p. 369). The navy did not accept Black nurses until 1945. Kalisch and Kalisch (2004) note that, had both military branches taken advantage of the numbers of Black nurses in the Cadet Nurse Corps, each would have enlisted at least 1,520 nurses.

Organizing for Strength

Barred from professional affiliation or membership, especially in the Southern states, Black nurses as early as 1901 realized that the problems of discrimination and segregation they faced could only be overcome through collective action. In 1901, Black graduates of established schools in New York, Washington, D.C., and Chicago organized alumnae associations. By 1908, under the leadership of Martha Franklin, Black nurses organized at the national level (Carnegie, 1992). The organization, which came to be known as the National Association of Colored Graduate Nurses (NACGN), lasted from 1908 until 1951. The organization's goals were to (Pitts-Mosley, 1995),

- Achieve higher professional standards for Black nurses
- Break down discriminatory practices in schools of nursing, in jobs, and in nursing organizations
- Develop leadership among Black nurses

By the time the NACGN was dissolved in 1951, because its leaders felt that the organization had accomplished its mission and there was no justification for its continued existence, its members had fought discrimination on all fronts. It had fought especially hard for the integration of Black nurses into the ANA (Carnegie, 1992).

Another recognizable strength of the NACGN, although little recognized by prominent White nursing leaders during its early years, was its ability to form alliances with and gain the support of powerful groups and individuals able to further the cause of the Black nurse. For example, Lillian Wald displayed her faith in Black nurses by hiring three Black nurses in the Visiting Nursing Service in New York (Staupers, 1961). Other support for the NACGN came from the National Medical Association (NMA), the Black physicians' professional organization. The NMA invited the NACGN to hold meetings simultaneously in the same cities and published nurses' articles in its journals (Davis, 1999).

Lowering the Racial Barriers

The 1950s through the early 1970s was one of the most turbulent periods in American history. Hallmarked by the enactment of antidiscrimination and civil rights legislation, beginning with the Eisenhower administration in the 1950s and the Civil Rights Movement in the 1960s, parts of American society were ready and willing to embrace desegregation and observe antidiscriminatory laws. The South, however, remained highly resistant to change. The Civil Rights Act of 1964, passed by the Johnson administration, which prohibited racial discrimination in institutions receiving federal funding, dealt a blow to the segregationists.

Within nursing, the winds of change sweeping the nation also were being felt. The gains that had been achieved by Black nurses up to that point, such as the establishment of the NACGN, collaboration with the NMA, acceptance into the military, and integration into the ANA, were about to be expanded. These gains were consistent with the steady and purposeful strides nursing was making toward establishing itself as a profession. This included the initiation of nursing research and nursing theory development (Schultz, 1990). The profession not only backed away from its previous separatist policies, but took decisive action to lower racial barriers and integrate Black nurses into hospitals. Unprecedented studies on the integration of Black nurses into the workforce were undertaken. Several research articles and editorials addressing civil rights and integration issues were published in some of nursing's most prestigious journals (Goldstein, 1960). In an *American Journal of Nursing* article, for example, Goldstein studied how the services of Black nurses were being utilized on the nursing staffs of several hospitals. The study findings suggested that technological know-how and specialized skills were more of a determinant for employment in hospitals than race. Goldstein went on to note that as educational standards in

professional nursing were raised, the Black nurse with special preparation could qualify for a position for which preferred personnel (White nurses) were scarce. As such, the technical competence stressed in all nursing jobs became almost the sole criterion for acceptability in highly skilled specialties.

Goldstein made clear, however, that the Black nurse, as a less-preferred type, would lose out on promotions. She went on to assert that the trend toward specific educational requirements for particular positions, such as head nurse, would work to the ultimate advantage of those Black nurses who took advantage of training. Yet in the hospitals studied, Black nurses still faced a status dilemma that needed to be solved in order for the hospitals to function smoothly. Goldstein urged a deemphasis on race and a greater focus on professional status and skills.

A July 1964 article appearing in the *American Journal of Nursing* entitled, "Problems of Integration" reported on the difficulty of the ANA to get certain districts, such as the New Orleans district, to comply with the ANA's admission policy and practices. The New Orleans district still barred Black nurses from membership. Issuing an ultimatum, the ANA warned the Louisiana State Nurses Association that the state would be disqualified as an ANA constituent if its practices in the New Orleans district were not corrected by January 1, 1965 (Staupers, 1961). Further, advocating on behalf of the Black nurses, a delegate from Michigan called on the ANA to help districts not only to admit Black nurses, but to help them participate. Staupers also examined the integration of Black nursing in the United States. The April 1965 copy of the *American Journal of Nursing* included an article on how two nurses had integrated a nursing staff that had long been completely segregated.

From the 1950s to the 1970s, there was a significant shift in nursing's race and race relations policies, which had once intentionally erected barriers that excluded Black nurses from membership in professional nursing organizations, from participation in the mainstream of nursing, and from equal access to hospital-based employment.

The Nursing Shortage and Minority Considerations

The new millennium has brought with it a tremendous shift in the demographics of the nursing workforce. Just as nursing has seemed to be emerging as a true science- and research-based profession, evidenced by the successful integration of nursing theory, research, and practice (Schultz, 1990), it is now experiencing one of the largest and most serious nursing shortages ever.

In 2002, the Health Resources and Services Administration estimated that 30 states had shortages of registered nurses in 2000. It predicted that these shortages will intensify over the next 20 years. In February 2004, the U.S. Bureau of Labor Statistics predicted that more than 1 million new and replacement nurses will be needed by 2012. In a similar vein, reports from the American Association of Colleges of Nursing (AACN) have predicted a 20% shortage of registered nurses by 2020, translating into a shortage of over 400,000 registered nurses nationwide (AACN, 2004).

Factors contributing to this gloomy outlook include: (1) lower enrollments in schools of nursing (enrollments in 2001 were 17% lower than in 1995); (2) a shortage of faculty in schools of nursing, which is expected to increase dramatically in the next decade; (3) the increasing age of nurses due to the aging baby boom generation and the lowered numbers of people entering the profession; and (4) burnout and dissatisfaction, as reported in several studies (AACN, 2004).

Evidence shows that staffing shortages contribute to increased mortality. A landmark study by Aiken, Clarke, Cheung, Sloane, and Silber (2003) found that nurses reported greater job dissatisfaction and emotional exhaustion when they were responsible for more patients than they could care for safely. They also found that burnout and job dissatisfaction predicted nurses' intentions to leave their jobs within a year. Similarly, Goodin (2003) conducted an integrative review of the literature and found that, in addition to the reasons for the shortage presented earlier, the lingering poor image of nursing and the wide range of professional occupations now open to women also contribute to the nursing shortage. Substantiation of Goodin's findings came from the National Sample Survey of Registered Nurses (U.S. Department of Health and Human Services, 2001). The National Sample Survey showed that in March 2000, a total of 135,696 registered nurses were not employed in nursing, with a total of 72,568, or 53%, employed in non–health-related occupations. This survey found that the two most important reasons for the prevailing nursing shortage were inconvenient working hours (44.9%) and poor salaries (35.4%).

To fill the nursing gap, the recruitment of minorities into the profession seems a logical step.

However, because of the many career options now available to women and the public's unfavorable perception of nursing as a career choice, particularly in minority communities, few minority youngsters are choosing nursing as a career. In fact, statistical data emanating from the U.S. Department of Health and Human Services (U.S. DHHS, 2003) show that members of minority groups, although accounting for about 30% of the U.S. population, make up a mere 12% of the current nursing workforce. These dismal minority statistics, viewed in light of existing nurse shortages and the recognition of minorities as viable additions to the nursing workforce, have prompted legislative action at several governmental levels aimed at narrowing the remaining racial disparities in professional nursing.

Government Intervention

Corrective actions aimed at increasing the number of minorities choosing to pursue nursing as a career came in the form of 16 nursing workforce diversity grant awards from the DHHS in June 2003, totaling nearly $3.5 million to support nursing education opportunities for individuals from disadvantaged backgrounds. The grants were slated to fund scholarships or stipends and preentry preparation and retention activities for disadvantaged students, including students from racial and ethnic minority groups that are underrepresented among registered nurses. Minority enrollment in the nursing schools that received the grants averaged 38%, about double the national average of 19%. According to U.S. DHHS Secretary Tommy G. Thompson, "these schools and programs have proven their ability to enroll and graduate competent, skilled health care workers, which is important in expanding access to health care for all Americans" (U.S. DHHS, 2003, p. 1). He

went on to note that the grants would encourage minority students to enter the field of nursing and help alleviate the critical shortage. In July 2004, DHHS announced an additional $15.5 million to expand and strengthen the nursing workforce, with $5.4 million earmarked for the Nursing Workforce Diversity Program (U.S. DHHS, 2004).

Nursing Intervention

Several prominent nursing organizations are at the forefront of this move toward increasing minority recruitment into professional nursing. The AACN declared that as the United States struggles to find solutions to the current nursing shortage, nursing schools need to strengthen their efforts to attract more men and minority students (AACN Bulletin, 2001). To these ends, the NLN also has been very active by way of its legislative agenda. One element of its legislative package has been asking for increased funding for minority and disadvantaged students.

In an April 26, 2001 testimonial before the National Advisory Council on Nurse Education and Practice (NACNEP), Ruth D. Corcoran, chief executive officer of the NLN, pointed to the NLN's joint and dedicated effort in concert with that of the NACNEP in awakening healthcare stakeholders in academia, the industry, and government to the long-term effects of leaving major portions of our population substantially out of nursing—primarily, ethnic/racial minorities as well as males (Corcoran, 2001).

Further, statistical data emanating from DHHS, Health Resources and Service Administration Bureau of Health Professions shows that even when these underrepresented groups (minorities and men) pursue a nursing education, associate degree programs attract a great percentage of them (U.S. DHHS, HRSA, 2000).

Accordingly, Corcoran proposed several recommendations for improving access to nursing education programs for groups traditionally underrepresented in nursing. Among these were:

1. Creating partnerships among colleges and universities, precollege and college institutions, industry, professional societies, and communities that formulate and maintain effective grassroots career awareness activities for K–12 and reentry students, as well as their teachers, parents, and professional mentors.
2. Commitment in resources and the will to establish the networks and academic enrichment services, which have proven to be labor and time intensive, for successful academic advising, tutoring, and general nurturing of the student.
3. Financial assistance to enable disadvantaged students to pursue nursing studies (Corcoran, 2001).

The Importation of Foreign Nurses

One solution to nursing shortages in the United States has historically been the importation of foreign nurses, the majority of whom are people of color coming from underdeveloped and developing countries, such as India, the Philippines, and the Caribbean. Concordant with these recruitment efforts, Congress has passed needed legislation to facilitate the immigration of foreign nurses. For example, the Immigration Nursing Relief Acts of 1986, 1989, and 1990 provided nonimmigrant visas (H-1A) to international nurses hired to fill vacancies in U.S. hospitals (Flynn & Aiken, 2002). Also, the Nursing Relief to Disadvantaged Areas Act of 1999 addressed the nursing shortage in underserved

rural and urban areas that are generally difficult to staff. This piece of legislation allowed for the issuance of a maximum of 500 nonimmigrant visas (H-1C) per year to international nurses employed in designated health professional shortage areas, as defined by the U.S. DHHS. Unlike this legislative action, which was viewed as essential and needed, the Immigration Nursing Relief Act, because of political pressure, was allowed to "sunset" (Flynn & Aiken, 2002).

Admittedly, the importation of foreign nurses is a short-term solution to a much larger problem inherent in the U.S. healthcare system (Joel, 1996). Critics, such as the ANA, also question the ethics of importing nurses from other countries during a global nursing shortage. Luring skilled nurses from other countries robs their native countries of talented nurses and increases the global nursing shortage. Additionally, the ANA is concerned about exploiting workers once they begin working in substandard conditions, because many of them are hired to replace American nurses who leave due to deteriorating working conditions (Trossman, 2003).

Facing the Challenges of Tomorrow

Gone are the days of Jim Crow and state-mandated segregation laws that curtailed the professional training, practice, and earnings of Black nurses. The major challenge confronting professional nursing today and tomorrow is the disappearance of a qualified replacement nursing workforce to replace the aging baby-boom generation of nurses, the majority of whom are at, or rapidly approaching, retirement age.

Today more than ever before, the doors of opportunity are open to African Americans and other minorities interested in pursuing a nursing career or advanced preparation in nursing. However, the question that remains is whether White nurses and the power structure within nursing are committed and/or prepared to share the power base in professional nursing with African Americans and other minority nurses. The Cleveland Council of Black Nurses (CCBN) believes that old habits and racial stereotypes are hard to kill. Pointing to the high attrition rates among African American nursing students around the country, the CCBN describes a revolving door syndrome, and notes that the growing body of literature documents the difficulties of African American nursing students. They report feelings of estrangement and isolation on campus; pressure to conform to stereotypes; less equitable treatment by faculty, staff, and teaching assis-

tants; and more faculty racism than other students of color. The CCBN noted a parallel between the occurrences of today and those of yesterday, when White nurse educators and administrators took no responsibility for negative attitudes and discriminatory practices that excluded Blacks from admission into nursing programs and limited their employment opportunities (George, Bradford, & Battle, 1995).

Many predict that the appearance of the future nursing workforce will look quite different. In the final analysis, this may indeed be true. George, Bradford, and Battle (1995) remind us that our tomorrow rests in the minds, hearts, commitments, motivation, and achievements of African American nursing students and nurses, along with the commitment of all nurses, to the values and ideals of the nursing profession.

Discussion Questions

1. How have the social and nursing histories in the United States intersected to result in current statistics related to minorities in the profession?
2. Discuss future initiatives to increase the numbers of minorities in nursing in general and advanced practice nursing in particular.
3. Discuss future initiatives for decreasing healthcare disparities for the United States.

References

AACN Bulletin. (2001). *Effective strategies for increasing diversity in nursing programs*. Retrieved October 7, 2004, from www.aacn.ncheedu/publications/issues/dec01

AACN. (2004). *Nursing shortage resource*. Retrieved January 12, 2005, from www.aacn.nche.edu/Media/shortageresource.htm#about

Aiken, L. H., Clarke, S. P., Cheung, R. B., Sloane, D. M., & Silber, J. H. (2003). Educational levels of hospital nurses and surgical patient mortality. *JAMA, 290*(12), 1617–1623.

Bellafaire, J. A. (2000). *Black nurses in WWII*. Retrieved January 12, 2005, from www.ww2medicine.org/black.html

Bullough, V. L., & Bullough, B. (1978). *The emergence of modern nursing*. New York: MacMillan.

Carnegie, M. E. (1986). *The path we thread: Blacks in nursing, 1854–1984.* New York: J. B. Lippincott Company.

Carnegie, M. E. (1992). Black nurses in the United States: 1879–1992. *Journal of National Black Nurses' Association, 6*(1), 13–18.

Champinha-Bacote, J. (1988). The Black nurses' struggle toward equality: An historical account of the National Association of Colored Graduate Nurses. *Journal of National Black Nurses' Association, 2*(2), 15–25.

Corcoran, R. D. (2001, April 26). Testimony of the NLN before the National Advisory Council on Nurse Education and Practice. Silver Spring, MD.

Davis, A. T. (1999). *Early Black American leaders in nursing: Architects for integration and equality.* Sudbury, MA: Jones and Bartlett.

Elmore, J. A. (1976). Black nurses: Their service and their struggle. *American Journal of Nursing, 76*(3), 435–437.

Flynn, L., & Aiken, L. H. (2002). Does international nurse recruitment influence practice values in U.S. hospitals? *American Journal of Nursing Scholarship, 34*(1), 67–72.

George, V. D., Bradford, D. M., & Battle, A. (1995). Yesterday, today & tomorrow. *Nursing and Health Care Perspectives, 21*(5), 219–227.

Goldstein, R. L. (1960). Black nurses in hospitals. *American Journal of Nursing, 60*(2), 215–218.

Goodin, H. J. (2003). The nursing shortage in the United States of America: An integrative review of the literature. *Journal of Advanced Nursing, 43*(4), 335–343.

Hine, D. C. (1989). *Black women in white: Racial conflict and cooperation in the nursing profession, 1890–1950.* Bloomington: Indiana University Press.

Institute of Medicine. (2003). *Unequal treatment: Confronting racial and ethnic disparities in healthcare.* Washington, DC: Institute of Medicine.

Joel, L. A. (1996). Immigration: Why is it still up for discussion? *American Journal of Nursing, 96*(1), 7–8.

Kalisch, P. A., & Kalisch, B. J. (2004). *American nursing, a history* (4th ed.). Philadelphia: Lippincott Williams & Wilkins.

Massey, E. (1934). The Black nurse student. *American Journal of Nursing, 34*, 608–610.

Pitts-Mosley, M. O. (1995). Despite all odds: A three-part history of the professionalization of Black nurses through two professional nursing organizations, 1908–1995. *Journal of National Black Nurses' Association, 7*(2), 10–19.

Schultz, P. R. (1990, Winter). Milestones in the success of nursing as an emerging discipline. *American Journal of Pharmaceutical Education, 54*, 370–373.

Smith, D. B. (1999). *Health care divided: Race and healing a nation.* Ann Arbor: University of Michigan Press.

Staupers, M. K. (1961). *No time for prejudice: A story of the integration of Negroes in nursing in the United States.* New York: MacMillan.

Sullivan Commission. (2004). *Missing persons: Minorities in the health professions.* Washington, DC: The Sullivan Commission.

Trossman, S. (2003). The global reach of the nursing shortage: The American Nurses' Association questions the ethics of luring foreign-educated nurses to the United States. *Nevada RNformation, 12*(1), 25.

U.S. DHHS. (2001). *The registered nurse population: Findings from the 2000 national sample survey.* Retrieved January 12, 2005, from http://bhpr.hrsa. gov/healthworkforce/reports/rnsurvey/default.htm

U.S. DHHS. (2003). *HHS awards nearly $3.5 million to promote diversity in the nursing workforce.* Retrieved October 7, 2004, from http://www.os.hhs.gov/news/ press/2003pres/20030602.html

U.S. DHHS. (2004). *HHS awards $15.5 million to expand, strengthen nursing workforce.* Retrieved October 7, 2004, from http://www.hhs.gov/news/press/ 2004pres/20040722.html

U.S. DHHS, HRSA. (2000). *The registered nurse population: Findings from the national sample survey of registered nurses.* Retrieved October 4, 2004, from http://bhpr.hrsa.gov/healthworkforce/reports/ rnsurvey/rnss1.htm

Introduction to Ethics

George D. Pozgar

CHAPTER OBJECTIVES

1. Apply basic ethical concepts to advanced nursing practice.
2. Discuss important historical events that have influenced biomedical ethics.
3. Develop an understanding of relevant ethical theories and principles, person values and beliefs, and the concepts of morality that provide a framework for advanced nursing practice.
4. Apply the concept of situational ethics to the practice of advanced nursing.

Introduction

This chapter provides the reader with an overview of ethics and moral principles. Ethics and morals are derivatives from the Greek and Latin terms (roots) for custom. The intent here is not to burden the reader with the philosophy and arguments surrounding ethical theories, morality, principles, virtues, and values. However, as with the study of any new subject, words are the tools of thought. Therefore, some new vocabulary will be presented to the reader in order to apply the abstract theories and principles of ethics. One needs to understand the words and the concepts in order to make practical use of them.

Ethical dilemmas arise when values, rights, duties, and loyalties conflict, and consequently not everyone is satisfied with a particular decision. An understanding of the concepts presented here will help to reduce conflict when addressing ethical dilemmas and making difficult decisions.

Chapter 27

Ethics

How we perceive right and wrong is influenced by what we feed on.

AUTHOR UNKNOWN

Ethics, also referred to as moral philosophy, is the discipline concerned with what is morally good and bad, right and wrong. The term is also applied to any theoretical system of moral values or principles. Ethics is less concerned with factual knowledge than with virtues and values—namely, human conduct as it ought to be, rather than as it actually is.

Ethics is the branch of philosophy that seeks to understand the nature, purposes, justification, and founding principles of moral rules and the systems they comprise. Ethics deals with values relating to human conduct. It focuses on the rightness and wrongness of actions as well as the goodness and badness of motives and ends. Ethics encompasses the decision-making process of determining ultimate actions. It involves how individuals decide to live within accepted and desirable principles and how they live in harmony with the environment and one another.

Microethics involves an individual's view of what is right and wrong based on personal life experiences. Macroethics involves a more global view of right and wrong. Although no person lives in a vacuum, solving ethical dilemmas involves consideration of ethical issues from both a micro and macro ethical perspective.

The term *ethics* is used in three different but related ways, signifying (1) a general pattern or way of life, such as religious ethics (e.g., Judeo-Christian ethics); (2) a set of rules of conduct or moral code, which involves professional ethics and ethical behavior; and (3) philosophical ethics, which involves inquiry about ways of life and rules of conduct.

The scope of healthcare ethics encompasses numerous issues, including the right to choose or refuse treatment and the right to limit the suffering one will endure. Incredible advances in technology and the resulting capability to extend life beyond what would be considered a reasonable quality of life have complicated the process of healthcare decision making. The scope of healthcare ethics is not limited to philosophical issues but embraces economic, medical, political, social, and legal dilemmas as well.

Bioethics addresses such difficult issues as the nature of life, the nature of death, what sort of life is worth living, what constitutes murder, how we should treat people who are in especially vulnerable and painful circumstances, and the responsibilities we have to other human beings. The following events are some of many that have had a significant impact on healthcare ethics.

1932–1972: Tuskegee Study of Syphilis

The purpose of the Tuskegee study, involving African American men, was to analyze the natural progression of untreated syphilis. The study was conducted from 1932 through the early 1970s. The participants were not warned during the study that there was a cure for syphilis (i.e., penicillin). They believed that they were receiving adequate care and unknowingly suffered unnecessarily. The Tuskegee syphilis study used disadvantaged, rural black men to investigate the untreated course of a disease, one that is by no means confined to that population. We know now that the selection of research subjects must be closely monitored to ensure that specific classes of individuals (e.g., terminally ill patients, welfare patients, racial and ethnic minorities, or persons confined to institutions) are not selected for research studies because of their easy availability, compromised position, or manipulability. Rather, they must be selected for reasons directly related to the research being conducted.

1946: Military Tribunal for War Crimes

In 1946, a military tribunal began criminal proceedings against 23 German physicians and administrators for war crimes and crimes against humanity. As a direct result of these proceedings, the Nuremberg code was established, which made it clear that the voluntary and informed consent of human subjects is essential to research, and that benefits of research must outweigh risks to human subjects involved (Eastern Michigan University, n.d.).

1949: Nuremberg Trials: International Code of Medical Ethics

This code was adopted following numerous experiments conducted by the Nazis on prisoners in concentration camps. Prisoners were exposed to cholera, diphtheria, malaria, mustard gas, yellow fever, typhus, and other horrendous experiments, ultimately claiming thousands of lives. This exploitation of unwilling prisoners as research subjects in Nazi concentration camps was condemned as a particularly flagrant injustice.

1954: First Kidney Transplant

The National Institutes of Health published guidelines on human experimentation. The transplantation of human organs has generated numerous ethical issues (e.g., the harvesting and selling of organs, who should have first access to freely donated human organs, and how death is defined) (*A science odyssey*, 1998).

1960s: Cardiopulmonary Resuscitation

Prolonging life beyond what reasonably would be expected has generated numerous ongoing ethical dilemmas. Should limited resources, for example, be spent on those who have been determined to be in a comatose vegetative state with no hope of recovery? Or should limited resources be spent on preventive medicine that would improve the quality of life for all?

1964: World Medical Association

In 1964, the World Medical Association established guidelines for medical doctors doing biomedical research involving human subjects. The Declaration of Helsinki is the basis for good clinical practices today (Eastern Michigan University, n.d.).

1968: Harvard Medical School Report on Brain Death Criteria

How does one determine when brain death occurs? In 1968, the Harvard Ad Hoc Committee on Brain Death published a report describing the following characteristics of a permanently nonfunctioning brain, a condition it referred to as "irreversible coma," now known as brain death:

1. Patient shows total unawareness to external stimuli and unresponsiveness to painful stimuli.
2. No movements or breathing: All spontaneous muscular movement, spontaneous respiration, and response to stimuli are absent.
3. No reflexes; fixed, dilated pupils; no eye movement even when hit or turned, or when ice water is placed in the ear; no response to noxious stimuli; no tendon reflexes.

In addition to these criteria, a flat electroencephalogram was recommended (Harvard Ad Hoc Committee, 1968).

1970: Paternalism Questioned

As physicians are faced with many options for saving lives, transplanting organs, and furthering research, they also must wrestle with new and troubling choices—for example, who should receive scarce and vital treatment, how to determine when life ends, and what limits should be placed on care for the dying.

1971: Kennedy Institute of Ethics at Georgetown University

In 1971, the Joseph P. and Rose F. Kennedy Institute of Ethics was founded at Georgetown University and became the first academic bioethics center in the world. The Institute provides a comprehensive resource for academicians, ethicists, policy makers, and the general public through its library, programs, and publications. The library can be accessed through its Web site at http://bioethics.georgetown.edu/databases/.

In addition, it is the home to ethical scholars who lecture at conferences, seminars, symposia, and special programs worldwide. They also serve as consultants on government commissions or committees and testify at government hearings on a wide range of ethical issues. Emerging areas of research and study include racial and gender equality, international justice and peace, and other issues affecting vulnerable populations (Kennedy Institute of Ethics, 2007).

1972: Informed Consent

The case of *Canterbury v. Spence* (1972), set the "reasonable man" standard requiring informed consent for treatment. Patients must be informed of the risks, benefits, and alternatives associated with recommended treatments.

1974: National Research Act

Due to publicity from the Tuskegee Syphilis Study, the National Research Act of 1974 was passed. This act created the National Commission for the Protection of Human Subjects of Biomedical and Behavioral Research. One of the commission's charges was to identify the basic ethical principles that should underlie the conduct of biomedical and behavioral research involving human subjects and to develop guidelines to ensure that such research is conducted in accordance with those principles (Belmont Report, 2004).

The commission was directed to consider:

- the boundaries between biomedical and behavioral research and the accepted and routine practice of medicine
- the role of assessment of risk-benefit criteria in determining the appropriateness of research involving human subjects
- appropriate guidelines for the selection of human subjects for participation in such research
- the nature and definition of informed consent in various research settings (National Institutes of Health, 1979)

The Food and Drug Administration and the National Institutes of Health internal policy guidelines became federal regulation. As a result of the National Research Act, the National Commission for the Protection of Human Subjects in Biomedical and Behavioral Research was established.

1976: Substituted Judgment

In *In the Matter of Karen Ann Quinlan* (1976), the Supreme Court rendered a unanimous decision providing for the appointment of Joseph Quinlan as personal guardian of his daughter

Karen, with full power to make decisions regarding the identity of her treating physicians. Upon the concurrence of the guardian and family, if Karen's physicians concluded that there was no reasonable possibility of her emerging from her comatose condition to a cognitive, sapient state and that her life support apparatus should be withdrawn, they were to consult with the ethics committee of the institution where Karen was then hospitalized. If that consultative body concurred in the prognosis, the life support system could be withdrawn without any civil or criminal liability on the part of any participant, whether it be the guardian, physician, hospital, or others. In addressing itself to the question of possible homicide, the court concluded that there is a valid distinction between withdrawing life support systems in cases such as Karen's and the infliction of deadly harm either on one's self or another. It saw a difference between Karen's situation and the unlawful killing that is condemned in statutory law. The court denied that the death following withdrawal of treatment would be homicidal. Rather, it would be the result of previously existing natural causes, not from the withdrawal of treatment; and, even if it were considered homicide, it could not be unlawful if done pursuant to the exercise of an explicitly recognized constitutional right.

1978: Establishment of the President's Commission for Study of Ethical Problems in Medicine

The duties of the commission include conducting studies of the ethical and legal implications of the requirements for informed consent to participate in research projects and to otherwise undergo medical procedures; the matter of defining death, including the advisability of developing a uniform definition of death; voluntary testing, counseling, and information and education programs with respect to genetic diseases and conditions, taking into account the essential equality of all human beings, born and unborn; the differences in the availability of health services as determined by the income or residence of the persons receiving the services; current procedures and mechanisms designed to safeguard the privacy of human subjects of behavioral and biomedical research, to ensure the confidentiality of individually identifiable patient records, and to ensure appropriate access of patients to information; and such other matters relating to medicine or biomedical or behavioral research as the president may designate for study by the commission (42 U.S. Code 6A [XVI]).

1990: Physician-Assisted Suicide

Jack Kevorkian, a physician, assisted terminally ill patients in suicide outside the boundaries of the law.

1990: Patient Self-Determination Act

The Patient Self-Determination Act of 1990 was enacted to ensure that patients are informed of their rights to execute advance directives and accept or refuse medical care.

1994: Oregon's Death with Dignity Act

Physician-assisted suicide became a legal medical option for terminally ill Oregonians. The Oregon Death with Dignity Act allows terminally ill Oregon residents to obtain from their physicians and use prescriptions for self-administered, lethal medications.

1996: Health Insurance Portability and Accountability Act

The Health Insurance Portability and Accountability Act of 1996 (Public Law 104-191) was designed to protect the privacy, confidentiality, and security of patient information.

2001: President's Council on Bioethics

The President's Council on Bioethics was created by President George W. Bush in 2001. The council was charged with advising the president on bioethical issues that may emerge as a consequence of advances in biomedical science and technology (President's Council on Bioethics, n.d.).

2003: Human Genome System Became Fully Sequenced

The Human Genome Project, sponsored by the National Institutes of Health, completed the sequencing of the full human genome sequence in April 2003. The next phase in the project is research aimed at improving human health and fighting disease (National Human Genome Research Institute, 2007). The expectation is that genetic and medical research will accelerate at an unprecedented rate with ethical implications and dilemmas arising such as cloning, stem cell transplants, and others.

Ethical Theories

Ethics, too, are nothing but reverence for life. This is what gives me the fundamental principle of morality, namely, that good consists in maintaining, promoting, and enhancing life, and that destroying, injuring, and limiting life are evil.

ALBERT SCHWEITZER (SCHWEITZER, 1949)

Ethics seeks to understand and to determine how human actions can be judged as right or wrong. Ethical judgments can be made based upon our own experiences or based upon the nature of or principles of reason. Those who study ethics believe that ethical decision making is based upon theory. Ethical theories attempt to introduce order into the way people think about life and action. The following paragraphs provide a review of the more commonly discussed ethical theories.

Normative Ethics

Normative ethics is the attempt to determine what moral standards should be followed so that human behavior and conduct may be morally right. Normative ethics is primarily concerned with establishing standards or norms for conduct and is commonly associated with general theories about how one ought to live. One of the central questions of modern normative ethics is whether human actions are to be judged right or wrong solely according to their consequences.

General normative ethics is the critical study of major moral precepts of such matters as what things are right, what things are good, and what things are genuine. General normative ethics is the determination of correct moral principles for all autonomous rational beings.

Applied ethics is the application of normative theories to practical moral problems. It attempts to explain and justify specific moral problems such as abortion, euthanasia, and assisted suicide.

Consequential or Teleological Ethics

The consequential or teleological ethics theory emphasizes that the morally right action is whatever action leads to the maximum balance of good over evil. From a contemporary standpoint, theories that judge actions by their consequences have been referred to as consequentialism. Consequential ethics theories revolve around the premise that the rightness or wrongness of an action depends upon the consequences or effects of an action. The theory of consequentialism is based on the view that the value of an action derives solely from the value of its consequences. The goal of a consequentialist is to achieve the greatest good for the greatest number. It involves asking:

- What will be the effects of each course of action?
- Will they be positive or negative?
- For whom?
- What will do the least harm?

Nonconsequential Ethics

The nonconsequential ethics theory denies that the consequences of an action or rule are the only criteria for determining the morality of an action or rule. In this theory, the rightness or wrongness of an action is based on properties intrinsic to the action, not on its consequences.

Deontological Ethics

Deontological theory focuses on one's duties to others. It includes telling the truth and keeping one's promises. Deontology involves ethical analysis according to a moral code or rules, religious or secular, as presented below.

RELIGIOUS ETHICS

The Great Physician
Dear Lord, You are the Great Physician, I turn to you in my sickness asking for your help.

I place myself under your loving care, praying that I may know your healing grace and wholeness.

Help me to find love in this strange world and to feel your presence by my bed both day and night.

Give my doctors and nurses wisdom that they may understand my illness.

Steady and guide them with your strong hand.

Reach out your hand to me and touch my life with your peace. Amen.

UNIVERSITY OF PENNSYLVANIA
HEALTH SYSTEM

Religious ethics, as it relates to character and morality, varies from person to person based on one's religious beliefs. Religious beliefs are heavily influenced by the family within which one is born. The more dogmatic the belief, the more likely one will adopt the family's religious beliefs and values.

Often one's religious beliefs can change as circumstances change. What is troublesome to one individual may not be to another. One's need to survive can change his or her moral character. The extent to which one will adapt in order to survive can take on the extremes of who we really are and how far we will go in order to survive.

Religious codes of ethics are based on a particular religion. Biblical ethics, for example, is God centered. Judaism is based on Old Testament scriptures. Christianity is based on both Old and New Testament scriptures. The notion of right and wrong is not so much an object of philosophical inquiry as an acceptance of divine revelation. Moses, for example, received a list of 10 laws directly from God. These laws are known as the Ten Commandments. Some of the commandments are related to the basic principles of justice that have been adhered to by society since they were first proclaimed and published. For some societies, the Ten Commandments were a turning point where essential commands such as "thou shalt not kill" or "thou shalt not commit adultery" were accepted as law.

The Ten Commandments

1. I am the Lord thy God, which have brought thee out of the land of Egypt, out of the house of bondage. Thou shalt have no other gods before me.
2. Thou shalt not make unto thee any graven image, or any likeness of anything that is in heaven above, or that is in the earth beneath, or that is in the water under the earth. Thou shalt not bow down thyself to them, nor serve them.
3. Thou shalt not take the name of the Lord thy God in vain.
4. Remember the Sabbath day, to keep it holy.
5. Honor thy father and thy mother: that thy days may be long.
6. Thou shalt not kill.
7. Thou shalt not commit adultery.
8. Thou shalt not steal.
9. Thou shalt not bear false witness against thy neighbor.
10. Thou shalt not covet thy neighbor's house, thou shalt not covet thy neighbor's wife, nor his manservant, nor his maidservant, nor his ox, nor his ass, nor anything that is thy neighbor's.

Spirituality in the religious sense implies that there is purpose and meaning to life; spirituality generally refers to faith in a higher being. For a patient, injury and sickness is a frightening experience. This fear is often heightened when the patient is admitted to a healthcare facility. Healthcare organizations can help reduce patient fears by making available to them appropriate emotional and spiritual support and coping resources. It is a well-proven fact that patients who are able to draw upon their spirituality and religious beliefs tend to have a more comfortable and often improved healing experience. To assist both patients and caregivers in addressing spiritual needs, patients should be provided with information as to how their spiritual needs can be addressed.

Difficult questions regarding a patient's spiritual needs and how to meet those needs are best addressed upon admission by first collecting information about the patient's religious or spiritual preferences. Caregivers often find it difficult to discuss spiritual issues for fear of offending a patient who may have beliefs different from their own. If caregivers know from admission records a patient's religious beliefs, the caregiver can share with the patient those religious and spiritual resources available in the hospital and community.

SECULAR ETHICS

Unlike religious ethics, secular ethics are based on codes developed by societies that have relied on customs to formulate their codes. The Code of Hammurabi, for example, carved on a black Babylonian column, 8 feet high, now located in the Louvre in Paris, depicts a mythical sun god presenting a code of laws to Hammurabi, a great military leader and ruler of Babylon (1795–1750 BC). Hammurabi's code of laws is an early example of a ruler proclaiming to his people an entire body of laws. The following excerpts are from the Code of Hammurabi.

Code of Hammurabi

5

If a judge try a case, reach a decision, and present his judgment in writing; if later error shall appear in his decision, and it be through his own fault, then he shall pay twelve times the fine set by him in the case, and he shall be publicly removed from the judge's bench, and never again shall he sit there to render judgment.

194

If a man give his child to a nurse and the child die in her hands, but the nurse unbeknown to the father and mother nurse another child, then they shall convict her of having nursed another child without the knowledge of the father and mother and her breasts shall be cut off.

215

If a physician make a large incision with an operating knife and cure it, or if he open a tumor (over the eye) with an operating knife, and saves the eye, he shall receive ten shekels in money.

217

If he be the slave of some one, his owner shall give the physician two shekels.

218

If a physician make a large incision with the operating knife, and kill him, or open a tumor with the operating knife, and cut out the eye, his hands shall be cut off.

219

If a physician make a large incision in the slave of a freed man, and kill him, he shall replace the slave with another slave.

221

If a physician heal the broken bone or diseased soft part of a man, the patient shall pay the physician five shekels in money.

Principles of Healthcare Ethics

You cannot by tying an opinion to a man's tongue, make him the representative of that opinion; and at the close of any battle for principles, his name will be found neither among the dead, nor the wounded, but the missing.

E.P. WHIPPLE (1819–1886)[1]

Ethical principles are universal rules of conduct that identify what kinds of actions, intentions, and motives are valued. Ethical principles core to the ethical practice of medicine are discussed next. These principles assist caregivers in making choices based on moral principles that have been identified as standards considered worthwhile in addressing healthcare-related ethical dilemmas. Ethical principles provide a generalized framework within which particular ethical dilemmas can be analyzed. Caregivers, in the study of ethics, will find that difficult decisions often involve choices between conflicting ethical principles.

Autonomy

. . . no right is held more sacred, or is more carefully guarded, by the common law, than the right of every individual to the possession and control of his own person.

UNION PACIFIC RY. CO. V. BOTSFORD (1891)

The principle of autonomy involves recognizing the right of a person to make one's own decisions. *Auto* comes from a Greek word meaning self or the individual. In this context it means recognizing an individual's right to make his or her own decisions about what is best for himself or herself. Autonomy is not an absolute principle. The autonomous actions of one person must not infringe upon the rights of another.

Respect for autonomy has been recognized in the 14th amendment to the Constitution of the United States. The law upholds an individual's right to make his or her own decisions about health care. A patient has the right to refuse to receive health care even if it is beneficial to saving his or her life. Patients can refuse treatment, refuse to take medications, refuse blood or blood by-products, and refuse invasive procedures regardless of the benefits that may be derived from them. They have a right to have their decisions followed by family members who may disagree simply because they are unable to let go.

What has been mandated by law has been reflected in bioethical thinking. Although patients have a right to make their own decisions, they also have a concomitant right to know the risks, benefits, and alternatives to recommended procedures.

When analyzing an ethical dilemma, caregivers must consider how autonomy and the respect for a patient's wishes affect the caregivers' decision-making processes. Is, for example, the patient's right to self-determination being compromised because of a third party's wishes for the patient?

The caregiver respects the mentally competent decision-making capabilities of autonomous persons and that right of an individual to make his or her own decisions. The eminent Justice Cardozo, in *Schloendorff v. Society of New York Hospital* (1914), stated:

Every human being of adult years and sound mind has a right to determine what shall be done with his own body and a surgeon who performs an operation without his patient's consent commits an assault, for which he is liable in damages, except in cases of emergency where the patient is unconscious and where it is necessary to operate before consent can be obtained.

What happens when the right to autonomy conflicts with other moral principles, such as beneficence and justice? Conflict can arise, for example, when a patient refuses a blood transfusion considered necessary to save his or her life while the caregiver's principal obligation is to do no harm.

Autonomous decision making can be affected by one's disabilities, mental status, maturity, or incapacity to make decisions. Although the principle of autonomy may be inapplicable in certain cases, one's autonomous wishes may be carried out through an advance directive and/or an appointed healthcare agent in the event of one's inability to make decisions.

Beneficence

Beneficence describes the principle of doing good, demonstrating kindness, showing compassion, and helping others. In the healthcare setting, caregivers demonstrate beneficence by providing benefits and balancing benefits against risks. Beneficence requires one to do good. Doing good requires knowledge of the beliefs, culture, values, and preferences of the patient—what one person may believe to be good for a patient may in reality be harmful. For example, a caregiver may decide that a patient should be told frankly, "there is nothing else that I can do for you." This could be injurious to the patient if the patient really wants encouragement and information about care options from the caregiver. Compassion here requires the caregiver to tell the patient, "I am not aware of new treatments for your illness; however, I have some ideas about how I can help treat your symptoms and make you more comfortable. In addition, I will keep you informed as to any significant research that may be helpful in treating your disease processes."

Paternalism is a form of beneficence. People, often believing that they know what is best for another, often make decisions that they believe are in another person's best interest. It may involve, for example, withholding information from someone, believing that the person would be better off that way. Paternalism can occur due to one's age, cognitive ability, and level of dependency.

Medical paternalism involves making choices for (or forcing choices on) patients who are capable of choosing for themselves. This directly violates patient autonomy. Physicians are often in situations where they can influence a patient's healthcare decision simply by selectively telling the patient what he or she prefers based on personal beliefs. The problem of paternalism involves a conflict between principles of autonomy and beneficence, each of which is conceived by different parties as the overriding principle in cases of conflict. Conflict between the demands of beneficence and autonomy underlies a broad range of controversies.

Nonmaleficence

Nonmaleficence is an ethical principle that requires caregivers to avoid causing patients harm. Nonmaleficence is not concerned with improving others' well-being but rather with avoiding the infliction of harm. Medical ethics require healthcare providers to first, do no harm. In *In re Conroy*, 464 A.2d 303, 314 (N.J. Super. Ct. App. Div. 1983), "the physician's primary obligation is . . . First do no harm." Telling the truth, for example, can sometimes cause harm. If there is no cure for a patient's disease, a healthcare provider may have a dilemma. Should he tell the patient and possibly cause serious psychological harm, or should he give the patient what he considers false hopes? Is there a middle ground? If so, what is it? To avoid causing harm, alternatives may need to be considered in solving the ethical dilemma.

The caregiver, realizing that he or she cannot help a particular patient, attempts to avoid harming the patient. This is done as a caution against taking a serious risk with the patient, or doing something that has no immediate or long-term benefits.

The principle of nonmaleficence is broken when a physician is placed in the position of ending life by removing respirators, giving lethal injections, or by writing prescriptions for lethal doses of medication. Helping patients die violates the physician's duty to save lives. In the final analysis there needs to be a distinction between killing patients and letting them die.

Justice

Justice is the obligation to be fair in the distribution of benefits and risks. Justice demands that persons in similar circumstances be treated similarly. A person is treated justly when he or she receives what is due, is deserved, or can legitimately be claimed. Justice involves how people are treated when their interests compete with one another.

Can the Physician Change His Mind?

Walls had a condition that caused his left eye to be out of alignment with his right eye. Walls discussed with Shreck, his physician, the possibility of surgery on his left eye to bring both eyes into alignment. Walls and Shreck agreed that the best approach to treating Walls was to attempt surgery on the left eye. Prior to surgery, Walls signed an authorization and consent form that included the following language:

   a. I hereby authorize Dr. Shreck . . . to perform the following procedure and/or alternative procedure necessary to treat my condition . . . of the left eye.
   b. I understand the reason for the procedure is to straighten my left eye to keep it from going to the left.
   c. It has been explained to me that conditions may arise during this procedure whereby a different procedure or an additional procedure may need to be performed, and I authorize my physician and his assistants to do what they feel is needed and necessary.

During surgery, Shreck encountered excessive scar tissue on the muscles of Walls's left eye and elected to adjust the muscles of the right eye instead. When Walls awoke from the anesthesia, he expressed anger at the fact that both of his eyes were bandaged. The next day, Walls went to Shreck's office for a follow-up visit and adjustment of his sutures. Walls asked Shreck why he had operated on the right eye, and Shreck responded that he reserved the right to change his mind during surgery.

Walls filed a lawsuit. The trial court concluded that Walls had failed to establish that Shreck had violated any standard of care. It sustained Shreck's motion for directed verdict, and Walls appealed. The court stated that the consent form that had been signed indicated that there can be extenuating circumstances when the surgeon exceeds the scope of what was discussed presurgery. Walls claims that it was his impression that Shreck was talking about surgeries in general.

Roussel, an ophthalmologist, had testified on behalf of Walls. Roussel stated that it was customary to discuss with patients the potential risks of a surgery, benefits, and the alternatives to surgery. Roussel testified that medical ethics requires informed consent.

Shreck claimed that he had obtained the patient's informed consent not from the form but from what he discussed with the patient in his office. The court found that the form itself does not give or deny permission for anything. Rather, it is evidence of the discussions that occurred and during which informed consent was obtained. Shreck therefore asserted that he obtained informed consent to operate on both eyes based on his office discussions with Walls.

Ordinarily, in a medical malpractice case, the plaintiff must prove the physician's negligence by expert testimony. One of the exceptions to the requirement of expert testimony is

(continues)

Can the Physician Change His Mind? (continued)

the situation whereby the evidence and the circumstances are such that the recognition of the alleged negligence may be presumed to be within the comprehension of laymen. This exception is referred to as the "common knowledge exception."

The evidence showed that Shreck did not discuss with Walls that surgery might be required on both eyes during the same operation. There is evidence that Walls specifically told Shreck he did not want surgery performed on the right eye.

Expert testimony was not required to establish that Walls did not give express or implied consent for Shreck to operate on his right eye. Absent an emergency, it is common knowledge that a reasonably prudent healthcare provider would not operate on part of a patient's body if the patient told the healthcare provider not to do so.

On appeal, the trial court was found to have erred in directing a verdict in favor of Shreck. The evidence presented established that the standard of care in similar communities requires healthcare providers to obtain informed consent before performing surgery. In this case, the applicable standard of care required Shreck to obtain Walls's express or implied consent to perform surgery on his right eye (*Walls v. Shreck*, 2003).

1. Discuss the conflicting ethical principles in this case.
2. Did the physician's actions in this case involve medical paternalism?

Explain your answer.

Distributive justice is a principle requiring that all persons be treated equally and fairly. No one person, for example, should get a disproportional share of society's resources or benefits. There are many ethical issues involved in the rationing of health care. This is often due to limited or scarce resources, limited access due to geographic remoteness, or a patient's inability to pay for services combined with many physicians who are unwilling to accept patients who are perceived as "no pays" with high risks for legal suits.

Justice and Government Spending

Scarce resources are challenging to the principles of justice. Justice involves equality. Yet equal access to health care, for example, across the United States does not exist. How do you think the government should spend a trillion dollars? With 45 million Americans without healthcare insurance, describe the value of the one-time $300–$600 per household giveback from the United States treasury under the George W. Bush administration. Consider the following questions:

- Should the money have been distributed equally among families?

- Should the money have been distributed equally among all citizens?

- Should the money have been invested and saved for a rainy day?

- Should the money have been used to improve educational programs, build libraries, build state-of-the-art hospitals, or fund after-school programs for disadvantaged youths?
- Should the money have included both savings for that rainy day and funding for the programs described above?
- What would have been the greater good for all?

Injustice for the Insured

Even if you're insured, getting ill could bankrupt you. Hospitals are garnishing wages, putting liens on homes and having patients who can't pay arrested. It's enough to make you sick.

SARA AUSTIN

Hospitals are receiving between 4 million and 60 million dollars annually in charity funds in New York alone according to Elizabeth Benjamin, director of the health law unit of the Legal Aid Society of New York City. However, even the insured face injustice. In 2003, almost 1 million Americans declared bankruptcy because of medical issues, accounting for nearly half of all of the bankruptcies in the country. When an insured patient gets ill and exhausts his or her insurance benefits, should the hospital be able to:

- garnish the patient's wages?
- place liens on homes?
- arrest patients who cannot pay?
- block patients from applying for the hundreds of millions of dollars in government funds designated to help pay for care for those who need it?

Age and Justice

- Should an 89-year-old patient get a heart transplant because he or she is higher on the waiting list to receive a heart transplant than a 10-year-old girl?
- Should a 39-year-old single patient get a heart transplant because he or she is higher on the waiting list to receive a heart transplant than a 10-year-old boy?
- Should a 29-year-old mother of three get a heart transplant because she is higher on the waiting list to receive a heart transplant than a 10-year-old girl?
- Should a 29-year-old pregnant mother with two children get a heart transplant because she is higher on the waiting list to receive a heart transplant than a 10-year-old boy?

Emergency Care

When two patients arrive in the emergency department in critical condition, consider who should get treated first. Should the caregiver base his or her decision on the

- first patient who arrives?
- age of the patients?
- likelihood of survival?
- ability of the patient to pay for services rendered?
- condition of the patient?

Patients are to be treated justly, fairly, and equally. Yet what happens when resources are scarce and only one patient can be treated at a time? What happens if caregivers decide that age should be the determining factor as to who is treated first? One patient is saved and another dies. What happens if the patient saved is terminal and has an advance directive in his wallet requesting no heroic measures to save his life? What are the legal issues intertwined with the ethical issues in this case?

Justice describes how people are treated when their interests compete. Distributive justice implies that all are treated fairly; no one person is to get a disproportional share of society's resources or benefits. This principle raises numerous issues, including how limited resources should be allocated.

When there is a reduction in staff, managers are generally asked to eliminate nonessential personnel. In the healthcare industry this translates to those individuals not directly involved in patient care (e.g., environmental services employees). Is this fair? Is this justice? Is this the right thing to do?

Morality

Aim above morality. Be not simply good; be good for something.

HENRY DAVID THOREAU

Morality implies the quality of being in accord with standards of right and good conduct. Morals are deeply ingrained into a culture or religion and are often part of its identity. Morals are ideas about what is right and what is wrong; as examples, killing is wrong, helping the poor is right, easing pain is right, and causing pain is wrong. Morals should not be confused with cultural habits or customs, such as wearing a certain style of clothing. Morality is a code of conduct. It is a guide to behavior that all rational persons would put forward for governing their behavior.

It is important not only to examine what one considers the right thing to do in a given situation, but why it is the right thing to do. Being morally responsible requires that a person look inward and question his or her own values.

Morality describes a class of rules held by society to govern the conduct of its individual members. A moral dilemma occurs when moral ideas of right and wrong conflict.

Moral judgments are those judgments concerned with what an individual or group believes to be the right or proper behavior in a given situation. It involves assessing another person's moral character based on how he or she conforms to the moral convictions established by the individual and/or group. Lack of conformity typically results in moral censure, condemnation, and possibly derision of the violator's character. What is considered right varies from nation to nation, culture to culture, religion to religion, and person to person. There is no universal morality.

When it is important that disagreements be settled, morality is often legislated. Law is distinguished from morality by having explicit rules and penalties and officials who interpret the laws and apply the penalties. There is often considerable overlap in the conduct governed by morality and that governed by law. Laws are created to set boundaries for societal behavior. They are enforced to ensure that the expected behavior happens (Morality, 2005).

Virtues and Moral Values

The term virtue is normally defined as some sort of moral excellence or beneficial quality. In traditional ethics, virtues are those characteristics that differentiate good people from bad people. Virtues, such as honesty and justice, are abstract moral principles. Properly understood, virtues serve as indispensable guides to our actions. However, they aren't ends in themselves. Virtues are merely abstract means to concrete ends. The ends are values: the things in life that we aim to gain or keep. Most individuals have a tendency to focus on values and not virtues. Simply stated, most individuals find it difficult to make the connection between abstract principles (virtues) and that which has value. The relationship between means and ends, principles (virtues) and practice (values) is often difficult to grasp.

A moral value is the relative worth placed on some virtuous behavior. What has value to one person may not have value to another. A value is a standard of conduct. Values are used for judging the goodness or badness of some action. Ethical values imply standards of worth. They are the standards by which we measure the goodness in our lives. Intrinsic value is something that has value in and of itself. Instrumental value is something that helps to give value to something else (e.g., money is valuable for what it can buy).

Values may change as needs change. If one's basic needs for food, water, clothing, and housing have not been met, one's values may change such that a friendship, for example, might be sacrificed if one's basic needs can be better met as a result of the sacrifice. If a mom's estate is being squandered at the end of her life, a financially well-off family member may want to take more aggressive measures to keep the mom alive despite the financial drain on her estate. Another family member who is struggling financially may more readily see the futility of

expensive medical care and find it easier to let go. Values give purpose to each life. They make up one's moral character.

All people make value judgments and make choices among alternatives. The values one so dearly proclaims may change as needs change. Values are the motivating power of a person's actions and are necessary to survival, both psychologically and physically.

We begin our discussion here with an overview of those virtues commonly accepted as having value when addressing difficult healthcare dilemmas. The reader should not get overly caught up in the philosophical morass of how virtues and values differ, but should be aware that virtues and values have been used by many interchangeably. Whether we call compassion a virtue or a value or both, the importance for our purposes in this text is to understand what compassion is and how it is applied in the healthcare setting.

Commitment

I know the price of success: dedication, hard work, and an unremitting devotion to the things you want to see happen.

FRANK LLOYD WRIGHT

Commitment is the act of binding oneself (intellectually or emotionally) to a course of action. It is an agreement or pledge to do something. It can be ongoing or a pledge to do something in the future.

Compassion

Compassion is the basis of morality.

ARNOLD SCHOPENHAUER

Compassion in the healthcare setting means a deep awareness of and sympathy for another's

---

Who Makes the Rules?

Mr. Jones was trying to get home from a long trip to see his ailing wife, who had been ill for several years, suffering a great deal of pain. His flight was to leave at 7:00 p.m. Upon arrival at the airport in New York at 4:30 p.m., he inquired at the ticket counter, "Is there an earlier flight that I can take to Washington?" The counter agent responded, "There is plenty of room on the 5:00 p.m. flight but you will have to pay a $200 change fee." The passenger inquired, "Could you please waive the change fee? I need to get home to my ailing wife." The ticket agent responded, "Sorry, your ticket does not allow me to make the change."

The passenger made a second attempt at the gate to get on an earlier flight but the manager at the gate was unwilling to authorize the change, saying, "I don't make the rules."

Mr. Jones decided to give it one more try. He called the airline's customer service center. The customer service agent responded to Mr. Jones's plea: "We cannot overrule the agent at the gate. Sorry, you just got the wrong supervisor. He is going by the book."

1. Should rules be broken for a higher good?
2. Who decides?

---

suffering. The ability to show compassion is a true mark of moral character. There are those who argue that compassion will blur one's judgment. Detachment, or lack of concern for the patient's needs, however, is what often translates into mistakes that often result in patient injuries. Caregivers need to show the same compassion for others as they would expect for themselves or their loved ones. Those who have excessive emotional involvement in a patient's care may be best suited to work in those settings where patients are most likely to recover and have good outcomes (e.g., maternity units). As with all things in life, there needs to be a comfortable balance between compassion and detachment.

Never apologize for showing feeling. When you do so, you apologize for the truth.

BENJAMIN DISRAELI

Conscientiousness

A conscientious person is one who has moral integrity and a strict regard for doing what is considered the right thing to do. An individual acts conscientiously if he or she is motivated to do what is right, believing it is the right thing to do. Conscience is a form of self-reflection on and judgment about whether one's actions are right or wrong, good or bad. It is an internal sanction that comes into play through critical reflection. This sanction often appears as a bad conscience in the form of painful feelings of remorse, guilt, shame, disunity, or harmony as the individual recognizes that his or her acts were wrong. Although a person may conscientiously object and/or refuse to participate in some action (e.g., abortion), that person must not obstruct others from performing the same act if the others have no moral objection to it.

Cooperativeness

Cooperativeness is the willingness and ability to work with others. In the healthcare setting, it is important that caregivers work cooperatively as a team.

Courage

Courage is the greatest of all virtues, because if you haven't courage, you may not have an opportunity to use any of the others.

SAMUEL JOHNSON

Courage is the mental or moral strength to persevere and withstand danger. "Courage is the ladder on which all the other virtues mount" (Luce, 1979).

Discernment

Get to know two things about a man—how he earns his money and how he spends it—and you have the clue to his character, for you have a searchlight that shows up the innermost recesses of his soul. You know all you need to know about his standards, his motives, his driving desires, and his real religion.

ROBERT J. MCCRACKEN

The virtue of discernment is the ability to make a good decision without personal biases, fears, and undue influences from others. A person who has discernment has the wisdom to decide the best course of action when there are many possible actions to choose from.

Fairness

Do all the good you can, By all the means you can, In all the ways you can, In all the places you can, At all the times you can, To all the people you can, As long as you ever can.

JOHN WESLEY[2]

In ethics, fairness means being objective, unbiased, dispassionate, impartial, and consistent with the principles of ethics. Fairness is the ability to make judgments free from discrimination, dishonesty, or one's own bias.

Fidelity

Nothing is more noble, nothing more venerable, than fidelity. Faithfulness and truth are the most sacred excellences and endowments of the human mind.

CICERO

Fidelity is the virtue of faithfulness, being true to our commitments and obligations to others. A component of fidelity, veracity, implies that we will be truthful and honest in all our endeavors. It involves being faithful and loyal to obligations, duties, or observances. The opposite of fidelity is infidelity, meaning unfaithfulness.

Freedom

Freedom is the quality of being free to make choices for oneself within the boundaries of law. Freedoms enjoyed by citizens of the United States include the freedom of speech, freedom of religion, freedom from want, and freedom from physical aggression.

Honesty/Trustworthiness/Truth Telling

Lies or the appearance of lies are not what the writers of our Constitution intended for our country—it's not the America we salute every Fourth of July, it's not the America we learned about in school, and it is not the America represented in the flag that rises above our land.

MESSAGE FROM THE INTERNET

The virtue of honesty is possessed by those who do not lie, resulting in their being good. Trust involves confidence that a person will act with the right motives. It is the assured reliance on the character, ability, strength, or truth of someone or something. To tell the truth, to have integrity, and to be honest are most honorable virtues. Veracity is devotion to and conformity with what is truthful. It involves an obligation to be truthful.

Truth-telling involves providing enough information so that a patient can make an informed decision about his or her health care. Intentionally misleading a patient to believe something that the caregiver knows to be untrue may give the patient false hopes. There is always apprehension when one must share bad news; the temptation is to gloss over the truth for fear of being the bearer of bad news. To lessen the pain and the hurt is only human. But in the end, truth must win over fear.

At the end of our days, the most basic principles of life, trust and survival, are on trial.

AUTHOR UNKNOWN

Healthcare Morass

The declining trust in the nation's ability to deliver quality health care is evidenced by a system caught up in the morass of managed care companies, which have in some instances inappropriately devised ways to deny healthcare benefits to their constituency. In addition, the continuing reporting of numerous medical errors serves only to escalate distrust in the nation's political leadership and the providers of health care.

Physicians find themselves vulnerable to lawsuits, often because of misdiagnosis. As a result, patients are passed from specialist to specialist in an effort to leave no stone unturned. Fearful to step outside the boundaries of their own specialties, physicians escalate the problem by ineffectively communicating with the primary care physician responsible for managing the patient's overall healthcare needs. This can also be problematic if no one physician has taken overall responsibility to coordinate and manage a patient's care.

Politics and Discerning Truth

Truthfulness is just one measure of one's moral character. Unfortunately, politicians don't always set good examples for the people they serve. The following are but a few examples of how political decisions have caused, or have given the appearance of causing, division to the detriment of unity. Discuss the following political decisions and how they have helped to divide the nation by political party.

1964: GULF OF TONKIN

Did President Johnson order U.S. bombers to retaliate for a North Vietnamese torpedo attack that never happened (Cohen & Solomon, 1994)?

2003: PERSIAN GULF WAR

Did President George W. Bush have legitimate reasons to believe that Saddam Hussein had weapons of mass destruction? If so, was there a real threat that he would use them against the United States?

2004: PRESCRIPTION DRUGS

Senior citizens who did not have prescription drug coverage through Medicare, found that needed medications were unaffordable. Has this issue been honestly and effectively addressed by our government, or must many of the nation's aging population substitute drugs for food?

Hopefulness

Hope is the last thing that dies in man; and though it be exceedingly deceitful, yet it is of this good use to us, that while we are traveling through life, it conducts us in an easier and more pleasant way to our journey's end.

FRANÇOIS DE LA ROCHEFOUCAULD

Hopefulness in the patient care setting involves looking forward to something with the confidence of success. Caregivers have a responsibility to balance truthfulness while promoting hope. The caregiver must be sensitive to each patient's needs and provide hope.

Integrity

Integrity involves a steadfast adherence to a strict moral or ethical code and a commitment to not compromise this code. A person with integrity has a staunch belief in and faithfulness to, for example, his or her religious beliefs, values, and moral character. Patients and professionals alike often make healthcare decisions based on their integrity and their strict moral beliefs. For example, a Jehovah's Witness will refuse a blood transfusion because it is against his or her religious beliefs, even if such refusal may result in death. A provider of health care may refuse to participate in an abortion because it is against his or her moral beliefs. A person without personal integrity lacks sincerity and moral conviction, and may fail to act on professed moral beliefs.

Preservation of Life

Medical ethics do not require that a patient's life be preserved at all costs and in all circumstances. The ethical integrity of the profession is not threatened by allowing competent patients to decide for themselves whether a particular medical treatment is in their best interests. If the doctrines of informed consent and right of privacy have as their foundations the right to bodily integrity and control of one's own fate, then those rights are superior to the institutional considerations of hospitals and their medical staffs. A state's interest in maintaining the ethical integrity of a profession does not outweigh, for example, a patient's right to refuse blood transfusions.

Kindness

When you carry out acts of kindness, you get a wonderful feeling inside. It is as though something inside your body responds and says, yes, this is how I ought to feel.

HAROLD KUSHNER

Kindness involves the quality of being considerate and sympathetic to another's needs.

Respect

Respect for ourselves guides our morals; respect for others guides our manners.

LAURENCE STERNE

To give and show respect is to show special regard to someone or something. Caregivers who demonstrate respect for their patients will be more effective in helping them cope with the anxiety of their illness. Respect helps to develop trust between the patient and caregiver, and improve healing processes. If caregivers respect the family of a patient, cooperation and understanding will be the positive result, encouraging a team effort to improve patient care.

Situational Ethics

A person's moral values and moral character can be compromised when faced with difficult choices. Why do good people behave differently in different situations? Why do good people sometimes do bad things? The answer is fairly simple: One's moral character can sometimes change as circumstances change; thus the term situational ethics.

> Situational ethics refers to a particular view of ethics, in which absolute standards are considered less important than the requirements of a particular situation. The standards used may, therefore, vary from one situation to another, and may even contradict one another (Situational ethics, n.d.).

For example, a decision not to use extraordinary means to sustain the life of an unknown 84-year-old may result in a different decision than it would if the 84-year-old is one's mother. To better understand this concept, consider the desire to live, and the extreme measures one will take in order to do so. Remember that ethical decision making is the process of determining the right thing to do in the event of a moral dilemma. For example, those who survived the crash of a Fairchild FH-227 twin turboprop airplane on Friday, October 13, 1972, were faced with some difficult survival decisions. The plane, which was crossing the Andes Mountains carrying 40 passengers and 5 crew, disappeared from the modern world, and everyone on board was thought to be dead. However, 72 days later, 16 emerged alive and told their story ("Alive," 2001). They chose to live by feeding off of those who did not live. This is a gruesome picture indeed, but it illustrates to what lengths one may go in certain situations (situational ethics) in order to survive.

Here are some situational issues to think about:

1. Describe how what you believe to be the right thing to do might change as circumstances change.
2. Describe how your consultative advice might change based on a patient's needs, beliefs, and family influences.

The Final Analysis

People are often unreasonable, illogical and self-centered;
> *Forgive them anyway.*

If you are kind, people may accuse you of selfish, ulterior motives.
> *Be kind anyway.*

If you are successful, you will win some false friends and some true enemies;
> *Succeed anyway.*

What you spend years building, someone may destroy overnight;
> *Build anyway.*

The good you do today, people will often forget tomorrow;
> *Do good anyway.*

Give the world the best you have, and it may never be enough;
> *Give the world the best you have anyway.*

You see, in the final analysis, it is between you and God;
> *It was never between you and them anyway.*

AUTHOR UNKNOWN

Summary Case: Honesty

Annie, a 23-year-old woman with two children, began experiencing severe pain in her abdomen while visiting her family in May 2002. After complaining of pain to Mark, her husband, in June 2002, he scheduled an appointment with Dr. Roberts, a gastroenterologist, who ordered a series of tests. While conducting a barium scan, a radiologist at Community Hospital noted a small bowel obstruction. Dr. Roberts recommended surgery, and Annie agreed.

Following surgery on July 7, Dr. Brown, the operating surgeon, paged Mark over the hospital intercom as he walked down a corridor on the ground floor. Mark, hearing the page, picked up a house phone and dialed zero for an operator. The operator inquired, "May I help you?"

"Yes," Mark replied. "I was just paged."

"Oh, yes. Dr. Brown would like to talk to you. I will connect you with him. Hang on. Don't hang up," the operator instructed.

Mark's heart began to pound.

"Mark?" Dr. Brown asked.

"Yes."

"Well, surgery is over," Dr. Brown informed him. "Your wife is recovering nicely in the recovery room."

Mark was relieved, but for a moment. "That's good," he said.

Dr. Brown continued, "I am sorry to say that she has carcinoma of the colon."

Mark replied, "Did you get it all?"

"I am sorry, but the cancer has spread to her lymph nodes and surrounding organs," the doctor said.

Mark asked, "Can I see her?"

Dr. Brown replied, "She is in the recovery room but I am sure it will be okay to see her."

Before hanging up, Mark told Dr. Brown, "Please do not tell Annie that she has cancer. I want her to always have hope."

Dr. Brown agreed, "Don't worry, I won't tell her. You can tell her that she had a narrowing of the colon."

Mark hung up the phone and proceeded to the recovery room. Upon entering the recovery room, he spotted his wife. His heart sank into his stomach. Tubes seemed to be running out of every part of her body. He walked to her bedside. His immediate concern was to see her wake up and have the tubes pulled out so that he could take her home.

Later, in a hospital room, Annie asked Mark, "What did the doctor find?"

Mark replied, "He found a narrowing of the colon."

Annie asked, "Am I going to be okay?"

(continues)

Summary Case: Honesty (continued)

"Yes, but it will take a while to recover," Mark replied.

"Oh, that's good. I was so worried," said Annie. "You go home and get some rest."

"I'll see you in the morning," he said as he left.

Mark left the hospital and went to see his friends, Jerry and Helen, who had invited him for dinner. As Mark pulled up to Jerry and Helen's home, he got out of his car and just stood there looking up a long stairway leading to Jerry and Helen's home. They were standing there looking down at Mark. It was early evening, the sun was setting, a warm breeze was blowing, and Helen's eyes were watering. But for a few moments, it seemed like a lifetime. Mark discovered a new emotion as he stood there speechless. He knew then that he was losing a part of himself. Things would never be the same.

Annie had one more surgery 2 months later in a futile attempt to extend her life.

By November 2002, Annie was admitted to the hospital for the last time. Annie was so ill that even during her last moments she was unaware that she was dying. Dr. Brown entered the room and asked Mark, "Can I see you for a few moments?"

"Yes," Mark replied. He followed Dr. Brown into the hallway.

"Mark, I can keep Annie alive for a few more days or we can let her go."

Mark, not responding, went back into the room. He was now alone with Annie. Shortly thereafter a nurse walked into the room and gave Annie an injection. Mark asked, "What did you give her?"

The nurse replied, "Something to make her more comfortable."

Annie had been asleep; she awoke, looked at Mark, and said, "Could you please cancel my appointment at the university? I will have to reschedule my appointment. I don't think I will be well enough to go tomorrow."

Mark replied, "Okay, try to get some rest."

Annie closed her eyes, never to open them again.

Ethical and Legal Issues

1. Do you agree with Mark's decision not to tell Annie about the seriousness of her illness? Explain your answer.

2. Should the physician have spoken to Annie as to the seriousness of her illness? Explain your answer.

3. Describe the ethical dilemmas in this case (e.g., how Annie's rights were violated). Place yourself in Annie's shoes, the physician's shoes, and Mark's shoes, and then discuss how the lives of each may have been different if the physician had informed Annie as to the seriousness of her illness.

4. In the final analysis, is it possible to say who is right?

Discussion Questions

1. Discuss the questions posed throughout this chapter.
2. What common ethical dilemmas do you foresee facing in your new role as an advanced practice nurse?
3. What ethical theories and principles reviewed in this chapter apply to recent or current ethical issues you have faced in your practice?
4. Apply the ethical decision-making process to these issues.
5. How can the principle of justice raise ethical dilemmas?
6. How can the meaning of virtues and personal values and beliefs influence advanced practice?
7. Identify a situation in which a personal conflict of interest may arise and propose a resolution or actions to resolve the conflict.
8. Investigate the ethics committee in your organization and review its purpose, membership, and recent issues discussed in the committee. Attend a meeting and report to your classmates.
9. Discuss the ethical dilemmas involved in the allocation of scarce resources. How would the ethical principles, virtues, and values discussed in this chapter affect how you would allocate scarce resources? How might resolving this issue cause conflict between your personal values and beliefs and organization perspective?

Notes

1. American essayist.

2. Evangelist and founder of Methodism (1703–1791).

References

The Kennedy Institute of Ethics at Georgetown University. (2007, August). *The Kennedy Institute of Ethics*. Retrieved November 2, 2007, from http://kennedyinstitute.georgetown.edu/index.htm

Alive: The Andes Survivors. (2001). Retrieved November 2, 2007, from http://members.aol.com/porkinsr6/alive.html

Belmont Report. (2004, October). *Presentation for IRB Members*. Retrieved November 9, 2007, from www.rgs.uci.edu/ora/rp/hrpp/BelmontReport.ppt

Canterbury v. Spence, 464 F.2d 772 (D.C. Cir. 1972).

Cohen, J., & Solomon, N. (1994). *30-year anniversary: Tonkin Gulf lie launched Vietnam war.* Retrieved

November 2, 2007, from http://www.fair.org/
media-beat/940727.html

Eastern Michigan University. (n.d.). *Protection and use of human
subjects in research.* Retrieved November 2, 2007, from
http://www.rcr.emich.edu/module1/a_7part1.html

Harvard Ad Hoc Committee on Brain Death. (1968).
Brain death. Retrieved November 2, 2007, from
http://www.ascensionhealth.org/ethics/public/
issues/harvard.asp

In re Conroy, 464 A.2d 303, 314 (N.J. Super. Ct. App.
Div., 1983).

In the Matter of Karen Ann Quinlan, 70 N.J. 10 (1976).

Intute: Health and Life Sciences. Retrieved from
http://bioresearch.ac.uk/browse/mesh/C0020125L
0020125.html

Luce, C. B. (1979). *Reader's Digest.*

Morality. (2005). In *Stanford encyclopedia of philosophy.*
Retrieved November 2, 2007, from http://
plato.stanford.edu/entries/morality-definition/

National Human Genome Research Institute. (2007).
The large-scale genome sequencing program: History.
Retrieved December 10, 2007, from http://www.
genome.gov/25521731

National Institutes of Health. (1979, April). *The Belmont
Report: Ethical principles and guidelines for the protection of human subjects of research.* Retrieved
November 9, 2007, from http://ohsr.od.nih.gov/
guidelines/belmont.html

Patient Self-Determination Act of 1990, 42 U.S.C.
1395cc(a)(1).

President's Council on Bioethics. (n.d.). Retrieved
November 2, 2007, from http://www.bioethics.gov/
reports/past_commissions/index.html

Schloendorff v. Society of New York Hospital, 105 N.E.
92, 93 (N.Y. 1914).

Schweitzer, A. (1949). *Civilization and ethics.* New York:
Macmillan.

*A science odyssey—People and discoveries: First kidney trans-
plant performed.* (1998). Retrieved November 2,
2007, from http://www.pbs.org/wgbh/aso/
databank/entries/dm54ki.html

Situational ethics. (n.d.). *Wikipedia.* Retrieved November
2, 2007, from http://en.wikipedia.org/wiki/
Situational_ethics

Union Pacific Ry. Co. v. Botsford; 141 U.S. 250, 251
(1891).

United States Code, Title 42—The Public Health and
Welfare, Chapter 6A—Public Health Service,
Subchapter XVI—President's Commission for the
Study of Ethical Problems in Medicine and
Biomedical and Behavior Research, Section 300v-1.
Retrieved November 2, 2007, from http://
caselaw.lp.findlaw.com/casecode/uscodes/42/
chapters/6a/subchapters/xvi/sections/section_
300v-1.html

Walls v. Shreck, 658 N.W.2d 686 (2003).

Chapter 28

The Role of Codes of Ethics in Nursing's Disciplinary Knowledge

John G. Twomey

CHAPTER OBJECTIVES

1. Trace the historical developments of the code of ethics for nursing.
2. Apply ethical theories specific to health care to the role of the advanced practice nurse.

Introduction

Since the inception of modern nursing in the 19th century, considerable thought has been paid to the moral nature of the discipline. A cursory review of the writings of early leaders such as Nightingale highlights efforts to increase the numbers of qualified applicants into nursing. Although the call for "sober, honest, truthful, trustworthy applicants" (Dossey, 2000, p. 222) was based on an emotional desire to keep the ranks of the developing discipline free from scandal, it is now more accurate to describe the ethical core of nursing as being part of its intellectual heritage.

To fully appreciate the role of moral and ethical knowledge in nursing, it is necessary to examine the evolving development of ethics within the greater domain of disciplinary nursing knowledge. This examination requires a familiarity of how a distinct nursing ethic has emerged within the greater umbrella of bioethics. This historical occurrence cannot be fully comprehended without an appreciation of how the intellectual leaders of the discipline centered this development around an informal code of ethics for the profession that eventually became formalized into the current *Code of Ethics for Nurses* (American Nurses Association, 2001). Additionally, an ongoing issue within this profession of multiple subspecialty practices is whether a single code of ethics can serve a group of professionals with multiple interests and obligations that can pose intriguing individual moral challenges.

Views of Ethics for Nursing

Founders' Views

Florence Nightingale, the intellectual matriarch of modern nursing, set strict standards of behavior for the women she recruited to her radical model of care. Her then-modern concept of nursing went beyond the traditional view of nursing that was inured with the notion that personal care was limited to the intimate. Generally, such care was delivered by the family or by those in society, usually women, who were forced to provide such intimate care for pay. These circumstances often were shameful for both caregiver and patient, for it meant that either had to leave the familiar bosom of the family and seek or provide services, through pecuniary means, that should have been given, not paid for (Rothman, 1990). Not surprisingly, premodern nursing, for pay, was considered in many societies to be on par with prostitution.

Nightingale's efforts often have been portrayed as persuading society, as well as the group of women recruited to her cause, to accept a notion of women who shared a devotion of intimate caring that divorced the emotion of caring from the physical. Nightingale's best-known works emphasize her drive to merge her strong belief in the emergent 19th century principles of public health and the scientific basis that such health was founded on with an interesting insistence on behavior that married military discipline with a fervor such as one could find in contemporary religious orders (Church, 1990).

It is not surprising that most accounts of Nightingale's views on moral behavior centered on her beliefs that nurses' personal behaviors were the most important part of the ethical role. Therefore, dress, decorum, and devotion were considered within the auspices of virtue and came to be how the public perceived how a professional nurse should be judged. But recent examination of Nightingale's correspondence suggests that she struggled to reconcile her public and private personas. Nightingale's much-touted public persona as a woman who sought to consolidate nursing's position through connections with powerful men has come into question. Widerquist (1990) has challenged F. B. Smith's widely accepted characterization of Nightingale's relationships as only being based on a need for power, stating, ". . . they [her relationships] resulted not in a need for power, but from her idealized need for perfection and mutuality, i.e., sympathy, a quality of fellow feeling, with others before she was able to sustain a relationship" (p. 303). This interpretation may provide some evidence that although Nightingale seemed to prefer attention to rule in her nurses, she also viewed the perfect world as one based on virtues that included a spirituality that was embedded in an ethic of nursing care.

Nightingale's views almost completely dominated the vision of professional nursing that immigrated to the United States and elsewhere. Not until well into the 20th century did nursing practice based on her methods go much beyond education and practical nursing interventions. Subsequent American nursing leaders worked with little success to move nursing into modern professional reforms, such as control of entry into practice and nursing knowledge development, during the early genesis of nursing. However, they did confront the need to go beyond the concepts of duty and service as the core values of nursing. Early prominent American nurses such as Lavinia Dock and

Annie Goodrich wrote persuasively of the need for nurses to go beyond etiquette in their practice. They called for nurses to recognize that the intimate nature of their practice was a basic ethical concept, and therefore a core value that necessitated more than superficial physical care (Hamilton, 1994). Hamilton argues that these beliefs ultimately were transformed into the concepts of compassion and caring. However, before they could become the core values of modern nursing, they needed to be separated from their original interpretations of being religious values. The development of ethical knowledge in nursing continually focused on virtues as well as principles. As will be discussed, the evolution of the current *Code of Ethics* for Nurses is a reflection of this intellectual tradition.

Views on Codes of Ethics

Early nursing leaders did not believe that ethical codes were necessary for the emerging profession. As has been noted, this was not from lack of interest in nurses' behaviors. In fact, leaders' attention focused heavily on nurses' behaviors, but their dictums to both their students and nurses under their direction focused on proper behavior when providing care, not of care directed by ethics. During much of the 20th century, the result was that nursing practice was rule bound in both scientific principles and professional behaviors. This devotion to policy was less the result of proven data, but rather emerged from the inability of nursing to successfully ingrain itself in the developing healthcare system with its members as leaders rather than servants (Ashley, 1976).

Codes of ethics were not a primary part of the emergent health professions in the 19th century. The Hippocratic oath offered a list of behaviors for healers. Historically, its use was limited to those who had knowledge of foreign languages and access to books. The Nightingale pledge (n.d.) offered a similar listing of virtuous behaviors. Some of these behaviors appeared in future nursing codes. Nightingale had no hand in writing the Nightingale pledge, and she herself was famously opposed to external vehicles for guiding nursing behavior, such as licensure by government agencies. Finally, the lack of ethical codes for health professions during the 19th century reflected the absence of formal collective organizations. As professional organizations gained in size and power, their role in the development of ethical codes also increased.

Early American nursing leaders did address the issue of ethical codes, but found the argument for them to be unconvincing. Lavinia Dock and Annie Goodrich argued that ethical behavior was an essence of nursing and could be found within its practice of compassion and human interaction, not slavish devotion to rules. It is not surprising that Dock, with her experience at the Henry Street Settlement House, viewed nursing as a vibrant force that was attributable to the individual care that each nurse gave to her patients (Hamilton, 1994). Goodrich also rejected a code of ethics on the grounds that it took nurses away from compassion as a means and instead directed their efforts toward etiquette (Goodrich, 1932). Presumably, Goodrich did not agree with the code of ethics espoused by Isabel Hampton Robb (1900), as it was clearly a creed of etiquette.

A Code of Ethics for Nursing

Ethical codes reflect a range of ethical theories and guidelines. Given the versions that have been presented to nurses, it is useful to consider how those who would use them should interpret the contents of such codes. Ethical guidelines are derived from bioethics. Bioethics draw on the knowledge and processes of ethics to examine health care; as such they apply to the moral behavior of any person performing actions because he or she has chosen to be a healthcare professional. It may or may not involve patients directly. Nursing ethics and medical ethics are subsets of bioethics that apply to those in the specific professions. All bioethical codes share many similar concepts.

Metaethics—Where Theories Live

The term *metaethics* refers to ethical theories that are applicable to bioethics. Two familiar broad ethical theories that most nurses recognize include deontology and utilitarianism (Beauchamp & Childress, 2001). Deontology grounds the ethical value of one's actions on the value of the act itself. If an act, like truth telling, is good as a goal itself, then not adhering to that good is unethical. Therefore, telling a lie is unethical, even if it might ultimately provide a result that most reasonable people would define as good. Utilitarianism states that an act should be judged on how much good it produces. Contrast this view using the prior example.

A number of theories derive some of their base concepts from deontology and utilitarianism. These theories also fit under the metaethical framework. The most commonly recognized theory of bioethics is principled theory. Common concepts or principles such as patient autonomy, risk of harm, or provision of benefits have their base in principled theory. For example, the principle of autonomy has its theoretical underpinning in deontological thought. This thinking holds that a primary good is the

respect for personhood, therefore all patients are given respect by allowing them to make fully informed decisions about their care. Principled theory is employed when those people making bioethical decisions weigh the varied principles to assess which principle is most applicable in a particular situation. This theory, though not perfect in its ability to answer all bioethical questions, became the most applied bioethical theory in Western medical culture in the later half of the 20th century and continues to be an important part of contemporary bioethical discourse (Evans, 2000).

Recently, other theories have ascended in their contributions to ethical discussions, particularly in nursing ethics. Communitarianism is a framework of ethical thought that changes the locus of moral deliberation from the individual (as in the previously discussed theories) to the group within which the decision will be made. Therefore, the patient is recast from being an autonomous individual who is an isolated decision maker to one whose existence is made meaningful by being a member of a group. According to this theory, input from group members in decision making is just as important as that from the individual patient, because group members will be affected by the decision (Beauchamp & Childress, 2001).

Caring, or contextual, ethics provides a framework of ethical thought that grants insights into moral decision making that is appealing to many nurses. According to the theory of caring ethics, bioethical decisions are viewed through the prism of the relationship between the caregiver and the care recipient. Decisions are looked on as a means of maintaining the interdependent bond that a provider has with the patient (Noddings, 2003). Whereas principled theories tend to emphasize patient rights, caring and communitarian theories see the individual as existing more within a nurturing role. This caring relationship places the provider on equal footing with the patient in the decision-making process.

The metaethical level of theories provides the basic reference point for any ethical consideration. It is important to recognize that this level is often unspoken when people put forward their beliefs in a moral discussion. When someone states, "I feel that we should do this because ..." he or she is saying, "I believe this is an underlying core consideration." The core often lies within a broad theory. Such beliefs can also derive from other theoretical beliefs, such as religious theories on behavior, that often share the same values, such as the importance of providing justice to people.

For metaethical theories to be relevant to practice, their concepts need to be narrowed so that they can be applied to specific situations. The process of bringing theory to practice begins at the next level of analysis: descriptive ethics.

Descriptive Ethics— Where Codes Live

The descriptive level of ethical analysis is best understood as being juxtaposed between the metaethical (theory) level and the level below it, which is referred to as normative ethics, which can be likened to specific rules. Descriptive ethics provides broad descriptions of moral behaviors that are recognizable as coming from the theoretical frameworks already discussed. However, the guidelines that come from this level often have wide latitude and can be interpreted differently by the varied decision makers who use them, particularly when those decision makers approach the frameworks from different perspectives. For instance, both the nursing and medical codes of ethics have proscriptions from abandoning patients that are interpreted differently. Physicians, who have a legacy of operating their practices as businesses, are expected to continue to care for patients under many circumstances, but are allowed to refuse to care for patients who cannot pay them. By contrast, nurses, who come from a legacy of accepting patients who are assigned to them by their employers, have an ethic that only allows them to leave the care of a patient when another nurse will substitute and provide the needed care.

Descriptive ethics interpret the broad theories into understandable language so that the professions can adapt them to their professional needs. Therefore, the principle of justice, which states that people should be given what they deserve, is represented in the first provision of the *Code of Ethics for Nurses* (ANA, 2001), which states that nursing care is delivered without regard to economic status. Obviously, this statement is open to many interpretations, and how any individual nurse will abide by it depends on the specific professional situation. Indeed, this phrase within the first provision is not elaborated on further by the accompanying interpretive statement, whereas other pieces of the provision are interpreted in detail.

Descriptive ethical statements are heard widely when one is in professional training through formal and informal means of acculturation. New nurses are socialized through the use of such phrases as "to preserve confidentiality," "not to harm patients," "to make sure patients make informed decisions," and other slogans. When examined, such broad sayings provide little direction for the professional, for they are generally presented without context.

In the reality of everyday practice, nurses and other healthcare professionals do share information without patients' permission, sometimes do inflict some harm when doing painful procedures, and may purposely allow patients to make decisions that are not fully informed because they agree with the patients' decisions.

However, descriptive ethics are important for several reasons. They provide the professions with valuable weapons in their efforts to win the public's trust and to legitimate the professions as forces in a society's health. The use of descriptive ethics helps the professions to maintain a dynamic legacy of continuous ethical thought by leaving open the predominant theories to interpretation in ways that the professions want their members to present themselves. For example, the 2001 ANA code contains phrases that can be traced back to the original code ratified by the membership over a half century ago. The current code uses ethical referents that are well recognized by society and its members to draw attention to the newer, more modern and relevant interpretations that the profession needs in the 21st century (Daly, 1999).

Ethical codes also straddle the third level of ethical analysis—normative ethics. It is important to understand how such movement across the levels of analysis works to provide flexibility for professions as they address issues in their practice.

Normative Ethics— Where Codes Are Interpreted

Normative rules dominate our private and professional lives. They are seen in many forms, from civil regulations, such as traffic laws, to rules and regulations within our work settings. Normative rules can take the form of policies that govern professional practice, such as specifying which professionals can prepare drug preparations and which ones can administer them. Professional standards of care also can be stated in normative fashion, for example, as evidenced by clinical pathways that dictate specific action given a patient scenario.

It is not difficult to recognize the form that normative ethics takes within the healthcare setting. Specific rules that limit accessibility to patient records, policies that define how much free care will be given to indigent clients, and other written guidelines exemplify normative ethics and display how broader forms of ethics are grounded in practice. Generally, clinicians are comfortable with normative ethical rules because they are easy to understand and can be amended when it appears that contemporary patient care dictates such changes. Consider informed consent policies in today's hospitals that dictate many more points within a stay where patients are asked to give permission for different procedures. The underlying concept of autonomy has a much stricter interpretation today than a generation ago when patients rarely were approached to give consent after signing a general consent form at the admitting office.

Ethical codes are not generally written at the normative level, but because members of professions seek specific guidelines, many professions provide interpretations of the descriptive ethics that codes reflect. As illustrated later in the chapter, the ANA code provides a clear example of how a profession uses its professional code and adjunct policy statements to meet the needs of its members.

The Role of Codes

The existence of ethical codes for healthcare professionals is a relatively unquestioned phenomenon in current society. A listing on the Illinois Institute of Technology Web site (http://ethics.iit.edu/codes/health.html) contains dozens of links, some of them going to the base moral code of a given profession or professional sub-group, and others providing interpretations of the individual code. However, one simply cannot accept the premise that such codes exist because each health profession has such distinct ethical positions that they need to articulate them. Instead, codes must be seen as a vehicle for the legitimacy of a health profession itself.

Any group that claims to be a profession will exhibit a number of characteristics. The most common ones are claims to (1) a distinct body of knowledge, (2) control over the entry of members into the profession, and (3) a legitimacy and accountability of the professional group as it serves the needs of the society within which it exists. The latter is represented by the profession having leaders whose main responsibility is to help create an environment in which the profession can: (1) educate its members, (2) create knowledge through research that the profession can claim and pass on to its practicing members, and (3) participate in the policy process that society uses to negotiate relationships with the professions.

The means by which a profession accomplishes these tasks is through a leadership group. The collective action and influence of professional organizations are essential to the survival and advancement of a profession. Membership in a professional organization may be voluntary or mandatory. Whether or not a majority of the members have an active bond with the leadership organization, most professional organizations share the following features:

- Support through membership dues
- Some form of acceptance by government

authorities as being a legitimate voice for its members
- A relationship with the institutions that prepare and employ its members
- A governance model that allows participation by its members in its decision process
- A permanent staff that conducts the daily business of the profession

The professional group has many challenges when trying to maintain the profession's recognized legitimacy, and an ethical code is often one of the tools it employs. Whereas one might assume that a code is simply the list of directions for a given professional, examination of any professional code provides evidence that part of being a professional in that given field is to accept the values that the group espouses. For example, the third provision of the current ANA code states, "The nurse promotes, advocates for, and strives to protect the health, safety, and rights of the patient." The main goal of this statement is to focus the reader on the object of the sentence, the patient. When this statement was written, the goal of the authors, which was accepted by the professional group, was to underscore that the nursing profession was primarily responsible to its patients, not employers nor third-party payers. In a time of complex professional relationships, the one person a patient can rely on is the (registered) nurse. This is a value that the profession wants the public to see that it strongly embraces.

Thus, it is essential to recognize that the code of nursing ethics is commissioned, accepted, and owned by the professional group. It reflects not just moral values, but also the ethical face that the professional wants to present to current society.

The ANA Code of Ethics

The current code of ethics for nursing was published in 2001. The development of this version of the code began at least 6 years earlier (Daly, 1999). The code's roots are embedded in a half century of efforts at promulgating an ethical code. Early leaders of American nursing debated the need for a code of ethics for nurses, and early versions of nursing codes of ethics were proposed but not accepted (Fowler, 1999). In 1950, a formal code for nurses was accepted by the ANA (Fowler, 1992). During the next quarter century, this code was modified several times. For example, the ideas of etiquette and loyalty evolved over time into more professional concepts of professional autonomy and accountability (Scanlon & Glover, 1995). The code was again revised in 1969, and minor revisions occurred in 1976 and 1985 (Daly, 1999).

In 1995, the ANA called together a group of prominent nurse ethicists and asked them whether the 1985 version of the code needed further revision. When they replied affirmatively, the association appointed a task force of practicing and academic nurses to do a total revision of the code (Daly, 1999). The group convened in 1997, and by the time the task force was done and the current code was accepted by the house of delegates of the ANA in 2001, the code had a new title and the 11 provisions of the 1985 code had been reduced to 9. The preface and the interpretive statements had all been rewritten, and an afterword was added. The task force not only debated and rewrote multiple iterations of the new code, but at every stage input was sought from interested parties, such as the state associations that make up the federal structure of the ANA, prominent nurse leaders in nursing education and practice,

as well as subspecialty nursing organizations outside the ANA.

At one point, the adoption of the new code was held up by debate and politics within the organization's house of delegates. A temporary roadblock was generated by a deep schism between the state groups that formed this governance group over issues that the new code addressed, particularly the role of the nurse in collective actions within employment settings. This dispute caused the code to be sent back to the task force for further revision. As evidenced by this example, codes of ethics reflect more than the moral beliefs of the profession; they also are seen as powerful vehicles for professing the values of the profession—which are not always unanimous amongst the members of a given group.

Reading the Code

When anyone, nurse or layperson, reads the ANA code, it is necessary to remember that it is a descriptive ethical document. This code is not unlike many other professional codes in that it attempts to voice the ethics and values of the profession. All professions have to go beyond the descriptive nature of their codes. These groups get to the normative level whereby their audiences can more easily understand the practicality of their code's messages in several different ways.

The ANA has long chosen to portray its ethical assertions through a three-level mechanism. The first level is the code, with its nine provisions (see Figure 28–1). If one retrieves the code online or acquires a copy of the ANA code booklet, then one immediately has access to the accompanying interpretive statements, which offer more specific information to help to bridge the gap to the normative level. Provision 3, mentioned earlier, has six interpretive statements

Figure 28–1 ANA Code of Ethics

The ANA house of delegates approved these nine provisions of the new *Code of Ethics for Nurses* at its June 30, 2001 meeting in Washington, D.C. In July, 2001 the Congress of Nursing Practice and Economics voted to accepted the new language of the interpretive statements resulting in a fully approved revised *Code of Ethics for Nurses with Interpretive Statements*.

1. The nurse, in all professional relationships, practices with compassion and respect for the inherent dignity, worth and uniqueness of every individual, uniqueness of every individual, unrestricted by considerations of social or economic status, personal attributes, or the nature of health problems.

2. The nurse's primary commitment is to the patient, whether an individual, family, group, or community.

3. The nurse promotes, advocates for, and strives to protect the health, safety, and rights of the patient.

4. The nurse is responsible and accountable for individual nursing practice and determines the appropriate delegation of tasks consistent with the nurse's obligation to provide optimum patient care.

5. The nurse owes the same duties to self as to others, including the responsibility to preserve integrity and safety, to maintain competence, and to continue personal and professional growth.

6. The nurse participates in establishing, maintaining, and improving healthcare environments and conditions of employment conducive to the provision of quality health care and consistent with the values of the profession through individual and collective action.

7. The nurse participates in the advancement of the profession through contributions to practice, education, administration, and knowledge development.

8. The nurse collaborates with other health professionals and the public in promoting community, national, and international efforts to meet health needs.

9. The profession of nursing, as represented by associations and their members, is responsible for articulating nursing values, for maintaining the integrity of the profession and its practice, and for shaping social policy.

Source: Reprinted with permission from American Nurses Association. *Code of Ethics for Nurses with Interpretive Statements*. © 2001 nursebooks.org, American Nurses Association, Silver Spring, MD.

that begin to detail that the services that nurses provide to their patients include protection of sensitive information (3.1, 3.2) and extend to safeguarding the patient from impaired colleagues (3.6). If one reads any of those interpretive statements, it is clear that they are more specific than the parent provision, but that there is still a lot of latitude and room for interpretation within them.

The ANA also has a third category of statements, which are very normative, called position statements. These statements are policy statements that the organization promotes in several clinical and policy areas, including the areas of ethics and human rights. For example, the position statement on assisted suicide (http://www.nursingworld.org/readroom/position/ethics/etsuic.htm) begins with a strong declaration that nurses should not participate in acts aimed at helping patients end their lives prematurely through any means. However, another position statement on pain relief (http://www.nursingworld.org/readroom/position/ethics/etpain.htm) provides support for nurses to titrate narcotic pain relief to levels that might be lethal if the express goal of the act is to relieve pain, not cause death. The message is that individual nurses will never be able to ask their professional organization to completely answer all ethical questions. What will be found within the code, the interpretive statements, and the position statements are mixes of ethical theory, professional values, and discussions of the competing issues within a given topic so that nurses can apply this guidance to their specific context.

As previously stated, the 2001 code consists of nine provisions. The first three provisions describe the central nursing ethic as being that of the individual nurse providing care to patients. The first provision centers on social justice; the nurse is linked with providing care in an indiscriminate fashion, no matter the economic, racial, social, or value system of the patient he or she encounters. The second provision defines fidelity as a significant value of nursing, but it makes clear in no uncertain terms that the relationship most important to nurses is that with patients. The third provision focuses on the ethical duties of the nurse and specifies that protection of the patient is a major part of nursing. To fully understand these provisions, one must go to the individual interpretive statements. But if one stops momentarily to look closely at these introductory provisions, evident in these three statements of just 75 words, the professional organization puts forth a clear and cogent statement of philosophy. Nurses act without reflecting on the nature of

their patient, they protect the patient, and, most importantly, they center their actions around a relational ethic that harkens back to the original nursing value of caring, which does not reduce the patient to just a body with an illness, but views the patient as a holistic being with complex needs that nurses can address (Bishop & Scudder, 1990).

The first three provisions also perform another task for the nursing profession. The 2001 code is another step in the development of nursing's value system, particularly its beliefs about its own moral self. Earlier codes, formal and informal, moved from etiquette to duty. The emphases of such duties often were toward supposed colleagues, particularly physicians, who were actually superiors, if not employers. As social values changed, nursing's attention turned to values such as racial justice, and it shifted its loyalties in directions that allowed its members to focus on the objects of their care, the patient. The value of duty evolved into the concept of advocacy for the patient. But as bioethical views of the nurse–patient relationship moved away from the paternalism of the past, advocacy had to be modified. So the interpretive statements accompanying the first three provisions now hold language that emphasizes that equal relationship between nurses and their patients. For example, interpretive statements 1.1 through 1.5 focus on issues of human dignity and describe the topic as accommodating issues as specific as pain relief and end-of-life care to such general issues as self-determination. Interpretive statement 1.5 also notes that such respect extends to relations between all professionals, therefore placing nurses alongside all health colleagues in mutually supporting roles. This theme continues in interpretive statements 2.1 through 2.4. These statements play off the provision's broad dictum that the nurse primarily serves the patient by recognizing that a practicing clinician has many claims to his or her time. The statements discuss how to identify and work with possible conflicts of interest and very pointedly note that any party to an ethical problem involving the nurse must have an equitable voice in a proposed solution.

Provision 3 reflects the historical threads that have made up the fabric of the ANA's ethical codes over the years. Over the years, many strong statements about confidentiality have been made at the provision level. The task force working on the 2001 code decided that many patient rights deserved the same level of protection as patient information, and provision 3 addresses the need for nurses to also help to protect the autonomy of subjects in research as well as actively shield patients from impaired professionals or improper practice. Interpretive statement 3.5 is the longest of the interpretive statements; it lays out a clear duty for the nurse to be a whistle-blower, despite the acknowledged risks that acting in such a role places the nurse. This interpretive statement is written in such normative language that it could stand alone as a position statement on this topic.

In provisions 4, 5, and 6, the code shifts a bit as it addresses the nurse as a moral agent who has responsibilities of duty that provide good care in ways that go beyond direct patient care but that are truly within the venue of the profession. Provision 4 is very simple: Nursing care is delivered by nurses, and only nurses are responsible for nursing care that is delivered, even if that care comes from someone else. Anyone with the faintest familiarity with the history of professionalism in nursing knows that the profession has struggled to control a crucial piece of its discipline, that of entry into practice.

The result is that not only are there multiple pathways of entry to the status of a registered nurse, much nursing care is and has been given by nonregistered nurses. All four of the interpretive statements in provision 4 directly state that the ANA claims responsibility for maintaining the professional and ethical standards that define good nursing practice. In response to calls by other allied medical groups to be involved in providing semiprofessional nursing care, interpretive statement 4.4 directly notes that nursing responsibilities can never be delegated, only specific nursing tasks, and only nurses can do that delegating. The ultimate responsibility for any nursing care is always owned by the nurses involved in that care, including those nurse administrators who provide the setting where care is given.

Provision 5 is a new and unique addition. For the first time in an ANA code of ethics, a statement that the individual nurse has moral worth is proclaimed in a provision. This represents the progression of nursing values through the years and shows that the profession feels comfortable in its development as a scientific discipline. As such, the profession can now more forthrightly assert its humanistic values, not just vis-à-vis the patient, but also as a part of the individual nurse's devotion to the profession, harkening back to the values of nursing's early leaders.

Provision 6 continues this theme of the nurse's responsibility for establishing the proper ethical milieu for the delivery of care, but what happens in this provision is evidence of the moral maturation of modern nursing, as the profession claims once and for all that nurses are not beholden to any other group to prepare the environment where they provide care nor will they take an ethical back seat to any profession in the overall moral milieu of the healthcare setting. A subtle shift occurs within provision 6. Whereas the focus earlier in the code is on the individual nurse, this provision begins to assign the broader responsibilities that the professional group wishes to claim. Although all of the first eight provisions begin with the statement "The nurse . . . ," the later part of the code focuses more on the profession of nursing and the relationship of the individual nurse to the discipline.

The interpretive statements within provision 6 begin to discuss the duties of the nurse that are not directly patient centered. Interpretive statements 6.1 and 6.2 reiterate that the central virtues of the nursing profession cannot be imparted by the individual nurse without support. Therefore, the code now addresses how the nursing profession must provide assistance to the nurse in ways that allow the nurse to practice in an ethically appropriate manner. The code also makes it clear that the verb *to nurse* applies to the relationship of any nurse in any working relationship. So the nurse educators have duties to their students just as nurse administrators have responsibilities to the staff nurses under their authority. Consequently, staff nurses on a chronically understaffed unit have a moral responsibility to provide care that meets acceptable professional and ethical standards. If the usual pattern of care on the unit does not meet these standards, then the nurse administrator has at least equal responsibility to change the situation so that patients are treated safely and with respect.

Interpretive statement 6.3 represents probably the most contentious issue that the profession currently faces. The topic of collective action rights and the role of the ANA in assisting nurses who choose to exercise those rights has rent the fabric of the professional organization within the past decade. Professional nurses have claimed the right to collective bar-

gaining for over a half-century, with the ANA supporting this right by allowing each state unit to decide individually as to the level of involvement it will have in the matter. However, there is a sharp divide between those state nurses associations that reject this as a part of professional nursing and those that see it as an absolute good. This disagreement has escalated in recent years as a minority of registered nurses have come to believe that not only do nurses have a right to collective bargaining, but that professional nursing organizations should make representing nurses in collective bargaining a primary service. Despite the fact that the ANA has a stated goal and a defined subunit that addresses this issue, the disagreement over this issue has caused some state nurses associations to break away from the parent professional group and create their own group that does not accept the ANA's positions nor its code of ethics.

Therefore, interpretive statement 6.3 should be read as a policy statement from the ANA. It clearly supports the right to collective action and grounds that right within the duties of the registered nurse to ensure good patient care through the creation of a safe and nurturing environment as well within the right of the nurse to practice in a way so that the nurse is not continually morally degraded by having to work in substandard conditions. Between the lines is a belief that nurses deserve appropriate compensation and humane workloads. But because the definition of such terms is never clear cut and because the professional organization also must represent nurse executives and administrators, provision 6.3 has language that matches the general descriptive tone of the overall code and that leaves the topic of collective action somewhat understated.

The last three provisions of the code should be read as disciplinary statements that continue to claim the place of nursing as a leader in healthcare policy and delivery. The profession, through the ANA, made very determined efforts to place itself in the forefront of such efforts in the last quarter of the 20th century. Through documents such as *The Bill of Rights for Registered Nurses*, *Nursing's Social Policy Statement*, and the *Code of Ethics for Nurses*, the profession provides evidence of its leadership in providing ethical approaches to patient care (Know Your Rights, 2002).

Provisions 7 through 9 contain much material from past codes. Provision 7 synthesizes material from two of the provisions of the 1976 code regarding nursing's duties to make ongoing contributions to the profession's body of knowledge. The interpretive statements of this provision try to balance the nursing profession's need for sophisticated knowledge through research and expert clinical experience without either shutting the staff nurse out of this dynamic role or by putting the onus on that same person to be super nurse. Provision 7 reflects that the profession is moving forward and expects its members to make significant efforts toward disciplinary growth, even if by devoting oneself to personal professional growth at the bedside or just paying dues to the professional organization and attending local organizational meetings.

Provision 8 is a restatement of nursing's historical involvement in worldwide health. But the 2001 code goes further and says that this commitment is made as a full partner with other health professions.

Provision 9, the final statement in the code, is a self-reflective assertion that the ANA is the legitimate voice for the nation's registered nurses and that its current vehicles for portraying the face of nursing are well grounded. The three interpretive statements strongly declare that the association has done its job of providing a forum of debate that continues to provide a voice for the disparate viewpoints of the nation's largest group of healthcare providers. It also finishes laying out the case for the areas of interest in which nurses should have input. Interpretive statement 9.4 stakes the claim that the professional organization rightfully speaks from valid nursing disciplinary interests when it engages in activities such as lobbying for changes in laws that affect patient health, such as domestic violence laws.

In summary, the *Code of Ethics for Nurses* is best read as a descriptive document that provides basic guidelines for ethical conduct of nurses engaged in patient care and professional growth. Its equal purpose, like that of other professional ethical codes, is to lay the groundwork for a claim to legitimacy for the profession as a respected group with equal moral standing within the nation's healthcare workforce.

Alternative Codes

A continuing question nurses must consider is the need for alternative codes of ethics within the profession. It is certainly understandable when foreign nursing groups (e.g., the Canadian Nurses Association and the International Council of Nurses) wish to state their own views on nursing ethical standards and develop their own codes that have limited applicability to American registered nurses. But many subspecialty nursing organizations in the United States have considered the issue of whether a code of ethics for their group would advance their agenda as well as the welfare of the patients they serve (Peterson & Potter, 2004).

It is debatable whether specialized registered nurses experience ethical issues differently than their colleagues in other areas. In a series of surveys across several nursing specializations, reports from nurses in different clinical specialties did not reflect striking differences between the ethical issues they experienced or how they were resolved. Instead, any differences could be predicted by the type of practice setting (Redman & Fry, 1996, 1998a, 1998b). For example, pediatric nurses were concerned about child abuse (Butz, Redman, Fry, & Kolodner, 1998), whereas dialysis nurses reported the topic of ending treatment as a common ethical issue (Redman, Hill, & Fry, 1997).

Where specialty codes may have some contribution to an increased moral climate is when the descriptive level of the proposed code is minimized and the normative guidance to the specialty group and its outside audience is pronounced (Scanlon & Glover, 1995; Scanlon, 2000). An example of such a pathway is the program of the International Society of Nurses in Genetics (ISONG, 2007), which periodically prepares and releases position statements on discrete ethical issues that arise because of advances in genomic knowledge and subsequent impacts on genetic nursing practice, such as in the area of access to genetics services (ISONG, 2003).

Conclusion

Codes of ethics for health professionals provide guidance for conduct in patient encounters and justify the discipline's role as professional purveyors of care. The current ANA *Code of Ethics for Nurses* represents a much needed upgrade of the profession's moral guidelines that strongly states the group's just place as the spokesman for its members. The code stakes the claim to the emergence of nursing as a scientific but humanistic health group that constantly strives to update its knowledge base and has rightfully taken its place within the nation's accepted healthcare leaders. The nursing profession, guided by the *Code of Ethics for Nurses*, maintains a pursuit of excellence in practice, research, and education. This is evidenced by the accomplishments of the National Institute of Nursing Research at the National Institutes of Health, as well as the many respected colleges of nursing and magnet hospital nursing organizations.

Discussion Questions

1. What are the historical roots that have led to the development of the current *Code of Ethics for Nurses*?
2. Read each of the nine provisions and provide examples of how each affects ethical decision making for the advanced nursing practitioner.
3. What are the advantages and disadvantages of nursing subspecialty groups having separate codes of ethics?

References

American Nurses Association. (ANA). (2001). *Code of ethics for nurses with interpretive statements*. Washington, DC: American Nurses Association.

Ashley, J. (1976). *Hospitals, paternalism, and the role of the nurse*. New York: Teachers College Press.

Beauchamp, T. L., & Childress, J. F. (2001). *Principles of biomedical ethics* (5th ed.). New York: Oxford University Press.

Bishop, A., & Scudder, J. (1990). *The practical, moral, and personal sense of nursing*. New York: SUNY Press.

Butz, A. M., Redman, B. K., Fry, S. T., & Kolodner, K. K. (1998). Ethical conflicts experienced by certified pediatric nurse practitioners in ambulatory settings. *Journal of Pediatric Health Care, 12*(4), 183–190.

Church, O. (1990). Nightingalism: Its use and abuse in lunacy reform and the development of nursing in psychiatric care at the turn of the century. In V. Bullough, B. Bullough, & M. Stanton (Eds.), *Florence Nightingale and her era: A collection of new scholarship* (pp. 229–244). New York: Garland Publ., Inc.

Daly, B. J. (1999). Ethics. Why a new code? Code for nurses. *American Journal of Nursing, 99*(6), 64, 66.

Dossey, B. (2000). *Florence Nightingale: Mystic, visionary and reformer*. Philadelphia: Lippincott Williams & Wilkins.

Evans, J. H. (2000). A sociological account of the growth of principlism. *Hastings Center Report, 30*(5), 31–38.

Fowler, M. D. (1992). A chronicle of the evolution of the code for nurses. In G. B. White (Ed.), *Ethical dilemmas in contemporary nursing practice* (pp. 149–154). Washington, DC: American Nurses Association.

Fowler, M. D. (1999). Relic or resource? The code for nurses. *American Journal of Nursing, 99*(3), 56–57.

Goodrich, A. (1932). *The social and ethical significance of nursing: A series of lectures*. New York: Macmillan Company.

Hamilton, D. (1994). Constructing the mind of nursing. *Nursing History Review II*, 3–28.

International Council of Nurses. (2005). *The ICN code of ethics for nurses*. Retrieved November 2, 2007, from http://www.icn.ch/icncode.pdf

International Society of Nurses in Genetics (ISONG). (2007). *Position statements*. Retrieved November 2, 2007, from http://www.ISONG.org/about/position.cfm

International Society of Nurses in Genetics (ISONG). (2003). *Position statement: Access to genomic healthcare: The role of the nurse*. Retrieved November 2, 2007, from http://www.ISONG.org/about/ps_genomic.cfm

Know Your Rights. (2003). Available at http://nursingworld.org/tan/novdec02/rights.htm

Nightingale Pledge. (n.d.). Available at http://www.accd.edu/sac/nursing/honors.html

Noddings, N. (2003). *Caring: A feminine approach to ethics and moral education*. Berkeley: University of California Press.

Peterson, M., & Potter, R. L. (2004). A proposal for a code of ethics for nurse practitioners. *Journal of the American Academy of Nurse Practitioners, 16*(3), 116–124.

Redman, B. K., & Fry, S. T. (1996). Ethical conflicts reported by registered nurse/certified diabetes educators. *The Diabetes Educator, 22*(3), 219–224.

Redman, B. K., & Fry, S. T. (1998a). Ethical conflicts reported by rehabilitation nurses. *Rehabilitation Nursing, 26*(4), 179–184.

Redman, B. K., & Fry, S. T. (1998b). Ethical conflicts reported by registered certified diabetes educators: A replication. *Journal of Advanced Nursing, 28*(6), 1320–1325.

Redman, B. K., Hill, M. A., & Fry, S. T. (1997). Ethical conflicts reported by certified nephrology nurses (CNNs) practicing in dialysis settings. *American Nephrology Nurses Association Journal, 24*(1), 23–33.

Robb, I. H. (1900). *Nursing ethics for hospitals and private use*. Cleveland, OH: E. D. Kloeckert Publishing.

Rothman, D. J. (1990). *The discovery of the asylum: Social order and disorder in the new republic* (rev. ed.). Boston: Little, Brown.

Scanlon, C. (2000). A professional code of ethics provides guidance for genetic nursing practice. *Nursing Ethics, 7*(3), 262–286.

Scanlon, C., & Glover, J. (1995). A professional code of ethics: Providing a moral compass for turbulent times. *Oncology Nursing Forum, 22*(10), 1515–1521.

Widerquist, J. G. (1990). Dearest Rev'd Mother. In V. Bullough, B. Bullough, & M. Stanton (Eds.). *Florence Nightingale and her era. A collection of new scholarship* (pp. 288–308). New York: Garland Publ., Inc.

Index

A

AACN. *See* American Association of Colleges of Nursing

AALL. *See* American Association of Labor Legislation

AAMC. *See* Association of American Medical Colleges

AANA. *See* American Association of Nurse Anesthetists

ABCX model, 387

Abdellah, Faye, 475

Abdominal aneurysms, endovascular placement of grafts for, 267

Abortion, 522

Abraham, I. L., 446

Academy of Nursing Ad Hoc Group on Knowledge Generation, 471

Acceptance techniques, stress management and, 64

Access
  to nursing education programs, 512, 513
  partial, in United States, 81
  to preventive and curative healthcare services, 109

Accountability, 300
  ANA Code of Ethics and, 550
  autonomy and, 8
  customer service and, 265
  fiscal responsibilities and, 203, 204
  future of managed care and, 250
  Loeb model of care and, 13
  organizational, 283

Accounting concepts, 210–211

Accreditation
  educational standards and, 26
  patient safety and, 354–355
  regulatory focus on quality and, 339–343

Acculturation, 497, *497*

ACNM. *See* American College of Nurse Midwives

Acquired immune deficiency syndrome, 119, 121, 142, 221, 258, 292, 296, 340, 464
  CNSs and persons with, 24
  globalization and, 158

Activism, educators and modeling of, 295

Actors, policy process and, 290

ACTUP. *See* AIDS Coalition to Unleash Power

Acute care model, 88*t*
  move from, to chronic care model, 255

Acute disease, 98

Acute myocardial infarction, Hospital Quality Initiative and focus on, 342

Adaptation model, 387, 411

Administrative Procedures Act, 289

Administrative systems, 368–370
  categories of, and their uses, 369*t*

Adult education, 280

Advanced, defined, 23

Advance directives, 521, 531

Advanced nurse practitioner, quality of culture and, 323

Advanced Nursing Curriculum Guidelines and Program Standards for Nurse Practitioner Education (NONPF), 27

Advanced nursing practice
  information technology for, 361–371
  models and theories applicable in, 385–389
    community models, 388–389
    family models, 387–388
    nursing models and theories, 385, 387

Advanced practice nurses, 24
  as case managers, 286
  definition of, 296
  designation of, as providers, 280
  expanded scope of nursing and, 287–288
  financial management for, 209–216
    budget cycle, 213–216
    elements of financial management, 210–211
    managerial accounting and financial analysis, 211–213
  financial roles and responsibilities of, 215–216
  finding foundation in theory and research, 280–282
  healthcare problems defined by, 292
  multiple roles of and bright future for, 295–300
  new organizational paradigm and, 282–284
  political system and engagement by, 300
  public policy and, 275–301

Advanced practice nursing, 23–29
  definition of, 23
    as adopted by International Council of Nurses, 27–28
  description of, 23–25
  educational standards and, 26–27
  redefining, 29
  self-assessment of development needs in, 50*t*
  theoretical issues and challenges in, 27–29

Advanced practice role, international evolution of, 27–28

Advertising, pharmaceutical, 83

Advocacy organizations, 306

Affinity diagrams, 332, 334*t*
Affirmations, 64
Affordability, 247
Africa, medical resources distribution in, 110
African American men, Tuskegee study of syphilis and, 518
African American nurses, opportunities for, 513–514
African immigrants, 492
AFT. *See* American Federation of Teachers
Agan, R. D., 427
Age, justice and, 530
Ageism, 430
Agency for Healthcare Policy and Research, 268, 282, 336–337, 354, 455
    components within, 456–457
    mission of, 456
    patient safety and response by, 351
Agency policies, 288
Agenda for Change (JCAHO), 339–340
Agendas, 334
    setting of, policy process and, 290, 292
Agents, epidemiology triangle and, *97, 98*
Aggleton, P. J., 380
Aggregate community model, 388–389
Aging population
    growth in healthcare expenditures and, 166
    number of persons 65 or older in millions, 1900-2030, *167*
    shrinking workforce and, 257
AHA. *See* American Hospital Association
AHCPR. *See* Agency for Healthcare Policy and Research
AIDS. *See* Acquired immune deficiency syndrome
AIDS activists, 306
AIDS Coalition to Unleash Power, 292
Aiken, L. H., 8, 349, 511
Air pollution, 106
Alarm systems, improving effectiveness of, 356
Alerts, laboratory, 368
Alfano, Gwenrose, 475
"Alive," 537
Allergy profiles, 368
Alligood, M. R., 380
All payer rate systems, 183
Almshouses, 133
Altering techniques, stress management and, 62
Alternative codes of ethics, 555–556

Alternative therapies, 158
Altman, S. H., 184
Altruism, 300
Alzheimer's disease, genetic mapping and, 267
AMA. *See* American Medical Association
Ambulatory settings, patient safety and, 355
America
    alternative treatments and healthcare in, 158
    expansion of social entitlements in, 158
    medical care in corporate era, 155–158
        corporatization of healthcare delivery, 155–156
        globalization, 156–158
        information revolution, 156
    postindustrial, medical services in, 135–155
        birth of Blue Shield, 145
        birth of Medicaid and Medicare, 151–153
        birth of workers' compensation, 143
        Blue Cross plans, 144–145
        combined hospital and physician coverage, 145
        development of public health, 141–142
        early blanket insurance policies, 144
        economic necessity and Baylor Plan, 144
        employment-based health insurance, 145–146
        failure of national healthcare initiatives, 146–151
        growth of professional sovereignty, 135–141
        health services for veterans, 143
        prototypes of managed care, 153–155
        regulatory role of public health agencies, 153
        rise in chronic conditions, 142–143
        rise of private health insurance, 143
        specialization in medicine, 141
        technological, social, and economic factors, 143–144
    preindustrial, medical services in, 130–135
        medical practice in disarray, 131
        missing institutional core, 132–133

        primitive medical procedures, 131–132
        substandard medical education, 134–135
        unstable demand, 133–134
American Academy of Nursing, 19, 472, 475, 477, 479, 482
American Association of Colleges of Nursing, 2, 36, 280, 511
American Association of Labor Legislation, 146, 147
American Association of Nurse Anesthetists, 26
American College of Nurse Midwives, 26
American College of Surgeons, 460
American culture, beliefs and values predominant in, 110–111
American Federation of Labor, 148
American Federation of Teachers, 15
American Heart Association, Council on Cardiovascular Nursing, 477
American Hospital Association, 19, 144, 173
    national healthcare initiatives and, 148
American Indians, 501
American Journal of Nursing, 510
American Managed Care and Review Association, 234
American Medical Association, 117, 152, 159, 172, 176, 294, 343
    Blue Shield and, 145
    contract practice and, 153
    formation of, 131, 139
    national healthcare initiatives and, 146, 147, 148, 149, 176
    patient safety and response by, 349
American Nurses Association, 12, 278, 279, 299, 309, 473, 507
    Cabinet on Nursing Research, 477
    Code of Ethics for Nurses, 488, 549, 550–555, *551*
        reading, 550–555
    Commission on Research, 475
    Nursing Safety & Quality Initiative, 355
    patient safety and response by, 348–349
    Political Action Committee of, 312
    research conferences of, 475
American Nurses Association Commission, research agendas and priorities of, 471
American Nurses Foundation, grants program, 474

American Organization of Nurse
Executives, 2, 3
American Psychological Association,
Committee on Religion and
Psychiatry, 96
American Red Cross, 259
American Society of Superintendents of
Training Schools of Nurses. *See*
Superintendents' Society
AMI. *See* Acute myocardial infarction
ANA. *See* American Nurses Association
Analytic studies, 453
Anderson, E. T., 389
Anderson, G., 428
Anesthesia, 136
discovery of, 137 (exhibit)
Angioplasty, 165
Anthrax, 103, 259
Anthropology, 280, 281, 440
Antibiotic resistance, 258, 466
Antifraud and abuse provisions, Balanced
Budget Act of 1997 and, 189
Antiseptic surgery, 136, 137 (exhibit)
AONE. *See* American Organization of
Nurse Executives
APA. *See* Administrative Procedures Act
APNs. *See* Advanced practice nurses
Apollo hospital chain (India), 157
Application passwords, 363
Applied ethics, 522
Appreciation, 283
Apprenticeships, medical, in
preindustrial America, 134
Appropriateness studies, 463
Appropriations process, legislation and,
293
Aristotle, 404
Army Nurse Corps, Black nurses in, 509
Ashley, Jo Ann, 16
Asian immigrants, 492
Asians, 501
Assertiveness, 300
communication and, 62
nurses, patient safety and, 354, 355
training in, 277
Assessment
application of, to nursing process,
386*t*
theory-based nursing practice and,
394*t*
Assets, 212
Assimilation, 497
Assisted suicide, 522
ANA position statement on, 551
Association Medical Care Plans, 172
Association of American Medical
Colleges, 140

Assurance, insurance *vs.,* 173
Auerbach, D., 262
Aukerman, M., 286
Austin, Sara, 530
Authorization process, legislation and, 293
Autonomy, 8, 300, 525–526, 548
ANA *Code of Ethics* and, 550
Loeb model of care and, 13
magnet hospitals and, 19
nurses and, 277, 280
Avoidance techniques, stress
management and, 62–64

B

Baby boomers
aging of, 166
nursing shortages and, 511, 513
public entitlement programs
and, 247–248
direct care worker pool and, 257
hospital demand and, 260
Medicare system and, 186
Baccalaureate programs in nursing,
creation of, 34
Bachelor of Arts, 32
Bachelor of science degrees in nursing
education, 276
Bacterial genetics, 466
Bacteriology, advances in, 136
Bad apple theory, 458
Baicker, K., 248
Balanced budget, 214
Balanced Budget Act of 1997, 164,
185–191, 232, 233, 342
child health initiative within, 195
major provisions of, 188–189
Medicaid and, 194–197
projected savings, 1998-2002, *187*
sources, percent, and dollar amount
in billions, of contributions
toward, 188, *188*
Balanced Budget Refinement Act of
1999, 164, 191
Balanced life, 3, 53
Balanced scorecard, 216, 217*t*
Balance sheet, 212, 212*t*
Bankruptcies, medical issues and, 530
Bar code readers, 362
Barker, A. M., 3, 58
Barker-Sullivan model of mentor
partnerships, 44, *44*
Barnard, K., 480
Barsamian, E. M., 460
Bartleby, the Scrivener (Melville), 283
Basic science research, 452, *452*
Basic social structures, 441

Batey, M., 474, 480
Battle, A., 506, 514
Baylor Plan, economic necessity and, 144
Baylor University Hospital (Dallas), 144,
172
BBA. *See* Balanced Budget Act of 1997
Beavers system model, 388
Bed alarms, improving effectiveness of,
356
Behavior, model of career development
and, 49*t*
Behavioral risk factors, 98, 108
percentage of population with, 99*t*
Behavioral systems model, 387, 393
Beijing United Family Hospital and
Clinics, 157
Beliefs, cultural, healthcare delivery and,
109–111
Benchmarking, 216–217, 335–336
Beneficence, 526–527
Benefit buydowns, 229
Benefits Improvement and Protection
Act of 2000, 191, 194
Benjamin, Elizabeth, 530
Benner, P. G., 281, 423, 424, 425, 427,
428
Bernstein, R. J., 404
Berthold, J. S., 415
Betts, Virginia Trotter, 279
Bevis, E. O., 16
Bias
clinical trials and reduction of, 453
evidence-based practice and
minimizing of, 403
transcultural nursing and, 499
Biblical ethics, 523
Billings, 387
Bill of Rights for Registered Nurses, 555
Bills, legislative process and, 278
Bioethics, 518, 543, 546
Bioinformatic research, 465–466
Biological weapons, 259
Biomedical science, 130
Biomedicine, 111
Biometrics scans, 362
Biotechnology, 466
Bioterrorism, 103–104, 158, 267, 269,
300
transformation of public health
and, 258–260
Bipartisan Patient Protection Act of
2001, 230
"Birth" (Nin), 426
Bishop, A., 423, 424
Bismarck, Otto von, 305
Black nurses
collective action by, 509

segregation during Civil War era and, 506
segregation laws and, 508
Black-operated schools, 507
Blacks, 501
Blancett, S. S., 286
Blank, A.E., 281
Blanket insurance policies, early, 144
Blood pressure cuffs, 368
Blood transfusions, fluid substitutes and, 267
Blue Cross, 143, 144, 172, 183
Medicare policies and, 177
Blue Cross Association, 145
Blue Cross/Blue Shield, 72
merger of, 145
Blue Cross Commission, 145
Blue Cross movement, lasting impact of, 173
Blue Cross plans
successful private enterprise and, 144–145
uniform features of, 173
Blueprint for a Healthy Community: A Guide for Local Health Departments, 259
Blue Shield, 143, 172
self-interest of physicians and birth of, 145
Blum, H. L., 105
Blum's model, cultural beliefs and values and, 109
Boland, S., 286
Borges, J. R., 46
Boston University, 35
Boston University School of Nursing, early training grants for, 473
Bottorff, J., 428
Bowers, B., 493
Bowman, A., 294
Bradford, D. M., 506, 514
Brain death criteria, Harvard Medical School report on, 519
Brainstorming, 295, 331–332, 334t
Brain surgery, image-guided, 267
"Breakthroughs in Nursing Research" (Donaldson), 482
Breast cancer, 100, 296
annual percent decline in, 101t
Brewster, L. R., 206
Britain, general practitioners in, 141
Brooten, D., 281, 479
BRT. *See* Business Roundtable
BSNE. *See* Bachelor of science degrees in nursing education
BSP. *See* Basic social structures
Buber, M., 414
Buchmueller, T., 242

Budget cycle, 213–216
budget development, 213–214
Budgets
development of, 213–214
padding, 214
review process for, 213–214
types of, 214
Budget variance report, 214
sample, for a clinical area, 215t
Budget variance reports, review of, 216
Budget variances, monitoring, 214–215
Burden of care, 483
Burdick, Quentin, 279
Bureau of Health Professions, 512
Bureau of Indian Affairs, 292
Bureau of Labor Statistics, 511
Burke, Sheila, 279
Burnout, 511
Bush, George H. W., 149, 221
Bush, George W., 103, 104, 118, 248, 309, 522, 535
Business cards, 311
Business Roundtable, 351
Byrnes, John W., 152
Bytes, 362

C

CAA. *See* Consolidated Appropriations Act for Fiscal Year 2000
Cabinet on Nursing Research, 471
Cadet Nurse Corps, 508, 509
Calgary family model, 387, 388
California, play-or-pay mandate in, 253
California Medical Association, 145
California Physicians Service, 145
Cambodians, newborn-naming customs of, 501
Cameras, 362
Campaigns, political, direct mail strategies and, 311–312
Canada
health services delivery in, 110
universal health care in, 118
Canadian Nurses Association, 555
Canales, M., 493
Cancer, 121
diet and, 108
early detection of, 100
genetic mapping and, 267
Cancer mortality, annual percent decline in, 101t
Canterbury v. Spence, 520
Capital budgets, 214
Capital Gang, The, 298
Capitalism, 282
culture of, in United States, 111

Capitation, 78–79, 154, 222
package pricing *vs.,* 83
Capitation grants, for nursing education programs, 297
Capps, Lois, 300, 309
Cardiac monitors, 368
Cardiac problems, in women, 296
Cardiac procedures, minimal access, 267
Cardiopulmonary resuscitation, 519
Care, 404–405
ANA *Code of Ethics* and, 552
culturally competent, 496–498, 497, 501
differentiating practice and, 405–406, 405t
Career development
model of, 48–50, 49t
planning process for, 50–51
Career ladders, 18, 28
Caregivers, empowering, 296
Care protocols, nursing information systems and, 366
Caring, 120
Native American point of view and, 496
Carnegie, M. E., 506
Carnegie Foundation for the Advancement of Teaching, 140
Carotid endarterectomy, 268
Carper, Barbara, 375, 419, 420, 421, 422, 424, 426, 427, 428, 430, 439
Carve-outs, 233–234
Casalino, L. P., 206
Case-based nursing, 13
Case studies, early, 472
Cash flow statements, 212, 212t, 213
Catholic Church, 32
Catholic University of America, 35
Caucasians, 501
Cause and effect (fishbone) diagrams, 330, 334t
CBO. *See* Congressional Budget Office
CCBN. *See* Cleveland Council of Black Nurses
CCIP. *See* Chronic Care Improvement Program
CCNE. *See* Commission on Collegiate Nursing Education
CDC. *See* Centers for Disease Control and Prevention
CDs, 363
Center for Patient Safety, 351
Centers for Disease Control and Prevention, 104, 105, 259, 466
Centers for Medicare and Medicaid Services, 192, 194, 197, 232, 245, 249, 340, 352

quality initiatives by, 342–343
Web site for, 68–69
Central processing unit, 362
Centrifugal families, 388
Centripetal families, 388
Certification
nurse specialty areas and, 277
reframing, 29
Certified nurse midwives, 2, 23, 24
educational standards and, 26–27
policy process and, 279
Certified registered nurse anesthetists, 2, 23, 24
educational standards and, 26–27
policy process and, 279
Cervical cancer, 100
annual percent decline in, 101*t*
Chalmers, H., 380
Champion, 333, 334, 335*t*
Champy, J., 325
Chaplains, 96
Charity funds, to hospitals, 530
Charles, S. C., 283
Chase Capital Partners, 247
Checksheets, 331, 334*t*
Chemical weapons, 259
Chen, Y., 496
Cheung, R. B., 511
Cheyovich, Theresa, 478
Child abuse, 296
Child care, 101
Children
health insurance coverage of, by income, 2003, *196*
uninsured, 195
China, tobacco industry and, 157–158
Chindex International, 157
Chinese culture
experience of nursing practice in, 496
gender and, 110
Chinn, P., 419, 420, 421, 422, 424, 426, 428, 429
Chit economy, politics and, 313
Cholera, 102, 133, 141, 142
Chopoorian, T., 430
Christianity, 523
Chronic care, 88*t*
Chronic Care Improvement Program, 255–256
Chronic illness, 98, 269
future of and challenges with, 255–256
high-risk pools and, 249
rise in, in postindustrial America, 142–143
Chrysler Corporation, 221

Cicero, 534
Cigarette smoking, health promotion strategies and, 100
City of Hope, 475
Civil defense agencies, 259
Civil Rights Act of 1964, 510
Civil rights legislation, 510
Civil Rights Movement (1960s), 510
Civil War, 24, 32, 131, 135
race, nursing profession and, 505
Claims, multiple payers of, 85–86
Claims processors, within U.S. healthcare delivery system, 72, 73*t*
Clarity of mind, time management and, 53–54
Clark, R. L., 208
Clarke, S. P., 8, 511
CLAS. *See* Culturally and linguistically appropriate standards
Classism, 430
Clergy, early practice of medicine in America by, 131
Cleveland Council of Black Nurses, 514
Client focus, selecting models and theories for nursing practice and, 392
Client outcomes, selecting models and theories for nursing practice and, 392
Client type, selection of models and theories and, 390
Clinical alarm systems, improving effectiveness of, 356
Clinical doctorates, 39–40
programs for, 36–38
as requirement for advanced clinical practice nursing, 2
Clinical guidelines, AHCPR, 456
Clinical judgment, 458
Clinical medicine, advances in, 466
Clinical nurse leader, educational requirements for, 3
Clinical nurse specialists, 2, 23, 24
policy process and, 279
role of, 26
Clinical nursing research, 281
Clinical pathways, 281
Clinical practice guidelines, managed care organizations and, 227–228
Clinical problems, identification of, 296
Clinical-process improvement, 336–337
Clinical research, *452,* 452–453
Clinical science, 479
Clinical systems, 366–368
clinical information processing systems, 366–368
laboratory, 368

order entry, 366–367
patient monitoring, 368
pharmacy, 368
radiology, 368
nursing information systems, 366
Clinical technology, new frontiers in, 266–267
Clinical therapy, forms of, in preindustrial America, 131–132
Clinical trials, 453
Clinical uncertainty, 467
Clinton, Bill, 117, 118, 149, 150, 189, 221, 350
Clinton, Hillary Rodham, 117
Clinton administration, national healthcare proposals during, 149, 150, 176, 185, 204, 241–242, 250, 252, 308
Clock speed, of computer, 362
Closed panel HMOs, 224
CMS. *See* Centers for Medicare and Medicaid Services
CNM. *See* Certified nurse midwife
CNS. *See* Clinical nurse specialist
COBRA. *See* Consolidated Omnibus Budget Reconciliation Act
Coddington, D. C., 208
Code of Ethics for Nurses (ANA), 488, 543, 545, 547, 549, 550–555, *551*
provisions in 2001 code, 552–555
Code of Hammurabi, 524, 525
Codes of ethics
alternative, 555–556
ANA *Code of Ethics for Nurses,* 488, 542, 546, 547, 549, 550–555, *551,* 556
for nursing, 545–549
religious, 523–524
views on, 545
Cody, W. K., 374, 375, 382
COGME. *See* Council on Graduate Medical Education
Cognitive development, in children, 389
Cohen, H., 356
Cohesiveness and organization, growth of professional sovereignty and, 135, 138–139
Coile, R. C., 254
Coinsurances, 229
high-risk pools and, 249
Medicare, 177
Cold War, 148
Coleman-Miller, B., 494
Collaboration, 286, 479
problem solving and, 446
Collaborative interdependence, 300
Collaborative team approach, 264–265

Colleagueship, 479

Collection agencies, 86

Collective action rights, ANA *Code of Ethics* and, 554

Collective bargaining, 14, 15, 16, 153, 299
    group health insurance and, 145

College of Philadelphia, 134

Colon cancer, exercise and reducing risk of, 108

Color printing, 363

Columbia University, 134
    doctoral programs in nursing at, 34, 35
    school of nursing at, 11

Commercialism, research and, 465

Commission on Collegiate Nursing Education, 2

Commitment, 532

Committee on Religion and Psychiatry (APA), 96

Committee on the Quality of Care in America, 353

Communicable diseases, of childhood, 472

Communication
    with immigrants, 492
    with legislators, 309–310
    managing, 61–62

Communitarianism, 546, 547

Community health, 94
    assessment of, 121
    integration of individual health and, 119–124

Community health center program, 118

Community hospitals, 121

Community models, 388–389, 395

Community nursing process model, 389

Community rating, Blue Cross plans and, 173

Compassion, 527, 532–533, 545

Competency, educational applications and determination of, 370–371. *See also* Cultural competency

Competition
    among healthcare providers in U.S., 83
    customer service and, 265–266
    managed, 252–253

Complex health care systems model, 387

Comprehensive Health Planning Act, 179

Compromise, politics and, 307

Computerized medical records, security and, 319

Computerized technology, 165

Computers
    hardware, 362–363
    software, 362, 363

Conceptual nursing theories, 383

Conference committees, 293

Confidentiality, 522
    ANA *Code of Ethics* and, 553
    information technology and, 364–365
    medical errors and, 348

Confirmability, qualitative methodologies and, 441

Conflict management, 62
    delegation and, 59
    politics and, 307

Conflict resolution, 300

Confusion, perspective transformation and, 384

Congestive heart failure, 107

Congress, 147, 150, 151, 289, 293, 313

Congressional Budget Office, 185, 256

Congressional Nursing Caucus, 300

Congruence, selecting models and theories for nursing practice and, 391–392

Conrad, Pete, 279

Conscientiousness, 533

Consequential (or teleological) ethics, 522–523

Consolidated Appropriations Act for Fiscal Year 2000, significant provisions of, 189–190

Consolidated Omnibus Budget Reconciliation Act, 183

Constancy of purpose, total quality management and, 324

Constitution (U.S.), 289
    Fourteenth Amendment to, 526

Consumer choice, 247

Consumers
    alternative health care and, 158
    managed care, marketplace power and, 156

Consumer sovereignty, evolution of U.S. healthcare delivery system and, *159*

Contextual ethics, 546

Continued education, quality leadership and, 326*t*, 328

Continuous quality improvement, 325

Continuum of services, healthcare delivery and, 87

Contract practice, 153–154

Contractual allowances, 211

Control, 16
    empiricism and, 439
    financial management and, 210
    freedom through, quality improvement and, 326–327, 326*t*

Control charts, 330–331, 334*t*

Cooper, M., 423

Cooperation, 424

Cooperativeness, 534

Co-payments, 223, 225, 227
    benefit buydowns and, 229
    managed care and, 227, 249
    point-of-service plans and, 225

Coping skills, purpose of, 62

Corcoran, Ruth D., 512, 513

Core-care-cure model, 385

Coronary care units, 276

Coronary heart disease, 121

Corporate dominance, evolution of U.S. healthcare delivery system and, *159*

Corporate era, 130

Corporate practice doctrine, 139

Corporate practice of medicine, 153

Corporatization, of healthcare delivery, 155–156, 160

Cost centers, 210

Cost containment, 282, 284
    clinical nurse specialists and, 24
    realignment of nursing roles and, 25

Cost effectiveness, 247

Costs
    shifting of, 151, 220
        in fragmented market, 208
        Medicaid and, 248
    types of, 211
    utilization and, 79

Coughlin, T. A., 248

Council of Nurse Researchers, 475

Council on Graduate Medical Education, 261, 262

Council on Graduate Schools, 37

Council on Medical Education, 140

Courage, 534

Court system, 289

Cowan, Marie, 477, 479

CPU. *See* Central processing unit

CQI. *See* Continuous quality improvement

Cradock, S., 385

Creativity, multiple paradigms and, 444

Credibility
    of health professionals, 310
    qualitative methodologies and, 441

Criteria for Evaluation of Nurse Practitioner Programs, 27

Critical care pathways, 383

Critical theory, 479

Critical thinking, 395
    advanced practice nurses and, 275
    application of, to nursing process, 386*t*
    models, theories and, 384–385

Criticism
    empathy and, 428

political process and, 314
Critique, developing art of, 475
CRNAs. *See* Certified registered nurse anesthetists
Crossfire, 298
Crossing the Quality Chasm: A New Health System for the 21st Century (IOM), 318, 341, 353
Cross-subsidization, 151
Cross-training, of health service workers, 265, 270, 285
Crowley, D., 478, 480
Cultural authority, 136
    dependency and, 138
Cultural autonomy, 497, 497
Cultural beliefs and values, healthcare delivery and, 109–111
Cultural competence, 488, 491–501
    development of, 264, 270
    diaspora and, 492–494
    human migration patterns and, 492
    multiple definitions of, 496–497
Cultural diversity, 501
Cultural domains model, 500, 500t
Cultural imposition, 497, 497–498, 499
Culturally and linguistically appropriate standards, 493t
Culturally competent care, 496–498, 497, 501
Cultural pain, 499
Cultural sensitivity training, 494
Culture
    group identity and, 496
    identity and, 501
    Western health care and, 494–496
Culture care preservation, defined, 497
Culture of quality
    building, 323, 326
    leadership and, 318
    team effectiveness and, 332
Culture shock, 497
Curative health care services, 87
Curative medicine, 93
Curran, 388
Curtis, Namahyoke Sockum, 506
Customer focus, quality improvement and, 325, 326t
Customer service, enhanced focus on, 265–266

D

Dartmouth College, 134
Dashboard report, 327
Data analysis, 441
Data integrity, 338
Davis, Carolyne, 279

Day planners, 57, 58
DBA. *See* Doctor of business administration
DC. *See* Doctor of chiropractic medicine
DDS. *See* Doctor of dental surgery
Death
    defining, 521
    leading causes of, 2003, 103t
    medical errors and, 318, 340, 350, 461
Death with Dignity Act (Oregon), 521
Debate, practicing rules of, 298
Decision making, financial management, 210
Decision support systems, 369
Declaration of Helsinki, 519
Deductibles, 223, 225, 227
    high, health plans with, 243–244
    high-risk pools and, 249
    managed care and, 249
De facto segregation, 507
Defensive medicine, 87
Deficit Reduction Act of 2005, 249, 256
Defined contribution plans, 246–247
Delegation
    process of, 60
    time management and, 59–60
Delivering Health Care in America: A Systems Approach (Shi and Singh), 68
Delivery, within healthcare delivery system, 75–76, 76, 78
Demand. *See also* Supply and demand
    free-market conditions and, 82, 82
    health care and, 84
    unstable, in preindustrial America, 133–134
Demand-side rationing, of health care, 114
Deming, W. E., 324, 327, 335
Democracy, 306
Democratic party, 308
Demographics, of nursing workforce, 511
Demonstration projects, Balanced Budget Act of 1997 and, 189
Denial claims, rebilling and, 86
Dentists, in preindustrial America, 134
Dent v. West Virginia, 140
Deontological ethics, 523–524
Deontology, 114, 546
Department of Defense, 175, 197, 292
Department of Health, Education, & Welfare, 15
Department of Health and Human Services, 93, 197, 340, 352, 455, 512
    Office of Minority Health, 493
Department of Justice, 259

Department of Veterans Affairs, 143
Dependability
    qualitative methodologies and, 441
    reputations and, 313
Dependency, growth of professional sovereignty and, 135, 138
Depersonalization, traditional medical model and, 266
Depression, diabetes management and, 264
Descarte, René, 437
Descriptive ethics, 547–548
Descriptive studies, 453
Descriptive theories, 374
Desegregation, 510
Detachment, 533
Developed countries, national health insurance in, 71
Developmental health, 101
    environment and, 108
Devers, K. J., 206
Dewey, J., 412, 413
Diabetes, 430
    collaborative team approach to, 264
    genetic mapping and, 267
Diagnosis
    application of, to nursing process, 386t
    theory-based nursing practice and, 394t
Diagnosis-related groups, 25, 181, 183–184, 185, 284, 457
    advent of, 205–207
Diagnostic and treatment technology, new, growth in healthcare expenditures and, 165–166
Diagnostic techniques, advances in, 136
Diaphragmatic breathing, 64
Diaspora, 492–494
Dickoff, J., 415
Diers, D., 430
Diet, health problems and, 108
Dietary consults, 501
Dietitians, 141
Digitization, of healthcare documentation, 402
Direct costs, 211
Directions for Nursing Research: Toward the 21st Century, 477
Direct mail campaigning, 311–312
Direct-to-consumer advertising, 166
Disability insurance, 148
Discernment, 534
Discipline, defined, 433
"Discipline of Nursing, The" (Donaldson and Crowley), 478
Discounted fees, 79, 154

Discrimination, collective action by
  Black nurses and, 509
Disease
  acute, subacute, and chronic, 98
  germ theory of, 137 (exhibit)
  illness and, 97–98
  prevention of, 99–100, 120
    public health and, 102
Disease vectors, 106
Disks, 363
Disparities in health care, 488, 494, 505
Dispensaries, 132
Disraeli, Benjamin, 533
Dissertations, 281
Dissonance, perspective transformation
  and, 384
Distance learning programs, 36
Distributional efficiency, 118–119
Distributive justice, 529, 531
Diversity, 488, 501
  disparities in health care and, 494
  future of healthcare workforce and,
    263–264, 269
  transcultural nursing and, 498
Division of Nursing fellowships, 35
DMD. See Doctor of dental medicine
DNP. See Doctorate of Nursing Practice
DNSc. See Doctor of nursing science
Dock, Lavinia, 11, 544, 545
Doctoral education, 3, 281
  brief history of, 32–34
  future of, 38–39
  in nursing, evolution of, 31–40
Doctoral programs
  broad purposes of, 31
  clinical, 36–38
  early, 14
  historical development of, 3
  in and for nursing, 34–36, 277, 400
  political leadership training and, 295
Doctorate of Nursing Practice, 2, 3
Doctor of business administration, 33
Doctor of chiropractic medicine, 34
Doctor of dental medicine, 34
Doctor of dental surgery, 33, 34
Doctor of education, 33, 34
Doctor of medicine (MD), 33, 34
Doctor of nursing practice, 37, 38
Doctor of nursing science, 33, 34, 36, 37
Doctor of optometry, 34
Doctor of osteopathy, 34, 363
Doctor of pharmacy, 34, 38
Doctor of podiatric medicine, 34
Doctor of public health, 33
Doctor of science in nursing, 35, 36
Doctor of veterinary medicine, 34
Doctors in roentgenology, 137 (exhibit)

Dodd, 69
Dole, Bob, 279
Domains and Competencies of Nurse
  Practitioner Practice, 27
Donabedian, Avedis, 459
Donaldson, S., 472, 474, 478, 479, 482
DOS. See Doctor of osteopathy
Doubiago, Sharon, 426
Double-blind studies, 453
Downsizing, 282, 285
DPH. See Doctor of public health
DPM. See Doctor of podiatric medicine
DRA. See Deficit Reduction Act
Dracup, 479
DRGs. See Diagnosis-related groups
Drills and practice sessions, education
  applications and, 370
Drucker, Peter, 283
Drug administration, tracking, 368
Drug dependence, 430
Drug trials, 465
DSN. See Doctor of science in nursing
Duvalle, M., 387, 388
DVDs, 363
DVM. See Doctor of veterinary medicine
Dzurec, L. C., 446

E

E. coli, 100
Early childhood development, 101
Early detection, of cancer, 100
Early-warning systems, 260
EBM. See Evidence-based medicine
Ebola, 104
EBP. See Evidence-based practice
EBRI. See Employee Benefit Research
  Institute
Eclecticism, nursing theories and, 382
Ecology, 120
Economic factors in health care, in
  postindustrial America, 143–144
Economic incentives
  for physicians, 166
  rising health care costs and,
    168–169
Economic resources, scarcity of, 112
EdD. See Doctor of education
Eden, M., 460
Eden Alternative model, 257
Education. See also Medical education
  health status and, 106–107
  in hospital-based schools of
    nursing, 11
  of political selves, 295–296
  quality and, 329
Educational applications, 370–371

  competency determinations with,
    370–371
  education evaluated with, 370
  education provided by, 370
Educational institutions, within U.S.
  healthcare delivery system, 72, 73t
Educational reform, growth of
  professional sovereignty and, 135,
  140–141
Educational requirements, for advanced
  practice nursing, 2–3
Educational standards, nursing
  specialties and, 26–27
Education funding, problem
  identification and, 296–297
Effectiveness research, 463
Efficiency, 282
  budget variance for nursing and, 215
e-health, 156, 160, 247
80/20 rule (Pareto principle), 58, 327, 330
Eisenberg, B., 265
Eisenberg, D. M., 131
Eisenhower, Dwight D., 149
Eisenhower administration, civil rights
  legislation and, 510
Elderly population
  chronic care environment and, 269
  demand for physicians and, 262
  geriatrics training and care for, 263
  Medicare and, 151–152
  public entitlement programs and,
    247–248
Electronic medical records, 338
Eliot, Charles, 140
Ellis, R., 480
Elmore, J. A., 506
e-mail, 61, 363
Emergency care, 530–531
Emergency departments
  partial access and, 81
  uninsured population seeking care
    in, 168
EMILY'S list, 312
Emotional dissatisfaction, 511
Empathy, 413, 427–428, 501
Empirical knowledge, 414
Empirical standards, quality assessment
  and, 460–461
Empiricism, 435, 479
  criticism of, 439–440
Empiricist paradigm, 438, 444
  interpretative paradigm vs.,
    436–437t
Empirics, 375, 409, 419, 420, 421t, 439
  Carper's description of, 420
  essential elements, 423t
  personal knowing and, 427t

science of nursing, 410, 420–422
Employee Benefit Research Institute, 151
Employee Retirement and Income
  Security Act of 1974, 174, 175, 237,
  254
Employer-based health insurance, 75, 77,
  80, 242
Employer-based regulatory approach, for
  health care financing, 252*t*
Employer mandates, 254
Employers
  power balancing and, 86
  self-funded insurance and, 174
Employment-based health insurance,
  145–146
  trends in, 242–243
Empowerment, through perspective
  transformation, 395
Encouragement, 283
End-of-life care, 88*t*
Enemies, politics and, 307
Energy conservation, personal, time
  management and, 54
Enforcement rule, HPAA, 364
England, national health program
  history in, 147
English language proficiency, limited,
  healthcare services and, 492, 493
Enriched living environments, in
  nursing homes, 257
Environment
  determinants of health and, 105,
    105, 106–108
  developmental health and, 108
  epidemiology triangle and, *97*, 98
  holistic health and, 120
  model of career development and, 49*t*
Environmental health, 102
Environmental Protection Agency, 102
Environment concept, nursing
  metaparadigm and, 383
EPA. *See* Environmental Protection
  Agency
Epidemics, public health and, 141
Epidemiologic methods, applications of,
  454
Epidemiology, 453–454, 467
  experimental, 454
Epidemiology triangle, *97, 97*
Equality
  hospital-based employment and, 511
  justice and, 529–530
Equitable distribution of health care,
  112–116
  market justice, 113–114
  social justice, 114–116
Equity, 117–119

distributional efficiency and, 118–119
  in health care, 94
  limitations of market justice and, 119
Erikson, Erik, 389, 393
ERISA. *See* Employee Retirement and
  Income Security Act of 1974
Errors. *See* Medical errors
*Essentials of Baccalaureate Education for
  Professional Nursing* (AACN), 29
*Essentials of Doctoral Education for
  Advanced Nursing Practice* (AACN), 2
*Essentials of Master's Education for Advanced
  Practice Nursing* (AACN), 29
Estes, C. L., 204
Esthetic pattern of knowing, 413
Esthetics, 375, 409, 419, 420, 421*t,* 439
  art of nursing, 411–412, 427–429
  essential elements of, 429*t*
  scientific meaning *vs.,* 412–413
Ethical codes, role of, 548–549
Ethical theories, 522–524
  consequential or teleological ethics,
    522–523
  deontological ethics, 523–524
  nonconsequential ethics, 523
  normative ethics, 522
Ethics, 375, 410, 419, 420, 421*t,* 439,
  488, 517–540
  applied, 522
  cardiopulmonary resuscitation and,
    519
  consequential, 522–523
  contextual, 546
  deontological, 523–524
  descriptive, 547–548
  essential elements in, 425*t*
  experimental epidemiology and, 454
  first kidney transplant and, 519
  Harvard Medical School report on
    brain death criteria, 519
  Health Insurance Portability and
    Accountability Act and, 522
  Human Genome Project and, 522
  informed consent case (1972), 520
  Kennedy Institute of Ethics
    (Georgetown), 520
  military tribunal for war crimes
    (1946), 519
  as moral component, 415–416,
    422–424
  nonconsequential, 523
  normative, 522, 547, 548
  Nuremberg Trials, 519
  Oregon's Death with Dignity Act,
    521
  paternalism questioned, 520
  Patient Self-Determination Act, 521

physician-assisted suicide and, 521
  President's Commission for Study
    of Ethical Problems in
    Medicine, 521
  President's Council on Bioethics, 522
  program evaluation and, 294
  research, 464–465
  secular, 524
  situational, 537
  substituted judgment, 520–521
  Tuskegee Study of syphilis, 518
  use of term, 518
  views of, for nursing, 544–545
    codes of ethics, 545
    founders' views, 544–545
  World Medical Association, 519
Ethnic identity, nursing domains and, 496
Ethnicity, healthcare workforce and, 264
Ethnography, 440
Euro-American culture, shift to
  pluralism and, 491
Europe
  healthcare delivery system in U.S.
    vs., 129
  hospitals in, 132
  institutional dissimilarities
    between U.S. and, 147
  medical schools in, 134
  national health program history in,
    147
  universal health care in, 118
Euthanasia, 522
Evaluation
  application of, to nursing process,
    386*t*
  of education, 370
  policy process and, 290, 294–295
  theory-based nursing practice and,
    394*t*
Evidence, grading of, 337
Evidence-based health care
  era of, 267–269, 270
  values-based practice and, 406–407
Evidence-based medicine, 336
  defined, 461
  research findings and, 461–462
Evidence-based practice, 286, 324,
  337–338
  clarion call for, 402–403
  clinical process improvement and,
    336–339
  summary of, and five-step process,
    337*t*
Executive branch of government, 289
Exercise
  reducing risk of colon cancer and,
    108

stress management and, 64
Expanding consciousness, health as, 387
Expenses, 211
Experimental epidemiology, 454
Explanatory theories, 374
Explicit standards, quality assessment and, 460

F

Facilitator, 334, 335t
Faculty development grants, nursing research and, 298
Faculty qualifications, nursing education and, 34–35
Faculty Research Development Grants Program, 35
Fadiman, A., 495
Fagin, C., 430, 483
Fairness, 534
Faith, 96, 524
Faithfulness, 534
Family development models, 387
Family health promotion model, 389
Family interactional models, 387–388
Family medicine, proportion of women in, 262
Family models, 393, 395
    types of, 387–388
Family structural-functional models, 388
Family systems models, 388
Faults in systems, looking for, quality leadership and, 326t, 327
Fawcett, J., 375, 383, 384, 389, 390, 434, 443
Faxing, 363
Federal Employee Health Benefits program, 250
Federal government, biomedical research funding and, 464
Federally qualified health center, 81
Federal Register, 352
Federal Trade Commission, 293
Fee-for-service payment era, 205
Fee-for-service payments, 222
Fein, R., 198
Fellowships, nursing research and, 298
Feminism, 479
Feminist consciousness raising, 15–16
Feminization, of physician workforce, 262
Fidelity, 534
    ANA Code of Ethics and, 552
Field, Justice Stephen J., 140
Financial analysis statements, 212
    standard, 212t
Financial resources management, 203–217

accounting concepts, 210–211
for advanced practice nurses, 209–216
financial results and quality outcomes, 216–217
healthcare environment: deciding whether health care is a right or a privilege, 204–209
introductory remarks on, 203–204
Financial terms, relationship among, 212t
Financing health care, 163–198
    Balanced Budget Act of 1997, 185–191
    components of healthcare expenditures, 169–170
    concluding remarks on, 198
    evolution of health insurance: third-party payment, 171–174
    expenditures in perspective, 164–169
        aging population, 166
        economic incentives that fuel rising costs, 168–169
        growth of specialized medicine, 166–167
        labor-intensive industry, 168
        new diagnostic and treatment technology, 165–166
        uninsured and underinsured, 168
    future of: continuing change, 197–198
    future options in, 246–249
    government as a source of payment, 175–176
    within healthcare delivery system, 75, 76, 78
    introductory remarks about, 163–164
    long-term care challenges and, 256–257
    Medicaid, 192–197
        Balanced Budget Act of 1997, 194–197
    Medicare, 176–185
    Medicare Prescription Drug, Improvement, and Modernization Act of 2003, 191–192
    other government-funded services, 197
    self-funded insurance programs, 174–175
    sources of healthcare payment, 170–171
Finer, H., 473
Fiscal year, 213
Fishbone diagrams, 330, 334t

Fitzpatrick, J. J., 477
Fixed costs, 211
Flarey, D. L., 286
Flash drives, 363
Fleming, Alexander, 137 (exhibit)
Flexner, Abraham, 33, 140
Flexner Report, 140
Flip charts, 333
Flowcharts, 330, 334t
Folkman, 387
Food and Drug Administration, 259, 520
Food contaminants, 106
Food safety, 100
Forand, Aime, 152
Force field, 105, 106
Ford, 478
Forecasting and projecting, budget planning and, 213
Foreign direct investment, in health services enterprises, 157
Foreign nurses, importation of, 512
Forgiveness, practicing, 64
Formal mentorship programs, 45
For profit organizations, accounting and, 210
Fourteenth Amendment, to Constitution, 526
FQHC. See Federally qualified health center
Framingham (Mass.) heart disease study, 453–454
Frances Payne Bolton School of Nursing (Case Western Reserve University), 36–37
Franklin, Martha, 509
Fraud, healthcare, HIPAA and prevention of, 364
Freedom, 534
Freedom through control, quality improvement and, 326–327, 326t
Free market approach, to health care financing reorganization, 251t
Free-market conditions
    health care in United States and, 81–84, 89–90
    price, supply, and demand under, 82, 82, 83–84
Freire, P., 404
Friedman, M. M., 388, 393
Friends, politics and, 307
From Novice to Expert (Benner), 425
FTC. See Federal Trade Commission
FTE. See Full-time equivalent
Full-risk HMOs, 233
Full-time equivalent, 261
Functional nursing, 13
Functional status, components of, 463

"Fundamental Patterns of Knowing in Nursing" (Carper), 419, 420
Fund balance, changes in, 212, 212*t*
Funding
  of doctoral studies, 35
  of education, problem identification and, 296–297
  of nurse scientist graduate training grants, 36
  of nursing education, 14
Funeral benefits, 148
Future of health services delivery, 241–270
  bioterrorism and transformation of public health, 258–260
  challenges for managed care, 249–250
    accountability, 250
    management of risk, 249
  comprehensive reform, 250, 252–254
    employer mandates, 254
    managed competition, 252–253
    play-or-pay coverage, 253
    single-payer health plans, 250, 252
  concluding remarks about, 269–270
  enhanced focus on customer service, 265–266
  evidence-based health care and, 267–269
  financing and insurance options, 246–249
    defined contribution plans, 246–247
    high-risk pools, 249
    public entitlement programs, 247–248
    tax credits and vouchers, 248–249
  healthcare workforce and, 261–264
    deficits in geriatric training, 263
    supply and demand for nurses, 262–263
    supply and demand for physicians, 261–262
    workforce diversity, 263–264
  hospitals in U.S. and, 260–261
  introductory remarks about, 241–242
  national and global challenges, 254–258
    challenges of chronic illness care, 255–256
    infectious diseases and globalization, 257–258
    long-term care challenges, 256–257
    wellness, prevention, and health promotion, 254–255
  new frontiers in clinical technology, 266–267
  trends in private and public health insurance, 242–246
    for employment-based insurance, 242–243
    high-deductible health plans, 243–244
    insurance restructuring in Massachusetts, 244–245
    for Medicare and Medicaid, 245–246
  work organization, 264–265
    collaborative team approach, 264–265
    cross-training, 265
FY. *See* Fiscal year

G

Gadow, 424
Gamel, C., 28
Gaming, education applications and, 370
Gap analysis, 331
GATS. *See* General Agreement on Trade in Services
Gay Men's Health Crisis, 292
GDP. *See* Gross domestic product
Gebbie, Kristine, 279
Gender
  pay disparities and, 264
  roots of nursing and, 9–10
General Agreement on Trade in Services, 155
General Electric, 335
Generalists
  proportion of specialists to, 141
  shortage of, 262
Generalizability, empirical research and, 438
General practitioners, in Britain, 141
Gene therapy, 109, 267, 270
Genetic engineering, 267
Genetic makeup, as health determinant, 105, *105*
Genetic mapping, 267
Genomics research, 466
George, V. D., 506, 514
Georgetown University, Kennedy Institute of Ethics at, 520
Geriatricians, 263
Geriatric training, deficits in, 263, 270
German graduate school model, 33
Germany
  compulsory sickness insurance in, 146
  national health program history in, 147
Germ theory of disease, 137 (exhibit)
Geyman, J. P., 218
GI bill, 297
Gigahertz, 362
Gilligan, C., 423
Gladwell, Malcolm, 27
Glaser, B. G., 474
Glass ceiling, 19
Globalization, 130, 156–158, 160
  infectious diseases and, 257–258
GMHC. *See* Gay Men's Health Crisis
Goals, 289
  ethics and, 415
  policy and, 288
  within Professional Development Plan, 51*t*
Goal setting
  benefits of, 51
  time management and, 57–58
Godin, 318
Goeppinger, J., 389
Goggin, M. L., 294
Goldmark report, 11
Goldstein, R. L., 510
Goodin, H. J., 511
Goodman, K. W., 403
Goodrich, Annie, 545
Gortner, S. R., 438
Goverde, K., 28
Government
  executive branch of, 289
  health planning and, 116
  legislative branch of, 289
  nursing shortage, minorities and intervention by, 512
  as payment source, 175–176
  policy process and response by, 292–293
Government agencies, U.S. healthcare delivery system and, 72, 74
Government spending, justice and, 529–530
GPs. *See* General practitioners
Grading evidence, 337
Graduate degrees, education funding and, 296–297
Graduate education, 14
  for nurses, 277
  political self and, 295–296
Grand theories, 374, 383
Great Britain, national health insurance in, 175
Great Depression, 11–12, 13, 144, 148
  nursing procedures evaluation and, 472
Great Society, 24, 152
Green House Project, 257

Gross domestic product, 220, 246
    national health expenditures as
        share of, 164, *165*
Grossman, M., 113
Gross revenue, 211, 212*t*
Grounded theory, 440
Ground rules, 334–335, 335*t*
Group Health Association of America, 234
Group Health Cooperative of Puget
    Sound (Seattle), 154, 227
Group health insurance, collective
    bargaining and, 153
Group HMOs, 224
Group nursing, 13
Group practice, 153, 154
Group rates, health insurance, 77
Grypdonck, M., 28
Guba, E. G., 434
GUI, 363
Guidelines, improving, 268–269
Gulf of Tonkin incident (1964), 535
Gun laws, 306

H

Haas, J. E., 278
Habermas, J., 404
Haislmaier, E. F., 245
Haitian culture, 495
Hall, Lydia, 13, 16, 385
Halm, E. A., 268
Hamilton, D., 545
Hammer, M., 325
Hammurabi, 524, 525
Hamric, A., 23
Hand washing, 100
Hanson, C., 23
Hantavirus, 258
Happiness, time management and, 54
Hardware, 362–363
Hardy, M. E., 435, 444
Harrington, C., 204
Harvard College, 32
Harvard Medical School
    medical education reform and, 140
    report on brain death criteria by, 519
Harvard University, 134
Hassenplug, Lulu Wolf, 475
Hawaii, employer mandates in, 254
HCBW. *See* Home and Community
    Based Waiver
HDHPs. *See* High-deductible health
    plans
Healing
    cultural belief systems and,
        494–495
    spirituality and, 524

Health
    determinants of, 104–108
    developmental, 101
    holistic approach to, 93
    medical model and, 94–95
    medical sociology definition of,
        94–95
    public, 101–102
    social model of, 111–112
    varying definitions of, 94–95
    WHO definition of, 494
Health Affairs, 69
Health care. *See also* Financing health
    care
    changing paradigm in, 284–288
    continuous quality improvement
        introduced to, 324–328
    disparities in, 488, 494
    equitable distribution of, 112–116
    financing of, 208–209
    old paradigm *vs.* new paradigm of,
        287*t*
    rise in cost of, 135, 151, 163, 204,
        219–220, 242, 246
Healthcare delivery
    changing paradigm in and changes
        in nursing practice, 275–276
    complexity of, 75, 76
    corporatization of, 155–156
    organization of, in U.S., 117
    overarching factors and
        implications for, 109–111
    trends and directions in, 88
Healthcare delivery system
    basic components of, 75–77
        delivery, 75–76, 76
        financing, 75, 76, 78
        insurance, 75, 76, 78
        payment, 76, 76–77, 78
    blend of public and private
        involvement in, 74
    description of, 72, 74–75
    disenfranchised segment within,
        77–78
    external forces having effects on, 80
    objectives for, 75
    overview of scope and size of, 72
    primary characteristics of, in U.S.,
        79–87
        continuum of services, 79, 87
        high technology, 79, 87
        imperfect market, 79, 81–84
        legal risks, 79, 87
        multiple payers, 79, 85–86
        no central agency, 79–81
        partial access, 79, 81
        power balancing, 79, 86–87

    quest for quality, 79, 87
        third-party insurers and payers,
            79, 84–85
    quality of life and, 104
    significance for healthcare
        practitioners and policy
        makers, 88–89
    transition from traditional insurance
        to managed care, 78–79
    trends and directions, 87–88
    understanding, 68
    uniqueness of, in United States,
        71–90
Healthcare documentation, digitization
    of, 402
Healthcare dollar, national: where it
    came from (2003), *171*
Healthcare ethics, scope of, 518
Healthcare ethics principles, 525–531
    age and justice, 530
    autonomy, 525–526
    beneficence, 526–527
    emergency care, 530–531
    injustice for the insured, 530
    justice, 527, 529
        government spending and,
            529–530
    nonmaleficence, 527
Healthcare expenditures
    components of, 169–170
    factors related to growth in, 164–165
    national
        in perspective, 164
        as a share of the gross domestic
            product, 164, *165*
Health Care Financing Administration,
    236, 279
Health care financing reorganization,
    general approaches for, 251–252*t*
Healthcare morass, 535
Healthcare payments, sources of, 170–171
Healthcare problems, defining, 292
Healthcare quality, 323–344
    accreditation and regulatory focus
        on, 339–343
    clinical process improvement and
        evidence-based practice, 336–339
    continuous quality improvement
        and, 324–328
    quality improvement successes and,
        335–336
    tools and techniques for improving
        quality and performance,
        328–335
Healthcare Research and Quality Act of
    1999, 456
Healthcare services, continuum of, 88*t*

Healthcare setting, selection of models and theories and, 390

Healthcare systems in 21st century, factors related to changes in, 286

Healthcare systems model, 393

Health Care USA (Sultz and Young), 68

Health concept, nursing metaparadigm and, 383

Health Confidence Survey (2006), 151

Health determinants, relative contribution of, to premature death, 105, *105*

Health disparities, *Healthy People 2010* initiative and elimination of, 123–124

Health information technology, 118

Health insurance
access and, 81
coverage of children, by income, 2003, *196*
disenfranchised persons and, 77–78
employer-based, 75, 77
employment-based, 80, 145–146
future options in, 246–249
history behind, 172
lack of, growth of healthcare expenditures and, 168
moral hazard and, 84
in United States, 116–117

Health Insurance Experiment (RAND), 457, 458

Health insurance movement, technological, social, and economic factors related to, 143–144

Health Insurance Portability and Accountability Act of 1996, 186, 244, 361, 522
enactment of, 364, 365
enforcement of, 365
security rule control safeguards, 365*t*
Title I and Title II of, 364
Title I highlights, 364*t*

Health insurance premiums
increases in, compared to other indicators, *230*
rise in cost of, 242

Health Maintenance Organization Act of 1973, 155, 222, 223–225

Health maintenance organizations, 74, 78, 141, 155, 205
failures of, 208
managed care *vs.*, 222–223
outcomes research and, 467

Health plan, 78

Health Plan Employer Data and Information Set, 235, 236

Health plan enrollment, for covered workers, by plan type, 1988-2004, *227*

Health planning, government and, 116

Health plans, 82
performance rating of, 83
single-payer, 250, 251*t*, 252

Health policy, health services research and, 457–458

Health professionals, healthcare delivery system and, 88–89

Health promotion, 99–100, 120
future of, 254–255
secondary status of, in U.S., 94

Health protection, 102–104

Health reimbursement arrangements, 243, 244

Health Resources and Service Administration Bureau of Health Professions, 512

Health Resources and Services Administration, 263, 511

Health savings accounts, 118, 243, 244, 247

Health Security Act of 1993, 252

Health services research, 454–457
Agency for Healthcare Research and Quality and, 455–457
health policy and, 457–458

Health Services Utilization study, 458

Health status, education and, 106–107

Health status indicators, 121

Healthy People 2000: National Health Promotion and Disease Prevention, 121

Healthy People 2010: Healthy People in Healthy Communities, 121–124, *122,* 254

Healthy People 2010 focus areas, 123 (exhibit), 124

Healthy People initiatives, 93, 121–124

Heart disease, 107
diet and, 108
genetic mapping and, 267

Heart failure, Hospital Quality Initiative and focus on, 342

HEDIS. *See* Health Plan Employer Data and Information Set

Hegyvary, S., 281

Helton, A., 389

Henderson, Virginia, 13, 281, 473, 475

Henry Street Settlement House, 314, 508, 545

Henry Street Settlement Visiting Nursing Service, 508

Hepatitis B, 158

Hepatitis C, 158, 258

Heredity, health and, 108–109

Hermeneutics, 440, 479

Hewitt Associates, 247

HF. *See* Heart failure

HHS. *See* Department of Health and Human Services

Hierarchy of needs (Maslow), 389

High-alert medications, 356

High-deductible health plans, 243–244

High-risk pools, 249

High technology, 219
healthcare delivery and, 87

Hill, 488

Hill-Burton funds, 177

Hine, D. C., 506

HIPAA. *See* Health Insurance Portability and Accountability Act

HIP Health Plan of New York, 154

Hippocratic oath, 545

HIS. *See* Hospital information systems

Hispanics, 492, 501

Historicism, 438

HIT. *See* Health information technology

HIV. *See* Human immunodeficiency virus

HIV/AIDS epidemic, 258, 270

Hmong culture, 495

HMOs. *See* Health maintenance organizations

Hobbies, 64

Holism, 120
cultural competence and, 499
Native American point of view and, 496

Holistic health care, 68, 124
dimensions of, *95,* 95–96
integrated model for, 120, *120*

Home and Community Based Waiver, 257

Home health care, 87, 156, 277

Homeland security, public health and, 258

Homeland Security Act of 2002, 103

Homeopaths, 131

H-1A visas, for foreign nurses, 513

Honesty, 534–535
summary case, 538–539

Hope, 96, 536

Horizontal integration, 207, 208

Hospice care, by nurses, 277

Hospital administrators, cost containment and, 284

Hospital Association Act, 154

Hospital-based nursing schools, 11

Hospital care
healthcare expenditures and, 169, *170*
IOM study on medical errors and, 461
rise in expenditures for, 219

trends in, *220*
Hospital infections, staphylococcus and, 466
Hospital Insurance Trust Fund, 185
Hospital performance data, patient-severity adjusted, 461
Hospital Quality Alliance, 342
Hospital Quality Initiative (CMS), 342
Hospitals, 286
    charity funds to, 530
    community, 121
    equal access to employment in, 511
    future outlook for, in U.S., 260–261
    during Great Depression, 144
    information systems in, 365–366
    institutionalization and, 137–138
    merchant marine, 147
    new roles for nurses in, 277
    nursing expertise in, 276
    operating margin for, 208
    organizational culture of, 12
    outcomes research and, 467
    in preindustrial America, 132
    social reformism and growth of, 11
    specialty, 157
Hospital stays, shortened, 402
Hospital Trust Fund, 187
Host, epidemiology triangle and, 97, *97*
House of Representatives, 300, 308
HRAs. *See* Health reimbursement arrangements
HSAs. *See* Health savings accounts
HSIs. *See* Health status indicators
Hughes, C. E., 8
Human conservation principles, nursing activities and, 385
Human genome, commercialism, ethics and, 465
Human Genome Project, 522
Human genome sequence, 522
Human immunodeficiency virus, 142
    CNSs and persons with, 24
    globalization and, 158
Humanistic nursing model, 387
Human relations school of management, 13
Human subjects, National Research Act and, 520
Humor, 64
Huntington's disease, genetic mapping and, 267
Hurricanes, 259
Hussein, Saddam, 535
Hypertension, 97

dietary choices and treatment of, 108
screening for, 100

I

Iacocca, Lee, 221
Identity, culture and, 501
Ideological differences, failure of national healthcare intitatives and, 148–149
IDS. *See* Integrated delivery system
Illinois Institute of Technology Web site, 549
Illness
    behavioral risk factors and, 98
    disease and, 97–98
    wellness promotion and, 88
Imaging technologies, new frontiers in, 266–267
Immigration, 492
Immigration Nursing Relief Acts of 1986, 1989, and 1990, 513
Immunizations, 100, 101
Immunology, 136
Implementation
    application of, to nursing process, 386*t*
    policy process and, 290, 293–294
    theory-based nursing practice and, 394*t*
Important tasks, urgent tasks *vs.,* 58, 59
Incentive payments, Medicare beneficiaries and, 343
Income inequality, health indicators and, 107
Incrementalism, 280
India
    Apollo hospital chain in, 157
    tobacco industry and, 158
Indiana University, 38
Indian culture, gender and, 110
Indian Health Service, 175
Indirect costs, 211
Individual health, integration of community health and, 119–124
Individualism, national healthcare initiatives and, 148
Individual practice associations, 224, 226
Industrial accidents, 102
    workers' compensation and, 143
Industrial capitalism, 135
Industrialization, 11
Industrial management methods, 12
Industry performance metrics, 210
Infant mortality, 121
    partial access and, in United States, 81

redistributive policies and, 107
Infectious diseases, 269
    drug-resistant pathogens and, 466
    globalization and, 158, 257–258
    role of public health and, 142
Infectious waste, 102
Inflation, 164, 208, 220
Influenza epidemic of 1918, racial quotas and, 508
Influenza virus, new forms of, 258
Informal mentorship, 45
Information, 282
Information management, 338–339
Information revolution, 130, 156, 160
Information technology, 165
    administrative systems, 368–370
    for advanced nursing practice, 361–371
    clinical systems, 366–368
    educational applications, 370–371
    hardware, 362–363
    hospital information systems, 365–366
    long-term care challenges and, 257
    managing, 338–339
    patient data and, 361
    privacy and confidentiality issues, 364–365
    security considerations, 363–364
    software, 363
Informed consent, 520, 521, 528–529
    normative ethics and, 548
Infusion pumps, improving safe use of, 356
Injustice, for the insured, 530
Injustice, political participation and, 306
Inkjet printers, 363
INP/APNN. *See* International Nurse Practitioner/Advanced Practice Nursing Network
Input devices, 362
In re Conroy, 527
Institute for Healthcare Improvement Web site, 338
Institute for Safe Medication Practice, 354
Institute for the Future, 266
Institute of Medicine, 19, 101, 318, 354, 458, 505
    healthcare quality reports of, 340–342
    medical errors study by, 461
    patient safety and first report and responses by, 349–353
    patient safety and second report and responses by, 353–355
Institutional core, primitive, in preindustrial America, 132–133

Institutional dissimilarities, failure of national healthcare intitatives and, 147–148
Institutionalization, growth of professional sovereignty and, 135, 137–138
Instrumental value, 532
Insurance
    assurance *vs.*, 173
    within healthcare delivery system, 75, 76, 78
    intermediary role of, 85
    purpose of, 84
    self-funded, 174–175
Insurance companies, reimbursement through, 76–77
Insurance restructuring, in Massachusetts, 242, 244–245
Insured patients, injustice for, 530
Insurers, within U.S. healthcare delivery system, 72, 73*t*
Integrated delivery systems, 83, 207
Integration, 510
    multiple paradigms and, 445
Integration theory, 443
Integrity, 300, 415, 533, 536
Intensive care units, 276
Interdependent relationships, patient safety and, 347
Interdisciplinary teams, 285
Interest groups, 289
Internal Revenue code, employer-sponsored health insurance and, 146
Internal Revenue Service, health reimbursement arrangements and, 243
International Council of Nurses, 27, 28, 555
International Nurse Practitioner/Advanced Practice Nursing Network, 28
International Society of Nurses in Genetics, 555
Internet, 156, 338, 370
    e-health plans and, 247
    medical information on, 83
Internship programs, political, nurses participation in, 279
Interpersonal model, 385
Interpersonal Relations in Nursing (Peplau), 400
Interpretative paradigm, 444
Interpretative paradigm, 375, 440–441
    criticisms of, 441–442
    empiricist paradigm *vs.*, 436–437*t*
Interpretative statements, ANA *Code of Ethics* and, 552–555
Interpreter services, 493*t*

Interruptions, controlling, 60
Interventions, therapeutic, 100
In the Matter of Karen Ann Quinlan, 520–521
Intrinsic value, 532
Intuitive knowing, 427
IOM. *See* Institute of medicine
IPAs. *See* Individual practice associations
Irreversible coma (brain death), 519
Ischemic heart disease, 107
ISMP. *See* Institute for Safe Medication Practice
IT. *See* Information technology
Item-based pricing, 83
"I-Thou" encounter, personal knowledge and, 413–414
IV pumps, 368

J

Jacobs-Kramer, M., 419, 420, 421, 422, 424, 426, 428, 429
James, P., 415
Japan, total quality management approach and, 324
JCAHO, 354
    patient safety and, 357
Jenkins, J., 18, 477
Jim Crow, 506, 513
JNC-7, 403
Job dissatisfaction, 511
Job stress, 62
Johns Hopkins University, 38, 140
Johnson, 387, 393
Johnson, Lyndon B., 152, 535
Johnson, R. W., 242
Johnson, Samuel, 534
Johnson administration, civil rights legislation and, 510
Joiner, B. L., 324, 335
Joiner triangle, 328, *328*
Joint Commission on Accreditation of Health Care Organizations, 339–340, 459
    patient safety and, 348–349, 354–355
Joint Commission on Accreditation of Hospitals, 176
Journal of the American Medical Association, 475
Journals, 8, 64
Judaism, 523
Judeo-Christian ethics, 518
Judicial interpretations, 289
Julian, J., 474
Jump drives, 363
Juran, J. M., 324, 327, 335

Justice, 527, 529
    age and, 530
    distributive, 529, 531
    government spending and, 529–530
    in health care, 94
    in U.S. health delivery system, 116–117
        health insurance, 116–117
        organization of healthcare delivery, 117

K

Kaiser, Henry J., 154
Kaiser Family Foundation, Henry J., 192
Kaiser-Permanente Health Care System, 154, 155, 205, 224
Kalisch, B. J., 509
Kalisch, P. A., 509
"Kangaroo care," 481, 482
Kaptchuk, T. J., 131
Kassenbaum-Kennedy Bill, 186
Keen, D. J., 208
Keeping Patients Safe: Transforming the Work Environment of Nurses (IOM), 341–342
Kellogg Foundation Nursing Service Administration Research Project, 473
Kennedy, E., 283
Kennedy, M. S., 482
Kennedy Institute of Ethics (Georgetown University), 520
Kenney, J. W., 375, 380
Kerr-Mills Act of 1960, 152, 193
Kevorkian, Jack, 521
Keyboards, 362
Kidney transplants, first, 519
Kim, H. S., 389, 390, 434
Kimball, J. F., 144
Kindness, 536
King, I. M., 281, 387
King's College, 134
Kirkpatrick, C., 354, 355, 356
Klein, E., 48
Knights Templar, 10
Knowing, 375
    distinguishing patterns of, 417
    fundamental patterns of, in nursing, 409–417
    identifying patterns of, 409–416
        current stages, 411
        empirics, 410
        esthetic pattern of knowing, 413
        esthetics, 411–412
        esthetics *vs.* scientific meaning, 412–413
        ethics, 415–416

new perspectives, 410–411
personal knowledge and, 413–415
patterns of, 419
using, 416–417
Knowledge workers, 282
requirements for, 283
Kohlberg, L., 423
Kongstvedt, Peter, 225
Kramer, F. M., 37
Krysl, M., 426
Kuhn, T. S., 410, 422, 434, 435, 442, 443, 444
Kushner, Harold, 536

L

Labor
health care industry and, 168
instability in nursing labor force, 13–14
"Taylorism" and, 12
Laboratory, 368
Laboratory technologists, 141
Labor Health Institute (St. Louis), 154
La Guardia, Fiorello, 154
Langer, S. K., 413
Language, cultural competence and, 492, 493
Laparoscopic procedures, 165
Laser printers, 363
Lassiter, P. G., 389
Laudan, L., 447
Law(s), 289
government response to public problems and, 292
nursing practice and, 278
policy and, 289
Lawsuits, healthcare delivery and, 87
Layoffs, 285
Lazarus, 387
Leaders, team, 333, 335t
Leadership
new paradigms for, 283, 284
patient safety standards and, 357
promoting culture of quality and, 318
for quality, 329
Leahey, M., 388
Leapfrog Group, 286, 338, 351, 354
Legislation
majority rule and passage of, 309
policy process and, 290
Legislative branch of government, lawmaking and, 289
Legislative process, nurses, public policy and, 278, 290–291

Leininger, Madeleine, 281, 387, 488
transcultural model of, 496, 497, 498–500
Length of stay, 206
Leone, Lucile Petry, 472, 473, 474, 475
Lester, J. P., 294
Letters
to the editor, effectiveness of, 310
as lobbying tools, 309
Letting go, 62
Levine, 385
Lewis, Charles, 478
Liabilities, 212
Libertarianism, market justice and, 114
Licensing, 159
growth of professional sovereignty and, 135, 139–140
Licensure, 276
multistate, 299
Life, preservation of, 536
Life cycle, of families, 387
Life expectancy
chronic disorders and increase in, 255
Healthy People 2010 initiative and, 123, 124
increase in, 142
partial access and, in United States, 81
Lifestyle and behaviors, as health determinants, 104, 104
Lifestyle risk factors, 108
Light pens, 362
Lincoln, Y. S., 434
Lindeman, Carol, 475, 476
Lindsey, 479
Line item, 214
LINUX, 363
Lister, Joseph, 137 (exhibit)
Literature, nursing theoretical, 400
Literature criteria, selection of relevant models, theories and, 389
Lobbyists, 278, 280, 314
Local public health agencies, 260
Loeb Center, Montefiore Medical Center (New York City), 13, 16, 475
Logical empiricism, 402
Logical positivism, 402, 435–436, 439
Logs, time management, 56, 56t
Long-term care, 88t
future and challenges with, 256–257
financing, 256–257
information technology, 257
infrastructure, 257
regulation, 257
resources, 257

workforce, 257
insurance for, 171
projected expenditures for, 255
Long-term planning, 283
LOS. See Length of stay
Lo Sasso, A. T., 242
Louis Harris and Associates, 149
Louisiana State Nurses Association, 510
Loveland-Cherry, C. J., 389
Lowi, T., 293
LTC. See Long-term care
Luft, H., 222
Lumby, J., 428
Lung cancer, 107
Luther Hospital (Wisconsin), 475
Lyme disease, 258

M

Macroethics, 518
MADD. See Mothers Against Drunk Driving
Magnet Hospital program, 19
Magnet hospitals, attraction of, 19
Magnetic resonance imaging, 165
Mahoney, Mary, 507
Majority rule, 307–309
Major medical expense coverage, birth of, 146
Making Healthcare Safer: A Critical Analysis of Patient Safety (AHRQ), 351
Malloch, K., 350
Malone, Beverly, 279
Malpractice lawsuits, 87, 348
Mammograms, 100, 121
Managed care, 69, 120, 130, 160, 163–164, 219–238, 242, 243, 269
backlash to, 229, 230–231, 237
corporatization of health care and, 156
emerging developments in, 228–232
evolution of, 225–228
features of, 154
fundamentals of, 221–223
future challenges for, 249–250
accountability, 250
risk management, 249
future of, 237
healthcare expenditures and impact of, 164
health maintenance organizations vs., 222–223
HMO Act of 1973 and, 223–225
introductory remarks on, 219–221
Medicaid and enrollment in, 195, 195

Medicare and Medicaid and,
232–234
morass of, 535
nursing responses to, 286
performance measures and, 467
prices, payers and, 82
research studies and, 465
rise of, 155
technology and, 166
transition from traditional
insurance to, 78–79
Managed care enrollees, number of,
selected years, 1988-2000, *226*
Managed care organizations, 75, 135,
155, 223, 247
accountability and, 230
changes in, 231–232
mixed-model, 226
performance measures, categories
of, 235–236
power balancing and, 86
quality and, 234–237
reimbursement and, 76
risk management and, 249
trends with, 227
within U.S. healthcare delivery
system, 72, 73*t*
women workers in, 263
Managed care prototypes, 153–155
contract practice, 153–154
group practice, 154
prepaid group plans, 154–155
Managed competition, 252–253
Managerialism, 12
Managing accounting and financial
analysis, 211–213
basic financial terms, 211
financial analysis statements,
212–213
Mandrack, M. M., 356
Man–living–health theory, 387
Manthey, M., 16, 18
Marches, 292
Margin, 211, 212, 212*t*
Marginalization, 493
Market-based healthcare system,
outcomes of, 208
Marketing, of prescription drugs, 166
Market justice, 118, 124
equitable distribution of health
care and, 113–114
limitations of, 119
social justice *vs.*, 115*t*
Marram, G., 16
Maslow, Abraham, 389, 414
Maslow's hierarchy of needs, 389
Massachusetts

development of public health
system in, 142
health insurance market
restructuring in, 242,
244–245, 253
Massachusetts General Hospital, 18, 137
(exhibit)
Massage, 64
Massey, E., 506
Mass production, 135
Master of Science in Nursing
curriculum, research in, 375
Master's degrees, 2, 3, 27, 32, 38–39,
279, 281, 297
Master's programs in nursing, 400
political leadership training and,
295
Mature science, characteristics of,
442–443
Mayeroff, M., 424, 425, 430
Mayo Clinic, 154, 157, 247
McCarthy, Caroline, 306
McClellan, M., 248
McCracken, Robert J., 534
McCubbin, H. I., 387
McCubbin, M. A., 387
McFarland, M., 496, 499
McFarlane, J. M., 389
McKay, R., 388, 414
McKenna, H., 381, 382, 389, 390
McLaughlin Group, The, 298
MCOs. *See* Managed care organizations
MD. *See* Doctor of medicine (MD)
Meaning, 96
Means testing, 248
Media, healthcare agenda setting and, 292
Medicaid, 25, 72, 74, 77, 80, 82, 86,
111, 116, 117, 129, 172, 175, 186,
192–197, 205, 219, 250, 253, 256,
279, 454, 483
Balanced Budget Act of 1997 and,
194–197
Bush administration and cuts in, 118
creation of, 135, 151–153, 160
curtailed spending in future and, 248
enactment of, 192
future trends in, 245–246
growth in share of beneficiaries
enrolled in managed care,
1991-2000, *195*
healthcare payment and, 170, 171
hospital industry and enactment of,
220
intent of, 193
managed care and, 232–234
reasons behind growth in spending
on, 194

taxes on the middle class and, 242
Medicaid managed care enrollment
(1996-2003), Medicaid population
and numbers and percent of, 234*t*
Medical Assistance Act, 152
Medical care
health and, 109
as health determinant, 105, *105*
service categories, 87
Medical care delivery, 94
Medical discoveries, groundbreaking,
137 (exhibit)
Medical education
reform of, 140–141
standardization of, 139
substandard, in preindustrial
America, 134–135
Medical errors, 286, 348, 457
deaths related to, 318, 340
IOM definition of, 350
QuIC's expanded definition of, 352
research on, 461
Medical knowledge, growth in, 464
Medical model, 94–95, 124
wellness model *vs.,* 99
Medical nursing, 276
Medical Outcomes study, 458
Medical pluralism, in preindustrial
America, 131
Medical practice, free entry into, in
preindustrial America, 131
Medical procedures, primitive, in
preindustrial America, 131–132
Medical profession, cultural authority
and, 136
Medical savings accounts, 244, 247
Medical schools
establishment of, in America, 134
in preindustrial America, 134
Medical science, growth in, health
services delivery and, 130
Medical social workers, 141
Medical suppliers, within U.S. healthcare
delivery system, 72, 73*t*
Medical technologies, types of, and future
delivery of patient care, 266–277
Medical Treatment Effectiveness
Program, 456
Medicare, 25, 72, 74, 77, 81, 82, 86,
111, 116, 117, 129, 172, 175, 195,
205, 219, 250, 253, 256, 279, 462
Balanced Budget Act of 1997 and,
164, 185–191
chronology of significant changes
to, 178–179
claims data analysis and, 454

cost containment efforts and, 180–181
creation of, 135, 151–153, 160
diagnosis-related groups and, 181, 183–184, 185, 206, 284
enactment of legislation for, 176
funding of, *vs.* funding of Medicaid, 193
future spending patterns for, 247, 248
future trends in, 245–246
healthcare payment and, 170
hospital industry and enactment of, 220
hospitals, fiscal pressures and, 261
managed care and, 232–234
market forces, managed care principles and, 198
medical advancements and, 182
Part A of, 176–177
Part B of, 177, 184, 188, 245
Part C of, 188
Part D of, 158, 191, 245
patient safety and, 350, 353
pay for performance initiatives and, 343
physician price freeze and, 184
professional standards review organizations and, 179, 180
prospective payment system and, 181–182, 185
reimbursement mechanism for, 177
resource-based relative value scale system and, 184–185
services documentation and, 86
spending by at $85 billion less than projected (FYs 1998-2002), *190*
spending projections for, 177
taxes on the middle class and, 242
Medicare, Medicaid, and State Child Health Insurance Program Benefits Improvement and Protection Act, 164
Medicare Advantage Plan, 191, *233,* 245
Medicare+Choice Program, 187, 188, 190–191, 232
for 1990-2004, *233*
Medicare Conditions of Participation (CoP), 353
Medicare Payment Advisory Commission, 187
Medicare Prescription, Improvement, and Modernization Act of 2003, 191–192, 232, 243, 245, 255
Medication errors, preventing, 368
Medications, high-alert, 356
Medicine

early practice of, in America, 131
specialization in, in postindustrial America, 141
Medi-gap, 177, 185
Meditation, 64, 96
Megahertz, 362
Meleis, A. I., 380, 382, 389, 443, 478
Memory, computer, 362
Meningitis, 472
Mental health, holistic health and, 95, *95*
Mentor criteria, selection of relevant models, theories and, 389
Mentor-mentee relationship
within Barker-Sullivan model, 44, *44*
importance of, 43
stages of, 45–46, 48
development of role competencies (stage two), 46
dissolution of relationship (stage 4), 46, 48
growing independence (stage three), 46
selecting mentor and determining expectations (stage one), 45–46
Mentors, 3, 296
benefits with, 43
defined, 43
selecting, 45–46, 47*t*
Mentorship
Barker-Sullivan model of, 44, *44*
model for, 43–45
networking *vs.,* 48
Merchant marine hospitals, 147
Mergers and acquisitions, 285, 286
Merrill Lynch, 247
Meta-analyses, 456
outcomes research and, 463
Metaethics, 546–547
Metanarrative ideal, of nursing, 444
Metaparadigm concepts, of nursing, 433–434
Metaparadigms, for nursing theory, 375
Metatheory, 374
Metrics, 335
MHPs. *See* Multiskilled health practitioners
Microelectronics, in digital detectors, 266
Microethics, 518
Microphones, 362
Middle Ages, 32
Middle range theories, 374
Midwest Research Institute (Kansas City), 348
Midwifery, 483

Midwives, 131
Milio, N., 290
Militancy, rising expectations of professionalism and, 14–15
Military Health Service, 197
Military tribunal for war crimes (1946), 519
Miller, E. A., 256
Miller, R., 222
Milstead, J. A., 69
Minimally invasive surgery, 267
Minorities, 492
health care disparities and death rates among, 494
in healthcare workforce, 269
managed care workforce and, 264
mortality and morbidity rates and, 505
nursing shortage and, 511–513
Minority nurses, opportunities for, 513–514
Mishel, M., 477
Mission, organizational, 283
Mitchell, P. H., 413
Mixed-model managed care organizations, 226
MMA. *See* Medicare Prescription, Improvement, and Modernization Act of 2003
Mobility, types of, 8–9
Moch, S., 425
Models
appropriate, identification of, 390
relevant, selection of, 389–391
Molecular genetics, 267
Money, politics and, 311–313
Mongan, James J., 150
Moore, K. D., 208
Moos, R. H., 387
Mor, V., 256
Moral code, 415
Moral hazard, health insurance and, 84
Morality, 531
knowledge of, 415
Moral judgments, 531
Moral knowing, 423, 424
Moral philosophy, 517. *See also* Ethics
Moral values, virtues and, 531–537
Moral worth of nurse, ANA *Code of Ethics* and, 553
Morass of healthcare, 535
Morehead, M. A., 460
Morse, J., 425, 428
Mortality
disparities in health care and, 494
Medicare patients and, 182
staffing shortages and, 511

Moss, C., 423, 424
Mothers Against Drunk Driving, 306
Mouse (mice), computer, 362
MRI. *See* Midwest Research Institute
    (Kansas City)
MSAs. *See* Medical savings accounts
Multiculturalism, 498, 501
    limits of, 493–494
Multicultural professionals, nursing lens
    of, 495–496
Multicultural societies, beliefs, values in,
    110
Multifunctional devices, 363
Multinational corporations, 155, 160
Multiparadigmism, 447, 448
    implications of, for nursing
        science, 446–447
Multiple paradigms, single paradigms
    or?, 443–446
Multiple payers, 85–86
Multiskilled health practitioners, 265
Multivoting, 332, 334*t*
Murdaugh, C., 477
Music, 64
Mutchnick, J. S., 157

N

NACGN. *See* National Association of
    Colored Graduate Nurses
NACNEP. *See* National Advisory Council
    on Nurse Education and Practice
NACNS. *See* National Association of
    Clinical Nurse Specialists
Nahm, Helen, 475
National Advisory Council on Nurse
    Education and Practice, 512
National Association of Blue Shield
    Plans, 172
National Association of Clinical Nurse
    Specialists, 27
National Association of Colored
    Graduate Nurses, 509, 510
National Association of County Health
    Officials, core public health
    functions enumerated by, 259–260
National Bipartisan Commission on the
    Future of Medicare, function of,
    187–188
National Center for Health Services
    Research and Health Care
    Technology, 455
National Center for Health Statistics, 121
National Center for Nursing Research,
    471
    biological task force of, 482

national nursing research agenda,
    480
    precursors to, 473
National Commission for Quality Long-
    Term Care, 256
National Commission for the Protection
    of Human Subjects of Biomedical
    and Behavioral Research, 518, 520
National Commission on Nursing, 19
National Committee on Quality
    Assurance, 234, 235, 236, 343
National Database of Nursing-Sensitive
    Quality Indicators, 348, 349
National health care, 269
National healthcare expenditures, trend
    in, *220*
National healthcare initiatives
    Clinton administration and, 149,
        150, 204, 241–242, 250, 252,
        308
    failure of, 146–151, 176
        ideological differences,
            148–149
        institutional dissimilarities,
            147–148
        political inexpediency, 147
        tax aversion, 149–151, 159
National healthcare program, U.S.
    medical profession and organized
    blocking of, 135
National health insurance, 71, 221, 251*t*
    lack of, in United States, 209
National Health Security Act, 176, 185,
    186, 198, 221
National Institute for Health and
    Clinical Excellence, 268
National Institute for Nursing Research,
    298, 480, 481, 555
    precursors to, 473
    research agenda of, 472
    scientific goals set by, 481
National Institutes of Health, 298, 351,
    455, 473, 476, 477, 555
    human experimentation guidelines
        of, 519, 520
    Human Genome Project and, 522
National League for Nursing, 507, 512
National League for Nursing Education,
    472, 507
    grading committee report of, 11
National Medical Association, 509, 510
National Mental Health Act of 1946, 196
National Nursing Council for War
    Service, 509
National Organization of Nurse
    Practitioner Faculties, 27

National Patient Safety Goals (JCAHO),
    354
National provider identifier, 365
National Quality Forum, 353
National Quality Foundation, 342
National Research Act, 520
National Research Service Awards Act
    (1974), 476
National Rifle Association, 306–307
National Safety Council, 62
National Sample Survey of Registered
    Nurses, 511
Native American point of view, nursing
    from, 496
Natural disasters, 259
Naturalists, 131
Naylor, M. D., 281
NCLEX. *See* Nursing Competency
    Licensing Exam
NCQA. *See* National Committee on
    Quality Assurance
ND. *See* Doctor of nursing
NDNQI. *See* National Database of
    Nursing-Sensitive Quality Indicators
Needs, health care and, 84
Negative margin, 212
Negative yield, 211
Negotiated discount fees, preferred
    provider organizations and, 226
Negotiation skills, 300
Net revenue, 212*t*
Networking
    mentorship *vs.*, 48
    political process and, 311
    program planning and, 216
Net worth, changes in, 212, 212*t*
Neuman, 387, 393
New Deal, 148
New England Hospital for Women and
    Children (Boston), racial quotas at,
    507
Newman, M. A., 387, 434
New York City Health Department, 142
New York University
    doctoral programs in nursing at,
        34, 35
    early training grants for, 474
NHQI. *See* Nursing Home Quality
    Initiative
Nightingale, Florence, 9, 10, 20, 275,
    300, 374, 472, 543
    ethics views of, 544
    as first nurse theorist, 399
Nightingale pledge, 545
Nin, Anais, 426
NINR. *See* National Institute of Nursing
    Research

Nixon, A. J., 125
Nixon, Richard M., 155, 476
NLN. *See* National League for Nursing
NLNE. *See* National League for Nursing Education
NMA. *See* National Medical Association
Noddings, N., 423
Nominal group technique, 332, 334*t*
Noncompliance, 356
Nonconsequential ethics, 523
Nonmaleficence, 527
NONPF. *See* National Organization of Nurse Practitioner Faculties
Nonprice rationing, 116
Nonprofit health plans, 145
Nonprofit organizations, accounting and, 210
Norbeck, 479
Normative ethics, 522, 547, 548
Normative standards, quality assessment and, 461
Norrish, B., 207
Northern Pacific Railroad Beneficial Association, 153
Nosich, G. M., 384
NPI. *See* National provider identifier
NPs. *See* Nurse practitioners
NQF. *See* National Quality Forum; National Quality Foundation
NRA. *See* National Rifle Association
N-STAT. *See* Nurses Strategic Action Team
NTAs. *See* Nurse Training Acts
Nuremberg code, 519
Nuremberg Trials, 519
Nurse-agent, selection of models, theories and, 390
Nurse anesthetists, 141
"Nurse dose," outcomes and, 281
Nurse educators, educational requirements for, 3
Nurse empowerment, new systems of, 286
Nurse-midwives, politics and, 307–308
Nurse practice, guiding forces behind, 401
Nurse Practitioner Competencies in Specialty Areas, 27
Nurse practitioners, 2, 23, 277
  evolving role of, 24–25
  master's degree education for, 27
  policy process and, 280
Nurse Reinvestment Act, 299, 309
Nurse researchers, educational requirements for, 3
Nurses
  changing paradigm in health care and, 284–288

emerging political role of, 278–280
  expanding settings for, 277
  future supply and demand for, 262–263
  legislative process, public policy and, 290
  political appointments of, 279
  public policy and, 290–291
  racial quotas and, 508–509
Nurse scholars, 280
Nurse scientist graduate training grants, 36, 473
Nurses' Directory of Capitol Connections, 296
Nurse shortages, 262, 300
Nurses' roles, dimensions to, 278
Nurses Strategic Action Team, 279
Nurse staffing, professional nursing and, 19–20
Nurse–teachers, education funding and, 297
Nurse theorists, early, 281
Nurse Training Acts, 297, 475
Nursing
  Anglo-American tradition of, 399–400
  changes in practice of, 275–278
  during Civil War era, 505
  codes of ethics for, 545–549
  as culturally competent profession, 491–501
  defined, 23
  doctoral programs in, 34–36, 277
  expanding boundaries of, 277
  fundamental patterns of knowing in, 409–417
  metaparadigm concepts of, 433–434
  organizational, strengthening, 299
  paradigms in, 435, 437–439
  patient safety and role of, 355–357
  poor image of, and shortages in, 511
  as a profession: key ideas for integration, 7–9
  relevance of theory-based practice in, 380–381
  roots of contradictions in, 9–10
  segregation laws and, 506–509
  transcultural, 498–500, 501
  views of ethics for, 544–545
Nursing actions, selecting models and theories for nursing practice and, 392
Nursing administration, support for, 297
Nursing autonomy, 8
Nursing case management, 281
Nursing Competency Licensing Exam, 370

Nursing education, 276
  funding of, 14
Nursing home care
  healthcare expenditures and, 169, *170*
  Medicaid program and, 194
Nursing Home Compare Web site, 342
Nursing home payments, Medicaid and, 171
Nursing Home Quality Initiative (CMS), 342, 353, 355
Nursing homes
  enriched living environments in, 257
  patient safety and, 353
Nursing information systems, advantages and disadvantages with, 367*t*
"Nursing in the Year 2000: Setting the Agenda for Knowledge Generation and Utilization," 477
Nursing knowledge
  structure of, 383–385
  summary of essential elements: model of, 421*t*
Nursing labor force, instability in, 13–14
Nursing models and theories, 381–382, 385, 387, 400
Nursing organizations, minority recruitment and, 512–513
Nursing Organizations Alliance, 299
Nursing Outlook, 483
Nursing philosophy and theory, evolution of, 400–401
Nursing practice
  guidelines for selecting models and theories for, 391–392
  models for, 8
Nursing Relief to Disadvantaged Areas Act of 1999, 513
Nursing research
  advanced nursing practice and, 281
  future opportunities in, 482–483
  historical roots of, 472–475
  investment in, 297–298
  National Institute of Nursing Research definition of, 480
  as nursing science, 478–479
  transitional period in, 475–478
Nursing Research, 473
Nursing Research Emphasis Grant Program (Division of Nursing), 479
Nursing schools
  growth of, 11
  race and, 507
Nursing science
  coming of age for, 479–482
  as mature science?, 442–443
  multiparadigmism and, 446–447

multiple paradigms of, 433–448
nursing practice *vs.,* 28
nursing research as, 478–479
use of term, 410
Nursing-sensitive quality indicators,
defined, 348
Nursing shortages, 13, 14, 20, 270
career ladders and, 18
minorities and, 511–513
government intervention, 512
importation of foreign nurses,
513
nursing intervention, 512–513
Nursing's Safety & Quality Initiative, 348
Nursing's Social Policy Statement, 555
Nursing theoretical literature, 400
Nursing theory
cultural competence model, 500
transcultural nursing, 498–500
Nursing Workforce Diversity Program,
512
Nutrition
cancer prevention and, 108
counseling about, 100
stress management and, 64

O

OASIS. *See* Outcomes and Assessment
Information Set
Oberst, M. T., 477
Obesity epidemic, 254
Objectives, 289
Objectivity, empiricism and, 439
OBRA. *See* Omnibus Budget
Reconciliation Act of 1989
O'Brien, B., 428
Observational studies, 453, 454
Obstetrical nursing, 276
Occupational Safety and Health
Administration, 102
Occupational stress, 62
assessment tool for, 63*t*
Occupational therapists, 141
OD. *See* Doctor of optometry
Office of the Forum for Quality and
Effectiveness in Health Care
(AHCPR), 456
Olson, D. H., 388
Omnibus Budget Reconciliation Act of
1989, 184
Omnibus Budget Reconciliation Acts of
1980 and 1981, 180
Op-ed columns, 310
Open-door policy, 60
Operating budgets, 214
Operating margin, for hospitals, 208

Operating system, 363
Operational definitions, 330, 334*t*
Optimism, 64
Order entry, 366–367
Orders, patient safety and, 355
Oregon
Death with Dignity Act in, 521
Hospital Association Act passed in,
154
Orem, D. E., 281, 385, 393, 412, 427
Organizational culture, model of career
development and, 49*t*
Organizational integration, 130
Organizational paradigm, for the 21st
century, 282–284
Organizations, effective, frameworks for
in the 21st century, 284*t*
Organized nursing, strengthening, 299
Organizing and directing, financial
management, 210
Organizing structures, types of, 210
Organs, harvesting and selling of, 519
Organ transplantations, 267
transition years and research on, 477
Origins of theory, selection of models,
theories and, 390
Orlando, 385
ORYX initiative, 340
Osborne, D. E., 298
OSHA. *See* Occupational Safety and
Health Administration
Otherness, cultural mores and, 493
O'Toole, L. J., Jr., 294
Ottawa Charter for Health Promotion,
120
Outcomes, "nurse dose" and, 281
Outcomes and Assessment Information
Set, 342
Outcomes research, 462–463, 467
Outpatient surgery, 87, 156
Output devices, 362
Ovarian cancer, annual percent decline
in, 101*t*
Owcharenko, N., 245

P

Package pricing, 83
PACs. *See* Political action committees
Pagers, improving effectiveness of, 356
Pain, cultural, 499
Pain management theories, 394
Pain relief, ANA position statement on,
552
Pang, S., 496
Pap smears, 100
Paradigms

nature of, 434–435
in nursing, 435, 437–439
selection of models and theories
and, 390
Parent abuse, 296
Pareto charts, 330, 334*t*
Pareto principle (80/20 rule), 58, 327
Parse, R. R., 387, 442
Parsimony/simplicity, selection of
models, theories and, 390
Parsons, T., 112
Partisan idcology, 308–309
Partnerships, 283
Password security, 363
Pasteur, Louis, 137 (exhibit)
Pastoral leaders, 96
Patel, V., 248
Paternalism, 11, 12, 15, 266, 270, 286,
527, 552
questioning of, 520
Paterson, 387
Patient-centered approach, 8
Patient-centered care, emergence of
primary nursing and, 16–17
Patient dumping, 182, 183
Patient identifiers, 355, 356
Patient information, protecting, 363,
522
Patient monitoring, 368
Patient safety, 318, 340, 461
American Medical Association
response on, 349
American Nurses Association
response on, 348–349
first Institute of Medicine report
and responses on, 349–353
Agency for Healthcare
Research and Quality, 351
Leapfrog, 351
Quality Interagency
Coordination Task Force,
352–353
JCAHO response on, 354–355
joint efforts related to, 354
as national priority, 347
nursing's role in, 355–357
second Institute of Medicine report
and responses on, 353–355
joint efforts, 354
Medicare response, 353
National Nursing Home
Quality Initiative, 353
Patient Safety Organizational Assessment
Tool, The, 352–353
Patient satisfaction, 336, 463, 464
emphasis on, 265, 270
Patient scheduling systems, 369

Patient Self-Determination Act of 1990, 521

Patient-severity adjusted hospital performance data, 461

Paul, R. W., 384

Payers
mix of, 208
multiple, 85–86
prices determined by, 82
third-party, 84–85
within U.S. healthcare delivery system, 72, 73*t*

Payment, within healthcare delivery system, 75, 76, 76–77

PCPs. *See* Primary care physicians

PDAs. *See* Personal digital assistants

Pediatric nursing, 276

Peer mentors, 46

Peer review, quality improvement and, 458, 459

Peer review organizations, 180

Pelligrino, E., 423

Pender, N. J., 389

Penicillin, 137 (exhibit)

Peplau, Hildegarde, 281, 385, 400, 475

Perception, recognition and, 412

Perennial voters, 309

Perfectionism, 60–61

Performance improvement, 325
principles of, 325–328
tools and techniques for, 328–335

Performance initiatives, Medicare pay for, 343

Performance rating, of health plans, 83

Per member per month, 79

Perrow, C., 9

Persian Gulf War, 535

Persistence, politics and, 309–311

Personal criteria, selection of relevant models, theories and, 389

Personal digital assistants, 57, 58, 338, 362

Personal is political commandment, 306–307

Personal knowing, 375, 419, 420, 421*t*, 424–426, 439

Personal knowledge, 409, 413–415, 416

Personal resource management
stress management, 62–64
time management, 53–62

Personal values and beliefs, selection of models, theories and, 390, 391

Personal well-being, 463

Person concept, nursing metaparadigm and, 383

Perspectives on Nursing Theory, 445

Perspective transformation

empowerment of nurses through, 395
phases leading to, 384
structure of, 383–385

Persuasiveness, politics and, 309–311

Pesthouses, 133

Pesznecker, B., 388

Peters, T. J., 283

Peterson, Oscar, 459

Pew Health Professions Commission, 285

Phantom providers, 83

Pharmaceutical advertising, consumers and, 83

Pharmaceutical companies, research and, 465

Pharmacies, 368
national healthcare initiatives and, 148

Pharmacists, short supply of, 261

PharmD. *See* Doctor of pharmacy

PhD, 3

Phenomenology, 375, 421, 440, 479

Pheomelanin, 126, 127

PHI. *See* Protected health information

Philosophy, 440

Phinney, J., 496

Phone calls
to legislators, 309–310
managing, 61

Physical activity, increasing, 100

Physical examinations, clinical nursing practice and, 277

Physical functional, outcomes research and, 463

Physical health, holistic health and, 95, 95

Physical therapists, 141

Physician-assisted suicide, 521

Physician Consortium for Performance Improvement (AMA), 343

Physician expenditures, rise in, 219

Physician order entry, 367

Physicians
birth of Blue Shield and self-interest of, 145
consolidation of power of, 135
contract practice and, 153
corporatization of health care and, 156
cultural authority of, 136
demand creation and, 84
dependency and, 138
economic incentives for, 166
future supply and demand for, 261–262
geographical migration of, 157

group practice and, 154
healthcare delivery system controls and, 228
informed consent and, 528–529
licensing of, 139–140
power balancing and, 86
prepaid group plans and, 154–155
unstable demand for, in preindustrial America, 133–134
urbanization and, 136

Physician services
healthcare expenditures and, 169, *170*
trend in, *220*

Physician specialists, 166

PI. *See* Performance improvement

Piaget, Jean, 389

Picker Institute (Boston), patient satisfaction instruments of, 464

Pie charts, 330, 334*t*

Pillars of Excellence, 335

Pincus, T., 107

Pitts-Mosley, M. O., 507

Planned Parenthood, Inc., 277, 314

Planned rationing, 116

Planning
application of, to nursing process, 386*t*
financial management and, 210
long-term, 283
time management and, 57–58

Play-or-pay approach, 245
for health care financing reorganization, 252*t*

Play-or-pay coverage, 253

Plessy vs. Ferguson, 506

Pluralism, 491

PMPM. *See* Per member per month

Pneumonia (PNE), 107
Hospital Quality Initiative and focus on, 342

Poetry, 426

Point-of-service (POS) plans, 225

Polanyi, M., 414

Policy experts
advanced practice nurses as, 275

Policy(ies)
as entity, 288–290
procedures and, 289
as process, 288, 290

Policy makers, healthcare delivery system and, 88–89

Policy process, 291–295
agenda setting, 291–292
government response, 292–293

policy and program evaluation, 294–295
policy and program implementation, 293–294
stages of, 290
Polio, 258, 464
Politeness, politics and, 309–311
Political action committees, 278
Political activism, 278, 282
Political affairs, definition of, 305
Political decisionmaking, 305
Political inexpediency, failure of national healthcare intitatives and, 147
Political process, making it work, 305–314
Political roles, of nurses, emerging, 278–280
Political science, 276
Political system, advanced practice nurses working with, 300
Politics
    definition of, 305
    discerning truth and, 535
    money and, 311–313
    ten universal commandments of, and reasons to obey them, 306–314
    visibility and, 313
Poor houses, 133
Poor population, Medicaid and, 151
Population health, 94, 109
Population research, 453–454
Porter-O'Grady, T., 18, 286, 350
Position statements, 288, 289, 551
Positive margin, 212
Positive yield, 211
Positivism, 402, 437
POS plans. *See* Point-of-service (POS) plans
Postpositivism, 438
Poverty, 221
    roots of nursing and, 9–10
Power balancing, U.S. health services system and, 86–87
Pozgar, 488
PPOs. *See* Preferred provider organizations
Practice
    defined, 23
    differentiating care and, 405–406, 405*t*
    as praxis, 404
    research, theory and, 375
Practice of Value, The (Raz), 407
Practice theories, 374
Praxis
    practice as, 404

understanding, 403–404
Prayer, 96
    stress management and, 64
Preapprovals, 166
Preceptors, 134
Predictive theories, 374
Predoctoral Research Fellowship Program, 35
Preferred provider organizations, 78, 225–226
Prejudice, transcultural nursing and, 499
Premature death, relative contribution of four health determinants and, 105, *105*
Premiums
    cost sharing and, 77
    for employer-sponsored health plans, increases in, 174
    health insurance
        increases in, 229, 242
        increases in, compared to other indicators, *230*
Prenatal care, 100, 101, 472
Prepaid group plans, 154–155
Prepaid group practice, 153
Prepaid health plans, 144, 233
Prepayment, 222
Presbyterian-University of Pennsylvania Medical Center, 474–475
Prescription drug costs, Medicare Part D and, 158, 191
Prescription drugs
    healthcare expenditures and, 169, *170*
    marketing of, 166
    senior citizens and unaffordability of, 535–536
Prescriptive privileges, 26
Preservation of life, 536
President's Commission for Study of Ethical Problems in Medicine, 521
President's Council on Bioethics, 522
Prevention, future of, 254–255
Prevention initiatives, Balanced Budget Act of 1997 and, 189
Preventive care, 87, 88*t*
Price
    free-market conditions and, 82, *82*
    payers and determination of, 82
Price rationing, 114
Pricewaterhouse Coopers, 247
Pricing, item-based *vs.* package, 83
Primary care, 88*t*, 120, 156
    health indicators and, 107
    transition years and research on, 477–478
    uninsured persons and, 81

Primary care case management, 233
Primary care physicians, 138, 141, 228
Primary care providers, 78, 83
Primary nursing, patient-centered care and emergence of, 16–17
Primary prevention, 100
PRIMEX training, at UCLA, 478
Principled theory, 546
Printers, 363
Print media, direct-to-consumer marketing of prescription drugs via, 166
Priorities, identifying, 327
Privacy
    information technology and, 364–365
    patient information and, 522
Privacy rule, HIPAA, 364
Private duty nursing, 13
Private financing, of healthcare services, 80
Private insurance
    administration costs, healthcare expenditures and, 169–170, *170*
    funding of healthcare expenditures and, 170
Private medical practice, entrenchment of, in American system, 135
Private practice of medicine, public health separated from, 142
Private sector employers, trends in insurance and, 243
Private time, allowing for, 60
Problem identification, by advanced practice nurses, 296–298
Problem solving, 62
Procedure authorizations, 166
Procedure manuals, 288
Procedures, 289
Processing speed, computer, 362
Procrastination, 60–61
Professional associations, patient safety and responses by, 348–349
Professional Development Plan, 50–51, 51*t*
Professional dominance, evolution of U.S. healthcare delivery system and, *159*
Professionalism
    nursing scholarship and, 14
    primary nursing and, 17
    quest for, in nursing, 7
Professional nursing, nurse staffing and, 19–20
Professional organizations, 8
    features of, 549
Professionals, characteristics of, 549
Professional sovereignty

growth of, in postindustrial
America, 135–142
cohesiveness and organization,
135, 138–139
dependency, 135, 138
educational reform, 135,
140–141
institutionalization, 135,
137–138
licensing, 135, 139–140
science and technology, 135,
136–137
urbanization, 135, 136
Professional standards review
organization, 179, 180
Profit centers, 210
Profits, healthcare delivery and, 74
Program implementation, policy process
and, 293–294
Program integrity provisions, Balanced
Budget Act of 1997 and, 189
Programs, 289
government response to public
problems and, 292, 293
policy and, 288
Progressive movement, 146
Progressive muscular relaxation, 64
Proposals, policy and, 288
PROs. See Peer review organizations
Prospective Payment Assessment
Commission, 182
Prospective payment systems, 164, 183,
185, 221, 284, 402, 457
advent of, 205–207
Medicare and, 181–182
Prostate cancer, 296
annual percent decline in, 101t
Protected health information, 364
Protestantism, 10
Protocols, improving, 268–269
Provider networks, approved, 225
Providers, within health plan, 78
PSROs. See Professional standards review
organization
Psychiatric nursing, 24, 276
Psychologists, 141
Psychology, 280
Public entitlement programs, 247–248
Public health, 101–102
bioterrorism and transformation of,
258–260
development of, in postindustrial
America, 141–142
distinguishing characteristics of, 102
social justice and, 114, 142
Public health agencies, regulatory role
of, 153

Public health policy, foreign policy and,
258
Public health research, 467
Public Health Security and Bioterrorism
Act of 2002, 103
Public policy, 288–291
advanced practice nurses and,
275–301
nurses and, 290–291
policy as an entity, 288–290
policy as a process, 290
purpose of, 288
Public sector employers, trends in
insurance and, 243
Pulcini, J., 2
Pulse oximeters, 368
Purnell, Larry, 488
cultural competence model of, 500,
500t

Q

QA. See Quality assurance
QAIP. See Quality assessment and
improvement programs
QI. See Quality improvement
Qualitative methods, 446
Qualitative research, 440
Quality
aims for, 318
healthcare delivery and quest for, 87
leadership for, 329
obsession with, 326, 326t
tools and techniques for
improvement of, 328–335
Quality assessment and improvement
programs, 353
Quality assurance, 324
Quality improvement, 344
language of, 325
Medicare beneficiaries and, 343
principles of, 325–328
research and, 458–461
scientific method tools for,
329–331
success with, 335–336
summary of tools and techniques,
334t
Quality improvement team concepts,
summary of, 335t
Quality improvement team effectiveness
lessons learned during promotion
of, 332–335
ground rules, 334–335
member selection, 333
team charge, 332–333
team roles, 333–334

Quality Interagency Coordination Task
Force, patient safety and response by,
352–353
Quality leadership, principles of, 326t
Quality movement, translation of, into
health care, 324–325
Quality of health care, 83
cultural competence and, 501
patient satisfaction and, 464
Quality of life, 104
evidence-based medicine and, 462
Quality outcomes, financial results and,
216–217
Quantitative methods, 446
of epidemiology, 454
Quarantines, in preindustrial America,
133
QuIC. See Quality Interagency
Coordination Task Force
Quinlan, Joseph, 520
Quinlan, Karen Ann, 520–521
Quint, J., 474
Quota system, race and, 507

R

Race
healthcare workforce and, 264
nursing profession and, 505
nursing profession during Civil
War era and, 505
nursing schools and, 507
quota system and, 507
Racial barriers, lowering, 509–511
Racial discrimination, in health care, 505
Racial quotas, world wars and, 508–509
Racial stereotypes, 514
Racism, 430
Rader, M., 412
Radio, direct-to-consumer prescription
marketing via, 166
Radiological technologists, 141
Radiology, 368
history behind, 137 (exhibit)
Railroads, 135
RAM. See Random access memory
RAND Corporation, 247
Medicare studies and, 182
RAND Health Insurance Experiment,
457, 458
Random access memory, 362
Randomized controlled studies, 463
Rate variance, from budgeted amount, 215
Rational drug design, 266
Rawls, John, 113
Raz, J., 407

RBRVS. *See* Resource-based relative value scale
RCA. *See* Root cause analysis
Read-only memory, 362
Reagan administration, gag-rule policy and, 288
Reason, praxis and, 404
"Reasonable man" standard, 520
Received view, 435
Recognition, 18–19
  perception and, 412
Reconceptualization, perspective transformation and, 384
Recorders, team, 333, 335*t*
Redesign of healthcare system, IOM principles for, 341
Redistributive policies, health and, 107
Reed, P. G., 444
Reengineering and redesign, of healthcare systems, 207–208, 283, 286, 325
Reform, 290
  comprehensive (if and when it occurs), 250–254
  expanding framework for nurses and, 298–300
  in healthcare system, 284
  workplace, 14–16
Refrigeration of foods, 100
Refugees, 492
Refusal, right to, 526
Regional alliances, managed competition and, 253
Registered nurses, 553
  workforce shortages and, 262
Regulation, 288, 293
  government response to public problems and, 292
  long-term care challenges and, 257
  policy process and, 289, 290
Regulatory focus on quality, accreditation and, 339–343
Regulatory process, 293
Rehabilitation Act of 1973, 289
Rehabilitative care, 88*t*
Rehabilitative therapies, 100
Reimbursement, 76–77
Relational statements, 441
Religious ethics, 523
Religious involvement, all-cause mortality and, 96
Report cards, 286, 327
Republican party, 308
  national health insurance proposals and, 148–149
Reputations, politics and, 313–314

Research, 276, 451–468. *See also* Nursing research
  advanced nursing practice and, 281
  areas of success in, 443
  bioinformatic, 465–466
  epidemiology, 453–454
  ethics, 464–465
  evidence-based medicine, 461–462
  experimental epidemiology, 454
  future challenges, 465–467
  growth in, 451
  in health and disease, 452–453
  health services, 454–458
    Agency for Healthcare Research and Quality, 455–457
    health policy and, 457–458
  on medical errors, 461
  neglect of, in preindustrial America, 130
  nursing theories and, 277
  outcomes, 462–463, 467
  on patient satisfaction, 464
  public health, 467
  quality improvement and, 458–461
  theory, practice and, 375
  variations in focus of, 452, *452*
Research in Nursing and Health, 476
Research in Patient Care Review Committee, 475
Research institutions, within U.S. healthcare delivery system, 72, 73*t*
Resistance to antibiotics, 258, 466
Resistance to stress, building, 64
Resnick, B. A., 478
Resolutions, 289
  perspective transformation and, 384
Resource-based relative value scale, 184–185, 221
Resources, within Professional Development Plan, 51*t*
Respect, 300, 536–537
  politics and, 307
Restorative health care services, 87
Restrictive fee schedules, 164
Retention, magnet hospitals and, 19
Retiree health benefits, erosion of, 242
Revenue, 211
Revenue stream, 211
Revenue to expense ratio, 211
Reverby, S., 12
Rew, L., 427
Richmond, J. B., 198
Rightsizing, 282
Risk factors

disease and, 98
  health promotion, disease prevention and, 99
Risk management
  future of managed care and, 249
  patient safety and, 352
Robb, Isabel Hampton, 545
Robert Wood Johnson Community Tracking Study household survey, 107
Robotic pharmacy system, 368
Rochefoucauld, François de la, 536
Roentgen, Wilhelm, 137 (exhibit)
Rogers, M. E., 281, 381, 383, 385, 400
Role ambiguity, 278
Role competencies, mentorship and development of, 46
Role conflict, 278
Role functioning, outcomes research and, 463
Role taking, 278
Rolled up budget, 213
ROM. *See* Read-only memory
Roosevelt, Eleanor, 314
Roosevelt, Franklin D., 148
Roosevelt, Theodore, 146
Root cause analysis, 331, 334*t,* 354
Root cause summary table, 331
Rothstein, W. G., 140
Roy, 387, 393
Royal College of Nursing in England, Scotland, and Northern Ireland, 279
Rules, higher good and, 533
Run charts, 330, 334*t*
Rundall, T., 207
Rural hospital initiatives, Balanced Budget Act of 1997 and, 189
Rush University, 37
Russell, C. S., 388

S

Sacrifice of form, 414
Safety. *See also* Patient safety
  workplace, 296
Safety hazards, 106
Safety net coverage, gaps in, 208
Sanger, Margaret, 314
Sanitary regulation, public health and, 141
SARS. *See* Severe acute respiratory syndrome
Satcher, David, 254
Satir, 387
Scanners, 362
Scarlet fever, 472
Scheduling

systems for, 369
time management and, 58
SCHIP (State Children's Health Insurance Program), 74, 77, 81, 82, 86, 111, 116, 117, 158, 186, 196
Schlegel, M., 16
Schloendorff v. Society of New York Hospital, 526
Scholars, nurse, 280
Scholarships, for minority students, 512
Scholtes, P., 325, 329
Schopenhauer, Arnold, 532
Schorr, T., 482
Schuurmans, M., 28
Schweitzer, Albert, 522
Science, phases of, 442
Science and technology, growth of professional sovereignty and, 135, 136–137
Science-based medicine, 136
Scientific approach, 496
Scientific management method, 12, 13
Scientific meaning, esthetics *vs.,* 412–413
Scientific method
American culture and, 110–111
steps in, 329*t*
Scientific method tools for quality improvement, 329–331
cause and effect (fishbone) diagrams, 330
checksheets, 331
flowcharts, 330
gap analysis, 331
operational definitions, 330
pie charts and Pareto charts, 330
root cause analysis, 331
run charts (time plots) and control charts, 330–331
Scientific paradigm, 410
Scott, Jessie, 475
Screen display, 362
Screenings, secondary prevention and, 100
Scudder, J., 423, 424
Sean, 349
Secondary prevention, 100
Secular ethics, 524
Security
computerized medical records and, 319
computers and, 363–364
patient information and, 522
Security rule, HIPAA, 364
Segall, M., 388
Segregation laws, 513
nursing and, 506–509
nursing practice under, 508

Self aspects, model of career development and, 49*t*
Self-assessment
of advanced practice nursing development needs, 50*t*
time management and, 54, 55*t*, 56–57
Self-care model, 385, 387, 393
Self-care products, 158
Self-determination, national healthcare initiatives and, 148
Self-employed people, health insurance and, 77
Self-esteem, perfectionism and, 61
Self-funded insurance programs, 174–175
Self-governance, 283
Self-interest, professionalism and, 8
Semivariable costs, 211
Semmelweis, Ignaz, 137 (exhibit)
Senate (U.S.), 308
Seniority, politics and, 313
Senior leadership, quality and, 329
Sentinel Event Alert, 354
Sentinel events, 354
Separate but equal law, 506
Service lines, 210–211
Service orientation, health services and transition to, 265–266
SES. *See* Socioeconomic status
Severe acute respiratory syndrome, 104, 119, 158, 258
Sexism, 430
Sexually transmitted diseases, 142
Shamansky, S. L., 388
Shared governance, initiation of, in healthcare institutions, 17–18
Shattuck, Lemuel, 142
Shaver, J., 479, 480
Shi, L., 107
Shortages. *See* Nursing shortages
Sick role, dependency and, 138
Silber, J. H., 8, 349, 511
Silver, 478
Simpson, Roy, 286
Simulation, education applications and, 370
Simultaneity worldview, 442
Single paradigms, multiple paradigms or?, 443–446
Single-payer health plans, 85, 250, 251*t*, 252
SIP. *See* Surgical infection prevention
Sit-ins, 292
Situational ethics, 537
Six Sigma, 335
Skill development, patient safety and, 356

Sloane, D. M., 8, 349, 511
Slote, M. A., 416
Small businesses, health insurance issues and, 77
Smallpox, 133, 141
bioterrorism threat and, 158
Smart boards, 333
Smith, B. C., 46
Smith, F. B., 544
Smoking cessation, 100
Snow, John, 102
Sochalski, J., 8, 349
Social cohesion, health and, 107
Social consciousness, 282
Social factors in health care, in postindustrial America, 143–144
Social functioning, outcomes research and, 463
Social health
holistic health and, 95, 95
unemployment and, 107
Social justice, 118
equitable distribution of health care and, 114–116
market justice *vs.,* 115*t*
Social mobility, professionalization and, 8
Social model of health, 111–112
Social programs, 282
Social reformism, 11
Social roles, sick individuals and, 111–112
Social Security, 152
legislation, 148
system reforms for, 248
Social Security Act of 1935, 151, 178, 193, 219, 296
Social Security Administration, 176
Social Security Amendment (1965), Title XVIII of, 152
Social support network, 95
Society for Academic Emergency Medicine, health defined by, 95
Socioeconomic status
determinants of health and, 106, 107
health, health care and, 467
Sociology, 280, 440
Sociopolitical congruency, selection of relevant models and theories and, 390
Sociopolitical knowing
as context of nursing, 429–431
essential elements of, 431*t*
Software, 338, 362, 363
Solberg, S., 428
Sound bites, 292
"South American Mi Hija" (Doubiago), 426

Southern Illinois University School of Medicine, patient satisfaction questionnaire of, 464
Spanish-American War, 506
Special interest groups, 292, 299
Specialists
  growth in number of, 262
  proportion of, to generalists, 141
Specialized care, 88*t*
Specialized medicine, healthcare expenditures and growth of, 166–167
Specialty hospitals, 157
Specialty referrals, authorization of, by primary physicians, 228
Spending, on health care in U.S., 209
Spirit Catches You and You Fall Down, The (Fadiman), 495
Spiritual assessment instruments, 96
Spiritual caregivers, 501
Spiritual health, holistic health and, 95, 95, 96
Spirituality, 524
Spreadsheets, 363
Sprenkle, D. H., 388
Spross, J., 23
Stability, perspective transformation and return to, 384
Staffing and scheduling system, 369
Staff model HMOs, 224
Staff satisfaction, 336
Stakeholders, diversity of, in United States healthcare system, 68
Standardized protocols, patient safety and, 356
Standard of living, erosion in, 246
Standards
  for doctoral programs, 36
  medical education reform and, 140
Standards of care, evidence-based practice and, 403
Standing, T. S., 37
Staphylococcus, hospital infections and, 466
Starfield, B., 209
State boards of nursing, 288
  nurses on, 277
State Children's Health Insurance Program. *See* SCHIP
State Children's Health Insurance Program Benefits Improvement and Protection Act of 2000, 256
State legislatures, partisanship and, 308
State Medicaid programs, 197
  benefits through, 193
Statement of cash flows, 212, 213

Statement of revenue and expense, 212, 212*t*
Statement on Clinical Nurse Specialist Practice and Education, 27
State nursing organizations, ANA-associated, 15
State public health agencies, 260
States
  health insurance reforms and, 242
  loss of premium revenue taxes in, 174
  Medicare payment programs and, 183
  structural deficits and, 248
Statistical methods, 439
Statistical theory, epidemiology and, 454
Statistics, 276
Staupers, M. K., 506
Stereotypes, 493
  racial, 514
Sterilization techniques, 137 (exhibit)
Sterne, Laurence, 536
Stevens, P., 430
Stevens, Rosemary, 11, 130, 173, 176, 177, 221
Stevenson, J. S., 34, 387, 477
Stewart, Isabel, 11, 12
Storage devices, 363
Strategic planning, 283
Strauss, A. L., 474
Stress
  building resistance to, 64
  changing perceptions of, 64
Stress management, 3, 62–64
  acceptance techniques, 64
  altering techniques, 62
  avoidance techniques, 62, 64
  model for, 62
  occupational stress, 62
  purpose of, 62
Stroke, 107
  diet and, 108
Structured discussion, 334*t*
Struthers, R., 496
Student labor, 11
Studer Group, 335
Subacute care, 87, 88*t*
Subacute disease, 98
Substance abuse, 221
Substituted judgment, 519, 520–521
Success, areas of, in nursing research, 443
Suicide, physician-assisted, 521
Sullivan, 318
Sunrise model, within transcultural nursing, 498–499
"Sunshine Across Living Centre" (Krysl and Watson), 426

Superintendents' Society, purpose of, 507
Supplemental Security Income, 193
Supplier-induced demand, 84
Supply and demand
  free-market conditions and, 82, 82
  for nurses, 262–263
  for physicians, 261–262
Supply costs, 211
Supply-side rationing, 116
Supreme Court, 140, 145, 175, 237, 506, 520
Surgery
  item-based pricing and, 83
  minimally invasive, 267
  outpatient, 156
Surgical infections, preventing, 340
Surgical nursing, 276
Surgical safety procedures, 355, 356
Surveillance systems, 260
Swing districts, 308
Synthesis, perspective transformation and, 384
Syphilis, 121
  Tuskegee study of, 518, 520
Systematic analysis, total quality management and, 324
Systems model, 387
Systems thinking, 283

T

Taft-Hartley Act, 14
Tamm, M. E., 96
Tanner, C., 427
Tapes, 363
Target, selection of models, theories and, 390
Task prioritization, urgent *vs.* important, 58, 59
Tax aversion, failure of national healthcare initatives and, 149–151, 159
Tax credits, 248–249
Tax Equity and Fiscal Responsibility Act of 1982, 180, 181
Taylor, B., 425, 428
Taylor, Frederick, 12
"Taylorism," 12
Teachers College—Columbia University, early training grants for, 474
Team communication and decisions, 331–332
  affinity diagrams, 332
  brainstorming, 331–332
  multivoting, 332
  nominal group technique, 332
Team leaders, 333
Team members, selecting, 333, 335*t*

Team nursing concept, 13
Team roles
champion, 333, 334
facilitator, 333, 334
recorder, 333
team leader, 333
team member, 333
timekeeper, 333, 334
Teamsters union, quality of care study and, 460
Teamwork, quality leadership and, 326t, 327–328
Technical competence, advanced practice nurses and, 275
Technicians, short supply of, 261
Technology. *See also* Clinical technology; Information technology
healthcare delivery and, 87, 130
healthcare ethics and, 518
in postindustrial America, 143–144
Teen driver education, 100
TEFRA. *See* Tax Equity and Fiscal Responsibility Act of 1982
Telecommunications, 156, 157
Telehealth, 156, 160, 270, 299
Telemedicine, 156, 157, 160
Teleological (or consequential) ethics, 522–523
Telephone orders, patient safety and, 355, 356
Television
direct-to-consumer prescription marketing via, 166
politics and, 311
Ten Commandments, 523–524
Terrorism, 103
Terrorist attacks of 2001, 259
Tertiary prevention, 100
Thank-you notes, to elected officials, 309, 310
Theoretical unification, 444, 447
Theories
definition and types of, 374
practice, research and, 375
relevant, selection of, 389–391
Theorist criteria, selection of relevant models, theories and, 389
Theory-based advanced nursing practice, 379–395
application of, 392–394
conceptual models, 379
guidelines for selecting models and theories for nursing practice, 391–392
issues related to, 381–383
relevance of, 380–381

selection of relevant models and theories, 389–391
structure of nursing knowledge and perspective transformation, 383–385
Theory-based nursing practice, 394t
Theory-practice gap, 381
Therapeutic interventions, 100
Therapists, short supply of, 261
Theses, 281
Third-party insurers and payers, 84–85
Third-party payment, evolution of health insurance and, 171–174
Third-party reimbursement, theory-based practice, patient's quality of life and, 381
Thompson, Tommy G., 353, 512
Thoreau, Henry David, 531
Thornburgh, Richard, 149
3-D technology, 266
Timekeeper, 334, 335t
Timelines, within Professional Development Plan, 51t
Time management, 3, 53–62
allowing oneself private time, 60
benefits of, 53–54
communications management, 61–62
controlling interruptions, 60
delegation and, 59–60
goal setting and planning, 57–58
log for, 56, 56t
poor, consequences of, 54
prioritizing tasks: urgent *vs.* important, 58, 59
procrastination and perfectionism, 60–61
scheduling and, 58
self-assessment and, 54, 55t, 56–57
strategies for, 57
Time plots, 330
Tingen, 375
Tobacco industry, globalization and, 157–158
Tobacco-related deaths, 121
To do lists, 61
To Err is Human: Building a Safer Health System (IOM), 318, 340, 349–350
Totality paradigm, 442
Total patient care, 413
Total quality improvement, 318
Total quality management, 324
Touch screens, 362
Toxic chemicals, 106
Toxic substances, 102
TQM. *See* Total quality management

Trade Adjustment Assistance Act of 2002, 248, 249
Trade guilds, academic degrees as outgrowth of, 32
Tradesmen, early practice of medicine in America by, 131
Traditional bureaucratic structures, 210
Training, quality leadership and, 326t, 328
Transactions and code set rule, HIPAA, 364
Transcription errors, eliminating, 367
Transcultural nursing model, 387, 498–500, 501
Transferability, qualitative methodologies and, 441
Transparency in healthcare, 118
Transplantation biology, 267
Triangulation, 446
TriCare, 250
Tri-Council of Nursing, 299
Triple option, 227
Truman, Harry, national healthcare and, 148, 149
Trust
delegation and, 59
politics and, 307
Trustworthiness, 534
Truth, discerning, politics and, 535
Truth, Sojourner, 506
Truth-telling, 535
Tschudin, Mary, 475
Tuberculosis, 141, 472
Tubman, Harriet, 506
Turnover, 14
Tuskegee study of syphilis (1932-1972), 294, 518, 520
Tutorials, education applications and, 370
Twentieth century, environmental health during, 102
Twenty Thousand Nurses Tell Their Story (Hughes, et al.), 473
Twomey, 488
Typhoid, 133, 141

U

UAW. *See* United Auto Workers
UHC. *See* University Healthsystems Consortium
Understandability, selection of models, theories and, 390
Undocumented workers, 492
Unemployed individuals, lack of health insurance for, 77
Unemployment, social health and, 107
Unemployment compensation, 148

Unequal Treatment: Confronting Racial and Ethnic Disparities in Healthcare (IOM), 505
Unification, paradigms and, 444
Uninsured population, 77–78, 81, 163, 208, 209
    characteristics of, 2003, *169*
    children, 195
    growth in healthcare expenditures and, 168
Unionism, 9, 15
Unions, 14, 146
    group health insurance and, 145
    national healthcare initiatives and, 148
Unique identifiers rule, HIPAA, 364
Unitary man, science of, 385
United Auto Workers, 15
United States
    capitalist culture in, 111
    complexity of healthcare delivery in, 72, 73*t*
    doctoral education programs in, 31, 39
    equity in healthcare delivery system in, 118–119
    evolution of healthcare delivery system in, *159,* 205–208
        advent of prospective payment and diagnostic-related groups, 205–207
        fee-for-service payment, 205
        reengineering and redesign of healthcare system, 207–208
    evolution of health services in, 129–160
    foreign-born population growth in, 492
    institutional dissimilarities between Europe and, 147
    justice in health delivery system in, 116–117
    market-oriented economy in, 74
    medical model in, 94–95
    nursing takes root in, 10–12
    partial access to health care in, 81
    uninsured people in, 209
    unique system of healthcare delivery in, 71–90, 129–130
Unity of purpose, quality leadership and, 326*t,* 327
Universal access, 81
Universal health care, 118, 269
Universal health insurance, proposed options and problems with, 250

University Healthsystems Consortium, 336
University nursing schools, nursing science coming of age and, 479
University of Alabama (Birmingham), 35
University of Arizona, early training grants for, 474
University of Berlin, 134
University of California-Los Angeles
    PRIMEX training at, 478
    research publications of nursing school at, 471
University of California-San Francisco, 35, 38
    research publications from nursing school at, 471–472
University of California School of Nursing, early training grants for, 473
University of Colorado, 37
    early training grants for, 474
University of Illinois, early training grants for, 474
University of Kansas School of Nursing, 348, 349
    early training grants for, 474
University of Kentucky, 38
University of Maryland, research publications from nursing school at, 472
University of Pennsylvania, 38, 134
University of Pittsburgh, 35
    early training grants for, 474
University of South Carolina, 37
University of Tennessee Health Science Center, 38
University of Washington School of Nursing, 474
    early training grants for, 473
University schools of nursing, research initiatives and, 481
UNIX, 363
Urbanization, 137
    growth of professional sovereignty and, 135, 136
Urgent tasks, important tasks *vs.,* 58, 59
U.S. Administration on Aging, 166
U.S. Department of Labor, 168
U.S. Human Resources Administration, 177
U.S. Public Health Service, 35, 197
    Division of Nursing Resources, 473
    hospitals, 175
U.S. Senate Special Committee on Aging, 189
Utilitarianism, 546

    social justice and, 116
Utility criteria, selection of relevant models, theories and, 390
Utilization, cost controls and, 79
Utilization of health services, health status of population and, 94
Utilization review, preferred provider organizations and, 226
Utilization volume increases, 220

V

Vaccines, 260
    therapeutic use of, 267, 270
Value-free science, fallacy of, 401–402
Value-laden theory, 401–402
Values
    cultural, healthcare delivery and, 109–111
    ethics and, 518
    practice and, 406
Values-based practice, evidence-based care and, 406–407
Value scale research, resource-based, 457
Vance, C., 43
Variable costs, 211
Venegoni, S. L., 286
Ventilator alarms, 356
Verbal orders, patient safety and, 355, 356
Vertical integration, 207, 208
Veterans, health services for, in postindustrial America, 143
Veterans Administration. *See* Department of Veterans Affairs
Veterans Affairs hospitals, 175
Veterans Health Administration, 197
VHA, Inc., 336
Videoconferencing, 156
Vienna school of philosophers, 435
Violence, 221, 430
Violent deaths, 121
Virtues
    commitment, 532
    compassion, 532–533
    conscientiousness, 533
    cooperativeness, 534
    courage, 534
    discernment, 534
    ethics and, 518
    fairness, 534
    fidelity, 534
    freedom, 534
    honesty, 534–535
    hopefulness, 536
    ingegrity, 536
    kindness, 536
    moral values and, 531–537

respect, 536–537
Visas, for foreign nurses, 513
Visibility, politics and, 313
Vision, advanced practice nurses and, 275
Visiting Nurse Associations, 25
Visualization, 64
Vital statistics, public health and, 141
Voice mail, 61
Volume, budget variance for nursing
    and, 215
Voluntary health insurance, 143, 145
Volunteers
    clinical trials and, 453
    political campaign, 312
Vomiting, postoperative, Yale study of,
    474
Vote counting, legislation process and,
    307
Voters, perennial, 309
Voting, 306
Vouchers, 248–249
Vreeland, Ellwynne, 474, 475

W

Wages, race and, 508
Wagner-Murray-Dingell bill, 148
Wakefield, Mary, 279
Wald, Lillian, 314, 508, 509
Wallack, S. S., 184
War crimes, military tribunal for, 519
Washington, 488
Washington, George, 132
Water contaminants, 106
Water supply protections, 100
Watson, J., 281, 387, 423, 424, 425, 426
Weitz, M., 411
Welch, William H., 140
Well-being, 463
    paradigm for health, 105, *106*
    time management and, 54
Wellness, 269, 411
    future of, 254–255
    promotion of, 88
    Western philosophies of, 501
Wellness model, medical model *vs.,* 99
Wells, Horace, 137 (exhibit)
Wellspring, 257
Wennberg, John, 455, 457
Werley, John, 477
Wesley, John, 534
Western health care, culture and, 494–496
Western Interstate Commission on
    Higher Education, 476

Western Journal of Nursing Research, The, 476
Western Reserve University School of
    Nursing, 11
    early training grants for, 473–474
West Nile virus, 142, 258
Whipple, E. P., 525
Whistle-blower responsibilities, ANA
    Code of Ethics and, 553
Whitfield, Ed, 300
WHO. *See* World Health Organization
Wholeness, 415
Widerquist, J. G., 544
Wiedenbach, E., 412, 415, 427
Wilcox, B., 389
Wilson, J. Q., 286, 353
Wilson, Pete, 477
Wilson, Woodrow, 146
Wofford, Harris, 149
Wolf, G., 286
Wolf, Karen A., 2
Women
    cardiac problems in, 296
    in physician workforce, 262
    roots of nursing and, 9–10
    workforce diversity and, 263, 269
Women's movement, nursing roles and,
    25
Woods, N. F., 34, 477, 479
Work
    changing organization of, 12–13
    recognizing structure in, 326, 326*t*
Workers, health plan enrollment for, by
    plan type, 1988-2004, *227*
Workers' compensation, 135, 136, 146
    birth of, 143
Workforce
    healthcare, future of, 261–264
        deficits in geriatric training,
            263
        diversity in, 263–264
        supply and demand for nurses,
            262–263
        supply and demand for
            physicians, 261–262
        long-term care challenges and, 257
"Work in America," 15
Work life, national crisis in quality of,
    15–16
Work organization, 264–265
    collaborative team approach,
        264–265
    cross-training, 265
Work Out, 335
Work pace, increase in, 347

Workplace, health insurance issues and, 77
Workplace safety, 296
Workstations, security considerations
    and, 363
World Health Organization, health
    defined by, 95, 494
World health system outcomes,
    comparison of, 209
World Medical Association, 519
World Trade Center (New York),
    terrorist attacks on, 103
Worldview, orientational definition of,
    501
World War I, 135
    health services for veterans in wake
        of, 143
    racial quotas and, 508
    U.S. entry into, 147
World War II, 13, 33, 39, 143, 148, 464
    employment-based health
        insurance and, 145–146
    health insurance benefits in wake
        of, 174
    nursing education programs after,
        276
    nursing research during, 472–473
    racial quotas and, 508–509
Wright, Frank Lloyd, 532
Wright, L. M., 388
Wrubel, J., 423

X

Xenotransplantation, 267
X-rays, discovery of, 137 (exhibit)

Y

Yale University
    first PhDs in U.S. awarded at, 32
    school of nursing at, 11
Yellow fever, 133, 141, 142
Yoga, 64

Z

Zaner, R., 423, 424
Zderad, 387
Zero-based budgeting, 213
Zuckerman, S., 248